机械通气：从病理生理到临床证据
Mechanical Ventilation: from Pathophysiology to Clinical Evidence

主　编　Giacomo Bellani
主　译　王瑞兰　陈德昌
副主译　谢　晖　皋　源　刘　娇

上海科学技术出版社

图书在版编目（CIP）数据

机械通气：从病理生理到临床证据 /（意）贾科莫
·贝拉尼（Giacomo Bellani）主编；王瑞兰，陈德昌主
译. -- 上海：上海科学技术出版社，2025.1.
ISBN 978-7-5478-6800-3
Ⅰ. R459.6
中国国家版本馆CIP数据核字第2024XE8565号

First published in English under the title
Mechanical Ventilation from Pathophysiology to Clinical Evidence
edited by Giacomo Bellani
Copyright © Giacomo Bellani，2022
This edition has been translated and published under licence from
Springer Nature Switzerland AG.

上海市版权局著作权合同登记号　图字：09-2022-0655号
封面图片由上海市第一人民医院谢晖提供

机械通气：从病理生理到临床证据
主　编　Giacomo Bellani
主　译　王瑞兰　陈德昌
副主译　谢　晖　皋　源　刘　娇

上海世纪出版（集团）有限公司
上海科学技术出版社　出版、发行
（上海市闵行区号景路159弄A座9F-10F）
邮政编码 201101　www.sstp.cn
浙江新华印刷技术有限公司印刷
开本787×1092　1/16　印张 24.75　插页 10
字数 500千字
2025年1月第1版　2025年1月第1次印刷
ISBN 978-7-5478-6800-3/R·3090
定价：198.00元

本书如有缺页、错装或坏损等严重质量问题，请向印刷厂联系调换

内容提要

本书全面概述了使用机械通气治疗患者时医疗人员面临的挑战和解决方案，内容包括病理生理机制和临床应用两方面，对于复杂的机械通气技术而言，这种编写方式将更利于读者进行临床实践。因机械通气在COVID-19大流行中受到广泛关注，故本书还包含其在COVID-19、资源匮乏环境等不同领域中的应用。

本书旨在用最简练的语言提供更丰富的知识，故每章均有精心绘制的图表，可帮助读者更直观地理解复杂的理论和技术。总之，本书是一本实用性极强的学习机械通气技术的参考书，可供急诊科、重症医学科、呼吸科等专业的医务人员使用。

英文版序言

为新书《机械通气：从病理生理到临床证据》撰写序言是强调机械通气仍然是危重症患者救治中应用最广泛的生命支持技术。

每年有数百万人因机械通气获救。

1952年，基于Bjorn A Ibsen博士的方法，脊髓灰质炎患儿得到了必要的呼吸支持。自此，该方法从一种简单的技术发展逐渐发展为一个复杂的临床学科，因此需要具备扎实的病理生理学知识，熟悉相关技术和设备，以及了解大量临床背景知识（而不只是呼吸系统相关的）。

从哥本哈根的脊髓灰质炎流行开始，到最近的H1N1流感及最新的COVID-19大流行，机械通气已被证明是疫情中最重要的生命支持方式，也是重症医学专业的基石。

本书致力于系统地介绍机械通气这一广泛应用的临床技术，正如其书名所示，从病理生理到临床证据。主要涉及重症医学领域，从基本技术背景到病理生理监测，再到现实生活中的临床场景。这种编写方式能为读者了解机械通气相关知识提供有效的帮助。本书还提供了机械通气技术中的重要更新。

本书由强大的作者团队编写，注定将成为任何对该学科感兴趣的人的最重要的参考书之一。

感谢Giacomo Bellani主编和其他所有编者的贡献。

Antonio Pesenti
Department of Anesthesia and Critical Care
Fondazione IRCCS Ca' Granda-Ospedale Maggiore Policlinico
Milan
Italy

Department of Pathophysiology and Transplantation
Università degli Studi di Milano
Milan
Italy

英文版前言

我常被问及，是什么促使我决定撰写一本关于机械通气的书。答案与支撑这本书的核心思想一样，非常简单：我坚信，在临床实践中，虽然临床指南是必要的，治疗方案也是有用的，但如果缺少了医生对于生理学及疾病状态下的"病理生理学"的深刻理解和一定的知识储备，那么机械通气的治疗效果将难以达到最佳。这些从病理生理学中提炼出的理念，经过临床试验的验证，最终被纳入指南之中。

此外，多篇论文都是以"机械通气是对急性呼吸衰竭进行救治的一种挽救生命的治疗方法……"这样的句子开头的，这当然是事实。但我更想强调的是，机械通气的独特之处在于，它为我们理解患者疾病状况提供了特别的机会，并能够实时监测患者对临床干预措施的反应。只需观察波形和测量几个参数，我们便能判断呼气末正压是否设置得过高导致肺过度膨胀、新引入的支气管扩张剂是否有效，以及支持患者的辅助通气过多还是过少，是否因肌肉无力而无法撤机，这样的例子有很多。因此，机械通气确实也是一种诊断工具，而且是实时的。在个体化治疗的时代，这一点尤为重要。尽管指南和方案非常有用，但它们无法提供治疗特定患者所需的所有复杂信息。优化患者-呼吸机之间的相互作用，以达到最佳床旁治疗效果，正是个体化治疗的体现。再次强调，病理生理学的知识是实现这一目标的关键工具。

此外，我必须说，总体而言，这本书绝对超出了我的预期。多年来，我有幸结识了众多在这一领域具有深厚造诣的专家同行。通过阅读他们的论文和聆听他们的演讲，明显可以看出他们的知识也来自日常实践和经验。我感到非常自豪和荣幸，他们接受了在这个项目中合作的邀请，并且他们都提供了极高质量的内容。需要知道的是，我要求作者限制参考文献的数量——与其进行全面、详尽的文献综述，提供作者认为有价值的资源更有意义。因此，如果书中漏掉哪些重要的参考文献，请不要归咎于这些作者。

我真诚地希望这本书能帮助我们的同事（尤其是年轻的），不仅是"学习"，更重要的是"理解"机械通气，而且还能被它所"吸引"，从而能够发展和测试新的想法，进而向其他人传授。

Giacomo Bellani

Monza

Italy

中文版前言

近年来,机械通气技术在我国的临床医学领域得到了广泛应用并快速发展。作为一种重要的呼吸支持手段,机械通气在重症医学、急救医学和麻醉学等多个领域发挥着不可替代的作用。在中国,随着重症监护病房数量的增加和医疗水平的提升,越来越多的医务人员开始关注机械通气的最新进展与临床应用。然而,在实际操作中,由于患者病情的复杂性和机械通气策略的多样性,如何科学、合理地应用机械通气仍然是临床医生面临的巨大挑战。与此同时,COVID-19等呼吸道传染病的流行,也使得机械通气在应对突发公共卫生事件中的重要性愈发凸显。深入理解机械通气的理论与实践,已成为医务人员的迫切需求。

Mechanical Ventilation: from Pathophysiology to Clinical Evidence 由 Giacomo Bellani 教授编写,以系统化的循证医学为基础,为读者提供了机械通气领域的最新研究成果和实践指南。与其他机械通气相关书籍相比,本书有几个显著的特色。首先,它不仅涵盖了机械通气的基础理论和病理生理机制,还深入探讨了各种复杂临床场景中的应用策略,包括急性呼吸窘迫综合征、急性低氧性呼吸衰竭、慢性阻塞性肺疾病、哮喘等常见呼吸衰竭的机械通气管理。其次,本书注重将最新的临床研究和指南与实际病例相结合,使读者能够通过临床实践消化理论知识,达到学以致用的目的。本书每一章都含有详尽的图表,可帮助读者更直观地理解复杂的概念和技术。最后,本书邀请了多位国际知名专家撰写不同章节,确保了内容的广泛性和前沿性,也能反映机械通气技术的全球发展趋势。

在翻译过程中,我们充分考虑了读者的阅读习惯和临床实际需求。为了确保译文的准确性和可读性,翻译团队由重症医学相关领域的专家组成,他们不仅熟悉原著的专业内容,还具有丰富的临床经验。在翻译过程中,我们力求在保持原著科学性和严谨性的同时,增强了语言的流畅性和可读性,旨在帮助读者更好地理解和应用书中的内容,更贴近中国读者的日常实践。

我们希望,通过本书的出版,能够为医务工作者提供一本既具权威性又实用的机械通气参考书,帮助大家更好地掌握机械通气的原理与应用技术,提高临床决策能力和对患者治疗的效果。同时,我们也希望本书能够启发更多的研究者参与机械通气领域的研究,推动其不断创新与发展。相信本书不仅能够成为临床医生的重要参考书籍,也能成为医学教育中的宝贵资源,为下一代医学人才的培养提供有力支持。

最后，感谢所有为本书翻译与出版工作付出辛勤努力的同仁们，感谢他们在繁忙的临床工作之余，为本书的顺利出版做出的重要贡献。期待本书能为推动中国机械通气领域的发展贡献一份力量，助力提升中国重症医学的整体水平。

王瑞兰

译者名单

主　译
王瑞兰　陈德昌

副主译
谢　晖　皋　源　刘　娇

译　者（按姓氏汉语拼音排序）
陈　瑨　上海市第一人民医院急诊危重病科
陈德昌　上海交通大学医学院附属瑞金医院重症医学科
陈子阳　上海市第一人民医院急诊危重病科
戴清霞　上海市第一人民医院急诊危重病科
邓会标　上海市第一人民医院急诊危重病科
皋　源　上海交通大学医学院附属仁济医院重症医学科
高甜甜　上海市第一人民医院急诊危重病科
宫　晔　复旦大学附属华山医院重症医学科
计恩东　上海市第一人民医院急诊危重病科
金珊珊　上海市第一人民医院急诊危重病科
李慧敏　上海市第一人民医院急诊危重病科
刘　娇　上海交通大学医学院附属瑞金医院重症医学科
吕　慧　上海市第一人民医院急诊危重病科
马少林　同济大学附属东方医院重症医学科
瞿洪平　上海交通大学医学院附属瑞金医院重症医学科
王　蕊　上海市第一人民医院急诊危重病科
王瑞兰　上海市第一人民医院急诊危重病科
王伟琴　上海市第一人民医院急诊危重病科
魏东坡　上海市第一人民医院急诊危重病科
谢　晖　上海市第一人民医院急诊危重病科

于晨希　上海市第一人民医院急诊危重病科
钟　鸣　复旦大学附属中山医院重症医学科
张　媛　上海市第一人民医院急诊危重病科
赵立娜　上海市第一人民医院急诊危重病科
肇寅辉　上海市第一人民医院急诊危重病科
周　媛　上海市第一人民医院急诊危重病科
周芳庆　上海市第一人民医院急诊危重病科

目 录

第一部分 通 气 技 术

1 呼吸系统基础生理学：气体交换与呼吸力学 ⋯⋯⋯⋯⋯⋯⋯⋯⋯⋯ 3
   1.1 气体交换 ⋯⋯⋯⋯⋯⋯⋯⋯⋯⋯⋯⋯⋯⋯⋯⋯⋯⋯⋯⋯⋯⋯ 3
   1.2 呼吸力学 ⋯⋯⋯⋯⋯⋯⋯⋯⋯⋯⋯⋯⋯⋯⋯⋯⋯⋯⋯⋯⋯⋯ 6

2 机械通气简史 ⋯⋯⋯⋯⋯⋯⋯⋯⋯⋯⋯⋯⋯⋯⋯⋯⋯⋯⋯⋯⋯⋯ 11
   2.1 呼吸、循环及两者相互作用 ⋯⋯⋯⋯⋯⋯⋯⋯⋯⋯⋯⋯⋯⋯⋯ 11
   2.2 氧气,燃烧,代谢,稳态 ⋯⋯⋯⋯⋯⋯⋯⋯⋯⋯⋯⋯⋯⋯⋯⋯⋯ 12
   2.3 机械通气的黎明 ⋯⋯⋯⋯⋯⋯⋯⋯⋯⋯⋯⋯⋯⋯⋯⋯⋯⋯⋯ 12
   2.4 经验教训 ⋯⋯⋯⋯⋯⋯⋯⋯⋯⋯⋯⋯⋯⋯⋯⋯⋯⋯⋯⋯⋯⋯ 15

3 危重症患者的气道管理 ⋯⋯⋯⋯⋯⋯⋯⋯⋯⋯⋯⋯⋯⋯⋯⋯⋯⋯ 18
   3.1 引言 ⋯⋯⋯⋯⋯⋯⋯⋯⋯⋯⋯⋯⋯⋯⋯⋯⋯⋯⋯⋯⋯⋯⋯⋯ 18
   3.2 ICU 气管插管的适应证 ⋯⋯⋯⋯⋯⋯⋯⋯⋯⋯⋯⋯⋯⋯⋯⋯ 19
   3.3 气管插管的准备和流程 ⋯⋯⋯⋯⋯⋯⋯⋯⋯⋯⋯⋯⋯⋯⋯⋯ 20
   3.4 气管插管流程 ⋯⋯⋯⋯⋯⋯⋯⋯⋯⋯⋯⋯⋯⋯⋯⋯⋯⋯⋯⋯ 21
   3.5 挽救性给氧 ⋯⋯⋯⋯⋯⋯⋯⋯⋯⋯⋯⋯⋯⋯⋯⋯⋯⋯⋯⋯⋯ 26
   3.6 气管导管的护理 ⋯⋯⋯⋯⋯⋯⋯⋯⋯⋯⋯⋯⋯⋯⋯⋯⋯⋯⋯ 27
   3.7 气道管理中的人为因素 ⋯⋯⋯⋯⋯⋯⋯⋯⋯⋯⋯⋯⋯⋯⋯⋯ 27
   3.8 未来研究 ⋯⋯⋯⋯⋯⋯⋯⋯⋯⋯⋯⋯⋯⋯⋯⋯⋯⋯⋯⋯⋯⋯ 27
   3.9 总结 ⋯⋯⋯⋯⋯⋯⋯⋯⋯⋯⋯⋯⋯⋯⋯⋯⋯⋯⋯⋯⋯⋯⋯⋯ 28

4 控制性机械通气：模式和监测 ⋯⋯⋯⋯⋯⋯⋯⋯⋯⋯⋯⋯⋯⋯⋯ 33
   4.1 压力控制通气 ⋯⋯⋯⋯⋯⋯⋯⋯⋯⋯⋯⋯⋯⋯⋯⋯⋯⋯⋯⋯ 35
   4.2 容量控制通气 ⋯⋯⋯⋯⋯⋯⋯⋯⋯⋯⋯⋯⋯⋯⋯⋯⋯⋯⋯⋯ 35
   4.3 压力调节的容量保障通气 ⋯⋯⋯⋯⋯⋯⋯⋯⋯⋯⋯⋯⋯⋯⋯ 35
   4.4 完全控制模式的生理特征 ⋯⋯⋯⋯⋯⋯⋯⋯⋯⋯⋯⋯⋯⋯⋯ 36

4.5　自主吸气努力时的模式特点 ………………………………………………… 37
　　4.6　控制通气过程中的监测 …………………………………………………… 39
　　4.7　总结 ………………………………………………………………………… 42

5　辅助通气：压力支持和双水平正压通气模式 ……………………………………… 44
　　5.1　引言 ………………………………………………………………………… 44
　　5.2　压力支持通气 ……………………………………………………………… 45
　　5.3　双水平正压通气模式 ……………………………………………………… 48
　　5.4　总结 ………………………………………………………………………… 51

6　辅助通气过程中患者的监测 ………………………………………………………… 54
　　6.1　吸气努力 …………………………………………………………………… 55
　　6.2　呼吸系统扩张的总压力 …………………………………………………… 58
　　6.3　人-机不同步 ………………………………………………………………… 59
　　6.4　气体再分布和呼吸摆动 …………………………………………………… 60
　　6.5　呼吸肌的超声评估 ………………………………………………………… 61
　　6.6　总结 ………………………………………………………………………… 61

7　神经调节通气辅助 …………………………………………………………………… 66
　　7.1　工作原理 …………………………………………………………………… 66
　　7.2　NAVA 时如何设置辅助通气 ……………………………………………… 68
　　7.3　神经调节通气辅助下如何设置呼气末正压 ……………………………… 70
　　7.4　神经调节通气辅助如何撤机 ……………………………………………… 71
　　7.5　神经调节通气辅助的临床效果 …………………………………………… 71
　　7.6　神经调节通气辅助的局限性 ……………………………………………… 72
　　7.7　总结 ………………………………………………………………………… 72

8　成比例辅助通气 ……………………………………………………………………… 75
　　8.1　引言 ………………………………………………………………………… 75
　　8.2　工作原理 …………………………………………………………………… 75
　　8.3　PAV＋的优势 ……………………………………………………………… 78
　　8.4　PAV/PAV＋应用的局限 …………………………………………………… 79
　　8.5　PAV＋吸气辅助的滴定 …………………………………………………… 79
　　8.6　总结 ………………………………………………………………………… 80

9　无创通气：适应证和注意事项 ……………………………………………………… 82
　　9.1　引言 ………………………………………………………………………… 82

目 录

9.2	无创通气的接口	82
9.3	通气模式	84
9.4	无创通气的生理学效应	84
9.5	无创通气的指征	85
9.6	无创通气患者监测的重要性	87
9.7	总结	89

10 经鼻高流量氧疗：从生理学到临床实践 … 92

10.1	引言	92
10.2	无效腔，气体混合和冲刷	93
10.3	呼气末正压的产生（或无）	94
10.4	呼吸做功	95
10.5	注意事项	96
10.6	总结	96

11 机械通气和体外膜肺氧合患者的护理 … 100

11.1	机械通气	100
11.2	俯卧位	102
11.3	体外膜肺氧合	106
11.4	总结	110

12 闭环通气模式 … 114

12.1	引言	114
12.2	强制每分钟通气	115
12.3	Smartcare/PS	115
12.4	自适应支持通气	117
12.5	INTELLiVENT‐ASV	119
12.6	总结	121

13 气道压力释放通气 … 124

13.1	引言	124
13.2	生理学	124
13.3	指征	125
13.4	设置	125
13.5	自主呼吸	127
13.6	撤机	128
13.7	总结	128

第二部分 临 床 情 景

14 急性低氧性呼吸衰竭和急性呼吸窘迫综合征 ································· 133
  14.1 急性低氧性呼吸衰竭和急性呼吸窘迫综合征：定义的难题 ········· 133
  14.2 流行病学：已知与未知 ·· 137
  14.3 病理生理学：见解与分歧 ·· 137
  14.4 呼吸支持方式 ·· 138
  14.5 有创机械通气：从"保护性"到"个体化" ······································ 138
  14.6 通气支持的辅助手段 ·· 139
  14.7 急性低氧性呼吸衰竭和急性呼吸窘迫综合征的特殊治疗 ············ 139
  14.8 临床结局 ·· 140
  14.9 急性低氧性呼吸衰竭：改变范式 ·· 141
  14.10 总结 ··· 141

15 呼吸机诱发的肺损伤和肺保护性通气 ·· 146
  15.1 呼吸系统的机械敏感性 ·· 147
  15.2 呼吸机诱发的肺损伤的病理生理学 ·· 148
  15.3 呼吸机诱导肺损伤的床旁评估 ·· 149
  15.4 设计肺保护策略 ··· 150
  15.5 肺保护性通气的临床证据 ·· 152
  15.6 总结 ··· 152

16 健康肺的机械通气：在手术室和重症监护室中 ···································· 156
  16.1 引言 ··· 156
  16.2 潮气量 ··· 157
  16.3 手术室中的潮气量 ··· 157
  16.4 重症监护室中的潮气量 ·· 158
  16.5 呼气末正压 ·· 159
  16.6 手术室呼气末正压的选择 ·· 159
  16.7 在重症监护室中呼气末正压的设置 ·· 160
  16.8 总结 ··· 161

17 急性呼吸窘迫综合征的呼气末正压设置 ·· 165
  17.1 引言 ··· 165
  17.2 病理生理：呼气末正压的益处 ·· 165
  17.3 病理生理学：呼气末正压的危害 ·· 166

17.4 急性呼吸窘迫综合征中呼气末正压设置的建议 …………………………… 166
   17.5 床旁滴定呼气末正压的策略 ……………………………………………… 167
   17.6 总结 ………………………………………………………………………… 170

18 脑损伤患者的机械通气 ……………………………………………………………… 175
   18.1 引言 ………………………………………………………………………… 175
   18.2 脑损伤患者有创机械通气的适应证 ……………………………………… 175
   18.3 通气策略和目标 …………………………………………………………… 176
   18.4 难治性呼吸衰竭的抢救干预措施 ………………………………………… 177
   18.5 撤机和气管切开 …………………………………………………………… 178
   18.6 神经肌肉疾病的通气 ……………………………………………………… 178
   18.7 总结 ………………………………………………………………………… 179

19 心力衰竭患者的有创与无创通气 …………………………………………………… 181
   19.1 引言 ………………………………………………………………………… 181
   19.2 急性心力衰竭时呼吸衰竭的病理生理 …………………………………… 181
   19.3 心力衰竭患者气道正压的基本原理 ……………………………………… 182
   19.4 无创正压通气治疗心源性肺水肿：临床证据 …………………………… 184
   19.5 无创和有创正压通气治疗心源性休克 …………………………………… 185
   19.6 心脏停搏后的通气 ………………………………………………………… 185

20 慢性阻塞性肺疾病和严重哮喘 ……………………………………………………… 189
   20.1 病理生理学 ………………………………………………………………… 189
   20.2 通用呼吸支持策略 ………………………………………………………… 191
   20.3 阻塞性肺疾病患者的有创控制通气：目标、动态气体陷闭的监测和
        通气策略 …………………………………………………………………… 191
   20.4 阻塞性肺疾病患者的有创辅助通气及撤机策略 ………………………… 193

21 肥胖患者的通气 ……………………………………………………………………… 196
   21.1 引言 ………………………………………………………………………… 196
   21.2 肥胖患者的机械通气需要调整的呼吸机输入参数 ……………………… 196
   21.3 肥胖患者的机械通气需要监测的呼吸机输出参数 ……………………… 198
   21.4 总结 ………………………………………………………………………… 200

22 简单和复杂患者的撤机 ……………………………………………………………… 202
   22.1 引言 ………………………………………………………………………… 202
   22.2 撤机的定义和步骤 ………………………………………………………… 203

  22.3 尝试撤机步骤 ……… 206
  22.4 预防拔管失败 ……… 209
  22.5 总结 ……… 212

23　COVID-19 相关呼吸衰竭的无创氧疗策略 ……… 217
  23.1 引言 ……… 217
  23.2 无创氧疗策略：设备、生理学和非 COVID-19 证据 ……… 218
  23.3 COVID-19 大流行期间无创氧疗策略的注意事项 ……… 219
  23.4 总结 ……… 222

24　COVID-19 中的有创通气 ……… 225
  24.1 引言 ……… 225
  24.2 气管插管和时机选择 ……… 226
  24.3 机械通气设置 ……… 226
  24.4 挽救性治疗 ……… 228
  24.5 气管切开术 ……… 230
  24.6 总结 ……… 230

25　不同手术情境下的机械通气 ……… 233
  25.1 引言 ……… 233
  25.2 腹腔镜手术 ……… 237
  25.3 肥胖患者 ……… 238
  25.4 胸外科手术 ……… 239
  25.5 心脏手术 ……… 239
  25.6 神经外科 ……… 240
  25.7 总结 ……… 241

26　患者的长期随访 ……… 245
  26.1 引言 ……… 245
  26.2 随访门诊和 PICS 框架 ……… 246
  26.3 总结 ……… 250

27　有限资源环境下的机械通气 ……… 253
  27.1 引言 ……… 253
  27.2 有限资源环境下的机械通气设施 ……… 253
  27.3 资源可变环境下机械通气的适应证 ……… 254
  27.4 资源有限环境下的机械通气模式 ……… 255

27.5	资源有限环境下的机械通气并发症	256
27.6	长期机械通气患者气管切开的实践	256
27.7	总结	256

28 患者转运期间的机械通气 259

28.1	概述	259
28.2	转运对患者生理的影响	259
28.3	设置转运呼吸机	260
28.4	肺部和气道并发症	260
28.5	心血管并发症	261
28.6	设备故障、注意事项和人为错误	261
28.7	检查清单的重要性	262
28.8	总结	264

第三部分 机械通气的辅助手段

29 俯卧位通气 269

29.1	基本原理	269
29.2	俯卧位的启动时机	271
29.3	实际问题	273
29.4	临床证据	274
29.5	总结	274

30 静脉-静脉体外膜肺氧合和体外二氧化碳清除 277

30.1	严重呼吸衰竭的病理生理：肺内分流和肺泡无效腔	277
30.2	为什么要采用体外气体交换	277
30.3	"全"流量静脉-静脉体外膜肺氧合与低流量体外二氧化碳清除	279
30.4	急性呼吸窘迫综合征患者体外气体交换的循证证据	280
30.5	静脉-静脉体外膜肺氧合治疗急性呼吸窘迫综合征患者的预后	281
30.6	是否应该增加体外膜肺氧合中心的数量	282
30.7	总结	282

31 体外膜肺氧合时的机械通气参数设置 286

31.1	引言	286
31.2	总结	292

第四部分　机械通气监测

32　呼吸系统的超声评估 ... 297
- 32.1　引言 ... 297
- 32.2　肺部超声 ... 297
- 32.3　膈肌 ... 301
- 32.4　辅助呼吸肌 ... 304
- 32.5　局限性 ... 304
- 32.6　总结 ... 304

33　电阻抗体断层成像技术 ... 307
- 33.1　引言 ... 307
- 33.2　电阻抗断层成像的基础 ... 308
- 33.3　使用电阻抗断层成像监测患者 ... 310
- 33.4　电阻抗断层成像评估局部肺通气和通气变化 ... 310
- 33.5　电阻抗断层成像评估局部肺灌注 ... 313
- 33.6　总结 ... 314

34　食管压监测 ... 317
- 34.1　引言 ... 317
- 34.2　食管压衍生变量的测量 ... 319
- 34.3　监测食管压力指导机械通气 ... 321
- 34.4　总结 ... 325

35　肺容积和容积二氧化碳图 ... 328
- 35.1　引言 ... 328
- 35.2　肺容积 ... 328
- 35.3　容积二氧化碳图 ... 332

36　影像学监测 ... 337
- 36.1　引言 ... 337
- 36.2　我们能从 ICU 里的胸片检查中得到什么 ... 338
- 36.3　机械通气患者何时需要 CT 检查 ... 340
- 36.4　总结 ... 341

第五部分 教　育　资　源

37 机械通气的教学：在线资源和模拟教学 ┈┈┈┈┈┈┈┈┈┈┈┈┈┈ 347
　37.1　引言 ┈┈┈┈┈┈┈┈┈┈┈┈┈┈┈┈┈┈┈┈┈┈┈┈┈┈┈┈ 347
　37.2　在线资源和应用 ┈┈┈┈┈┈┈┈┈┈┈┈┈┈┈┈┈┈┈┈┈┈ 347
　37.3　机械通气模拟教学 ┈┈┈┈┈┈┈┈┈┈┈┈┈┈┈┈┈┈┈┈ 348
　37.4　总结 ┈┈┈┈┈┈┈┈┈┈┈┈┈┈┈┈┈┈┈┈┈┈┈┈┈┈┈┈ 352

38 案例教学：机械通气控制模式 ┈┈┈┈┈┈┈┈┈┈┈┈┈┈┈┈┈┈ 353
　38.1　引言 ┈┈┈┈┈┈┈┈┈┈┈┈┈┈┈┈┈┈┈┈┈┈┈┈┈┈┈┈ 353
　38.2　临床案例 ┈┈┈┈┈┈┈┈┈┈┈┈┈┈┈┈┈┈┈┈┈┈┈┈┈┈ 353

39 案例教学：机械通气辅助模式 ┈┈┈┈┈┈┈┈┈┈┈┈┈┈┈┈┈┈ 363
　39.1　引言 ┈┈┈┈┈┈┈┈┈┈┈┈┈┈┈┈┈┈┈┈┈┈┈┈┈┈┈┈ 363

彩　色　插　图

第一部分
通气技术

1 呼吸系统基础生理学：气体交换与呼吸力学
Basic Physiology of Respiratory System: Gas Exchange and Respiratory Mechanics

Khoi Do, Guido Musch

1.1 气体交换

气体交换是指大气中的氧气（O_2）通过肺泡转移到血液中，同时二氧化碳（CO_2）从血液转移至肺泡气体的过程。二氧化碳随后通过呼吸通气排出。气体交换发生在呼吸系统的过渡区和呼吸区，是肺组织中肺泡所包覆的区域。肺泡是被包绕在毛细血管床中的微小气囊（图1.1），肺泡内空气与血液毗邻，为气体交换创造了最佳环境。氧气与二氧化碳分别通过呼吸通气和血流灌注的方式进入气体交换部位，此后通过气体分压梯度驱动的简单扩散机制跨过气-血屏障（即肺泡-毛细血管膜）进行转移[1]。在本章中，我们将论述气体交换的各个环节：氧气输送、二氧化碳清除、通气-灌注匹配及气体弥散。

大气中的氧气通过呼吸通气被输送至肺泡，输送到肺泡内的氧气量主要取决于吸入氧浓度。这可以通过肺泡气体计算公式来理解。其中，P_AO_2 = 肺泡氧分压，P_{atm} = 大气压，P_{H_2O} = 体温下水蒸气分压，FiO_2 = 吸入氧浓度，P_ACO_2 = 肺泡二氧化碳分压，R = 进入肺泡排放的二氧化碳与离开肺泡被摄入的氧气的量的比值（即呼吸商）[1,2]。

$$P_AO_2 = [(P_{atm} - P_{H_2O}) \times FiO_2] - \left(\frac{P_ACO_2}{R}\right) \qquad (1.1)$$

一旦氧气进入肺泡，驱动它进入血液的主要动力是跨肺泡-毛细血管膜的分压梯度，也就是肺泡氧分压（P_AO_2）与回心混合静脉血氧分压间的差值。如公式所示：P_AO_2 由气

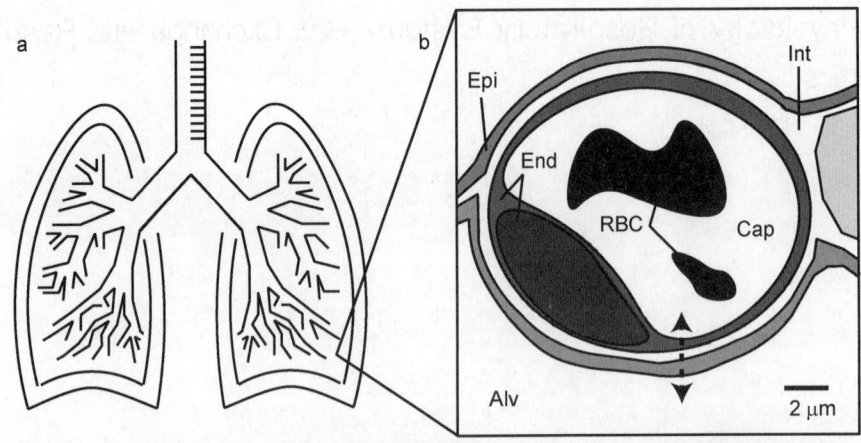

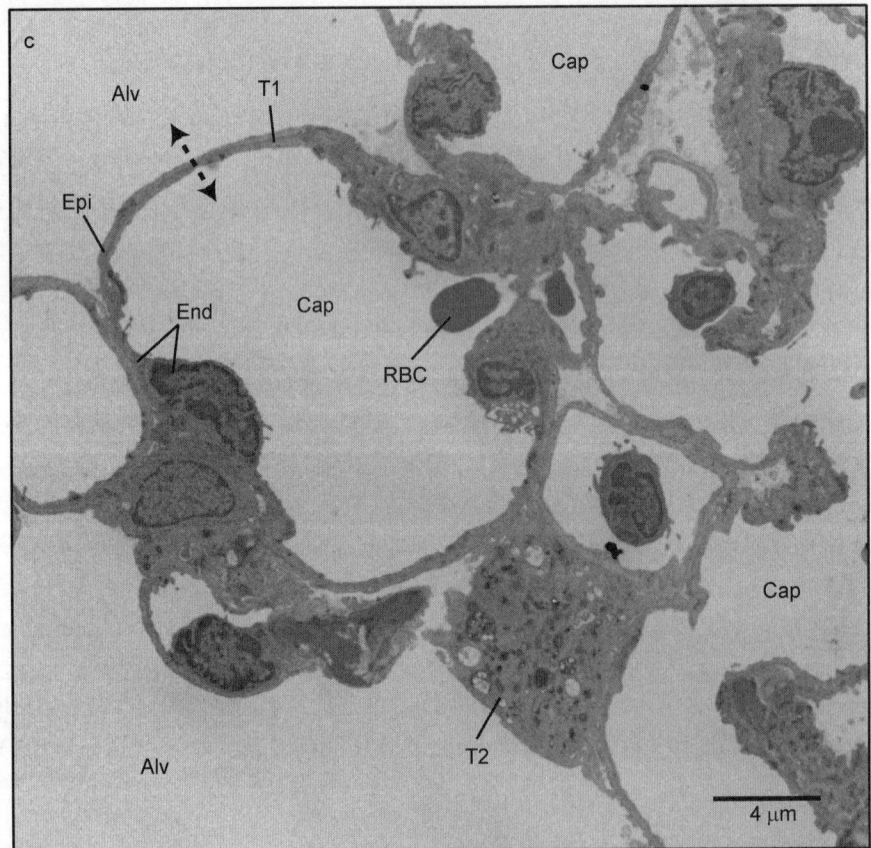

图1.1 a. 气体交换发生在远端气道,也称为过渡区和呼吸区。b和c分别以模式图和电子显微镜下图像展示了嵌入肺泡(Alv)内的肺毛细血管(Cap)的横截面。图中双箭头指示的是气体通过气-血屏障的弥散路径。这一界面也被称为肺泡-毛细血管膜,由肺泡上皮(Epi)和肺毛细血管内皮(End)相邻的基底膜组成。Ⅰ型(T1)和Ⅱ型(T2)肺泡细胞也可以在电子显微镜下看到。RBC,红细胞;Int,气-血交换界面

道吸入气体氧分压[$(P_{atm}-P_{H_2O})\times FiO_2$]与由于氧气弥散进入毛细血管导致的氧分压下降($P_ACO_2/R$)的差值所决定。除了吸入氧浓度,其他变量是相对固定的。通过增加吸入氧浓度,肺泡氧分压也会增加。同时,肺泡氧分压与混合静脉血氧分压差也会增大,故使氧气由肺泡向血液弥散的驱动力增加。

二氧化碳是细胞代谢的天然副产物,通过静脉系统被转运至肺毛细血管床,于此弥散到肺泡内并排放到大气中。与氧气的转运不同,二氧化碳的清除主要由呼吸通气所决定。肺泡平均二氧化碳分压由以下公式决定,其中 F_ACO_2=肺泡二氧化碳分数,$\dot{V}CO_2$=组织产生二氧化碳的速率,$\dot{V}_E$=每分钟通气量,$\dot{V}_d$=无效腔通气量[1,2]。

$$F_ACO_2=\frac{\dot{V}CO_2}{\dot{V}_E-\dot{V}_d} \tag{1.2}$$

($\dot{V}_E-\dot{V}_d$)代表肺泡通气速率或吸入空气中实际参加气体交换的气体量。在这个公式中,$\dot{V}CO_2$由代谢过程所决定,$\dot{V}_d$是解剖学参数,而$\dot{V}_E$是实际可调节的。每分钟通气量是潮气量与呼吸频率的乘积。通过改变这两个变量中的任意一个,可增加或减少二氧化碳的排出量。例如,潮气量或呼吸频率增加,F_ACO_2则下降,混合静脉血和肺泡间压力梯度差增加,进而驱动更多的二氧化碳进入肺泡。

如上所述,氧气通过呼吸通气被转运至气体交换的部位,通过血流灌注被摄取;相反,二氧化碳通过血流灌注被运输到气体交换的部位,经呼吸通气排出。为了达到最佳的气体交换效率,通气($\dot{V}$)与灌注($\dot{Q}$)必须匹配。理想的$\dot{V}/\dot{Q}$值是1,该值通常在直立个体的肺中部得以实现。从肺底部到肺尖部,$\dot{V}/\dot{Q}$值为 0.3~2.1[3]。$\dot{V}/\dot{Q}$值影响 P_AO_2和P_ACO_2的值,从而影响气体交换的效率(图1.2)。如果肺部某个区域有血流灌注但没有充气,如由于肺泡充满了液体,此时$\dot{V}/\dot{Q}$值为0,那么氧气就不能进入肺部,二氧化碳也不能被清除。因此,静脉血相当于绕过了所在区域的肺循环形成分流,不参与气体交换,从而混合静脉血的氧分压和二氧化碳分压得以保留。从生理学角度来看,这种分流造成的血液低氧和高碳酸的情况会严重降低动脉血氧饱和度和氧含量,导致肺泡-动脉氧分压(A-a)梯度增加。这种继发的低氧血症很难通过提高吸入氧浓度来纠正,分流的存在也会降低二氧化碳的排出效率。如果机体能够增加每分钟通气量来代偿,那么分流不会引起高碳酸血症。如果每分钟通气量是固定的,如患者采用了控制性机械通气,分流除了会引起低氧,还会引起二氧化碳潴留。另一方面,如果肺的局部没有血流灌注,如肺栓塞,但有充气,那么$\dot{V}/\dot{Q}$值趋于无穷大,功能上该区域构成无效腔通气,此时氧分压和二氧化碳分压与吸入气道的大气相同。生理学上,极高的$\dot{V}/\dot{Q}$值会导致肺泡无效腔和无效腔通气的增加。$\dot{V}/\dot{Q}$的不匹配会以不同方式显著影响肺泡内两种气体的浓度,并对气体交换产生显著的生理效应。

气体交换的最后一个步骤是氧气和二氧化碳分子在肺泡和毛细血管血液之间的弥散。气体分子按各自的压力梯度,以相反方向穿过气体-血液界面上菲薄的上皮-内皮层。气体流动速率($\dot{V}$)主要由菲克定律决定,其中 A=膜表面面积,ΔP=界面两侧的气体分压差,D=分子移动的距离[1,2]。

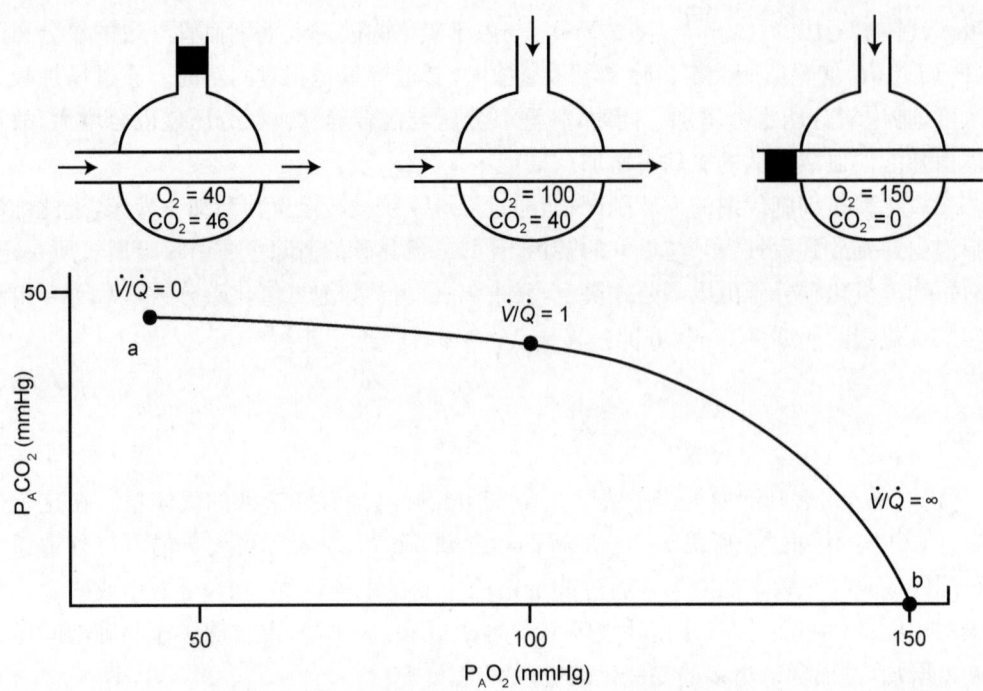

图1.2 氧气-二氧化碳图描述的是通气/灌注($\dot{V}/\dot{Q}$),以及一个肺单位内肺泡氧分压与肺泡二氧化碳分压的关系。肺单位包含肺泡及肺毛细血管。箭头指示的是气流和血流方向。曲线表示在 $\dot{V}/\dot{Q}$ 值为 0~∞ 时对应的 P_AO_2 和 P_ACO_2。a 点示分流,b 点示无效腔。P_AO_2,肺泡氧分压;P_ACO_2,肺泡二氧化碳分压;$\dot{V}/\dot{Q}$,通气/灌注。(经许可转载自参考文献[1])

$$\dot{V} = \frac{A(\Delta P)}{D} \tag{1.3}$$

氧气沿着分压差——100 mmHg(室内空气)的平均肺泡氧分压和 40 mmHg 的混合静脉氧分压,从肺泡向混合静脉弥散。二氧化碳从混合静脉(分压 46 mmHg)弥散到肺泡(平均分压 40 mmHg)中。机体通过优化菲克定律公式中的其余参数来使弥散效率最大化。气体-血液界面非常薄(0.2~0.3 μm);表面积巨大,可达 70~80 m²。这些优化条件使得即使在更高血流量下,也能实现气体迅速弥散。通常情况下,仅需血液通过肺毛细血管全长时间(0.75 s)的 1/3,气体弥散就达到了平衡状态[2]。

1.2 呼吸力学

呼吸力学指的是由压力、流速及容量间关系所描述的肺功能。理解呼吸力学需要掌握呼吸系统的大体解剖。呼吸系统由气道、肺及胸壁组成。胸腔由胸壁和膈围成。肺和胸壁之间的潜在腔隙称胸膜腔。胸膜腔内的液体有两种作用:润滑相邻滑动的胸膜,使肺附着于胸壁。

在呼吸系统中存在静态反向力,体现在肺和胸壁上。如图 1.3 所示,可以将其视为两根并联的弹簧,一根弹簧被压缩在其静息长度以下(胸壁),另一根弹簧则被拉伸至其静息长度以上(肺)[4]。肺自然地向内收缩,而胸壁则向外扩张。胸膜腔内的液体将两者相连,这些反向作用力有助于呼吸系统的结构完整性并对正常呼吸通气尤为重要。

肺的内向力主要来自两个因素:肺组织的弹性回缩和表面张力。弹性回缩主要是指物体在被拉伸或受压后恢复其自然形状的趋势,可以通过它的弹性系数来测量(如引起单位体积变化所需要的压力,$\Delta P/\Delta V$)。弹性系数的倒数就是顺应性,指的是物体在外力作用下发生形变的性质。例如,单位压力变化所带来的体积变化($\Delta V/\Delta P$)。肺的顺应性随肺容积而改变。一般在低容积时,肺组织表现出更好的顺应性和可扩张性;随着容积的增加,肺组织逐渐僵硬,顺应性下降[4]。这一现象可以通过吸气或呼吸时充气肺的压力-容积曲线来理解(图 1.3)。在低-中压力时,两条曲线相对陡峭,而在压力接近上限时曲线趋于平缓。较高肺容积时顺应性的下降与弹性回缩的增加主要是由于肺组织中的弹性蛋白及胶原纤维。高容积时弹性回缩增加是肺组织的固有特性,也是引起肺内向回缩的作用力之一。

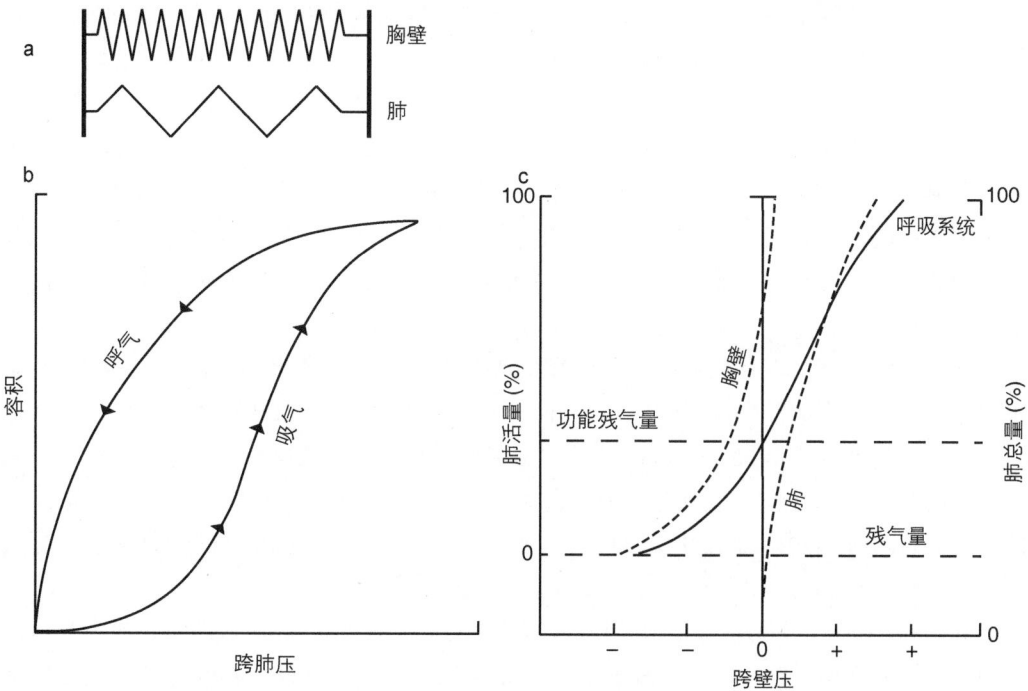

图 1.3 a. 两根平行的弹簧代表的是胸壁与肺之间的静态反向力。b. 吸气和呼气时充气肺的压力-容积曲线。c. 肺、胸壁及呼吸系统的压力-容积曲线。呼吸系统的曲线是肺与胸壁曲线的和。静态容积或平衡体积是指各曲线与 Y 轴的交点。呼吸系统在功能残气量(functional residual capacity,FRC)下处于平衡状态。b、c 经许可转载自参考文献[1]

第二个导致肺内向回缩的作用力是表面张力。表面张力是相邻液体或空气分子之间的引力。气道末端的肺泡表面覆盖着一层与空气接触的液体,形成气-液界面。由于这些液体分子较空气分子存在更强的引力,他们在黏附力的作用下紧密排列,形成内收压力来减少肺泡的体积。这些使肺泡塌陷的压力叠加在一起,最终使肺内向回缩[1]。

表面张力引起的主要问题是它降低了肺的顺应性,尤其在肺容积低的状态下,需要更强的吸气努力来启动吸气。这个现象可以在压力-容积曲线的吸气相中观察到(图1.3)。曲线起始段较为平坦,对应的是低顺应性。此时,肺需要克服表面张力来扩张。下呼吸道的Ⅱ型肺泡细胞会产生表面活性物质(一种磷脂)来减少这种初始的压力负荷,可以在低肺容积时缓解表面张力所带来的限制作用;并在吸气起始增加肺顺应性,而不损害肺的弹性回缩。表面活性物质还可以作为肺泡的"稳定剂",将肺泡塌陷压力(P_c)维持在最佳范围内[5]。根据拉普拉斯定律的定义,它通过调节表面张力(T)来做到这一点,其中P_c=塌陷压力,T=表面张力,r=半径[1,4]。

$$P_c = \frac{2T}{r} \tag{1.4}$$

根据拉普拉斯定律,减少肺泡半径会增加塌陷压力。这会使肺泡半径更小,并因此触发正反馈机制最终引起肺泡塌陷,实际上,肺泡的半径大小不一(0.1～0.25 mm)。在缺少肺泡表面活性物质的情况下,较小的肺泡会塌陷,塌陷的容积会转移到邻近的肺泡,相邻的肺泡反而增大,塌陷压力降低,进而倾向于进一步增大。理论上,这会显著增加整个肺部的肺泡容积差异。表面活性物质可以通过维持表面张力来防止肺泡塌陷及过度膨胀。这是因为当肺泡收缩时,表面活性分子会更加紧密地聚集在一起,从而相互排斥,降低表面张力;当肺泡扩张时,使得肺泡表面液体层的表面活性分子的排列变得稀疏,降低其相互作用的能力,导致表面张力增加,进而恢复高塌陷压力来对抗肺泡扩张。因此,肺泡表面活性物质的缺乏会导致肺部僵硬、肺充气不均匀,表现为充气不足和过度膨胀的区域交替分布[6]。

与肺组织的自然内收相对应的是胸壁的外扩趋势。相较于肺,胸壁有更大的静态容积。主要是由于胸壁存在自然外向弹性,该弹性主要由软骨、骨骼和肌肉产生。

肺内向的回弹力和胸壁外向的牵拉力由胸膜液联系在一起,建立起这两股反向力量之间的动态关系。这些反作用力达到平衡点时,呼吸系统即处于平衡状态。当呼吸系统偏离平衡状态时,会由校正力使其重新回到平衡状态。因此,这是个典型的稳定平衡的例子。

静态肺、胸壁及呼吸系统各自的压力-容积曲线可以很好地解释肺内向回弹力与胸壁外向牵拉力的平衡(图1.3)[1]。曲线显示了从残余容积(residual volume,RV)到总肺活量(total lung capacity,TLC)的容积范围内3个结构的跨壁压力。代表肺的曲线显示,即使在RV状态下,跨肺压(即肺泡内压减胸膜腔内压)依旧是正值,说明肺仍保持向内的回弹力。然而,胸壁曲线显示跨胸壁压在接近总肺活量前始终是负值(即胸膜腔内压低于大气压)。

呼吸系统曲线代表肺和胸壁曲线的总和,是通过计算不同容积下的跨肺压和跨胸壁压的总和而生成的。呼吸系统曲线穿过y轴的点,被标记为功能残气量(functional residual capacity,FRC),是呼吸系统达到平衡状态时的肺容积,肺内向的回弹力与胸壁外向的牵拉力相一致。高肺容积时,肺内(如肺泡)形成正压梯度促使气体排出,将曲线移回 FRC。当肺容积低于 FRC 时,则发生相反的过程。

通气发生于呼吸系统扩张或回缩后,然后返回至静息或平衡容积。大脑皮层和中脑通过延髓呼吸中枢的背侧和腹侧呼吸组(dorsal and ventral respiratory groups,DRG/VRG)来调节吸气。吸气分别由膈神经和肋间神经激活膈肌和肋间外肌而启动。吸气时,膈肌收缩、横膈下降,而肋间外肌向外上拉动肋骨和胸骨,增加胸腔容积。胸腔容积的增加降低了胸膜内压力,从而降低了肺内(如肺泡)压力(图1.4)。这样便形成相对于大气压的肺内负压,产生压力梯度,促进气体流入,直到肺内压力与大气压力相等。深吸气时需要额外的肌肉参与(如胸锁乳突肌、斜角肌和胸小肌),引起更大的胸廓扩张和压力梯度,从而增加吸入气体的流速和容积[1]。

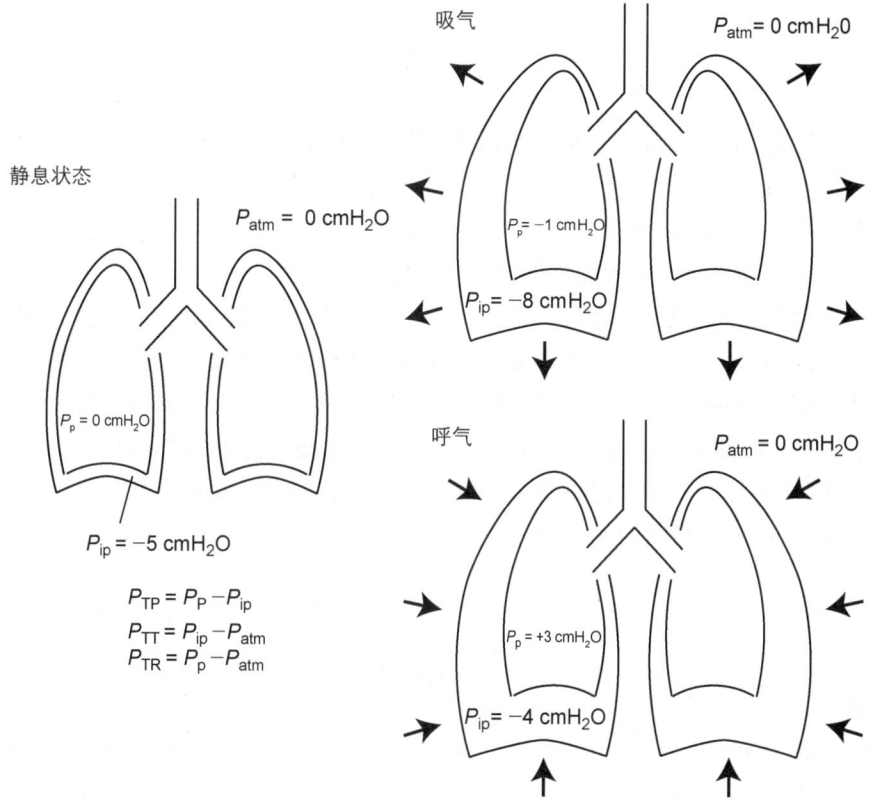

图1.4 吸气与呼气时的呼吸力学。吸气肌的收缩使压力发生变化,引起气体向内流动,从而增加肺容量。当吸气停止时,呼吸系统的弹性回缩力使肺内压力和大气压力之间的梯度发生逆转,从而产生呼气流。P_p,肺内压;P_{ip},胸膜腔内压;P_{atm},大气压;P_{TP},跨肺压;P_{TT},跨胸壁压;P_{TR},跨呼吸系统压

呼气通常是一个被动过程,不需要肌肉活动,仅基于肺的弹性回缩力。吸气结束时,胸腔内的拉伸感受器抑制 VRG,阻止其产生向膈肌和肋间外肌的动作电位。呼吸系统的弹性回缩使肺内压高于上呼吸道和大气的压力,形成相对于后者的正向压力梯度,促使气体向外流动(图1.4)。用力呼气涉及腹部肌肉(如腹内/外斜肌、腹横肌、腹直肌)和肋间

内肌,导致比单纯弹性回缩更大的肺内压增高。这些额外的压力增加了气体流速和呼出气体的量[1]。

吸气和呼气都涉及气体通过气道的流动。第一个描述该过程的近似模型是泊肃叶的层流模型,描述了管道内液体或气体的流动[6]。该模型基于下面的公式,其中 Q = 液体或气体流量,ΔP = 管道两端的压力梯度,R = 阻力。

$$\dot{Q} = \frac{\Delta P}{R} \tag{1.5}$$

根据这个公式我们可以推导出特定的关系。例如,对于特定的阻力,更大的压力梯度会产生更大的流量;或者更大的阻力会使流量减少。层流时阻力遵循下面的公式,其中 η 为黏度,l 为管道长度,r 为管道半径。

$$R = \frac{8\eta l}{\pi r^4} \tag{1.6}$$

由此可见,管道半径可显著地影响阻力,进而影响通过管道的流量,因为 r 在上述公式中以四次方的形式出现。传导气道(支气管)直径较大。细支气管直径小,但是它们的总横截面积很大。所以,支气管树中压力下降最大点在中等直径支气管处。在呼吸性细支气管中,气体不再流动,主要经弥散驱动气体穿过肺泡膜。

影响气道阻力的因素遵循泊肃叶定律所建立的原则。第一个因素是肺容积,肺容积增大阻力降低,肺容积减小则阻力增加。当肺扩张时,气道由于周围肺组织的牵拉而扩张。当肺容积很小时,气道可能会完全闭塞,尤其是在肺的下部。机体还可利用自主神经系统通过调节平滑肌张力改变气道直径。交感神经活动通过 β_2 肾上腺素受体引起支气管扩张,而副交感神经活动通过毒蕈碱受体引起支气管收缩。最后,吸入气体的黏度也会影响阻力,高黏度导致高阻力及低流速[1]。

(陈子阳,陈德昌 译)

参考文献

[1] West JB. Respiratory physiology: the essentials. 9th ed. Philadelphia: Lippincott Williams & Wilkins; 2012.

[2] Kreit JW. Gas exchange. In: Mechanical ventilation: physiology and practice. Oxford: Oxford University Press; 2017. https://doi.org/10.1093/med/9780190670085.003.0002.

[3] Wagner PD, Laravuso RB, Uhl RR, West JB. Continuous distributions of ventilation-perfusion ratios in normal subjects breathing air and 100 percent O_2. J Clin Invest. 1974;54(1):54-68.

[4] Kreit JW. Respiratory mechanics. In: Mechanical ventilation: physiology and practice. Oxford: Oxford University Press; 2017. https://doi.org/10.1093/med/9780190670085.003.0001.

[5] Macklem PT, Permutt S. The lung in the transition between health and disease. 1st ed. New York: Marcel Dekker; 1979.

[6] Cavagna G. Fundamentals of human physiology. 1st ed. Cham: Springer Nature; 2019.

2 机械通气简史

A Short History of Mechanical Ventilation

Philippe R. Bauer

2.1 呼吸、循环及两者相互作用

呼吸系统的重要性在《圣经》中已有体现，被描述为生命之气："耶和华神用地上的尘土造人，将生命之气吹进他的鼻孔"（创世纪 2：7）[1]。机械通气的相关探索实践跨越了两个世纪（图 2.1）。呼吸系统本身的发现归功于公元二世纪的希腊医生 Aelius Galenus。他在关于动物气管和肺的解剖文献《论身体各部分的功能》（*De usu partium corporis humani*）中首次报道了肺的人工送气，以及呼吸与循环间的相互作用。Leonardo da Vinci 证明了空气通过胸腔的风箱作用进入肺部。1543 年，Andreas Vesalius 最先在解剖文献《论人体的构造》（*De Humani Corporis Fabrica*）中记载了通过向动物气管插管实现正压通气[2]。1667 年，Robert Hook 成功地重复了 Vesalius 的实验[1]。当时是想通过进入肺部的空气使心脏降温，心脏泵出的血液进入动脉使身体降温[1]。

公元 200 年	呼吸系统的发现
1543 年	正压通气的概念
1670 年	负压通气的概念
1774 年	氧气的发现
1865 年	内环境稳定原理
1913 年	喉镜的发明

图 2.1　机械通气发展的时间轴

P. R. Bauer (✉)
Division of Pulmonary and Critical Care Medicine, Mayo Clinic, Rochester, MN, USA
e-mail: Bauer.Philippe@mayo.edu

G. Bellani (ed.), *Mechanical Ventilation from Pathophysiology to Clinical Evidence*, https://doi.org/10.1007/978-3-030-93401-9_2

1928 年	负压通气(铁肺)与脊髓灰质炎
1944 年	间歇性正压氧疗与胸部创伤
1952 年	正压通气与脊髓灰质炎
1963 年	Engström 通用呼吸机
1967 年	急性呼吸窘迫综合征
1970 年	体外膜肺氧合
1975 年	最佳呼气末正压
1987 年	婴儿肺的概念
2000 年	低潮气量策略
2015 年	驱动压的重要性
2019 年	COVID-19 与战略储备

图 2.1(续)

2.2 氧气，燃烧，代谢，稳态

尽管自公元前 200 年以来，在各种空气燃烧实验中(包括 Leonardo da Vinci 的实验)已有对存在氧气的怀疑，但直到 1774 年才被 Carl Wilhelm Scheele 和 Joseph Priestley 同时发现，Antoine Lavoisier 则证明了氧气对于燃烧和呼吸都是必不可少的[1]。两个主要的现象促成了他们的发现。血液从肺部流出时比其进入时的颜色更鲜红，表明"某样物质"(即氧气)在通过肺部时被带入血液。1865 年，Claude Bernard 根据从器官流出的血液温度较流入时更高的现象，发现了组织代谢、二氧化碳和水的产生，并提出内环境调节或稳态的概念。

2.3 机械通气的黎明

第一种机械通气呼吸机提供的是负压通气，利用了 Sauerbruch 的基于压差的方法[3]。外部负压通气的概念是 John Mayow 在 1670 年提出的，第一个模型是 John Dalziel 在 1832 年设计的。第一批原型机制造于 1876 年，人类首次应用罐式呼吸器或"铁肺"是在 1928 年，用于美国波士顿儿童医院一名患有脊髓灰质炎和呼吸衰竭的儿童(图 2.2a)。铁肺在脊髓灰质炎流行期间被广泛使用，而脊髓灰质炎随着接种疫苗而消失。有一种被称为"龟壳"的便携式铁肺得到了患者的欢迎，允许患者活动(图 2.2b)。有些患者长期依赖机械通气：一位患者在梅奥诊所接受了长达 16 年的负压通气。我还记得 20 世纪 80 年代在法国治疗那些接受气管切开术和使用传统正压呼吸机的患者，他们已经成为了医院的一部分。

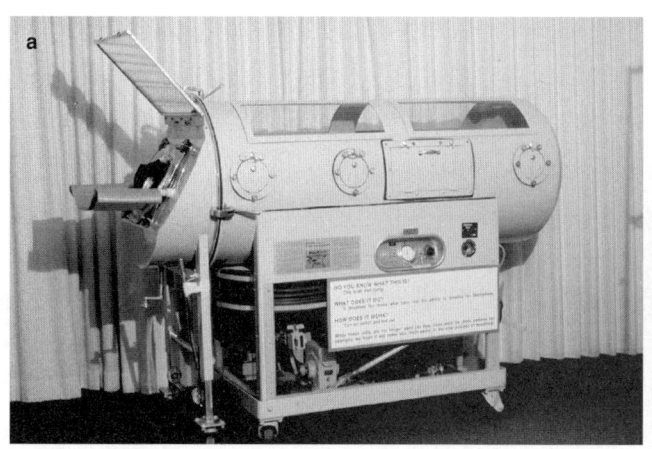
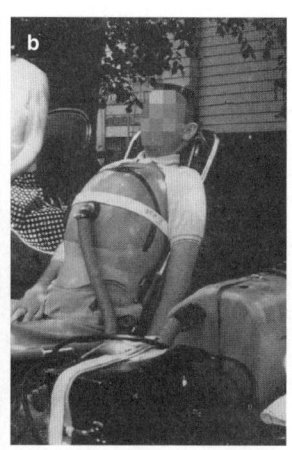

图2.2　a. 梅奥医学中心展示的一台负压通气机（铁肺）。b. 一名梅奥医学中心患者使用的便携式铁肺（龟壳）（见彩色插图）

当同时存在气体交换异常时，负压通气就显得效果不佳了[4,5]。间歇正压氧疗（intermittent positive pressure oxygen therapy，IPPOT），作为间歇正压通气（intermittent positive pressure ventilation，IPPV）的前身，在第二次世界大战期间被发现有益于治疗胸部创伤所致的湿肺（也被称为创伤后呼吸功能不全或呼吸窘迫综合征）[3]，Ashbaugh 在 1967 年将其命名为急性呼吸窘迫综合征（acute respiratory distress syndrome，ARDS）[4]。这推动了第二种机械通气机的产生，它可以实现正压通气。首次使用是在 1952 年，在丹麦脊髓灰质炎流行期间，用于哥本哈根布莱格丹医院的一例因"呼吸休克"而接受气管切开和正压通气的患者。使用正压通气后的病死率迅速下降，导致铁肺被迅速遗弃。Bennett 研制的给高空飞行员供氧的流量感应呼吸阀后来也被应用于机械通气机。1963 年，Engström 通用呼吸机问世：可以设置容积的、基于时间循环的并具有吸气末暂停功能的呼吸机[7]。第一代正压通气机需要电力驱动。除了爆炸危险，它们还因难以通过实际潮气量调整酸碱状态而闻名，有时会在调整慢性呼吸性酸中毒时出现代偿性代谢性碱中毒。我清楚地记得预防或纠正严重的碱中毒的困难。血气分析的发展使预防、检测和必要时纠正酸碱状态不再困难。第二代的正压通气机是气动装置。人们意识到呼气末正压（positive end-expiratory pressure，PEEP）在预防和纠正肺不张中的作用[8]，常常会使用叹息和吸气末暂停。我记得 Bennett MA-1 呼吸机[9]的 PEEP 设置限制在 17 cmH$_2$O 左右；西门子 Servo Ventilator 900 系列呼吸机的 PEEP 很容易在机器侧面进行调节，但可能会被呼出的雾化残留物堵塞。气管插管也是一个进展。最初人们通过颈部触诊进行盲插型插管，很有挑战性。Chevalier Jackson 和 Henry Harrington Janeway 在 1913 年发明喉镜后，其在气管插管时被广泛应用并减少了气管切开术的需求。在 1971 年，Servo 引入了电子反馈系统，建立了一个可靠的方式来设置呼吸机。最新一代的正压机械通气机配备了微处理器控制、各种通气模式，以及流量-容积环图及其他图示。随着时间的推移，研发重点转向呼吸机的同步性，包括触发、流量输送和呼吸驱动调节，也包括容量控制和压力控制通气、气道压力释放通气等完全呼吸支持通气模式，以及压力支持通气、成比例辅助通气、神经调节通气辅助等部分呼吸支持通气模式,还有一些其他专用通气模式。另外一种被称为高频震荡的技术,由于缺乏有效性,其存在的时间很短。20世纪70年代,Kolobow医生研制出一种高效的人工膜肺(被称为Kolobow肺),它在体外膜肺氧合(extracorporeal membrane oxygenation,ECMO)技术的发展中发挥了重要作用,当常规机械通气不足以纠正难治性低氧和高碳酸性呼吸性酸中毒时,就可以使用ECMO技术[10]。

除了有创的机械通气方式,无创通气也随着时间的推移而流行起来。20世纪40年代,它最初被用于治疗肥胖患者低通气综合征、阻塞性睡眠呼吸暂停和神经肌肉疾病等慢性疾病。间歇性正压呼吸(intermittent positive pressure breathing,IPPB)是一种压力循环模式的无创通气(IPPV),于1955年随着Bird呼吸机的出现而被广泛使用,用于限制性和慢性阻塞性肺疾病。尽管它存在的时间很短暂,但由于它发展出了压力支持通气模式[11]。20世纪90年代以来,无创通气在慢性阻塞性肺疾病急性期、急性充血性心力衰竭和急性低氧性呼吸衰竭等急性疾病中再次受到重视。随着对于有创机械通气潜在危害的逐步认识,无创通气变得越来越有吸引力。传统的无创通气界面是面罩或鼻罩,但因为在降低ARDS患者插管率和病死率方面的潜在益处,现在头罩被应用得更广泛(图2.3)。

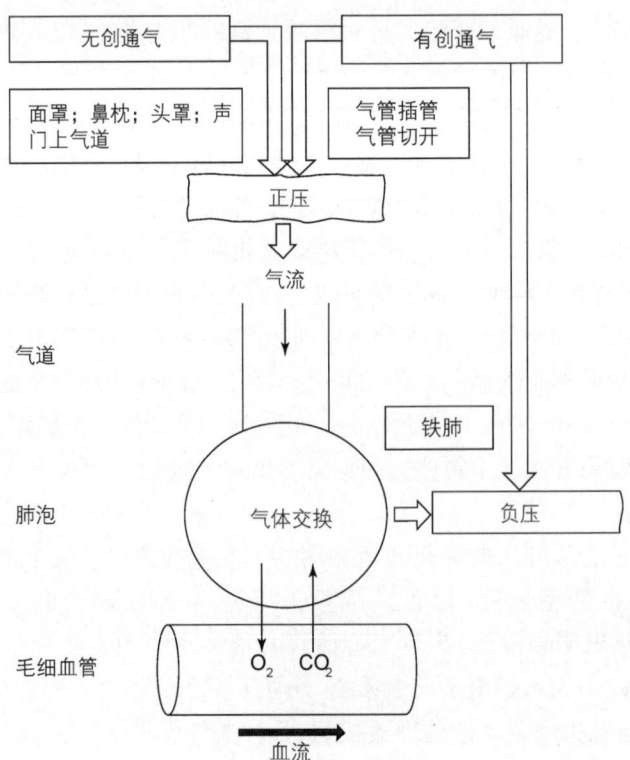

图2.3　不同机械通气模式下的呼吸系统与循环系统偶联

2.4 经验教训

机械通气在减少呼吸做功、提供充分的通气和氧合方面的好处，可能会被发生呼吸机诱导肺损伤[2]的风险抵消。呼吸机诱导肺损伤包括纵隔气肿、气胸和皮下气肿等气压伤，被描述为"通过损伤性通气策略释放介质，导致肺和远端器官损伤"[12]的生物伤，以及更广义上的与呼吸机相关的并发症。1944年，Macklin就报道了机械通气的有害影响，称肺部和纵隔的恶性间质性肺气肿是许多呼吸系统疾病和其他疾病的一个重要的隐匿并发症[13]。Ashbaugh在描述ARDS时着重强调了PEEP"有助于对抗肺不张和低氧血症"的作用[4]。1975年，Suter等提出"最佳呼气末气道压力"或"最佳PEEP"的概念，以获得最大的氧输送（心输出量乘以动脉血氧含量）、最低的无效腔分数，以及最大静态顺应性[14]。还需要预防低潮气量相关的肺不张，以及通过限制吸入氧浓度（FiO_2）来减少氧中毒的发生。随后的一段时间，插管的机械通气患者采用较大潮气量[10 mL/kg（实际体重）]及高PEEP的设定，常导致高气道峰压和高平台压。在COVID-19大流行中，紧急胸腔置管和巨大皮下肺气肿的情况再次频繁出现。

直到1987年，Gattinoni在对ARDS患者"不均一性肺"的观察中提出了"婴儿肺"的概念。随后，"萎缩的婴儿肺"概念定义了与肺损伤严重程度成比例减少的肺容积和气体交换的能力，并强调在急性呼吸衰竭中避免呼吸机相关肺损伤的重要性，方法是"遵循气体交换效率的趋势……，避免呼吸疲劳……，最小化氧需求和每分钟通气量……，优先低应力的潮气循环[15]"。

2000年，ARDSnet的一篇具有里程碑意义的研究证明了小潮气量和低平台压的益处。该研究发现初始潮气量设置为6 mL/kg（理想体重）、平台压设置为30 cmH_2O 或更低水平，与潮气量设置为12 mL/kg、平台压设置为50 cmH_2O 相比病死率下降[16]。在保持较低的潮气量和平台压的情况下，使用较高或较低的PEEP均可获得类似的结果[17]。伴随着驱动压概念的产生，呼吸机的设置得到了进一步的改进，其定义为驱动产生"符合内在功能性肺容积"的潮气量所需的压力，测量方式为平台压减去PEEP[18]。2015年，又一篇具有里程碑意义的论文发表，Amato等发现呼吸机设置相关的驱动压变化与ARDS患者生存率最相关，在设置呼吸机参数时应予以关注[18]。这些发现被LUNG SAFE研究证实，这项大型观察性研究表明插管后第1天驱动压超过14 cmH_2O 的患者预后较差[19]。

COVID-19大流行期间的实践表明肺保护性通气策略仍然适用。可使用持续气道正压通气（continuous positive airway pressure，CPAP）以降低气管插管率。神经肌肉阻滞剂和俯卧位已越来越频繁地被应用，ECMO也被用来进行挽救性治疗。然而，如何恰当地镇静仍然是个难题。最后，需要审慎地决定气管插管（和拔管）的时机以优化有创机械通气的风险获益比，同时应管理事实上有限的呼吸机供应或合理使用储备库存，如美国的国家战略储备呼吸机[20]（图2.4）。

美国国家战略储备所持有的呼吸机示例

柯惠 (Puritan Bennett) LP10　　　飞利浦EV300

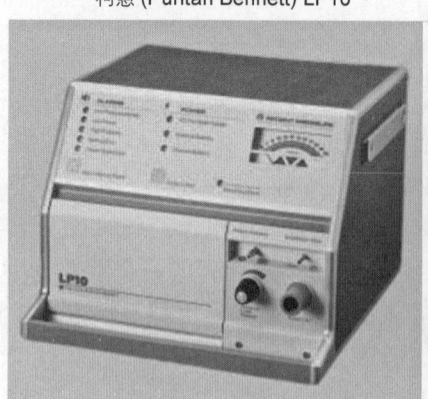
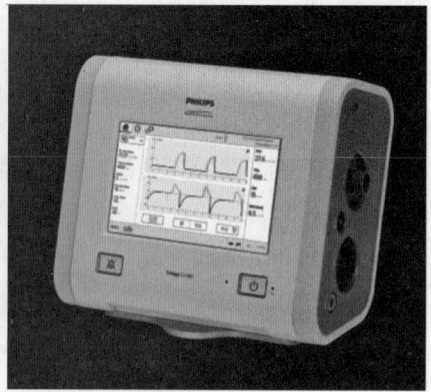

https://www.aarc.org/resources/clinical-resources/strategic-national-stockpile-ventilator-training-program/

图 2.4　COVID-19 大流行期间美国国家储备呼吸机示例

（陈子阳，刘娇　译）

参考文献

[1] Brewer LA Ⅲ. Respiration and respiratory treatment: a historical overview. Am J Surg. 1979; 138: 342-54. https://doi.org/10.1016/0002-9610(79)90262-9.

[2] Slutsky AS. History of mechanical ventilation. From Vesalius to ventilator-induced lung injury. Am J Respir Crit Care Med. 2015; 191: 1106-15. https://doi.org/10.1164/rccm.201503-0421PP.

[3] Grenvik A, Eross B, Powner D. Historical survey of mechanical ventilation. Int Anesthesiol Clin. 1980; 18: 1-10. https://doi.org/10.1097/00004311-198001820-00002.

[4] Ashbaugh DG, Bigelow DB, Petty TL, Levine BE. Acute respiratory distress in adults. Lancet. 1967; 2(7511): 319-23. https://doi.org/10.1016/s0140-6736(67)90168-7.

[5] Kacmarek RM. The mechanical ventilator: past, present, and future. Respir Care. 2011; 56: 1170-80. https://doi.org/10.4187/respcare.01420.

[6] Pallis CA. Poliomyelitis in Denmark: impressions from Blegdam Hospital, Copenhagen. Lancet. 1953; 265: 726-8. https://doi.org/10.1016/s0140-6736(53)90442-5.

[7] Engstrom CG. Treatment of severe cases of respiratory paralysis by the Engström universal respirator. Br Med J. 1954; 2: 666-9. https://doi.org/10.1136/bmj.2.4889.666.

[8] Hedenstierna G, Brismar B, Strandberg A, Lundquist H, Tokics L. New aspects on atelectasis during anaesthesia. Clin Physiol. 1985; 5(Suppl 7): 127-31. https://doi.org/10.1111/j.1475-097x.1985.tb00615.x.

[9] Bone RC, Eubanks DH. Understanding and operating the Bennett MA-1 ventilator. Tips on adjusting the controls to avoid problems. J Crit Illn. 1992; 7: 547-60.

[10] Gattinoni L, Pesenti A, Berra L, Bartlett R. Ted Kolobow. Intensive Care Med. 2018; 44: 551-2. https://doi.org/10.1007/s00134-018-5162-4.

[11] Handelsman H. Intermittent positive pressure breathing (IPPB) therapy. Health Technol Assess

Rep. 1991; 1: 1 - 9.

[12] Tremblay L, Valenza F, Ribeiro SP, Li J, Slutsky AS. Injurious ventilatory strategies increase cytokines and c-fos m-RNA expression in an isolated rat lung model. J Clin Invest. 1997; 99: 944 - 52. https://doi.org/10.1172/JCI119259.

[13] Macklin MT, Macklin CC. Malignant interstitial emphysema of the lungs and mediastinum as an important occult complication in many respiratory diseases and other conditions: an interpretation of the clinical literature in the light of laboratory experiment. Medicine. 1944; 23: 281 - 358.

[14] Suter PM, Fairley B, Isenberg MD. Optimum end-expiratory airway pressure in patients with acute pulmonary failure. N Engl J Med. 1975; 292: 284 - 9. https://doi.org/10.1056/NEJM197502062920604.

[15] Marini JJ, Gattinoni L. Time course of evolving ventilator-induced lung injury: the "shrinking baby lung". Crit Care Med. 2020; 48: 1203 - 9. https://doi.org/10.1097/CCM.0000000000004416.

[16] Acute Respiratory Distress Syndrome Network. Ventilation with lower tidal volumes as compared with traditional tidal volumes for acute lung injury and the acute respiratory distress syndrome. N Engl J Med. 2000; 342: 1301 - 8. https://doi.org/10.1056/NEJM200005043421801.

[17] Brower RG, Lanken PN, MacIntyre N, Matthay MA, Morris A, Ancukiewicz M, et al. Higher versus lower positive end-expiratory pressures in patients with the acute respiratory distress syndrome. N Engl J Med. 2004; 351(4): 327 - 36. https://doi.org/10.1056/NEJMoa032193.

[18] Amato MB, Meade MO, Slutsky AS, Brochard L, Costa EL, Schoenfeld DA, et al. Driving pressure and survival in the acute respiratory distress syndrome. N Engl J Med. 2015; 372: 747 - 55. https://doi.org/10.1056/NEJMsa1410639.

[19] Bellani G, Laffey JG, Pham T, Fan E, Brochard L, Esteban A, et al. Epidemiology, patterns of care, and mortality for patients with acute respiratory distress syndrome in intensive care units in 50 countries. JAMA. 2016; 315: 788 - 800. https://doi.org/10.1001/jama.2016.0291.

[20] Branson R, Dichter JR, Feldman H, Devereaux A, Dries D, Benditt J, et al. The US strategic National Stockpile Ventilators in coronavirus disease 2019: a comparison of functionality and analysis regarding the emergency purchase of 200,000 devices. Chest. 2021; 159: 634 - 52. https://doi.org/10.1016/j.chest.2020.09.085.

3 危重症患者的气道管理

Airway Management in the Critically Ill

Sheila Nainan Myatra

3.1 引言

气管插管（tracheal intubation，TI）是危重症患者中最常见的操作之一[1]。危重症患者存在生理性困难气道，可能出现低氧血症、低血压、代谢性酸中毒、神经功能损害和右心衰竭等生理功能紊乱，增加了TI过程中的出现并发症的风险[2,3]。与手术室气道管理相比，危重症患者气道管理紧迫性强、吸入风险高、插管条件复杂、高级气道设备有限，以及操作者水平参差不齐使得ICU中气道管理更具挑战[4]，详见表3.1。

表 3.1 对危重症患者气管插管的挑战

	ICU 环境因素
基础设施	难以靠近患者头部，患者周围空间不足
设备	高级气道设备，如纤维支气管镜、视频喉镜等在ICU不容易获得
监测	心电监护仪通常放在床的头端，背向操作者，导致无法看到
人员	在紧急TI时能否配置经过培训的熟练操作人员存在不确定性
时机	无论白天还是晚上，可能随时需要紧急TI
	患 者 因 素
气道评估	因为缺乏时间或患者不配合，可能难以进行气道评估或无法评估
解剖学挑战	颌面部外伤、颈椎损伤、气道损伤、烧伤等

S. N. Myatra (✉)
Department of Anesthesiology, Critical Care and Pain, Tata Memorial Hospital, Homi Bhabha National Institute, Mumbai, Maharashtra, India

© The Author(s), under exclusive license to Springer Nature Switzerland AG 2022
G. Bellani (ed.), *Mechanical Ventilation from Pathophysiology to Clinical Evidence*, https://doi.org/10.1007/978-3-030-93401-9_3

续　表

患者因素	
误吸风险	可能未禁食或者存在危重症导致的胃瘫
预充氧	预充氧时间不足,通气/灌注不匹配导致预充氧效率低下;生理储备的缺乏可能导致氧饱和度快速下降,从而减少 TI 的安全呼吸暂停时间
生理性困难气道	病情危重致生理储备差,存在低血压、低氧血症等,增加 TI 并发症风险
患者配合	患者可能因病情危重而无法配合
患者唤醒	与手术室不同的是,在 ICU 延迟气道管理是不可能的,因为对危重症患者需要立刻建立有效的人工气道
操作者因素	
训练、经验和技能的不确定性	插管人员可能只经过有限的气道管理训练,只有有限的技能,缺乏经验的初级医生可能需要单独 TI
人为因素	患者、ICU 或与操作者相关的因素,单独或综合起来可能会给操作者造成压力,从而影响操作水平 精神负荷过重、定式思维、视野狭窄、沟通不良等可能会增加犯错的风险

TI,气管插管。

一些国家的研究调查表明,在危重症患者 TI 过程中,包括低氧血症、低血压、心律失常、心脏停搏和死亡等在内的并发症发生率较高[5-12]。第四次英国国家调查结果表明,ICU 中 61% 的发生严重气道相关并发症的病例最终死亡或出现脑损伤,而麻醉期间这一比例仅为 14%[5]。未能使用二氧化碳描记、后备计划不周、对高风险气道认识不足、缺乏高级的气道管理技能和设备等是主要原因。在 INTUBE 研究,即一项纳入近 3 000 名危重症患者的大型国际气道管理前瞻性研究中,发现 45.2% 的患者至少经历过一次严重的插管相关的不良事件。其中,占比最高的不良事件是心血管功能不稳定,发生于 42.6% 的患者。发生过严重低氧血症和心脏停搏的患者分别占 9.3% 和 3.1%。根据潜在疾病严重程度进行校正后,经历过严重不良事件的患者在 ICU 和病程第 28 天死亡风险更高[13]。因此,对危重症患者的 TI 是一种高风险的操作[3]。

鉴于对危重症患者 TI 出现并发症的风险高,各个国际学会都制定了相关指南,用于管理危重症患者 TI 的指南,重点关注提高患者安全的措施[14-16]。最近的综述强调了减少此类患者出现并发症的重要管理策略[17-20]。本章将提供关于在对危重症患者 TI 过程中优化首次插管成功率,并最大限度增强患者安全的最新证据。拔管和气管切开不属于本章内容。

3.2　ICU 气管插管的适应证

常见适应证包括以下几条。

(1) 需要有创机械通气(氧合/通气不足、避免高碳酸血症、控制过度通气、需要神经肌肉麻醉、手术后选择性通气)。

(2) 保护气道,防止胃内容物误吸。
(3) 血流动力学不稳定,如休克、心脏停搏等。
(4) 缓解上气道阻塞。
(5) 气管支气管灌洗。

3.3 气管插管的准备和流程

3.3.1 临床病史及检查

对危重症患者进行 TI 往往为紧急性事件,可能没有足够的时间来获取完整的临床病史和进行全面检查。然而,在进行 TI 之前,仍要尽可能获取相关病史和检查结果。除了与当前疾病、合并症有关的病史,还应从患者或家属那里获取与气道管理相关的病史,如最近一次经口进食的时间,有无琥珀胆碱或其他药物禁忌,药物过敏史,有无义齿、松动或缺失的牙齿,有无睡眠呼吸暂停的病史,以及以往困难 TI 的病史。除了对心肺系统和其他系统进行检查,还应查阅相关实验室和影像学检查结果。

3.3.2 气道评估

由于时间紧迫或患者不配合,全面评估气道是不可行的。在一项对 30 000 余名手术室患者进行的系统性回顾和荟萃分析中,发现上唇咬合试验结果(下切牙不能咬住上唇)、短舌颌间距、下颌后缩、改良 Mallampati 分级预测困难气道的阳性似然比分别为 14、6.4、6 和 4.1[21]。针对危重症患者气道评估提出的 12 分 MACOCHA 评分(Mallampati 分级、阻塞性睡眠呼吸暂停、颈椎活动度、张口度、昏迷或低氧血症的存在,以及麻醉医师的存在)将解剖学、生理学和操作者技能考虑在内以预测困难气道[22]。该评分简单易行,可能更适用于危重症患者(表 3.2)。

表 3.2　MACOCHA 评分[22]

评分内容	分值
患者相关因素	
Mallampati Ⅲ级或Ⅳ级	5
阻塞性睡眠呼吸暂停综合征	2
颈椎活动度降低	1
张口受限	1
病理因素	
昏迷	1
严重低氧血症	1

续表

评 分 内 容	分 值
操作者因素	
非麻醉医生	1
总分	12

3.3.3 气道车和检查清单

在 TI 前,应在患者床边准备好一辆配备所有必需物品的气道车,以保证安全、便捷地进行 TI、改善氧合和血流动力学支持[14,16]。使用检查清单有助于确保在 TI 前按照指南推荐备好必需物品和完成准备工作[16]。然而,一项将对 ICU 患者 TI 前使用检查清单与常规流程进行比较的随机研究发现,在 TI 后,两组的最低血氧饱和度和最低收缩压没有差异[23]。然而,这项研究中使用的检查清单并未包括优化 TI 前生理状况的干预措施,如无创通气、液体负荷、早期使用升压药等,这可能解释了为什么结果没有受到影响。此外,参与研究的中心对于其他 ICU 工作流程有丰富的使用检查清单的经验,因此对照组可能已经准备好了大部分检查清单上的项目[23]。无论如何,在应用 Montpellier 插管集束化方案(旨在减少与 TI 相关的危及生命的并发症)后发现,在经验不足的情况下,一份包括优化生理状态必要措施的插管前检查清单是有帮助的[24]。

3.3.4 团队准备

考虑到 ICU 中 TI 的复杂性和高风险,提前进行团队准备和规划至关重要。研究表明,插管团队配备两名气管操作者,其中至少一名是有经验的人员,可以减少并发症[24]。在进行 TI 之前,团队成员间应就气道关注点、TI 方案、团队成员各自角色和责任、后备方案,以及抢救方案进行明确的沟通。

3.4 气管插管流程

危重症患者生理紊乱会增加 TI 并发症风险,因此必须优化患者生理状态,并采取措施提高首次 TI 成功率以避免并发症。表 3.3 概述了这些措施。

表 3.3 对危重症患者气管插管过程中的重要措施

气 道 干 预	重 要 措 施
气道评估	考虑使用 MACOCHA 评分[22]
团队准备	有两名操作者在场(至少有一名有气道管理经验) 成员之间就气道关注点、气管插管方案、后备和抢救方案中的角色和责任提前进行明确的沟通

续 表

气 道 干 预	重 要 措 施
患者体位	半直立或斜坡位 防止 FRC 下降来改善氧合,降低胃内容物误吸风险
预充氧和无呼吸氧合	与带阀储氧面罩相比,采用 HFNO 预充氧,在非严重低氧患者中能降低插管相关并发症 严重缺氧患者预充氧应选择 NIV 在充分预充氧后可采用无呼吸氧合和轻柔面罩通气来延长诱导和喉镜检查间的氧合维持时间,尤其对于低氧高风险的患者
快速程序化插管	考虑对所有患者应用
麻醉诱导	首选静脉注射氯胺酮或依托咪酯,除非禁忌
神经肌肉阻断剂	使用静脉注射罗库溴铵或琥珀胆碱,除非禁忌
血流动力学	围插管期通过补液或升压药维持血流动力学 可以考虑早期使用升压药
气管插管设备选择	初次气管插管时应考虑使用导芯或探条 配备视频喉镜,在预测为困难气道的情况下,如果可行,应首选带硬质导管针的超角度视频喉镜,而不是传统形状的视频喉镜
气管插管位置的确认	使用呼气末二氧化碳波形图确认
挽救性给氧	气管插管尝试次数限制在两次之内 尝试使用面罩或 SAD 改善氧合 插管失败时,如果使用面罩或 SAD 能恢复通气,则考虑行外科手术、经皮气管造口术,或者由气道专家经 SAD 通过纤维支气管镜进行气管插管 如果无法插管也无法给患者通气,必须紧急行环甲膜穿刺术;另外,如果有经验丰富的外科医生在场,也可以立即行气管切开造口术
困难气道管理之后	监测患者,注意并发症 如有必要,治疗气道水肿并评估气道 做好文字记录,如可行,为患者和家属提供咨询 团队内总结讨论
人为因素	使用团队共享心理模型进行交流 遵循流程图进行气管插管,以减少精神负荷,提高对气管插管失败的识别和管理能力 进阶培训需涵盖气道管理的技术和非技术能力两个方面

FRC,功能残气量;HFNO,经鼻高流量氧疗;NIV,无创通气;SAD,声门上气道装置。

3.4.1 患者体位

相较于完全平卧位,嗅探位或半直立位(斜坡位)是否有助于提高声门可视性、使 TI 更容易仍存在争议[25]。一项多中心研究表明,与嗅探位相比,斜坡位会增加 TI 难度。但是,该研究中采用的斜坡位可能是并非标准的体位,需要审慎地解读研究结果[26]。一项大型回顾性研究表明,斜坡位联合嗅探位能显著降低危重症患者并发症的发生率[27]。一项前瞻性观察研究表明,与仰卧位相比,斜坡位可提高急诊床首次 TI 成功率[28]。虽然缺乏随机临床试验,但直立位确实可以提升预充氧效果,防止功能残气量的减少,减少误吸入肺的风险,对高风险人群非常有帮助。最近的指南推荐采用头部抬高的体位,特别是对于有高误吸风险和低氧的患者[14,15]。

3.4.2 预充氧和无呼吸氧合

危重症患者在 TI 过程中有很高的低氧风险[2,3]。可以使用简单面罩、标准经鼻给氧或经鼻高流量氧疗(high flow nasal oxygen, HFNO)、无创通气(non-invasive ventilation, NIV)面罩或这些设备的组合来输送氧气。标准经鼻给氧或 HFNO 可在尝试 TI 期间持续输送氧气(无呼吸氧合)。除了给氧外,HFNO 还能产生 PEEP[29]。NIV 通过压力支持增加每分钟通气量,降低右心室前负荷和左心室后负荷来提高氧合、提供 PEEP 和改善通气[30]。

需要比较不同的预充氧和无呼吸氧合策略,以延长呼吸暂停安全时间(从呼吸停止到氧合下降的时间)。在 PROTRACH 研究中,将既往无低氧血症($PaO_2/FiO_2 \geqslant 200$ mmHg)的患者随机分配到应用 HFNO(从诱导至 TI)或面罩进行预充氧的两组中。虽然 HFNO 不能提高 TI 期间最低氧饱和度,但 HFNO 组患者 TI 相关并发症更少[31]。在内科 ICU 中进行的一项纳入 150 名成人的随机开放标签研究中,发现与标准治疗组相比,在 TI 时使用流量 15 L/min 的鼻导管不能提高 TI 期间的最低氧饱和度[32]。在 FLORALI 2 研究中,接受 TI 的危重成人患者被随机分为 NIV 组和 HFNO 组(从诱导到 TI),两组间严重低氧血症的发生率无差异。但是,在 $PaO_2/FiO_2 < 200$ mmHg 的亚组分析中发现 NIV 可能有益[33]。Jaber 等在一项概念验证研究中发现,与单纯 NIV 相比,通过 NIV 预充氧时联合采用 HFNO 的无呼吸氧合改善 TI 时严重低氧的效果更好[34]。当然,还需要更多的研究来证实这些研究结果。

根据最近的文献,NIV 似乎是预充氧的首选方法,特别是对于严重低氧患者。在非严重低氧患者中,与带阀储氧面罩相比,采用 HFNO 预充氧时 TI 相关并发症较少。

3.4.3 麻醉诱导

用于麻醉诱导的药物会增加血液动力学和呼吸相关并发症风险,对危重症患者,通常需要减少诱导药物的剂量[35]。危重症患者应优先选择氯胺酮和依托咪酯,因为它们具有良好的血流动力学特性[36]。在诱导期间减少患者的每分钟通气量可能会减弱代谢性酸中毒的呼吸代偿,使酸中毒和休克加重,TI 过程中呼吸代偿的丧失可能加剧诱导过程中本就存在的低氧血症[37]。

3.4.3.1 丙泊酚

即使不使用肌松剂,丙泊酚也能减弱气道反射,为 TI 提供良好条件。但它可能不适用于大多数休克、低血容量、存在心血管合并症导致生理储备下降的危重症患者,因为他们使用丙泊酚后血压会急剧下降甚至出现心动过缓。回顾性研究表明,当应用了各种防治低血压的策略,包括补液和给予升压药时,丙泊酚的使用仍是安全的[38,39]。虽然在多个气道管理指南中[14,16],氯胺酮和依托咪酯已被建议作为危重症患者 TI 诱导时的首选药物,但 INTUBE 研究中显示,丙泊酚仍是最常用(42%)的诱导药物[13]。

3.4.3.2　依托咪酯

依托咪酯会抑制肾上腺皮质的功能。一项 Cochrane 系统性评价和一项纳入观察性研究的荟萃分析表明,单剂依托咪酯与危重症患者的病死率升高不相关[40,41]。如果依托咪酯用于感染性休克患者,应考虑补充皮质醇[42]。

3.4.3.3　氯胺酮

除非存在禁忌证,氯胺酮是危重症患者常用的诱导剂,因为它可以维持血流动力学稳定。在一项对 655 名危重症患者进行的随机对照试验中,比较了依托咪酯或氯胺酮用于快速程序化插管(rapid sequence intubation, RSI)的效果,并未发现氯胺酮和依托咪酯在插管状态或严重不良事件方面存在差异。然而,依托咪酯组中肾上腺皮质功能不全的发生率更高[36]。一项比较两种诱导剂对成年创伤患者影响的研究中显示,在 RSI 中使用依托咪酯还是氯胺酮在首次插管成功率、非 ICU 住院天数、无机械通气天数和病死率上均没有差异[43]。

3.4.4　快速程序化插管的争议

危重症患者可能因为危重疾病出现胃排空障碍,或在 TI 时没有禁食。因此,常规 RSI 中包括使用快速起效的药物(诱导剂和肌肉松弛剂)、按压环状软骨,以及在诱导和 TI 之间中断通气(限制胃胀气,从而减少误吸入肺)。

3.4.4.1　使用神经肌肉阻滞剂或自主呼吸

危重症患者采用 RSI 有较高的首次插管成功率和较低的 TI 相关并发症发生率[44-46],因此所有患者都应考虑应用 RSI。使用神经肌肉阻滞剂可以改善面罩通气,松弛上呼吸道肌肉张力(包括喉痉挛),改善插管条件,以及优化胸壁顺应性。然而,在危重症患者中诱导呼吸暂停可能会导致氧饱和度快速下降(继发于 FRC 的丧失、高代谢率、生理性分流和通气/灌注不匹配),突出了围插管期氧合与挽救性给氧的重要性。由于担心使用神经肌肉阻滞剂后出现无法进行面罩通气的风险,因此使用这些药物存在顾虑。然而,最近的指南表示,即使在无法插管、无法通气的紧急情况下也建议使用这些药物[14,16]。一项比较给危重症患者使用琥珀胆碱和罗库溴铵的研究发现,两者在氧饱和度下降程度和首次 TI 成功率方面没有差异[47]。紧急情况下可以使用舒更葡糖快速逆转罗库溴铵的效应[48],但其对于危重症患者的安全性数据有限。琥珀胆碱可能导致高危患者出现危及生命的高钾血症,故应谨慎使用。

在手术室中使用视频喉镜(videolaryngoscope, VL)或纤维支气管镜进行清醒 TI 具有较高的成功率和安全性。然而,这需要患者的配合和临床医生的专业技术,因此可能不适用于那些病情不稳定或者不配合的危重症患者。

3.4.4.2　按压环状软骨

TI 时按压环状软骨仍存在争议。Cochrane 系统性评价的结论是还需要更多的证据[49]。最近的一项随机双盲研究表明,在误吸高危患者中,对照组预防误吸的效果并不劣于按压环状软骨组[50]。临床医生常常难以识别环状软骨位置。此外,有证据表明,按压环状软骨可能会恶化喉部视野,从而影响 TI 的成功,甚至会影响面罩通气[51,52]。尽管如此,一些学会指南仍然推荐在 RSI 时按压环状软骨[14,16]。

3.4.4.3 RSI 过程中的面罩通气

在 RSI 期间,由于神经肌肉阻滞和 TI 会使肺通气中断,导致危重症患者有较高的低氧血症风险。在 PREVENT 研究中,401 例危重症患者在麻醉诱导至 TI 期间被随机分配至面罩通气组或无通气组[53]。通气组患者严重低氧血症(氧饱和度<80%)的发生率较低且肺误吸风险无增加。虽然这项研究不是针对肺误吸的,但它提供了一些证据,即 RSI 期间温和面罩通气可以减少缺氧,尤其是在高风险患者中。

3.4.5 气管插管期间的血流动力学支持

在 INTUBE 研究中,危重症患者 TI 后循环不稳定的发生率为 42.6%[13]。麻醉诱导剂的使用、交感神经兴奋的丧失、低血容量和正压通气可能是造成这种后果的原因。血流动力学不稳定是包括病死在内不良结局的独立预测因素[12,13]。低血压和低氧同时发生更容易导致心脏停搏[12]。补液和升压药物常用于预防和治疗低血压。作为 TI 集束化管理的一部分,已证实 TI 前补液可以减少致死性并发症[24]。然而,最近的一项研究显示 TI 前的常规补液没有益处,但是该研究没有将患者按风险分层[54]。在 TI 期间早期使用升压药物替代补液来预防低血压的效果需要进一步研究。

3.4.6 气管插管的设备选择

3.4.6.1 使用视频喉镜

一项荟萃分析比较了直视喉镜(direct laryngoscopy,DL)和 VL 用于手术室外紧急 TI 的效果,结果显示在 ICU 患者亚组中,VL 下首次 TI 成功率较高,误入食管的发生率较低;至于总体成功率,两者没有区别。值得关注的是,VL 的使用与更多致死性并发症,包括低血压相关[55]。最近,一项比较 VL 和 DL 的荟萃分析纳入 9 个随机对照试验,包含 2 000 多名危重症患者。该研究发现,即使在评估这些研究时考虑操作者经验,使用 VL 也没有改进首次插管的成功率[56]。这些荟萃分析中的一些研究显示,使用 VL 时严重威胁生命的并发症的发生率更高。对这些结果的解释是,当 VL 观察到清晰的喉部时很难中止 TI 的尝试,导致呼吸暂停时间延长和发生并发症。此外,纳入的研究存在异质性,部分为低质量研究。然而,尽管最近的证据不支持在 ICU 的 TI 中常规使用 VL,但使用 VL 能比 DL 更好地显露声门,其仍是 ICU 困难气道管理中的重要工具[57]。在预测为困难气道的情况下,如果可以获得,带有导管针的超角度 VL 优于传统形状 VL。未来的研究将会更好地定义 VL 在 ICU 中的作用,这些研究需要将首次 TI 成功且无并发症复合临床结局作为主要研究终点而不是单一的首次 TI 成功率[57]。

3.4.6.2 使用探条

最近的一项随机试验纳入了急诊科至少有一种困难气道特征的患者,比较了使用探条和带导芯的气管导管进行 TI 的效果[58]。使用探条组的首次 TI 成功率明显更高。这是一项单中心研究,操作者具备使用探条的经验。因此,这个结论的普遍性是不确定的。尽管如此,对于那些具备经验的操作者而言,建议使用探条来进行首次 TI 是合理的。

3.4.6.3 使用导管针

导管针通常用于挽救困难气道的 TI。在危重症患者中,常规使用导管针对首次插管成功率的影响尚未得到研究。Jaber 等在一项多中心随机研究中纳入法国 32 个 ICU 的 999 名危重症成年患者,比较了在 DL 下带或不带导管针进行 TI 对首次插管成功率的影响。结果显示,在带导管针进行 TI 的分组中,首次尝试插管的成功率显著高于单独 TI 组,并未发现两组之间并发症的发生率存在差异[59]。

这两项研究的结果为给危重症患者进行 TI 时常规使用探条和导管针提供了有力的依据[60]。

3.4.7 确认气管插管位置

应使用二氧化碳波形图确认 TI 是否在位(5～6 个稳定波形且无下降趋势)[14,16]。在 NAP4 报告中,未使用二氧化碳波形图确认导管位置导致 ICU 中 17 例死亡或脑损伤事件[5]。插管进入食管和插管意外移位在死亡或脑损伤事件中的占比高达 82%。该报告强烈建议为所有危重症患者监测二氧化碳波形图来确认 TI[5]。然而,尽管 NAP4 报告显示,由于未监测二氧化碳波形图而导致的不良事件的发生率较高,但在该报告发表十年后,INTUBE 研究显示通过监测二氧化碳波形图来确认 TI 位置的患者仅占 25%。此外,该研究还显示有 70% TI 误入食管的患者未使用二氧化碳波形图监测来确认导管位置[13]。这凸显了增加全球对二氧化碳波形图监测的认识和使用的重要性,以提高气道管理安全。

3.5 挽救性给氧

如果在尝试 TI 时患者血氧饱和度下降,应该进行面罩通气以改善氧合。使用口咽气道、双手操作手法可优化面罩通气效率。如果面罩通气不足,可以插入声门上气道(supraglottic airway,SGA)装置[14-16]。这些装置被盲插至气道,在喉入口周围形成密封。应首选第二代 SGA 装置,因为它有助于胃减压并提供更好的喉部密封[14,16]。

对危重症患者使用 SGA 进行紧急通气往往能挽救他们的生命。所有从事危重症患者气道管理的临床医生都应该学习这项技能[61]。由于不用于 ICU 常规气道管理,重症专家对于使用这类设备通常不熟悉或未经过培训。NAP4 报告发现,在使用紧急手术开放气道的患者中,有一半病例没有插入 SGA 装置进行挽救性通气。此外,在行环甲膜切开术后插入 SGA 装置通常也能成功,这表明或许可以不行环甲膜切开术[5]。

在插入 SGA 装置,成功进行紧急通气并恢复血氧饱和度之后,危重症患者需要人工气道进行长期机械通气,应考虑后续人工气道建立的方法:应由气道专家在纤维支气管镜引导下通过 SGA 装置进行 TI,因为危重症患者需要一个确定的气道以保证后续通气[14]。

如果 SGA 装置插入不成功,而且使用不同技术手法和神经肌肉阻滞剂进行面罩通气也无法有效紧急通气时,即使氧饱和度保持不变,也应立即进行紧急环甲膜穿刺术[14-16]。

环甲膜穿刺术的最佳方法仍有争论。可以通过外科手术或采用宽口径环甲膜穿刺套管(商用套件)。采用细针进行环甲状膜穿刺后需要经转换装置接呼吸机进行通气,这在 ICU 通常是做不到的。

未预料的困难 TI 后,监测患者是否出现并发症是至关重要的。应关注并治疗气道水肿。可能需要专科医生进行进一步的气道检查,特别是在发生气道损伤时。记录困难气道的诊治经过,如有可能,向患者或家属提供咨询是非常重要的[14]。

3.6 气管导管的护理

TI 后应根据需要启动机械通气,适当镇静。应在气管导管上标记与切牙(或鼻子)的位置关系。最好在每个护理班次核对气管导管的位置并记录标记位置,以检查导管是否移位。TI 后应常规行胸部 X 线摄影检查,确认 TI 及鼻胃管位置。应该在确认位置后再开始鼻胃管喂养。根据需要使用密闭式吸痰装置引流痰液,以保持气管导管通畅。每日使用气囊压力计检查气管气囊压力,使其始终保持在 20~30 cmH$_2$O,以减少压力性损伤、黏膜缺血和误吸的风险。

3.7 气道管理中的人为因素

考虑到危重症患者气道管理过程的复杂性和挑战性,人为因素的考量变得极为重要。人为因素指的是个体、团队、患者、环境和机构特征如何影响人类行为,从而可能影响临床医生在气道管理过程中的技术和非技术能力。在高压的环境下,可能出现精神负荷过重、情境意识缺失、定式思维和低效决策等问题[14,16]。根据 NAP4 报告,至少 40% 的不良结局是人为因素导致的。导致不良结局的因素有培训和经验不足、不遵守指南和失败后无应急预案[5]。团队成员间需要提前沟通气道管理方案和应急预案,包括角色和责任分配,可能有助于解决其中一些问题。在模拟和实际场景中使用认知辅助工具,有助于在危急情况下提高技术能力和团队沟通效率;然而,这一领域需要进一步的研究[62]。涡流方法(Vortex Approach)[63]就是一种认知辅助工具,用于支持决策过程和帮助临床医生应对气道危机。

3.8 未来研究

未来的研究需要确定提高首次 TI 成功率的最佳干预措施,以及降低 TI 并发症高发生率(尤其是高频出现的血流动力学并发症)的最佳管理策略。旨在增加首次 TI 成功率的干预措施应与旨在优化生理学的措施相结合。未来的临床试验应着眼于更好地定义 VL 在 ICU 中的作用,特别是 VL 辅助 TI 成功所需的理想声门视图和气道辅助设备的合理使用。这些研究需要将首次 TI 成功且无并发症的复合临床结局作为主要研究终点,而不是单纯的首次 TI 成功率。床旁胃超声也有助于识别存在误吸高风险的患者,应在危重症患者中进一步研究其应用价值。

3.9 总结

危重症患者存在生理性困难气道,对于这类高危人群而言,TI 仍然是一项高风险操作,伴有高并发症风险。认识到这些患者 TI 过程中的各种挑战,并使用适当策略来提高首次插管成功率同时保证患者安全至关重要。进一步研究将有助于确定改善患者预后的最佳策略。

财务披露:无。

利益冲突:无。

(吕慧,皋源 译)

参考文献

[1] Russotto V, Myatra SN, Lafey JG. What's new in airway management of the critically ill. Intensive Care Med. 2019; 45: 1615-8.

[2] Mosier JM, Joshi R, Hypes C, Pacheco G, Valenzuela T, Sakles JC. The physiologically difficult airway. West J Emerg Med. 2015; 16(7): 1109-17.

[3] Vakil B, Baliga N, Myatra SN. The physiologically difficult airway. Airway. 2021; 4: 4-12.

[4] Divatia JV, Khan PU, Myatra SN. Tracheal intubation in the ICU: lifesaving or life threatening? Indian J Anaesth. 2011; 55: 470-5.

[5] Cook TM, Woodall N, Harper J, Benger J, Fourth National Audit Project. Major complications of airway management in the UK: results of the fourth National Audit Project of the Royal College of Anaesthetists and the difficult airway society. Part 2: intensive care and emergency departments. Br J Anaesth. 2011; 106: 632-42.

[6] Jaber S, Amraoui J, Lefrant JY, Arich C, Cohendy R, Landreau L, et al. Clinical practice and risk factors for immediate complications of endotracheal intubation in the intensive care unit: a prospective, multiple-center study. Crit Care Med. 2006; 34: 2355-61.

[7] Griesdale DE, Bosma TL, Kurth T, Isac G, Chittock DR. Complications of endotracheal intubation in the critically ill. Intensive Care Med. 2008; 34: 1835-42.

[8] Simpson GD, Ross MJ, McKeown DW, Ray DC. Tracheal intubation in the critically ill: a multi-centre national study of practice and complications. Br J Anaesth. 2012; 108: 792-9.

[9] Martin LD, Mhyre JM, Shanks AM, Tremper KK, Kheterpal S. 3,423 emergency tracheal intubations at a university hospital: airway outcomes and complications. Anesthesiology. 2011; 114: 42-8.

[10] Mayo PH, Hegde A, Eisen LA, Kory P, Doelken P. A program to improve the quality of emergency endotracheal intubation. J Intensive Care Med. 2011; 26(50-6): 12.

[11] Bowles TM, Freshwater-Turner DA, Janssen DJ, Peden CJ, RTIC Severn Group. Out-of-theatre tracheal intubation: prospective multicentre study of clinical practice and adverse events. Br J

[12] De Jong A, Rolle A, Molinari N, Paugam-Burtz C, Constantin JM, Lefrant JY, et al. Cardiac arrest and mortality related to intubation procedure in critically ill adult patients: a multicenter cohort study. Crit Care Med. 2018; 46: 532-9.

[13] Russotto V, Myatra SN, Laffey JG, Tassistro E, Antolini L, Bauer P, et al. Intubation practices and adverse peri-intubation events in critically ill patients from 29 countries. JAMA. 2021; 325: 1164-72.

[14] Myatra SN, Ahmed SM, Kundra P, et al. Republication: all India difficult airway association 2016 guidelines for tracheal intubation in the intensive care unit. Indian J Crit Care Med. 2017; 21: 146-53.

[15] Quintard H, I'Her E, Pottecher J, et al. Intubation and extubation of the ICU patient. Anaesth Crit Care Pain Med. 2017; 36: 327-41.

[16] Higgs A, McGrath BA, Goddard C, et al. Guidelines for the management of tracheal intubation in critically ill adults. Br J Anaesth. 2018; 120: 323-52.

[17] Sklar MC, Detsky ME. Emergent airway management of the critically ill patient: current opinion in critical care. Curr Opin Crit Care. 2019; 25(6): 597-604.

[18] Scott JA, Heard SO, Zayaruzny M, Walz JM. Airway management in critical illness: an update. Chest. 2020; 157(4): 877-87.

[19] De Jong A, Casey JD, Myatra SN. Focus on noninvasive respiratory support before and after mechanical ventilation in patients with acute respiratory failure. Intensive Care Med. 2020; 46(7): 1460-3.

[20] Mosier JM, Sakles JC, Law JA, Brown CA 3rd, Brindley PG. Tracheal intubation in the critically ill. Where we came from and where we should go. Am J Respir Crit Care Med. 2020; 201(7): 775-88.

[21] Detsky ME, Jivraj N, Adhikari NK, Friedrich JO, Pinto R, Simel DL, Wijeysundera DN, Scales DC. Will this patient be difficult to intubate? The rational clinical examination systematic review. JAMA. 2019; 321(5): 493-503.

[22] De Jong A, Molinari N, Terzi N, et al. Early identification of patients at risk for difficult intubation in the intensive care unit: development and validation of the MACOCHA score in a multicenter cohort study. Am J Respir Crit Care Med. 2013; 187(8): 832-9.

[23] Janz DR, Semler MW, Jofe AM, et al. A multicenter randomized trial of a checklist for endotracheal intubation of critically ill adults. Chest. 2018; 153: 816-24.

[24] Jaber S, Jung B, Corne P, et al. An intervention to decrease complications related to endotracheal intubation in the intensive care unit: a prospective, multiple-center study. Intensive Care Med. 2010; 36: 248-55.

[25] Myatra SN. Optimal position for laryngoscopy—time for individualization? J Anaesthesiol Clin Pharmacol. 2019; 35(3): 289-91.

[26] Semler MW, Janz DR, Russell DW, Casey JD, Lentz RJ, Zouk AN, deBoisblanc BP, Santanilla JI, Khan YA, Joffe AM, Stigler WS, Rice TW, Check UPI. Pragmatic critical care research G. a multicenter, randomized trial of ramped position vs sniffing position during endotracheal intubation of critically ill adults. Chest. 2017; 152: 712-22.

[27] Khandelwal N, Khorsand S, Mitchell SH, Joffe AM. Head-elevated patient positioning decreases complications of emergent tracheal intubation in the ward and intensive care unit. Anesth Analg. 2016; 122: 1101-7.

[28] Turner JS, Ellender TJ, Okonkwo ER, Stepsis TM, Stevens AC, Sembroski EG, Eddy CS, Perkins AJ, Cooper DD. Feasibility of upright patient positioning and intubation success rates at two academic EDs. Am J Emerg Med. 2017; 35: 986-92.

[29] Goligher EC, Slutsky AS. Not just oxygen? Mechanisms of benefit from highflow nasal cannula in hypoxemic respiratory failure. Am J Respir Crit Care Med. 2017; 195: 1128-31.

[30] Kallet RH, Diaz JV. The physiologic effects of noninvasive ventilation. Respir Care. 2009; 54: 102-15.

[31] Guitton C, Ehrmann S, Volteau C, Colin G, Maamar A, Jean-Michel V, Mahe PJ, Landais M, Brule N, Bretonniere C, Zambon O, Vourch M. Nasal high-flow preoxygenation for endotracheal intubation in the critically ill patient: a randomized clinical trial. Intensive Care Med. 2019; 45: 447-58.

[32] Semler MW, Janz DR, Lentz RJ, et al. Pragmatic critical care research group. Randomized trial of apneic oxygenation during endotracheal intubation of the critically ill. Am J Respir Crit Care Med. 2016; 193: 273-80.

[33] Frat J-P, Ricard J-D, Quenot J-P, et al. Non-invasive ventilation versus high-flow nasal cannula oxygen therapy with apnoeic oxygenation for preoxygenation before intubation of patients with acute hypoxaemic respiratory failure: a randomised, multicentre, open-label trial. Lancet Respir Med. 2019; 7: 303-12.

[34] Jaber S, Monnin M, Girard M, et al. Apnoeic oxygenation via high-flow nasal cannula oxygen combined with non-invasive ventilation preoxygenation for intubation in hypoxaemic patients in the intensive care unit: the single-centre, blinded, randomised controlled OPTINIV trial. Intensive Care Med. 2016; 42: 1877-87.

[35] Allaouchiche B, Duflo F, Debon R, et al. Influence of sepsis on minimum alveolar concentration of desflurane in a porcine model. Br J Anaesth. 2001; 87: 280-3.

[36] Jabre P, Combes X, Lapostolle F, et al. Etomidate versus ketamine for rapid sequence intubation in acutely ill patients: a multicentre randomised controlled trial. Lancet. 2009; 374(9686): 293-300.

[37] McKown AC, Casey JD, Russell DW, et al. Risk factors for and prediction of hypoxemia during tracheal intubation of critically ill adults. Ann Am Thorac Soc. 2018; 15: 1320-7.

[38] Koenig SJ, Lakticova V, Narasimhan M, Doelken P, Mayo PH. Safety of Propofol as an induction agent for urgent endotracheal intubation in the medical intensive care unit. J Intensive Care Med. 2015; 30(8): 499-504.

[39] Zettervall SL, Sirajuddin S, Akst S, et al. Use of propofol as an induction agent in the acutely injured patient. Eur J Trauma Emerg Surg. 2015; 41(4): 405-11.

[40] Gu WJ, Wang F, Tang L, Liu JC. Single-dose etomidate does not increase mortality in patients with sepsis: a systematic review and meta-analysis of randomized controlled trials and observational studies. Chest. 2015; 147(2): 335-46.

[41] Bruder EA, Ball IM, Ridi S, Pickett W, Hohl C. Single induction dose of etomidate versus other induction agents for endotracheal intubation in critically ill patients. Cochrane Database Syst Rev. 2015; 1: CD010225.

[42] Jung B, Clavieras N, Nougaret S, et al. Effects of etomidate on complications related to intubation and on mortality in septic shock patients treated with hydrocortisone: a propensity score analysis. Crit Care. 2012; 16(6): R224.

[43] Upchurch CP, Grijalva CG, Russ S, et al. Comparison of etomidate and ketamine for induction

during rapid sequence intubation of adult trauma patients. Ann Emerg Med. 2017; 69(1): 24 - 33 e22.

[44] Mosier JM, Sakles JC, Stolz U, Hypes CD, Chopra H, Malo J, Bloom JW. Neuromuscular blockade improves first-attempt success for intubation in the intensive care unit. A propensity matched analysis. Ann Am Thorac Soc. 2015; 12: 734 - 41.

[45] Okubo M, Gibo K, Hagiwara Y, Nakayama Y, Hasegawa K, Japanese Emergency Medicine Network Investigators. The effectiveness of rapid sequence intubation (RSI) versus non-RSI in emergency department: an analysis of multicenter prospective observational study. Int J Emerg Med. 2017; 10: 1.

[46] Wilcox SR, Bittner EA, Elmer J, Seigel TA, Nguyen NT, Dhillon A, Eikermann M, Schmidt U. Neuromuscular blocking agent administration for emergent tracheal intubation is associated with decreased prevalence of procedure-related complications. Crit Care Med. 2012; 40: 1808 - 13.

[47] Laurin EG, Sakles JC, Panacek EA, Rantapaa AA, Redd J. A comparison of succinylcholine and rocuronium for rapid-sequence intubation of emergency department patients. Acad Emerg Med. 2000; 7(12): 1362 - 9.

[48] Hristovska AM, Duch P, Allingstrup M, Afshari A. Efficacy and safety of sugammadex versus neostigmine in reversing neuromuscular blockade in adults. Cochrane Database Syst Rev. 2017; 8: CD012763.

[49] Algie CM, Mahar RK, Tan HB, Wilson G, Mahar PD, Wasiak J. Effectiveness and risks of cricoid pressure during rapid sequence induction for endotracheal intubation. Cochrane Database Syst Rev. 2015; (11): CD011656.

[50] Birenbaum A, Hajage D, Roche S, Ntouba A, Eurin M, Cuvillon P, Rohn A, Compere V, Benhamou D, Biais M, Menut R, Benachi S, Lenfant F, Riou B, Group II. Effect of cricoid pressure compared with a sham procedure in the rapid sequence induction of anesthesia: the IRIS randomized clinical trial. JAMA Surg. 2019; 154: 9 - 17.

[51] Allman KG. The effect of cricoid pressure application on airway patency. J Clin Anesth. 1995; 7: 197 - 9.

[52] Haslam N, Parker L, Duggan JE. Effect of cricoid pressure on the view at laryngoscopy. Anaesthesia. 2005; 60: 41 - 7.

[53] Casey JD, Janz DR, Russell DW, et al. Bag-mask ventilation during tracheal intubation of critically ill adults. N Engl J Med. 2019; 380: 811 - 21.

[54] Janz DR, Casey JD, Semler MW, Russell DW, Dargin J, Vonderhaar DJ, Dischert KM, West JR, Stempek S, Wozniak J, Caputo N, Heideman BE, Zouk AN, Gulati S, Stigler WS, Bentov I, Joffe AM, Rice TW, Pre PI, Pragmatic Critical Care Research G. Effect of a fluid bolus on cardiovascular collapse among critically ill adults undergoing tracheal intubation (PrePARE): a randomised controlled trial. Lancet Respir Med. 2019.

[55] Arulkumaran N, Lowe J, Ions R, et al. Videolaryngoscopy versus direct laryngoscopy for emergency orotracheal intubation outside the operating room: a systematic review and meta-analysis. Br J Anaesth. 2018; 120: 712 - 24.

[56] Cabrini L, Landoni G, Baiardo Redaelli M, Saleh O, Votta CD, Fominskiy E, Putzu A, Snak de Souza CD, Antonelli M, Bellomo R, Pelosi P, Zangrillo A. Tracheal intubation in critically ill patients: a comprehensive systematic review of randomized trials. Crit Care. 2018; 22(1): 6.

[57] Jaber S, De Jong A, Pelosi P, et al. Videolaryngoscopy in critically ill patients. Crit Care. 2019;

23: 221-7.
[58] Driver BE, Prekker ME, Klein LR, et al. Effect of use of a bougie vs endotracheal tube and stylet on first-attempt intubation success among patients with difficult airways undergoing emergency intubation: a randomized clinical trial. JAMA. 2018; 319: 2179-89.
[59] Jaber S, Rollé A, Godet T, Terzi N, Riu B, Asfar P, Bourenne J, Ramin S, Lemiale V, Quenot JP, Guitton C, Prudhomme E, Quemeneur C, Blondonnet R, Biais M, Muller L, Ouattara A, Ferrandiere M, Saint-Léger P, Rimmelé T, Pottecher J, Chanques G, Belafia F, Chauveton C, Huguet H, Asehnoune K, Futier E, Azoulay E, Molinari N, De Jong A, STYLETO Trial Group. Effect of the use of an endotracheal tube and stylet versus an endotracheal tube alone on first-attempt intubation success: a multicentre, randomised clinical trial in 999 patients. Intensive Care Med. 2021; 47(6): 653-64.
[60] Myatra SN, Sakles JC, Roca O. Maximizing first pass success when intubating the critically ill patient: use a stylet. Intensive Care Med. 2021; 47(6): 695-7.
[61] Thomsen JLD, Norskov AK, Rosenstock CV. Supraglottic airway devices in difficult airway management: a retrospective cohort study of 658,104 general anaesthetics registered in the Danish Anaesthesia database. Anaesthesia. 2019; 74: 151-7.
[62] Marshall S. The use of cognitive aids during emergencies in anesthesia: a review of the literature. Anesth Analg. 2013; 117(5): 1162-71.
[63] Chrimes N. The vortex: a universal 'high-acuity implementation tool' for emergency airway management. Br J Anaesth. 2016; 117(Suppl 1): i20-7.

4 控制性机械通气：模式和监测

Controlled Mechanical Ventilation: Modes and Monitoring

Eduardo L. V. Costa, Glauco M. Plens, Caio C. A. Morais

控制性机械通气（controlled mechanical ventilation，CMV）是指在吸气阶段，呼吸机控制运动方程（式 4.1）中的一个变量：流速（$\dot{V}$）或气道压力（P_{aw}）。只能控制一个变量（$\dot{V}$ 或 P_{aw}）的原因是，其他所有变量均为给定常数（R_{rs} 和 C_{rs} 是呼吸系统的固有特性）、衍生变量（体积是流速的积分）或由独立控制系统（吸气和呼气肌产生的压力）确定。

$$P_{aw}(t) = V(t)/C_{rs} + R_{rs} \times \dot{V}(t) + \text{PEEP} - P_{mus}(t) \tag{4.1}$$

其中，$V(t)$ 是呼气末容积基础上增加的瞬时容积，PEEP 是呼气末正压，P_{mus} 代表吸气肌和呼气肌产生的压力。在严格的 CMV 中，P_{mus} 为零，呼吸触发为单一模式。

控制不同变量可形成不同的控制模式，如经典的压力控制模式和容量控制模式。容量控制模式也可以（更为恰当地）称为流量控制模式，因为是通过控制流量以实现目标容积的，但前者更常用。

根据选择何种通气模式，控制系统接受目标参数所生成的不同任务，这些参数可由用户调整的呼吸机设置定义。在压力控制模式下，目标参数包括形成吸气压力的目标气道压力（包括可调斜率的压力上升波形）。然后呼吸机在设置的吸气时间内维持目标压力，随后压力快速降至用户定义的 PEEP 水平（图 4.1a）。

为了完成这项任务，呼吸机持续接收来自压力传感器的输入。通常使用"PID"控制器，该控制器根据与目标压力的三个预估距离决定吸气阀中产生的吸气流量：① 流量与实际气道压和目标气道压间的绝对差值成比例（proportional）；② 当这种绝对距离随时间持续存在，流量增加[积分（integral）]；③ 流量还取决于误差率[微分（derivative）]。这是压力控制模式下流量不确定的根本原因。

在容量控制模式下，PID 控制更为直接，因为控制的参数和目标参数相同。目标参数是吸气期间提前确定了波形的流量。这样，控制器将确定发送多少电流到比例流量阀，以达到目标流量波形(图 4.1b)。与压力控制模式类似，在呼气期间的目标参数是压力下降到设定的 PEEP 水平。

尽管在预后方面并没有证据表明哪种通气模式更好[1,2]，但临床上选择不同的模式肯定会产生不同的影响，我们将在本章中详细探讨。

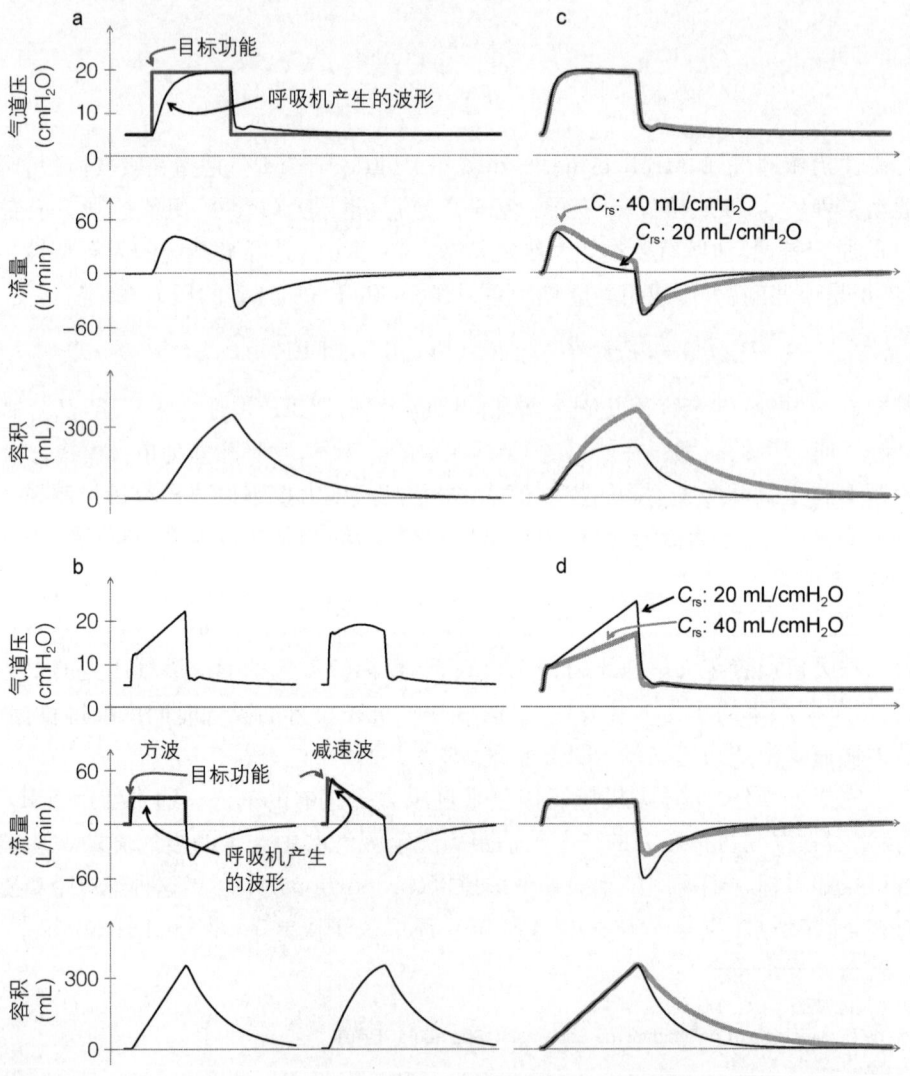

图 4.1　气道压力(P_{aw})、流量和容量波形在压力控制通气模式(PCV, a)和容量控制通气模式(VCV, b)过程中的表现。红色的线代表每种模式下的目标参数。c 和 d 分别说明了在压力控制和容量控制模式下呼吸系统顺应性(C_{rs})变化的影响。在 PCV(c)中，C_{rs} 的下降减少了输送的潮气量。相反，在 VCV(d)中，尽管 C_{rs} 有变化，但潮气量是相似的；然而，P_{aw} 与 C_{rs} 呈反向变化(见彩色插图)

4.1 压力控制通气

压力控制通气(pressure-controlled ventilation,PCV)是指呼吸机在吸气时按照预设压力波形升高气道内压(最常见的是方形或梯形)(图 4.1a)。这意味着最大气道压力由临床医生设定,这一特点在限制压力被认为是肺保护和避免血流动力学不稳定的优先考虑因素时受到特别关注。例如,在 PCV 时,可以限制平台压力和驱动压力,而不受呼吸力学变化的影响(图 4.1),但是这些变化会影响潮气量的输送。除了外源性 PEEP 和吸入氧浓度(所有模式通用的设置)外,只需设定三个目标参数:吸气压力(最大值或在外源性 PEEP 之上的增量)、吸气时间(绝对值或占总时间的比例,T_I/T_{TOT})和呼吸频率。

选择控制压力模式意味着必须放弃对流量的控制,需要密切监测潮气量和每分钟通气量(图 4.1c),这些容积指标不可避免地随呼吸系统阻力改变而变化。

4.2 容量控制通气

这种通气模式通过预设定的、用户选择的流量波形控制吸气时的流量进行通气,其中最常用的是方波(图 4.1b)。在这种情况下,气道压力随呼吸力学改变而变化(图 4.1d)。在一些调查中发现,尽管近年来压力控制和压力支持模式的应用有所增加,容量控制通气(volume-controlled ventilation,VCV)仍是重症监护中最常用的通气模式。VCV 的主要特点是输送由临床医生决定的固定潮气量。由于同时设定了呼吸频率,所以每分钟通气量也得到了保证。

除了外源性 PEEP,需设定的目标参数包括潮气量、吸气流速、流量波形(方波,在某些呼吸机上还有正弦波或减速波)和呼吸频率。

4.3 压力调节的容量保障通气

压力调节的容量保障通气(pressure-regulated volume-guaranteed ventilation,PRVG)是一种闭环模式,它提供了在压力控制模式下保持恒定潮气量的可能性。测量到的潮气量作为一个反馈控制变量,用于逐次自动调整压力控制。不同制造商对这种通气模式的命名不同,如压力调节的容量控制(pressure-regulated volume control,PRVC)、AutoFlow、自适应压力通气等。简而言之,在第一个周期中,呼吸机计算 VCV 周期内呼吸系统的顺应性。在随后的呼吸过程中,呼吸机根据计算的顺应性输送实现预设潮气量所需的吸气压力。PRVG 的这一特点有助于解决呼吸力学的持续变化带来的问题。在某些呼吸机上,可以设置一个高压限制,以避免使低顺应性患者出现损伤性肺泡峰压。但在有自主呼吸努力的情况下,潮气量可能经常增加或减少,导致呼吸机经常改变压力支持水平,影响患者的舒适度和呼吸做功。

4.4 完全控制模式的生理特征

4.4.1 肺保护

在患者没有呼吸努力的情况下，PCV 和 VCV 在肺保护方面是相当的。这两种模式都可以设置以避免过高的驱动压、平台压、潮气量和呼吸频率。在限制压力方面，PCV 的设置更直接，但需要密切监测潮气量，包括谨慎设置呼吸机报警参数（图 4.1c）。相反，在 VCV 中，定期测量平台压和设置压力报警参数非常重要（在监测章节中详细说明；图 4.3）。例如，C_{rs} 的降低，可能是由于肺不张或黏液痰栓，在固定潮气量的情况下导致气道压力升高（图 4.1d）。

这两种模式在气道峰压方面有一个重要的区别。由于典型的 PCV 流量波形为减速波形，与呈方波的 VCV 流量波形相比，即使吸气时间和潮气量相同，气道峰压也通常较低（图 4.1a，b）。这一特点背后的机制是，在 PCV 吸气开始时，气道流量即达到峰值，此时肺部刚开始充气。因此，与以恒定的气道阻力（P_{res}）和增加的弹性阻力（P_{el}）为特征的方波容量控制模式相反，PCV 模式下 P_{res} 随着 P_{el} 的上升而降低。当气体泄漏是一个重要关注点时（如喉罩通气），较低的气道峰压尤其重要[3]。然而，需要重点强调的是，在相同的潮气量下，VCV 和 PCV 中产生的平台压相同。

4.4.2 肺泡通气

在 P_{aw} 突然变化后，无论是在触发后还是在吸气结束后，肺泡压力达到再平衡都需要一段时间。利用时间常数，可以估算出肺部完全充气或排气所需的时间。简而言之，可将呼吸系统视为一个弹性组件和一个阻力元件，它们共同产生单指数衰减，时间常数可以定义为 R_{rs} 和 C_{rs} 的乘积。经过 3~4 个时间常数后，就能达成接近完全（95%~99%）的肺充盈或排空。

使用高呼吸频率时有两个主要原因使得这个概念至关重要。首先，在高呼吸频率下很少能实现完全的肺充盈。在 PCV 中，有时需要比肺泡压力高得多的吸气压力才能产生足够的吸气流量，方能在较短的吸气时间内输送足够的潮气量。即便达到目标潮气量，但是气道阻力突然降低（如在支气管扩张剂作用后）的情况下，可能存在输送潮气量过高的风险。在这种情况下，正确设置潮气量报警至关重要。在 VCV 中，通过直接控制潮气量，可以更容易地通过应用短吸气暂停来监测平台压，从而安全地设置较短的吸气时间。

其次，是为了适当设置呼吸机以避免内源性 PEEP 的发生（在监测章节中详细说明；图 4.3）。当呼气时间过短（小于 3 个时间常数）时，肺部排空不完全，导致产生内源性 PEEP。例如，当呼吸顺应性为 40 mL/cmH$_2$O 和气道阻力为 20 cmH$_2$O/(L·s)时，时间常数为 0.8 s，这意味着目标呼气时间大于 2.4 s。这里存在 PCV 和 VCV 间的一个重要区别。如果 VCV 下产生了内源性 PEEP，潮气量不会受影响（因为它是由呼吸机控制的），但平台压会上升；而在 PCV 下，由于平台压仍将受到限制，所以潮气量会减少。值得注意的是,当每分钟通气量较低时,特别是低于 10 L/min 时[4],对于自动 PEEP 或内源性 PEEP 的担忧应该是最小的。

4.5 自主吸气努力时的模式特点

自主吸气努力的存在会显著改变机械通气,因为一个独立的控制系统(延髓中的呼吸中枢)会将肌肉产生的压力(P_{mus})加入运动方程中。呼吸机如何应对吸气努力是压力和容量控制模式间的一个重要区别,特别是关于吸气流量的输送和跨肺压的变化。

4.5.1 满足吸气流量需求

在 VCV 过程中,吸气流量是临床医生预先设定的。因此,满足高吸气驱动力患者的流量需求可能会比较困难。低峰值吸气流量可能会增加呼吸做功并引起人-机不同步("流量饥饿")(图 4.2a)。

相反,在 PCV 中,呼吸机可以更自由地响应患者不同的吸气努力(图 4.2b)。因此,可以更容易地实现患者的舒适和与呼吸机的同步性[5]。如果在 VCV 中仔细地调整吸气流量峰值来满足患者需求,那么就可以克服 PCV 和 VCV 之间的差异,两者中呼吸做功就几乎没有区别了[2]。

4.5.2 跨肺压

跨肺压表示为呼吸机施加的正压与吸气肌产生的压力的绝对值(P_{mus})之和。吸气肌压力的存在将对 PCV 与 VCV 中的跨肺压产生不同的影响。

在 PCV 中,由膈肌引起的胸腔内压负向波动会导致呼吸机增加吸气流量和潮气量,以满足患者的需求并使气道压接近设定值(图 4.2b)。在这种情况下,跨肺泡的压力可能高于临床医生设定的吸气压力,因为 P_{mus}(未测量)将与呼吸机产生的压力叠加,可能导致肺损伤[6,7]。

相反,VCV 的一个可能的优势是在吸气努力时保持恒定的跨肺压。由于流量由临床医生预先确定,在患者努力存在的情况下,呼吸机施加的气道压将减小,维持预设的潮气量(图 4.2a)。然而,这一特点无法保证局部跨肺压不会增加。这种区域过度膨胀可以表现为不同肺区域之间的气体潮汐运动,导致 VCV 期间损伤性充气模式的持续存在(如潮汐复张和呼吸摆动现象)[8]。

4.5.3 呼吸叠加

当自主吸气时间长于设定的吸气时间时,PCV 和 VCV 之间的另一个重要区别就会显现出来。延长的吸气努力可能产生连续的吸气周期,称为双重触发不同步。在 VCV 中,双重触发可能会导致有害的潮气量"叠加",如果吸气周期间的呼气周期很短,那么叠加潮气量可能达到设定潮气量的两倍。PCV 模式可以将过度呼吸叠加的机会降至最低,因为输送的吸气流量取决于气道和肺泡之间的压力梯度(图 4.2)。

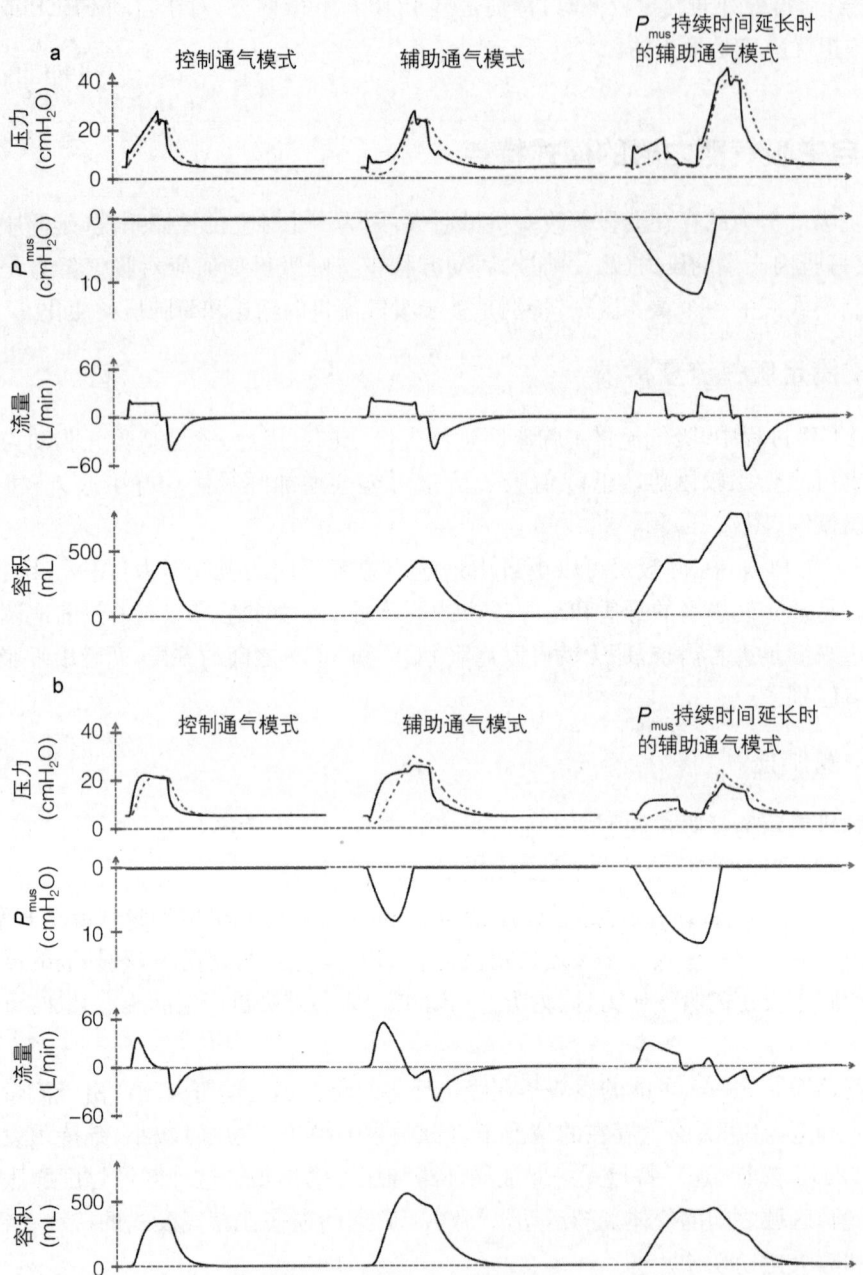

图4.2 在辅助通气/控制通气（A/C）时使用容量控制通气模式（VCV，a）和压力控制通气模式（PCV，b）的气道压、肺泡压（红色虚线）、肌肉压力（P_{mus}）、流量和容量波形。请注意，在 VCV 中，辅助通气时气道压下降，吸气流量和容量恒定。流量受限可能导致呼吸不耐受，被定义为"流量饥饿"，增加了双重触发的风险。相反，与完全控制通气相比，辅助通气 PCV 引起吸气流量增加，同时肺泡压力升高。P_{mus} 长于设定的吸气时间可能会导致双重触发不同步（a 和 b 中右侧的图）。注意在固定的 P_{mus} 下 VCV 和 PCV 之间的"叠加"潮气量的差异；真正的潮气量是通过连续吸气周期中的流量-时间波形积分来计算的（见彩色插图）

4.6 控制通气过程中的监测

在被动通气过程中监测呼吸系统的力学特性有助于了解呼吸衰竭的病理生理机制、设置机械呼吸机并尽量减少呼吸机相关肺损伤。有许多方法可以在静态(呼吸阻断技术)、准静态(低流量压力-容量曲线)和动态(应力指数)条件下评估呼吸力学。关于食管测压法和电阻抗断层成像等高级监测技术,请参考其他章节。

4.6.1 吸气阻力和呼吸顺应性的静态测量

如前所述,运动方程体现了克服 P_{res} 和 P_{el} 所需的机械力(式4.1)。在 VCV 期间,应用恒定流速时,吸气 P_{res} 将保持大致恒定(图 4.3a)。需要进行吸气末阻断(end-inspiratory occlusion,EIO)以中断气流并在吸气末维持肺容量。EIO 导致 P_{aw} 从吸气峰压(peak inspiratory pressure,PIP)迅速降至 P1,代表了流速依赖性阻力消耗的压力(图4.3a)。P_{aw} 快速下降后继续缓慢下降直至达到平台压(P_{plat})。第二次压力衰减的幅度取决于系统的黏弹性(图 4.3a)。至此,可以计算吸气时的气道阻力(R_{rs}):

$$R_{rs} = (PIP - P_{plat})/\dot{V}_i \qquad (4.2)$$

在控制通气时,健康成年人的平均 R_{rs} 约为 10 cmH$_2$O/(L·s)。由于支气管痉挛、肺容量减少和黏液生成,通气过程中 R_{rs} 可能发生变化,导致气道压增加(如果患者处于 VCV 模式下)或 V_T 减少(如果患者处于 PCV 模式下)。

C_{rs} 通常表示在准静态条件下从两个压力点计算出的顺应性。EIO 可以测出 P_{plat},即吸气末时的肺泡压力,代表呼吸系统的吸气末弹性回缩压。呼气末阻断(end-expiratory occlusion,EEO)可以测量呼气末肺泡压力($PEEP_{tot}$)(图 4.3a)。然后,即可以计算出 C_{rs}:

$$C_{rs} = V_T/(P_{plat} - PEEP_{tot}) \qquad (4.3)$$

延长的 EIO(>2 s)可能会因为黏弹性和呼吸回路中不易察觉的泄漏导致 P_{plat} 被低估。因此,建议使用较短的 EIO(≤0.5 s)[9]。

许多呼吸机还允许通过 EIO 在 PCV 中测量 C_{rs}(图 4.3b)。在没有 EIO 的情况下,只有在 PCV 期间吸气末流量接近零时,吸气压才会接近 P_{plat}。

4.6.2 低流量压力-容量曲线

早期获取 P-V 曲线的方法是将超大注射器连接到气管内导管,设备连接复杂且存在回路断开而导致肺塌陷的风险。如今,一些呼吸机提供了自动获取 P-V 曲线的工具(图 4.4a),通常在延长呼气后采用≤5 L/min 的恒定吸气流量获取。低吸气流量使得气道阻力降到最低,从而在充分镇静甚至肌松的患者中对弹性回缩压进行精确测量。

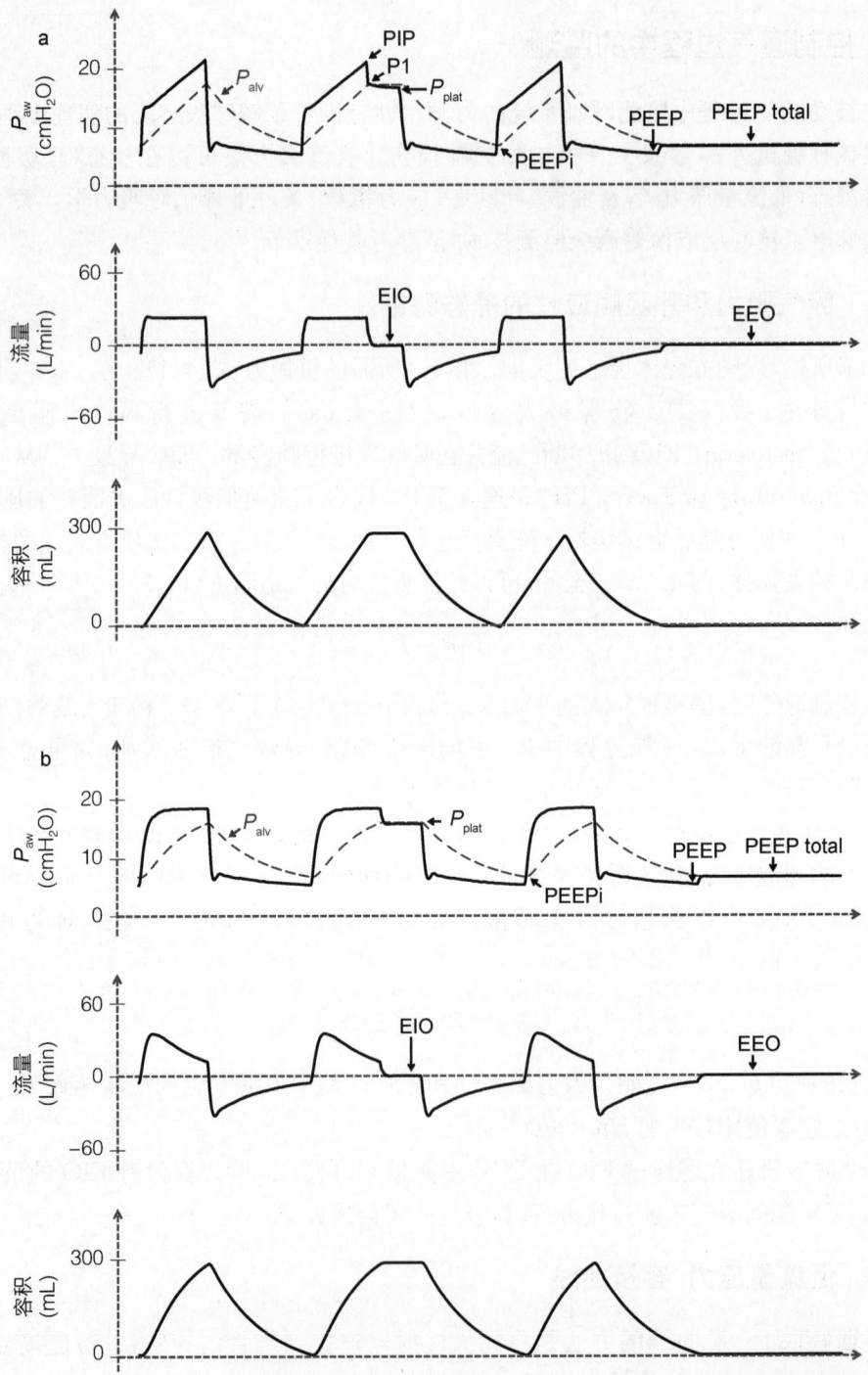

图 4.3 使用容量控制通气模式(VCV, a)以及压力控制模式(PCV, b)测量肺静态顺应性。P_{aw},气道压;P_{alv},肺泡压;P_{plat},平台压;PEEP,呼吸末正压;PEEPi,内源性 PEEP;EIO,吸气末阻断;EEO,呼气末阻断;PIP,吸气峰压;$PEEP_{total}$,总 PEEP

在 ARDS 患者中，P-V 曲线可能呈 S 形，在低吸气压时凹面向上，在较高吸气压时凹面向下（图 4.4a）。在对 ARDS 患者的生理研究中，压力水平在"下拐点"（lower inflection point，LIP）以下时存在肺塌陷的风险，在"上拐点"（upper inflection point，UIP）以上时存在肺泡过度膨胀（应变）的风险（图 4.4a）。一些研究建议应用 P-V 曲线来设置呼吸机，根据 LIP 设置 PEEP，使呼吸保持在高顺应性区域[10,11]。然而，没有证据表明 P-V 曲线法优于其他 PEEP 设置方法，如最大 C_{rs} 的 PEEP 递减法、呼气末跨肺压法和根据吸入氧浓度设置 PEEP（PEEP-FiO_2 表）。

最近，低流量 P-V 曲线已被用于识别完全气道陷闭[12]（图 4.4b）。作者观察到在控制机械通气时约四分之一中重度 ARDS 患者发生气道关闭。这一发现表明，当 PEEP 不

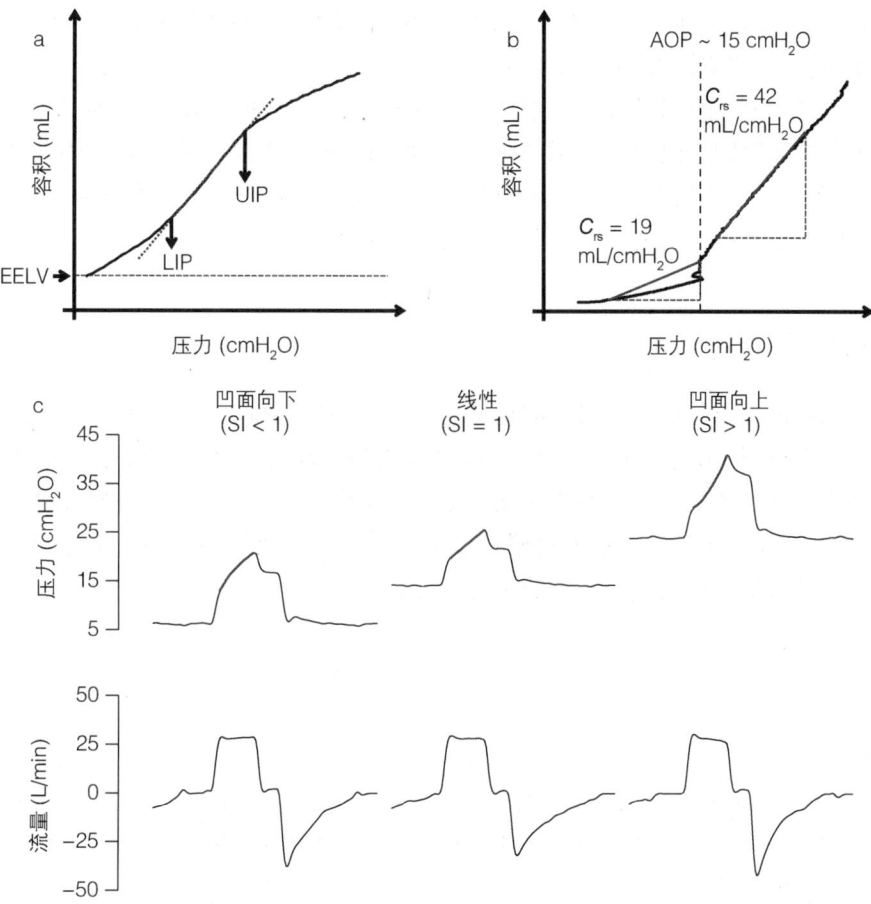

图 4.4 a. 急性呼吸窘迫综合征（ARDS）模型的压力-容积曲线。下拐点（LIP）和上拐点（UIP）定义为曲线开始偏离最大顺应线（红色虚线）的地方。b. 气道陷闭模型的低流量压力-容积曲线。注意压力-容积曲线起始段有一个极小的斜率，随后在压力达到气道开放压（AOP）（约 15 cmH₂O）以上后出现顺应性的突然改变。气道陷闭现象可导致呼吸系统顺应性（C_{rs}）计算错误。c. 吸气流量固定时动态压力-时间曲线示意图。左图为凹面向下（牵张指数 SI＜1），表示呼吸时有塌陷的肺泡复张。中间图中压力与时间呈线性关系（SI＝1），提示无肺复张或过度膨胀。右图，凹面向上（SI＞1），表示呼吸时存在肺泡过度膨胀。EELV，呼气末肺容积（见彩色插图）

足维持气道开放时,会增加对呼吸力学误判的风险。

4.6.3 牵张指数

牵张指数(stress index,SI)是在恒定吸气流量过程中,根据气道压与时间曲线计算出的一个值。假设在吸气过程中 R_{rs} 保持恒定,可以从压力-时间曲线的斜率识别出 C_{rs} 随肺容量增加的动态变化。SI 的计算基于应用于 P_{aw}-时间曲线的下述方程:

$$P_{aw}(t)=a \times t^b + c, \quad (4.4)$$

其中,b 是反映 P_{aw}-时间曲线形状的 SI 参数,a 表示在 $t=1\ s$ 时 P_{aw}-时间曲线的斜率;系数 c 是在 $t=0\ s$ 时的压力。当 $b<1$ 时,P_{aw}-时间曲线呈凹面向下的形状,表明顺应性随时间增加;当 $b>1$ 时,产生凹面向上的形状,表明顺应性随时间减少;$b=1$ 时,P_{aw}-时间曲线为直线,顺应性恒定(图 4.4c)。

在一个 ARDS 的实验模型中,在 SI 值为 0.90~1.10 时进行肺通气,所呈现的炎症标志物水平与未通气肺相似[13]。尽管 SI 作为一种识别损伤性通气模式的无创方法非常有前景,但之前需要专用软件来计算,限制了它的应用。然而,最近的一项研究发现,肉眼直接识别凹面向下和向上的波形具有良好的敏感性和特异性[14]。

4.7 总结

在对控制模式及其影响有很好的理解的情况下,PCV 和 VCV 在被动通气过程中非常相似。然而,如果出现自主吸气努力,这些模式会呈现出显著不同的特点,这可能会影响患者的舒适度和施加在肺部的跨肺压。尽管证据显示 PCV 和 VCV 在控制通气中具有临床等效性,但关注患者与呼吸机的相互作用以及在机械通气中监测自主呼吸的持续研究可能会为理解这些模式间的差异带来新的见解。

(吕慧,瞿洪平 译)

参考文献

[1] Esteban A, Alía I, Gordo F, Pablo R, Suarez J, Gonzá Lez G, Blanco JS. Prospective randomized trial comparing pressure-controlled ventilation and volume-controlled ventilation in ARDS. Chest. 2000;117:1690-6.

[2] Rittayamai N, Katsios CM, Beloncle F, Friedrich JO, Mancebo J, Brochard L. Pressure-controlled vs volume-controlled ventilation in acute respiratory failure: a physiology-based narrative and systematic review. Chest. 2018;148:340-55.

[3] Natalini G, Facchetti P, Dicembrini MA, Lanza G, Rosano A, Bernardini A. Pressure-controlled versus volume controlled ventilation with laryngeal mask airway. J Clin Anesth. 2001;13:436-9.

[4] Leatherman JW, McArthur C, Shapiro RS. Effect of prolongation of expiratory time on dynamic hyperinflation in mechanically ventilated patients with severe asthma. Crit Care Med. 2004;32:

1542-5.

[5] MacIntyre NR, McConnell R, Cheng KC, Sane A. Patient-ventilator flow dyssynchrony: flow-limited versus pressure-limited breaths. Crit Care Med. 1997; 25: 1671-7.

[6] Dreyfuss D, Soler P, Basset G, Saumon G. High inflation pressure pulmonary edema respective effects of high airway pressure, high tidal volume, and positive end-expiratory pressure. Am Rev Respir Dis. 1988; 137: 1159-64.

[7] Morais CCA, Koyama Y, Yoshida T, Plens GM, Gomes S, Lima CLAS, et al. High positive end-expiratory pressure renders spontaneous effort noninjurious. Am J Respir Crit Care Med. 2018; 197: 1285-96.

[8] Yoshida T, Nakahashi S, Nakamura MAM, Koyama Y, Roldan R, Torsani V, et al. Volume-controlled ventilation does not prevent injurious inflation during spontaneous effort. Am J Respir Crit Care Med. 2017; 196: 590-601.

[9] Henderson WR, Chen L, Amato MBP, Brochard LJ. Fifty years of research in ARDS: respiratory mechanics in acute respiratory distress syndrome. Am J Respir Crit Care Med. 2017; 196: 822-33.

[10] Dall'ava Santucci J, Armaganidis A, Brunet F, Dhainaut JF. Mechanical effects of PEEP in patients with adult respiratory distress syndrome. J Appl Physiol. 1990; 68: 843-8.

[11] Amato MBP, Barbas CSV, Medeiros DM, Magaldi RB, Schettino GPP, Lorenzi-Filho G, et al. Effect of a protective ventilation strategy on mortality in the acute respiratory distress syndrome. N Engl J Med. 1998; 338: 347-54.

[12] Chen L, Del Sorbo L, Luca Grieco D, Shklar O, Junhasavasdikul D, Telias I, et al. Airway closure in acute respiratory distress syndrome: an underestimated and misinterpreted phenomenon. Am J Respir Crit Care Med. 2018; 197: 132-6.

[13] Ranieri VM, Zhang H, Mascia L, Aubin M, Lin CY, Mullen B, et al. Pressure-time curve predicts minimally injurious ventilatory strategy in an isolated rat lung model. Anesthesiology. 2000; 93: 1320-8.

[14] Sun XM, Chen GQ, Chen K, Wang YM, Xuan H, Huang HW, et al. Stress index can be accurately and reliably assessed by visually inspecting ventilator waveforms. Respir Care. 2018; 63: 1094-101.

5 辅助通气：压力支持和双水平正压通气模式
Assisted Ventilation: Pressure Support and Bilevel Ventilation Modes

Irene Telias, Annemijn Jonkman, Nuttapol Rittayamai

5.1 引言

与完全控制通气相比，辅助通气时呼吸机和呼吸肌共同产生驱动力将气体输送到肺部：呼吸的总压力（P_{tot}）等于呼吸机压力（P_{vent}；或气道压，P_{aw}）和呼吸肌压力（P_{mus}）的总和。因此，潮气量受到呼吸机设置和患者自身因素的双重影响。在床旁安全地应用辅助通气模式需要了解其工作原理、生理效应、潜在的获益和风险，以及患者与呼吸机之间的相互作用。在本章中，我们将讨论辅助通气中的压力支持通气（pressure support ventilation, PSV）和双水平正压通气模式。

I. Telias (✉)
Interdepartmental Division of Critical Care Medicine, University of Toronto, Toronto, ON, Canada

Division of Respirology, Department of Medicine, University Health Network and Sinai Health System, Toronto, ON, Canada

Keenan Research Centre for Biomedical Science, Li Ka Shing Knowledge Institute, St. Michael's Hospital, Toronto, ON, Canada

A. Jonkman
Department of Intensive Care Medicine, Amsterdam University Medical Centers, location VUmc, Amsterdam, The Netherlands

N. Rittayamai
Division of Respiratory Diseases and Tuberculosis, Department of Medicine, Faculty of Medicine Siriraj Hospital, Mahidol University, Salaya, Thailand
e-mail: nuttapol.rit@mahidol.ac.th

© The Author(s), under exclusive license to Springer Nature Switzerland AG 2022
G. Bellani (ed.), *Mechanical Ventilation from Pathophysiology to Clinical Evidence*, https://doi.org/10.1007/978-3-030-93401-9_5

5.2 压力支持通气

5.2.1 流行病学和潜在的优缺点

PSV 是一种受限于压力和流量循环的自主通气模式。它的使用越来越普遍,可能是目前应用最广泛的自主通气模式。虽然最初常被用作撤机方法,但 PSV 也经常在疾病的急性期使用。在一项国际性队列研究中,至少有 10% 的患者在机械通气的最初 2 天内使用了自主通气模式,而 PSV 是最常用的模式[1]。

PSV 能减少呼吸肌的负担,同时保持一定的肌肉活动。患者可以在潮气量、吸气时间、吸气流量和呼吸频率上有一定的控制,所以提高了舒适度。然而,由于每次呼吸都施加相同的压力,不能根据患者的呼吸努力和代谢需求调整,也带来了支持不足或支持过度的风险。因此,理解 PSV 的工作原理并在监测患者反应的同时安全调整呼吸机参数至关重要。

5.2.2 压力支持通气的工作原理和生理学效应

5.2.2.1 触发灵敏度、吸气上升时间、压力支持水平和呼气切换

在使用 PSV 时,所有的自主吸气努力都会触发呼吸机送气。因此,患者的呼吸频率越高,呼吸机的支持频率就越高,反之亦然。通气辅助的水平和时机取决于各种参数设置,在大多数呼吸机上可以由临床医生进行设置,包括触发灵敏度、吸气上升时间、压力支持水平和呼气切换(图 5.1a)。

呼吸机通过流量或压力传感器,根据设置的触发灵敏度,检测患者的吸气努力。现代呼吸机能快速响应呼吸触发,触发延迟低于 100 ms[2]。一旦呼吸周期开始,呼吸机首先提供较高的吸气流量,然后在整个吸气周期中逐渐减少。吸气上升时间决定达到吸气峰值流量的速度,也就是达到气道峰压的速度。吸气上升时间应该设置得较短,因为更快的压力增加可以提升患者的舒适度并减少呼吸做功。吸气上升时间的默认值通常为 150 ms,很少有人调整这项参数,而且调整它没有临床意义。压力支持水平指由临床医师设置的高于 PEEP 的固定压力值,由呼吸机在每次吸气时输送。

当吸气流量下降到峰值流量的某一百分比(%峰值流量)时,就会切换到呼气相。通常默认为 25%,但在大多数呼吸机中,此参数可以在 1%~80% 的大范围内进行调整,从而分别延长和缩短吸气时间。在呼气肌活动或管路泄漏时,呼吸机有额外安全措施来进行呼气切换。可以通过设置呼气切换来调整吸气时间的长短,以更好地匹配患者中枢的吸气需求,避免吸气周期过短或过长(图 5.1b)。具体来说,对于阻塞性肺疾病患者使用较高的%峰值流量可以延长呼气时间,避免肺过度充气。

5.2.2.2 通气的决定因素和对呼吸模式的影响

通气机设置和患者因素(主要是呼吸努力和呼吸系统顺应性)共同影响潮气量、吸气时间和每分钟通气量。例如,更高的压力支持水平、更低的%峰值流量、更大的呼吸努力和更好的呼吸系统顺应性会导致更大的潮气量(图 5.1a)。较高的压力支持水平也会导致

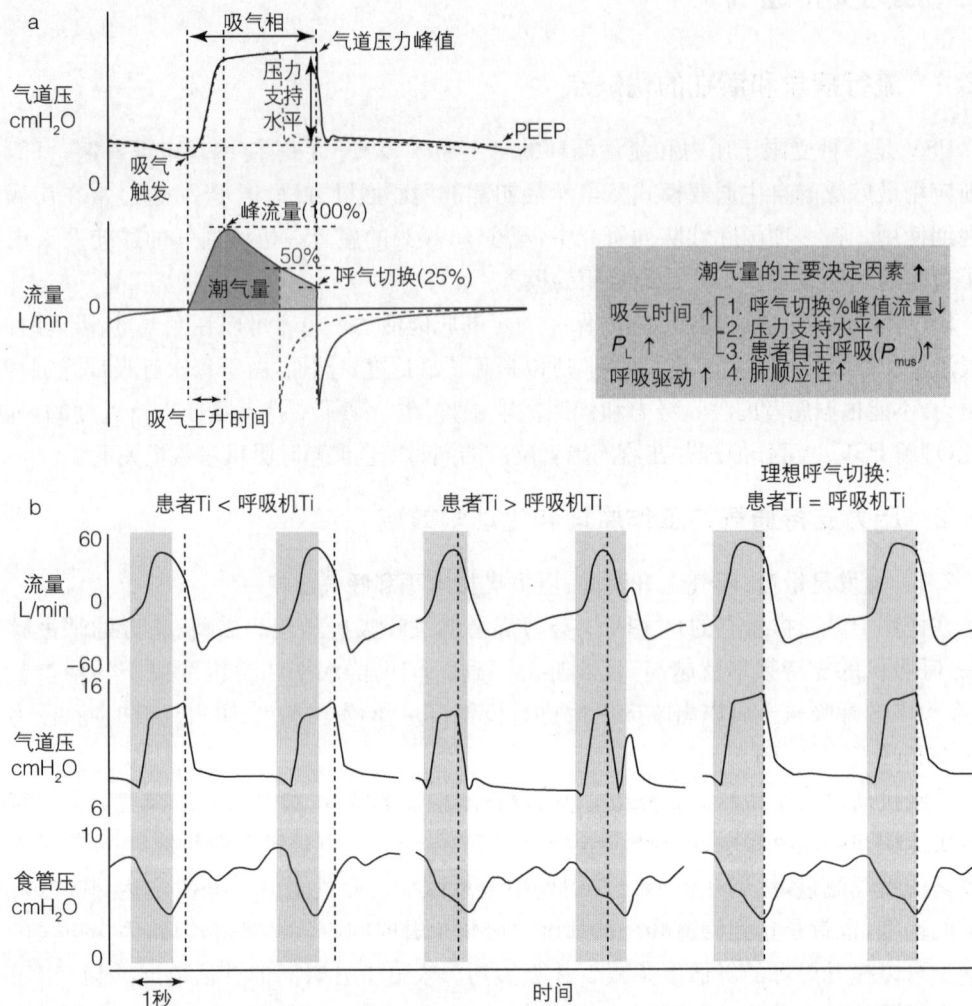

图5.1 压力支持通气工作原理及呼吸机吸气时间与患者吸气时间的关系。a. 压力支持通气模式下基本参数包括气道压力(P_{aw})、流量(Flow),以及单纯调整呼气切换设置(比如增加%峰值流量)对潮气量的影响。压力支持水平:设置的支持压力,即每次触发由呼吸机提供的高于 PEEP 的压力。吸气上升时间:从吸气开始到吸气峰值流量(也是气道峰压)的时间。通过增加%峰值流量(红色的虚线部分)来调整呼气切换可缩短呼吸机吸气时间(T_i),从而降低潮气量。在压力支持模式中,潮气量由呼吸机设置的参数(如呼气切换及压力支持水平)及患者自身因素(如患者呼吸肌压力及呼吸系统顺应性)共同决定。压力支持水平和呼吸肌压力共同决定了跨肺驱动压(P_L),而呼气切换及压力支持水平主要决定呼吸机 T_i,还受到患者吸气努力的强度及时机的影响。b. 显示了压力支持通气模式下呼吸机 T_i 与患者 T_i 不匹配情况(左图及中间图),以及呼气切换设置匹配患者 T_i 的例子(右图)。垂直虚线:呼吸机吸气周期末的呼气切换点。灰色区域:患者 T_i,将食管压力(P_{es})的最低点定义为患者吸气结束,说明不同呼气切换设置的效果。需要注意的是,患者吸气时间的确切定义存在争议(见彩色插图)

更长的吸气时间。相反,压力支持水平和呼吸努力越低,%峰值流量就越高,潮气量就越低。

在 PSV 期间,呼吸机设置也会对患者的呼吸模式产生影响。较高的支持会导致大多数患者吸气努力减少和自主吸气时间缩短[3]。由于较高的压力支持也会延长呼吸机的吸气时间,自主吸气缩短与呼吸机吸气延长之间的不匹配会经常发生。

5.2.3 压力支持模式中可能有害的患者–呼吸机相互作用

5.2.3.1 过度辅助引起的无效吸气努力及窒息事件

过度辅助指的是呼吸机支持过度,超过了患者的需求。通常发生在疾病恢复期,患者的代谢需求降低、呼吸力学改善,会导致多种容易被忽视的不良反应。第一,患者只需要付出最小的吸气努力就能够触发呼吸机,在剩余的吸气周期内进行被动吸气,存在膈肌萎缩的风险。这是由于 PSV 模式与按比例辅助通气模式不同,即使患者吸气努力很小也能获得(取决于压力支持水平和呼吸系统顺应性)相当量的潮气量。

第二,在吸气力度大幅下降时,可能会发生无效吸气,特别是在气流受阻的情况下(图 5.2a)。这是因为中枢控制的吸气时间缩短,在呼吸机未完成充分呼气之前就开始下一次

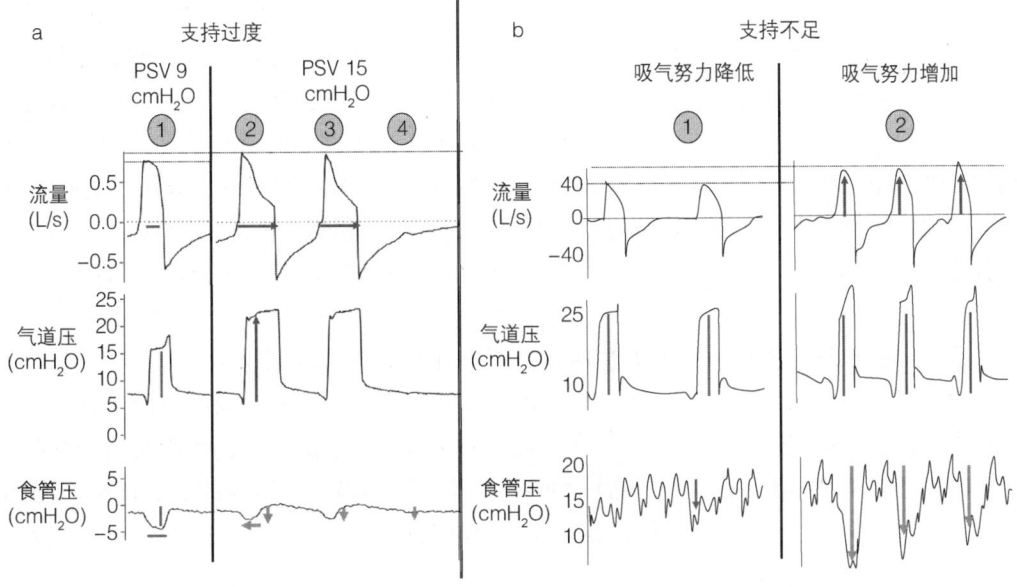

图 5.2 PSV 模式下支持过度和支持不足的机制和生理后果。a. 同一患者不同压力支持水平下流量、气道压(P_{aw})和食管压(P_{eso})波形图,左侧①中压力支持水平较低(支持压力=9 cmH$_2$O),右侧②③④中压力支持水平更高(支持压力=15 cmH$_2$O)。提高支持水平会引起吸气峰值流量、吸气时间(②中红色箭头)和潮气量(未显示)增加。增加辅助力度可以减少大多数患者的吸气力度和时间(食管压变化幅度更小、时间更短,②③中绿色箭头)。过度辅助会导致无效吸气,在呼吸机呼气相微小吸气努力(④绿色箭头)不足以触发呼吸机送气。b. 低吸气努力(左侧①)和吸气努力增加情况下(右侧②)患者的吸气峰值流量、气道压(P_{aw})和食管压(P_{eso})波形图,吸气努力增加可发生在新发感染导致代谢需求增加的情况下。在 PSV 模式下,即使患者付出更大的吸气努力,支持水平仍然保持不变。更高的吸气努力会导致食管压的下降幅度(绿色箭头)增加,同时也会导致更高的峰值流量(红色箭头)和更高的潮气量(未显示),并在气道压曲线中(红线)表现为流量饥饿。辅助不足可能导致过高呼吸驱动持续存在,并对肺和膈肌产生不利影响。PSV,压力支持通气。(见彩色插图)

吸气努力。当存在内源性呼气末正压的情况下,这些小的吸气努力在呼气相就无法触发呼吸机[4]。此时观察到的结果是实际呼吸频率低于患者努力的频率。改善无效呼吸最有效的策略是降低呼吸支持水平[5]。但需要注意的是,此时降低支持水平会导致患者呼吸频率大幅增加(通常增加一倍以上)且潮气量下降,这种变化反映的是患者自己的呼吸模式,不应该被认为是支持不足导致呼吸衰竭的标志。最后,过度辅助可能导致二氧化碳水平降低到驱动呼吸的阈值以下,进而引发睡眠期间的呼吸暂停事件,影响睡眠的连续性和质量[6]。这些窒息事件很容易被误解为是缺乏撤机的条件,而实际上它们是过度辅助的结果。

5.2.3.2 辅助不足导致流量饥饿和双重触发

相反地,如果在 PSV 时支持不足(图 5.2b),较强的吸气驱动和吸气努力形成过高的肺膨胀压力导致过度的应力和应变,会产生肺损伤的风险[7]。更重要的是,支持不足会导致流量饥饿、呼吸困难,以及持续的高呼吸驱动。同时,当吸气努力足够强时,会发生双重触发,导致吸入潮气量更大。需要注意的是,与成比例通气模式不同,PSV 模式不能适应患者呼吸需求的变化,所以在出现变化时及时调整呼吸机参数是至关重要的。

5.2.4 如何设置支持水平避免辅助过度或者不足

通常情况下,支持水平主要根据实际达到的潮气量、避免辅助呼吸肌的使用,以及呼吸频率来设置。初期研究以潮气量 8~12 mL/kg 为支持目标。然而,使用更低的潮气量(6 mL/kg)可更好地避免支持过度[5],并与更好的气体交换相关(更高效的一氧化碳弥散量)[8]。临床医生不应将降低呼吸频率视为目标,因为危重症患者静息状态下通常具有较高的呼吸频率。在 PSV 期间,呼吸频率低于 12 次/分可能提示支持过度,应该尽量避免[9]。研究发现当呼吸频率低于 30 次/分时,预示着压力-时间乘积低于 125 $cmH_2O \cdot s/min$(中低强度的吸气努力[10]),凸显出在 PSV 模式下,更高的呼吸频率是确保呼吸肌生理活动的最佳选择。

目前,滴定 PSV 支持水平的方法应包括测量呼吸驱动和呼吸努力。监测 P0.1、呼气末气道阻断压(P_{occ})、膈肌超声、食管压或膈肌电活动等。这些方法均可应用于临床决策过程中,将在第 6 章进行论述。然而,在使用 PSV 时,如何平衡患者的呼吸努力与呼吸机的支持仍然是挑战,因为不同的监测技术的目标值仍然不确定。目前的证据显示,保留中等强度的吸气努力、避免过强的跨肺驱动压和大潮气量更为合适。基于此,最近有文献给出了监测值的建议范围[11]。

5.3 双水平正压通气模式

5.3.1 双水平正压与其他压力控制模式对比

双水平正压通气是一种执行压力循环、时间控制、间歇性指令的通气模式,通过活动的呼气阀允许患者在任何时刻都能进行不受限制的自主呼吸。因此自主呼吸可以发生在呼吸机吸气-呼气循环中任意时间点(图 5.3a)[12]。双水平通气模式的优势之一是,即使没有任何呼吸驱动,仍然能保证一定程度的指令通气,但是仍允许患者自主呼吸。呼吸机可以设定两个水平的持续气道正压(continuous positive airway pressure,CPAP),包括高CPAP(P-high)和低CPAP(P-low)。在没有自主呼吸的情况下,这种模式类似于压力控制(pressure control,PC)通气,并且在常规设置的情况下,与压力控制反比通气(pressure control inverse ratio ventilation,PC-IRV)没有区别。当患者没有呼吸驱动时,呼吸机会从P-low升高到P-high吸气,再从P-high降低到P-low呼气。这种双水平正压通气可以根据患者与呼吸机呼吸同步程度[13]及呼吸机的高低压切换时间[14]进行分类,常见的包括双水平气道正压通气(BiPAP)和气道压力释放通气(APRV),如图5.3b所示。尽管如此,许多呼吸机厂家还是使用自己规定的术语来描述类似的模式(表5.1)。

所有压力控制通气模式,包括双水平正压通气模式,都涉及两个压力水平间的定时切换。根据与患者吸气努力的同步程度,这些模式可以分为全同步、部分同步和非同步模式[13](图5.3b)。在完全同步模式下,辅助呼吸完全由患者自主呼吸努力触发。而部分同步模式存在同步触发时间窗,允许患者在时间窗内触发辅助呼吸,同时在时间窗外还允许患者进行未经辅助的自主呼吸。最后,在非同步模式下,呼吸机会按照固定时间交替给予P-low和P-high,且在任何时间点都允许患者进行自主呼吸,但不能触发额外的压力支持。

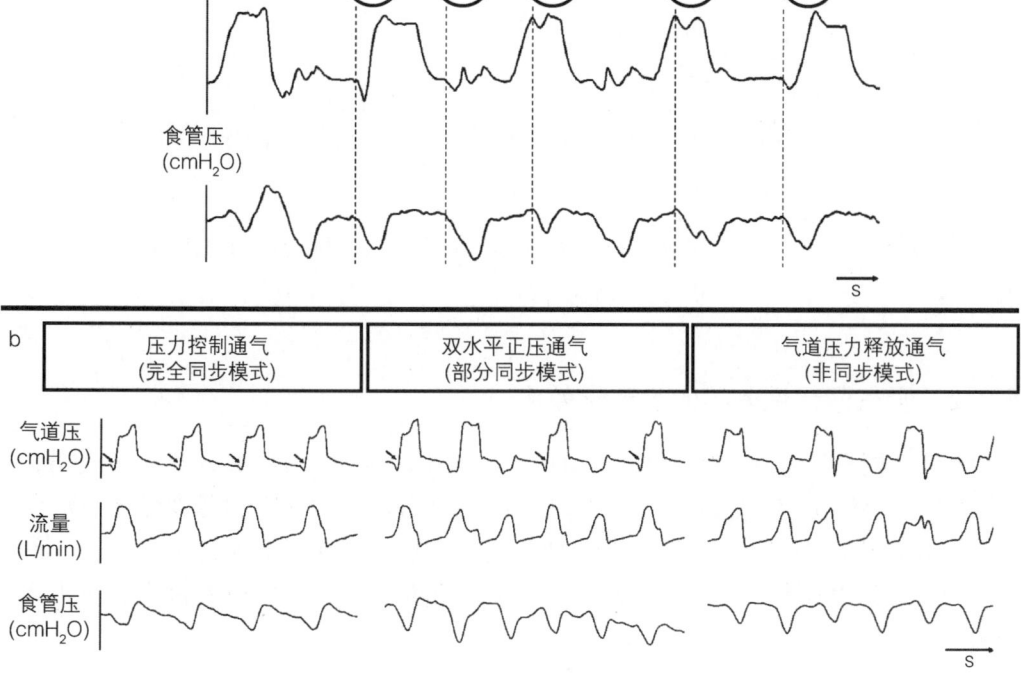

图5.3 a. 双水平正压通气的呼吸类型(由自主吸气位于呼吸机吸气-呼气周期的位置所决定)包括:① 同步呼吸;② 在P-low吸气;③ 在P-high吸气;④ 吸气从P-high持续到P-low;⑤ 呼气从P-low持续到P-high。虚线代表每次吸气努力的开始。b. 基于吸气同步程度的压力控制模式分类。黑色箭头表示患者的吸气努力与呼吸机同步

表 5.1 常见呼吸机品牌根据吸气的同步性对压力控制通气模式的不同命名

特 点	品 牌	模式名称
完全同步	Hamilton G5/S1	P-CMV
	Maquet Servo i/u	PC
	Drager Evita Infinity V500	PC-CMV
	Puritan Bennett 980	A/C PC
	GE Engström Carestation	PCV
	Vyaire AVEA/VELA	Pressure A/C
部分同步	Hamilton G5/S1	DuoPAP
	Maquet Servo i/u	Bi-Vent
	Drager Evita Infinity V500	PC-SIMV+
	Puritan Bennett 980	BiLevel
	GE Engström Carestation	BiLevel (Trigger window—on)
	Vyaire AVEA/VELA	BiPhasic
非同步	Hamilton G5/S1	APRV
	Maquet Servo i/u	APRV
	Drager Evita Infinity V500	PC-APRV
	Puritan Bennett 980	BiLevel
	GE Engström Carestation	BiLevel (Trigger window—off)
	Vyaire AVEA/VELA	APRV

5.3.2 吸气同步性差异的生理学效应

与完全同步的辅助压力控制模式(如 PCV)相比,非同步模式(如 APRV)和部分同步模式(如 BiPAP)更容易导致较低的潮气量和跨肺压,以及较大的潮气量变异度。另外,与 PSV 相比,非同步模式可以通过减少 ARDS 患者的肺不张而增加肺通气[15-17]。但是,与完全同步的压力控制模式相比,非同步或部分同步模式时需要患者付出更大的吸气努力[15-17]。

5.3.3 在辅助机械通气时设置双水平正压通气

双水平正压通气的呼吸机设置因人而异。在常规模式下,P-high 应根据平台压力来设置;然而,为了避免肺过度膨胀,一般建议限制 P-high<30 cmH_2O。P-low 通常设

置为 0 cmH$_2$O,由于 P-low 持续时间短,PEEPi 可以防止肺泡塌陷。有研究将 P-high 设置在 P-V 曲线上拐点下,将 P-low 设置在下拐点上,防止肺泡周期性的开放/塌陷。此外,其他设置 P-low 的方法,类似于 PEEP 的滴定,也是可行的[17]。

在机械通气早期,双水平正压通气通常设置长吸气时间(T-high)和短呼气时间(T-low)。BiPAP 和 APRV 的主要区别在于 P-high 的持续时间。一项先前的综述中发现,在使用 APRV 的研究中,有 46% 的患者采用了极端的吸呼比(I∶E),I∶E>2∶1,T-high 平均持续时间为 3.4 s±1.7 s;相比之下,在使用 BiPAP 的研究中,I∶E 设置为 1∶1 或轻度倒置(1∶1<I∶E<2∶1),T-high 平均持续时间为 2.4 s±0.9 s。此外,许多呼吸机还允许在患者每次自主吸气时增加额外压力支持以辅助自主呼吸。

5.3.4 辅助机械通气时双水平正压通气与常规通气模式比较的临床证据

许多临床试验对 ARDS 患者的双水平正压通气和常规通气策略进行了比较[18-20]。一项系统回顾和荟萃分析结果显示,双水平正压通气可缩短机械通气持续时间,并对血流动力学无不良影响。此外,一些研究还发现,与小潮气量的常规通气模式相比,双水平正压通气可以降低住院病死率[21]。

双水平正压通气也被应用于存在 ARDS 风险的患者。对高危创伤患者的观察性数据进行系统回顾分析表明,早期使用双水平正压通气可能有助于缓解 ARDS 的进展[22]。此外,一项纳入 63 例有 ARDS 风险创伤患者的随机研究表明,双水平正压通气和传统小潮气量肺通气策略具有相同的临床结局[23]。

5.4 总结

在辅助通气期间,呼吸机和呼吸肌共同提供压力驱动气体进入肺部。压力支持通气是最常用的辅助通气模式,可以减轻呼吸肌的负荷,让大多数患者感觉很舒适。但是,由于它提供的固定压力可能会带来支持过度或不足的风险,从而影响患者的临床预后。因此,在使用压力支持通气时需要密切监测患者并及时调整呼吸机的设置,以避免不良后果。双水平正压通气是一种执行压力循环、时间控制、间歇性指令的通气模式,通过活动的呼气阀允许患者在任何时刻都能进行不受限制的自主呼吸(非同步模式)。部分同步和非同步模式可以改善某些患者的肺通气,但与完全同步模式相比,吸气努力也会显著增加。因此,谨慎选择适当的患者人群非常重要。

(赵立娜,肇寅辉,马少林 译)

参考文献

[1] van Haren F, Pham T, Brochard L, Bellani G, Laffey J, Dres M, et al. Spontaneous breathing in early acute respiratory distress syndrome: insights from the large observational study to UNderstand the global impact of severe acute respiratory FailurE study*. Crit Care Med. 2019;

47(2): 229-38.

[2] Thille AW, Lyazidi A, Richard JCM, Galia F, Brochard L. A bench study of intensive-care-unit ventilators: new versus old and turbine-based versus compressed gas-based ventilators. Intensive Care Med. 2009; 35(8): 1368-76.

[3] Brochard L, Harf A, Lorino H, Lemaire F. Inspiratory pressure support prevents diaphragmatic fatigue during weaning from mechanical ventilation. Am Rev Respir Dis. 1989; 139(2): 513-21. http://www.ncbi.nlm.nih.gov/pubmed/2643905.

[4] Parthasarathy S, Jubran A, Tobin MJ. Cycling of inspiratory and expiratory muscle groups with the ventilator in airflow limitation. Am J Respir Crit Care Med. 1998; 158(5 Pt 1): 1471-8. http://www.ncbi.nlm.nih.gov/pubmed/9817695.

[5] Thille AW, Cabello B, Galia F, Lyazidi A, Brochard L. Reduction of patient-ventilator asynchrony by reducing tidal volume during pressure-support ventilation. Intensive Care Med. 2008; 34(8): 1477-86. https://doi.org/10.1007/s00134-008-1121-9.

[6] Parthasarathy S, Tobin MJ. Effect of ventilator mode on sleep quality in critically Ⅲ patients. Am J Respir Crit Care Med. 2002; 166(11): 1423-9.

[7] Yoshida T, Uchiyama A, Matsuura N, Mashimo T, Fujino Y. The comparison of spontaneous breathing and muscle paralysis in two different severities of experimental lung injury. Crit Care Med. 2013; 41(2): 536-45. http://eutils.ncbi.nlm.nih.gov/entrez/eutils/elink.fcgi?dbfrom=pubmed&id=23263584&retmode=ref&cmd=prlinks.

[8] da Costa NP, di Marco F, Lyazidi A, Carteaux G, Sarni M, Brochard L. Effect of pressure support on end-expiratory lung volume and lung diffusion for carbon monoxide. Crit Care Med. 2011; 39(10): 2283-9.

[9] Pletsch-Assuncao R, Caleffi Pereira M, Ferreira JG, Cardenas LZ, de Albuquerque ALP, de Carvalho CRR, et al. Accuracy of invasive and noninvasive parameters for diagnosing ventilatory overassistance during pressure support ventilation. Crit Care Med. 2017; 46(6): 1. http://insights.ovid.com/crossref?an=00003246-201803000-00009.

[10] Jubran A, van de Graaff WB, Tobin MJ. Variability of patient-ventilator interaction with pressure support ventilation in patients with chronic obstructive pulmonary disease. Am J Respir Crit Care Med. 1995; 152(1): 129-36. https://doi.org/10.1164/ajrccm.152.1.7599811.

[11] Goligher EC, Dres M, Patel BK, Sahetya SK, Beitler JR, Telias I, et al. Lung- and diaphragm-protective ventilation. Am J Respir Crit Care Med. 2020; 202(7): 950-61.

[12] Rittayamai N, Beloncle F, Goligher EC, Chen L, Mancebo J, Richard J-CM, et al. Effect of inspiratory synchronization during pressure-controlled ventilation on lung distension and inspiratory effort. Ann Intensive Care. 2017; 7(1): 100. http://www.ncbi.nlm.nih.gov/pubmed/28986852.

[13] Rittayamai N, Katsios CM, Beloncle F, Friedrich JO, Mancebo J, Brochard L. Pressure-controlled vs volume-controlled ventilation in acute respiratory failure: a physiology-based narrative and systematic review. Chest. 2015; 148(2): 340-55.

[14] Rose L, Hawkins M. Airway pressure release ventilation and biphasic positive airway pressure: a systematic review of definitional criteria. Intensive Care Med. 2008; 34(10): 1766-73. http://www.ncbi.nlm.nih.gov/pubmed/18633595.

[15] Yoshida T, Rinka H, Kaji A, Yoshimoto A, Arimoto H, Miyaichi T, et al. The impact of spontaneous ventilation on distribution of lung aeration in patients with acute respiratory distress syndrome: airway pressure release ventilation versus pressure support ventilation. Anesth Analg.

2009; 109(6): 1892 - 900. http://www.ncbi.nlm.nih.gov/pubmed/19923518.

[16] Calzia E, Lindner KH, Witt S, Schirmer U, Lange H, Stenz R, et al. Pressure-time product and work of breathing during biphasic continuous positive airway pressure and assisted spontaneous breathing. Am J Respir Crit Care Med. 1994; 150(4): 904 - 10.

[17] Daoud EG, Farag HL, Chatburn RL. Airway pressure release ventilation: what do we know? Respir Care. 2012; 57(2): 282 - 92.

[18] Putensen C, Zech S, Wrigge H, Zinserling J, Stüber F, von Spiegel T, et al. Long-term effects of spontaneous breathing during ventilatory support in patients with acute lung injury. Am J Respir Crit Care Med. 2001; 164(1): 43 - 9. http://www.ncbi.nlm.nih.gov/pubmed/11435237.

[19] Zhou Y, Jin X, Lv Y, Wang P, Yang Y, Liang G, et al. Early application of airway pressure release ventilation may reduce the duration of mechanical ventilation in acute respiratory distress syndrome. Intensive Care Med. 2017; 43(11): 1648 - 59. http://www.ncbi.nlm.nih.gov/pubmed/28936695.

[20] Varpula T, Valta P, Niemi R, Takkunen O, Hynynen M, Pettilä V. Airway pressure release ventilation as a primary ventilatory mode in acute respiratory distress syndrome. Acta Anaesthesiol Scand. 2004; 48(6): 722 - 31. http://www.ncbi.nlm.nih.gov/pubmed/15196105.

[21] Zhong X, Wu Q, Yang H, Dong W, Wang B, Zhang Z, et al. Airway pressure release ventilation versus low tidal volume ventilation for patients with acute respiratory distress syndrome/acute lung injury: a meta-analysis of randomized clinical trials. Ann Transl Med. 2020; 8(24): 1641. http://www.ncbi.nlm.nih.gov/pubmed/33490153.

[22] Andrews PL, Shiber JR, Jaruga-Killeen E, Roy S, Sadowitz B, O'Toole R, et al. Early application of airway pressure release ventilation may reduce mortality in high-risk trauma patients: a systematic review of observational trauma ARDS literature. J Trauma Acute Care Surg. 2013; 75(4): 635 - 41. http://www.ncbi.nlm.nih.gov/pubmed/24064877.

[23] Maxwell RA, Green JM, Waldrop J, Dart BW, Smith PW, Brooks D, et al. A randomized prospective trial of airway pressure release ventilation and low tidal volume ventilation in adult trauma patients with acute respiratory failure. J Trauma. 2010; 69(3): 501 - 10; discussion 511. http://www.ncbi.nlm.nih.gov/pubmed/20838119.

6 辅助通气过程中患者的监测
Monitoring the Patient During Assisted Ventilation

Alice Grassi, Irene Telias, Giacomo Bellani

在辅助机械通气期间，患者的呼吸肌与呼吸机共同完成呼吸。机械通气技术在过去十年中稳步发展，以改进患者-呼吸机相互作用为主要目标，开发出了不同的辅助通气模式(详见"5 辅助通气：压力支持和双水平正压通气模式")。辅助通气模式可以应用于疾病不同阶段：对于仍处于急性期的患者，可以作为控制通气的过渡；而在后期，可以作为撤机手段或长期带机模式。

允许患者在有创通气的情况下保持自主呼吸具有很多明显的生理优点。当所有呼吸功能都由患者的呼吸肌完成时，便向重建完全正常的呼吸生理迈出了重要的一步。相对于完全控制通气，辅助通气模式可以降低对镇静药物的需求（避免肌松药物）[1]，且可维持膈肌营养并预防其功能障碍[2,3]。但是，辅助通气与控制通气一样可能会使肺实质承受过度的应力和应变，导致肺损伤。但其机制较为特殊，被定义为"自发性肺损伤"[4]。强烈的自主吸气努力导致肺损伤的作用机制归纳如下：

A. Grassi
Department of Anesthesiology and Pain Medicine, University of Toronto, Toronto, ON, Canada

I. Telias
Interdepartmental Division of Critical Care Medicine, University of Toronto, Toronto, ON, Canada

Division of Respirology, Department of Medicine, University Health Network and Sinai Health System, Toronto, ON, Canada

Keenan Research Centre for Biomedical Science, Li Ka Shing Knowledge Institute, St. Michael's Hospital, Toronto, ON, Canada

G. Bellani (✉)
School of Medicine and Surgery, University of Milan-Bicocca, Monza, Italy
Department of Emergency and Intensive Care, ASST Monza, San Gerardo Hospital, Monza, Italy
e-mail: giacomo.bellani1@unimib.it

© The Author(s), under exclusive license to Springer Nature Switzerland AG 2022
G. Bellani (ed.), *Mechanical Ventilation from Pathophysiology to Clinical Evidence*, https://doi.org/10.1007/978-3-030-93401-9_6

(1) 不完全由临床医生控制的吸入潮气量过高。
(2) 呼吸摆动现象导致膈肌区域肺实质过度膨胀。
(3) 血管跨壁压力增加,增加肺水肿风险。
(4) 人-机不同步,特别是呼吸叠加导致肺过度膨胀。

除了肺损伤,还可能发生膈肌损伤,初步证据表明后者不仅可由膈肌废用引起,也可由过度收缩和(或)偏心收缩导致(肌肉损伤)[3]。

最后,自主吸气努力相关呼吸机送气引起胸腔内压力变化可以改善心脏前负荷,同时增加后负荷,在有利和不利的血流动力学效应间达到平衡[6]。

对于肺损伤患者来说,辅助通气是一种非常微妙的通气模式,因此,全面地监测以达到最大收益并避免风险至关重要。

6.1 吸气努力

进行辅助通气时监测患者的吸气努力有多种目的。第一,可评估呼吸支持水平和镇静深度是否恰当。第二,在撤机试验时呼吸努力的改变可预测此类试验成功与否[7]。第三,不足或过强的吸气努力可能与膈肌萎缩或功能障碍相关[3]。第四,在血流动力学不稳定时,吸气肌肉做功可能是主要的氧耗途径,因此需要使用镇静和(或)肌松剂减少氧耗[8,9]。最后,通过监测患者的吸气努力,还可计算施加于呼吸系统的总压力(后面会详细阐述)。

6.1.1 食管压力测量

为测量总呼吸做功(work of breathing,WOB)需要使用食管压力(P_{es})导管。尽管呼吸机 WOB 的是通过呼吸周期中压力-容积曲线所包围的面积来计算的(坎贝尔图,图6.1a),但这种方法并未考虑到呼吸肌的等长收缩和吸气努力的持续时间。食管压力时间乘积(esophageal pressure time product,PTP_{es})可以克服这一限制,它是吸气肌产生的压力(P_{mus})随时间变化曲线的积分(图6.1b),与呼吸肌的能量消耗密切相关。P_{mus} 等于胸壁静态回弹力与总 P_{es} 的差值。PTP_{es} 正常值为 50~150 $cmH_2O \cdot s/min$[10]。

在床边评估患者的吸气努力时,使用 P_{es} 摆动(从呼气末到最大吸气时 P_{es} 的下降值)更为实用,虽然它不如 WOB 或 PTP_{es} 精确但更为简便。将正常最大吸气的 P_{mus} 目标范围定为 5~10 cmH_2O(在胸壁回弹力较低的正常情况下对应的 P_{es} 摆动为 3~8 cmH_2O)是合理的,可以避免过度的肺应力和膈肌萎缩[11]。最近,一项旨在预测无创通气成败的研究中,发现无创通气后患者 P_{es} 摆动显著降低、更趋向于生理水平时,可以避免气管插管。

6.1.2 潮气量与呼吸频率

对于接受机械通气的患者来说,呼吸频率和潮气量并不是衡量其吸气努力的准确指标,因为它们容易受到呼吸力学和呼吸肌力量的影响。此外,危重症患者静息状态下的呼

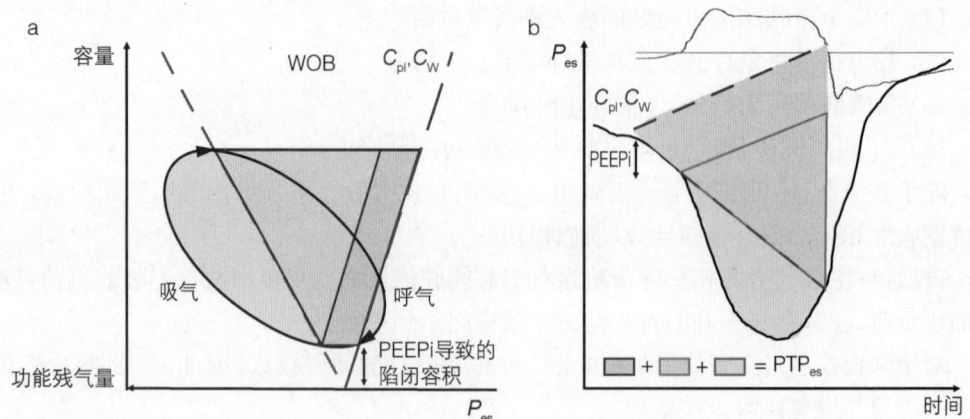

图 6.1 左图展示了以食管压力和肺容积绘制的坎贝尔图。内源性 PEEP(PEEPi)是指在没有吸入任何气体的情况下产生的压力。呼吸做功(WOB)是吸气肌压力(P_{mus})的积分。红色虚线表示胸壁的被动回弹力。WOB 有三个组成部分：阻力(吸气阶段的黄色区域)、弹性回缩力(绿色区域)和 PEEPi(蓝色区域)。呼气期的黄色小区域代表主动呼气 WOB。右图示压力-时间乘积(PTP)，即 P_{mus} 在吸气时间内的面积。作为 WOB，PTP 同样由三种成分组成：阻力(黄色)，弹性回缩力(绿色)和 PEEPi(蓝色)。PTP 是在吸气阶段计算的，即在两个零气流点之间。流量-时间曲线显示在 P_{es} 上方。C_{pl}，C_W：胸壁顺应性。(见彩色插图)

吸频率较高，在一定范围内($PaCO_2=23\sim45$ mmHg)不随呼吸驱动力而改变，还会受到其他因素的独立影响[14,15]。

但是在压力支持模式下，如果呼吸频率低于 17 次/分，则提示呼吸驱动和吸气努力低[16]。在不改变支持水平时潮气量增加，则表示吸气努力在增强。但是需要注意的是，在 PSV 时，即便吸气努力减小也不会导致潮气量降至某个特定的阈值以下。浅快呼吸指数(rapid shallow breathing index, RSBI)整合了这几项反映患者呼吸状态的变量，旨在早期预测 T 管自主呼吸试验期间[17]的撤机失败[RSBI>105/(min·L)]和提示呼吸疲劳[18]。

6.1.3 P0.1

P0.1 是指在短暂气道阻断时，患者吸气努力在前 100 ms 产生的压力下降值。在呼气末气道阻断切换至吸气初期，气道还未对吸气能量负荷产生反应(压力改变尚未产生气流)，所以 P0.1 可以定量反映患者中枢的呼吸驱动力。此外，P0.1 与气道阻力无关，因为其是在气流为零时进行测量的。由于 P0.1 的变异性较大，因此应该进行 3～4 次的测量并取平均值来准确反映呼吸驱动。健康人群中，P0.1 值为 0.5～1.5 cmH_2O[19]。P0.1 的优点之一是其易于测量，可以在大多数 ICU 呼吸机上进行，通过连续测定法(吸气努力过强时可能会低估实际值)和短暂呼吸末阻断法。最近的研究[20]证实了商用呼吸机测量 P0.1 的有效性，并证实其为评估患者呼吸驱动和呼吸做功的重要指标。研究结果表明，可以使用 1 cmH_2O 的阈值来定义低吸气努力(PTP/min<50 $cmH_2O\cdot s/min$)；而将 P0.1 高于 3.5～4 cmH_2O 定义为高吸气努力(PTP/min>200～300 $cmH_2O\cdot s/min$)。虽然高 P0.1 值或低 P0.1 值与撤机失败没有明显的相关性，但这些阈值在临床实践中可用于监测患者随呼吸支持变化而改变的吸气努力[20]。

6.1.4 气道阻断压

在较长时间的呼气阻断时（与P0.1相比），患者主动吸气引起气道压力下降（ΔP_{occ}），可作为评估吸气努力的另一个指标（图6.2a）。可以使用ΔP_{occ}，通过简单计算来准确预测P_{mus}（预测$P_{mus} = -3/4 \times \Delta P_{occ}$）。床旁测量时同样需要进行三次测量并计算平均值。为安全通气，预测P_{mus}的目标范围应与P_{mus}实际值相同，为5～10 cmH$_2$O[21]。

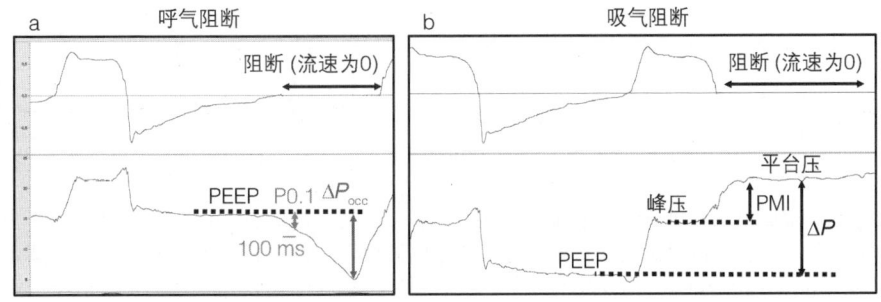

图6.2 a. 显示在压力支持通气期间进行的呼气末阻断。粉色的呼气末气道阻断压力变化（ΔP_{occ}）为PEEP和气道压最低点之间的差值。绿色的P0.1是在呼气末气道阻断期间，前100 ms内所产生的压力下降。b. 显示在压力支持通气期间进行的吸气末阻断。其间气道压稳定，气流为零，因此可以得到平台压的值。来自吸气末阻断的测量值有：平台压、压力肌肉指数（PMI＝平台压-气道峰压）、驱动压（ΔP）（见彩色插图）

6.1.5 压力肌肉指数

早在20世纪90年代就有通过吸气阻断的方法来估算吸气努力的技术[22,23]。这是因为，如果在吸气阻断期间患者呼吸肌松弛，这些肌肉在吸气末所产生的压力将"释放"在气道内；同时，在无气流时，在压力波形图上可见一个额外的压力，构成平台压（图6.2b）。为了更准确，需要待波形稳定后取值。平台压和气道峰压之间的差值为压力肌肉指数（pressure muscle index，PMI），与通过食管压导管测量的吸气末P_{es}摆动密切相关[23]。

6.1.6 膈肌电活动

膈肌电活动（electrical activity of diaphragm，EAdi）可以通过装有8个电极的营养管进行监测。尽管其主要用于神经调节辅助通气（见"7 神经调节通气辅助"），还是一个重要的监测工具。与监测呼吸机上的流量和压力波形图相比，EAdi明显在时间上离呼吸驱动释放更近，可以作为衡量呼吸驱动的指标[24]。而且EAdi与跨膈肌压密切相关，并与呼吸机辅助水平成比例变化[25]。EAdi可以通过"图形化"形式评估是否存在人-机不同步[26]、内源性PEEP[27]、反向触发[28]等情况（详见"37 机械通气的教学：在线资源和模拟教学"）。此外，在一次呼气阻断期间测得的ΔP_{occ}与EAdi的比值（有时也被称为神经肌肉偶联），使得在常规通气时可将EAdi进行转换，用以评估P_{mus}[29]，如图6.3所示。

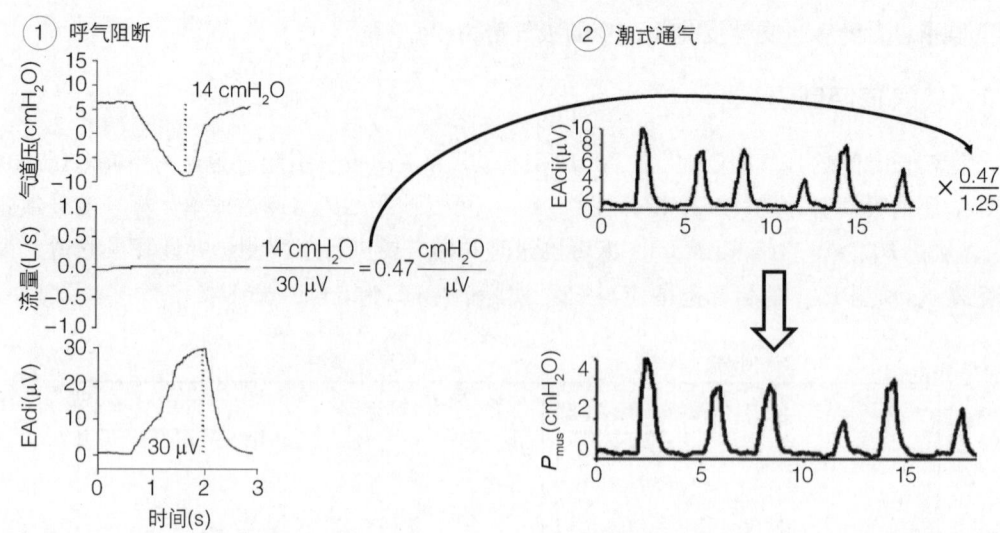

图 6.3 利用膈肌电活动（EAdi）评估肌肉压力（P_{mus}）。首先，在图①的呼气阻断期间，计算吸气努力产生的压力变化与相应 EAdi 变化的比值。这个比值被称为神经肌肉偶联或者压力-膈肌电活动比值指数（pressure/EAdi index，PEI），其单位为 $cmH_2O/\mu V$，代表患者呼吸肌每微伏电活动所产生的压力（以 cmH_2O 为单位）。该比值（考虑是等长收缩时膈肌收缩力更好，需要除以 1.25）经过转换后，可以在随后的呼吸监测中通过 EAdi 来评估 P_{mus}。

6.2 呼吸系统扩张的总压力

在辅助通气过程中，呼吸机产生的正压（由临床医生设置）和患者自身肌肉产生的负压，有助于克服呼吸系统的阻力和弹性回缩力，从而增加肺容积。因此，仅考虑呼吸机屏幕上显示的压力（气道峰压和 PEEP）并不能反映真实情况。

患者的吸气努力决定了每次呼吸中产生的胸腔负压，该负压会从外侧"牵拉"肺泡，使其充气。可以通过使用 P_{es} 导管直接测量的压力来替代胸腔负压进行监测。跨肺压（P_L）是 P_{aw} 和 P_{es} 之间的差值，可以用于估算在任何给定时刻肺泡所承受的压力。研究[30]表明，即使呼吸机施加的正压被限制在 $30\ cmH_2O$ 以下，强烈的吸气努力仍然会加重肺损伤，因为仅监测呼吸机显示的瞬时 P_{aw}（此时压力方程的部分变量无法被监测）不足以全面评估肺部承受的所有压力。

使用 P_L 作为肺应力的测量指标时，需要考虑许多影响因素。

动态 P_L 表示一次吸气努力时的最大 P_L，其包括克服气流阻力所产生的压力。但是，如果 P_L 无法抵消肺泡壁阻力，可能导致肺泡压变成绝对负值，可能会造成损伤。此外，P_L 通常是在控制通气的静态条件下计算出的，在比较辅助通气和控制通气时，应考虑到这一点[31]。此外，P_L 是一个衡量全局的指标，无法反映肺局部的不均一性（如后面章节中介绍的）。

虽然自主呼吸时 P_L 的安全限值尚未完全确定，但某些研究建议将 ΔP_L 不超过 $15\ cmH_2O$ 作为辅助通气的安全阈值[11]。

尽管 P_{es} 导管是最直接的测量 P_L 的方法，但在临床实践中并未普遍应用。现在已经发展出利用呼吸机压力波形估算呼吸系统扩张总压力的替代方法。使用上述吸气保持的方法，如图6.2b所示，可以测量PMI，也显示出平台压高于气道峰压，因为前者包括呼吸机产生的压力和吸气肌释放的肌肉压力[32-34]。该平台压与在控制通气时测量的意义完全相同，可以利用其计算静态驱动压（P_{plat}－PEEP）。与被动吸气相比，在辅助通气期间进行吸气保持更复杂和不确定，因为患者肌肉处于活动状态且肌肉没有松弛时平台压不可靠。约20%的患者在辅助通气过程中出现无法取值的情况，尤其是那些呼吸驱动强的患者[33,34]。目前，辅助通气时驱动压的安全限值尚未确定，但是一项使用与控制通气相同阈值的小型回顾性研究发现，驱动压同样与预后相关（<15 cmH_2O，越低越好）[35]。即使形成了水平稳定的平台波形，也不能排除呼气肌活动的存在[36]，这可能导致高估驱动压大小，反而会促使设置更安全的通气参数。

ΔP_{occ}可以通过PEEP与呼气保持时P_{aw}最低点的差值来计算（如前所述，是一种预测P_{mus}的方法），也可用于估算动态跨肺驱动压。相比于吸气保持法，通过ΔP_{occ}估算从技术上讲更易于执行，因为无须对呼吸机波形进行后续冻结解析。基于ΔP_{occ}估算动态跨肺驱动压的公式为：预计动态跨肺驱动压＝（气道峰压－PEEP）－2/3 ΔP_{occ}。使用此方法预测的压力在估计动态跨肺驱动压时的AUROC>0.9[21]。

需要特别注意的是，平台压和ΔP_{occ}的测量可以为临床医师提供补充信息，因此同时测量两者，尤其是在没有P_{es}导管的情况下，可以更全面地对呼吸力学进行描述。实际上，最近的一项在轻度ARDS动物模型中的研究表明，较高的潮气量和气道驱动压（而不是较高的动态驱动压）与更严重的肺和膈肌损伤有关[37]。

6.3 人-机不同步

人-机不同步现象发生于患者和呼吸机的吸气和呼气时间部分或全部不匹配时。人-机不同步是一个常见问题，可能会影响多达1/3的患者[38]。目前，一项多中心研究（BEARDS，NCT03447288）正在进行中，旨在研究ARDS患者机械通气时人-机不同步的发生率。一些研究表明，人-机不同步的发生率与结局事件（机械通气时间，ICU病死率）相关[39-41]。不过，人-机不同步可能是肺部疾病更严重的标志，而非导致不良结局的直接原因。这种不同步可能会让患者感到不适，导致镇静药物的剂量增加[38]。在机械通气期间，临床医生在床旁及时识别出人-机不同步的发生非常重要，此时需要优化呼吸机的设置，以减少不同步的发生率。识别和量化人-机不同步的自动化工具已经被开发出[42]。最常见的人-机不同步是无效触发，即患者的吸气努力未能触发呼吸机。这是患者肌肉产生的力量或气流不足以克服触发阈值所致，提示肌肉无力或存在内源性PEEP，可以通过P_{es}或EAdi等指标进行监测，因为在辅助通气期间，呼气肌活动的存在会导致内源性PEEP无法通过呼气阻断来测量。吸气气流产生前的P_{es}降低值或EAdi增加值可以用来估算吸气肌触发呼吸机所需克服的压力[27]。双重触发或双吸气是另一种常见的人-机不同步现象。发生该现象的原因是呼吸机设定的吸气时间短于患者的吸气时间，在未完全呼气的情况下患者再次触发呼吸[42]。这可能导致所谓的呼吸叠加，意味着输送的总潮气量高于预期目标，并可导致肺过度膨胀[43]。最后，自动触发是在没有患者吸气努力的情况下呼吸机自动送气，由心脏搏动引起的气流振荡或气体泄漏触发。而且同样会导致呼吸叠加。人-机不同步更完整的介绍请参阅相关文献[38]。如果配备 P_{es} 导管或 EAdi 监测设备,则能更容易地识别人-机不同步。利用这两种监测方法可以在呼吸周期中直接观察患者肌肉活动的强度和时间[8-10]。如果没有这些监测手段,临床医师应密切关注气道压力和呼吸机波形的变化,以识别人-机不同步的存在。第39章中包含了多种人-机不同步的图片,可以让读者对这个常见的问题有更多了解。

6.4 气体再分布和呼吸摆动

如前所述,P_{aw} 和 P_{es} 是呼吸系统膨胀压力的整体监测指标,不能区分不同区域。正常的肺具有类似于液体的表现,呼吸肌产生的压力均匀地作用于整个肺实质,而受损的肺则类似于"固体"[44]。这就意味着,在同样的扩张压力下,一些区域不会充气,而另一些区域会过度膨胀。然后,就会出现如图 6.4 所示的"呼吸摆动"现象。它指的是潮气量在不同

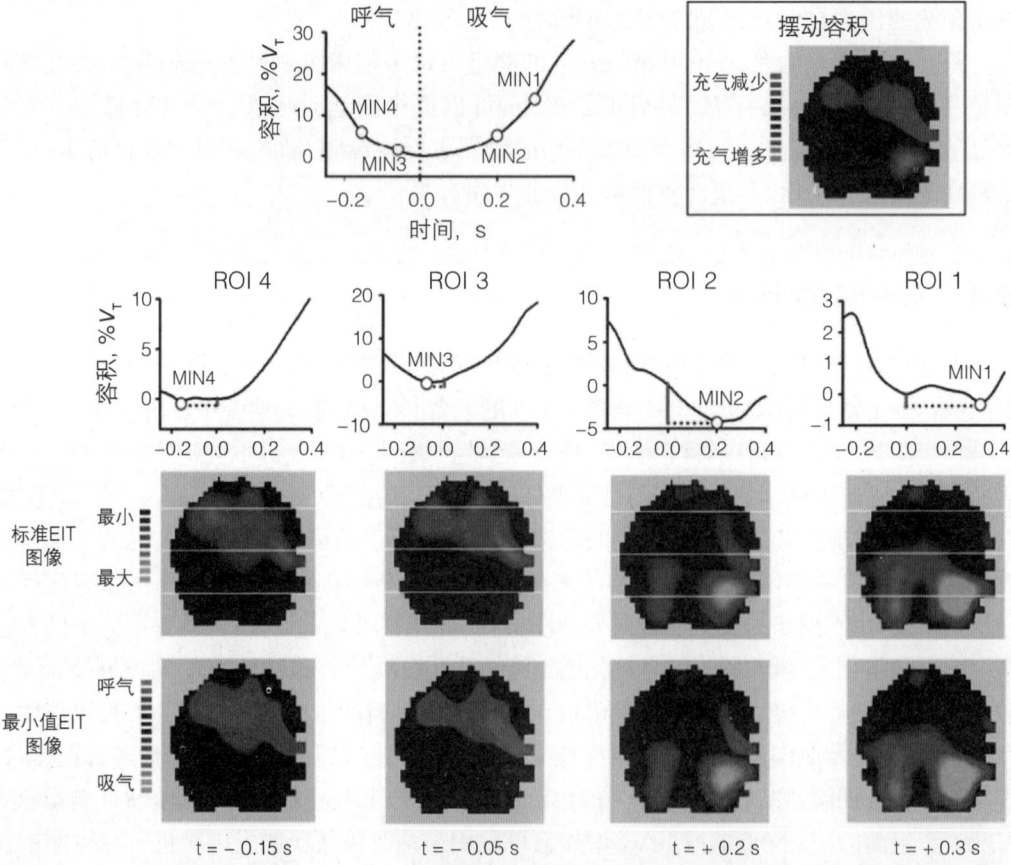

图 6.4 撤机试验中的呼吸摆动现象:观察到不同区域之间的不同步,背侧关注区域(ROI 3 和 ROI4)在呼气时显示出最小阻抗值(局部呼气),而腹侧区域(ROI1 和 ROI2)则在吸气时显示出最小阻抗值(吸气时最容易通气)。因此,一些进入 ROI 3 和 ROI4 的气体(红色)来自 ROI 1 和 ROI2;当背侧 ROI 开始吸气,腹侧 ROI 仍在呼气时(紫色区域)。摆动的气体从腹侧向背侧肺区域移动(方框图)。ROI,感兴趣区域(获得授权转载于参考文献[46])(见彩色插图)

时间常数肺组织之间的运动,监测呼吸机的波形变化或 P_L 均无法识别这种情况。最终导致充气肺区域的局部过度膨胀[45,46]。电阻抗断层成像(electrical impedance tomography,EIT)是一种床旁监测工具,可以通过可视化的方式识别不同肺区域间的通气差异(详见"33 电阻抗体断层成像技术")。EIT 是唯一能够识别"呼吸摆动"现象的监测手段,表现为一些肺区域膨胀,而另一些肺区域萎陷[45]。通气支持减少时,"呼吸摆动"现象会更明显,这可能与无效通气和肺局部过度膨胀有关[46]。此外,EIT 还可以提供关于吸气努力引起的局部通气分布变化的有用信息[47]。

6.5 呼吸肌的超声评估

呼吸肌超声是一种新兴的、快速发展的监测自主呼吸的方法[48]。膈肌厚度和功能已被广泛用于研究,并且显示与患者预后相关[2]。利用该技术具有非侵入性且床旁易用性的优势,最近辅助呼吸肌和腹肌已成为越来越多研究的研究对象。更多关于呼吸肌超声的详细信息请见"32 呼吸系统的超声评估"。

6.6 总结

在过去的十年中,更新了许多研究数据,使我们更好地理解允许自主呼吸的益处和风险,以及患者自主吸气努力的关键作用。除了 P_{es} 导管,还有很多技术可以在床旁应用。这些技术若要更广泛地应用于临床实践,需要临床研究不断跟进,以确定预防损伤并改善患者预后的目标。

(赵立娜,肇寅辉,钟鸣 译)

参考文献

[1] Chanques G, Constantin JM, Devlin JW, Ely EW, Fraser GL, Gélinas C, et al. Analgesia and sedation in patients with ARDS. Intensive Care Med. 2020;46:2342-56. https://doi.org/10.1007/s00134-020-06307-9.

[2] Goligher EC, Dres M, Fan E, Rubenfeld GD, Scales DC, Herridge MS, et al. Mechanical ventilation-induced diaphragm atrophy strongly impacts clinical outcomes. Am J Respir Crit Care Med. 2018;197:204-13. https://doi.org/10.1164/rccm.201703-0536OC.

[3] Goligher EC, Brochard LJ, Reid WD, Fan E, Saarela O, Slutsky AS, et al. Diaphragmatic myotrauma: a mediator of prolonged ventilation and poor patient outcomes in acute respiratory failure. Lancet Respir Med. 2019;7:90-8. https://doi.org/10.1016/S2213-2600(18)30366-7.

[4] Brochard L, Slutsky A, Pesenti A. Mechanical ventilation to minimize progression of lung injury in acute respiratory failure. Am J Respir Crit Care Med. 2017;195:438-42. https://doi.org/10.1164/rccm.201605-1081CP.

[5] Yoshida T, Fujino Y. Monitoring the patient for a safe assisted ventilation. Curr Opin Crit Care. 2021;27:1-5. https://doi.org/10.1097/MCC.0000000000000788.

[6] Pinsky MR. Cardiopulmonary interactions: physiologic basis and clinical applications. Ann Am Thorac Soc. 2018; 15: S45-8. https://doi.org/10.1513/AnnalsATS.201704-339FR.

[7] Jubran A, Tobin M. Pathophysiologic basis of acute respiratory distress in patients who fail a trial of weaning from mechanical ventilation. Am J Respir Crit Care Med. 1997; 155: 906-15. https://doi.org/10.1164/ajrccm.155.3.9117025.

[8] Mauri T, Yoshida T, Bellani G, Goligher EC, Carteaux G, Rittayamai N, et al. Esophageal and transpulmonary pressure in the clinical setting: meaning, usefulness and perspectives. Intensive Care Med. 2016; 42: 1360-73. https://doi.org/10.1007/s00134-016-4400-x.

[9] Akoumianaki E, Maggiore SM, Valenza F, Bellani G, Jubran A, Loring SH, et al. The application of esophageal pressure measurement in patients with respiratory failure. Am J Respir Crit Care Med. 2014; 189: 520-31. https://doi.org/10.1164/rccm.201312-2193CI.

[10] Pham T, Telias I, Beitler JR. Esophageal manometry. Respir Care. 2020; 65: 772-92. https://doi.org/10.4187/respcare.07425.

[11] Bertoni M, Spadaro S, Goligher EC. Monitoring patient respiratory effort during mechanical ventilation: lung and diaphragm-protective ventilation. Crit Care. 2020; 24: 106. https://doi.org/10.1186/s13054-020-2777-y.

[12] Tonelli R, Fantini R, Tabbì L, Castaniere I, Pisani L, Pellegrino MR, et al. Early inspiratory effort assessment by esophageal manometry predicts noninvasive ventilation outcome in de novo respiratory failure: a pilot study. Am J Respir Crit Care Med. 2020; 202: 558-67. https://doi.org/10.1164/rccm.201912-2512OC.

[13] Akoumianaki E, Vaporidi K, Georgopoulos D. The injurious effects of elevated or nonelevated respiratory rate during mechanical ventilation. Am J Respir Crit Care Med. 2019; 199: 149-57. https://doi.org/10.1164/rccm.201804-0726CI.

[14] Costa R, Navalesi P, Cammarota G, Longhini F, Spinazzola G, Cipriani F, et al. Remifentanil effects on respiratory drive and timing during pressure support ventilation and neurally adjusted ventilatory assist. Respir Physiol Neurobiol. 2017; 244: 10-6. https://doi.org/10.1016/j.resp.2017.06.007.

[15] Laghi F, Karamchandani K, Tobin MJ. Influence of ventilator settings in determining respiratory frequency during mechanical ventilation. Am J Respir Crit Care Med. 1999; 160: 1766-70. https://doi.org/10.1164/ajrccm.160.5.9810086.

[16] Pletsch-Assuncao R, Pereira MC, Ferreira JG, Cardenas LZ, De Albuquerque ALP, De Carvalho CRR, et al. Accuracy of invasive and noninvasive parameters for diagnosing ventilatory overassistance during pressure support ventilation. Crit Care Med. 2018; 46: 411-7. https://doi.org/10.1097/CCM.0000000000002871.

[17] Yang KL, Tobin M. A prospective study of indexes predicting the outcome of trials of weaning from mechanical ventilation. N Engl J Med. 1991; 324: 1445-50. https://doi.org/10.1056/NEJM199105233242101.

[18] Karthika M, Al Enezi FA, Pillai LV, Arabi YM. Rapid shallow breathing index. Ann Thorac Med. 2016; 11: 167-76. https://doi.org/10.4103/1817-1737.176876.

[19] Telias I, Damiani F, Brochard L. The airway occlusion pressure (P 0.1) to monitor respiratory drive during mechanical ventilation: increasing awareness of a not-so-new problem. Intensive Care Med. 2018; 44: 1532-5. https://doi.org/10.1007/s00134-018-5045-8.

[20] Telias I, Junhasavasdikul D, Rittayamai N, Piquilloud L, Chen L, Ferguson ND, et al. Airway occlusion pressure as an estimate of respiratory drive and inspiratory effort during assisted

ventilation. Am J Respir Crit Care Med. 2020; 201: 1086 - 98. https://doi.org/10.1164/RCCM.201907-1425OC.

[21] Bertoni M, Telias I, Urner M, Long M, Del Sorbo L, Fan E, et al. A novel non-invasive method to detect excessively high respiratory effort and dynamic transpulmonary driving pressure during mechanical ventilation. Crit Care. 2019; 23: 1 - 10. https://doi.org/10.1186/s13054-019-2617-0.

[22] Pesenti A, Pelosi P, Foti G, D'Andrea L, Rossi N. An interrupter technique for measuring respiratory mechanics and the pressure generated by respiratory muscles during partial ventilatory support. Chest. 1992; 102: 918 - 23. https://doi.org/10.1378/chest.102.3.918.

[23] Foti G, Cereda M, Banfi G, Pelosi P, Fumagalli R, Pesenti A. End-inspiratory airway occlusion: a method to assess the pressure developed by inspiratory muscles in patients with acute lung injury undergoing pressure support. Am J Respir Crit Care Med. 1997; 156: 1210 - 6. https://doi.org/10.1164/ajrccm.156.4.96-02031.

[24] Sinderby C, Navalesi P, Beck J, Skrobik Y, Comtois N, Friberg S, et al. Neural control of mechanical ventilation in respiratory failure. Nat Med. 1999; 5: 1433 - 6. https://doi.org/10.1038/71012.

[25] Beck J, Gottfried SB, Navalesi P, Skrobik Y, Comtois N, Rossini M, et al. Electrical activity of the diaphragm during pressure support ventilation in acute respiratory failure. Am J Respir Crit Care Med. 2001; 164: 419 - 24. https://doi.org/10.1164/ajrccm.164.3.2009018.

[26] Colombo D, Cammarota G, Alemani M, Carenzo L, Barra FL, Vaschetto R, et al. Efficacy of ventilator waveforms observation in detecting patient-ventilator asynchrony. Crit Care Med. 2011; 39: 2452 - 7. https://doi.org/10.1097/CCM.0b013e318225753c.

[27] Bellani G, Coppadoro A, Patroniti N, Turella M, Marocco SA, Grasselli G, et al. Clinical assessment of auto-positive end-expiratory pressure by diaphragmatic electrical activity during pressure support and neurally adjusted ventilatory assist. Anesthesiology. 2014; 121: 563 - 71. https://doi.org/10.1097/ALN.0000000000000371.

[28] Mellado Artigas R, Damiani LF, Piraino T, Pham T, Chen L, Rauseo M, et al. Reverse triggering Dyssynchrony 24 h after initiation of mechanical ventilation. Anesthesiology. 2021; 134: 760 - 9. https://doi.org/10.1097/ALN.0000000000003726.

[29] Bellani G, Mauri T, Coppadoro A, Grasselli G, Patroniti N, Spadaro S, et al. Estimation of patient's inspiratory effort from the electrical activity of the diaphragm. Crit Care Med. 2013; 41: 1483 - 91. https://doi.org/10.1097/CCM.0b013e31827caba0.

[30] Yoshida T, Uchiyama A, Matsuura N, Mashimo T, Fujino Y. Spontaneous breathing during lung-protective ventilation in an experimental acute lung injury model: high transpulmonary pressure associated with strong spontaneous breathing effort may worsen lung injury. Crit Care Med. 2012; 40: 1578 - 85. https://doi.org/10.1097/CCM.0b013e3182451c40.

[31] Bellani G, Grasselli G, Teggia-Droghi M, Mauri T, Coppadoro A, Brochard L, et al. Do spontaneous and mechanical breathing have similar effects on average transpulmonary and alveolar pressure? A clinical crossover study. Crit Care. 2016; 20: 1 - 10. https://doi.org/10.1186/s13054-016-1290-9.

[32] Bellani G, Grassi A, Sosio S, Foti G. Plateau and driving pressure in the presence of spontaneous breathing. Intensive Care Med. 2019; 45: 97 - 8. https://doi.org/10.1007/s00134-018-5311-9.

[33] Sajjad H, Schmidt GA, Brower RG, Eberlein M. Can the plateau be higher than the peak pressure? Ann Am Thorac Soc. 2018; 15: 754 - 9. https://doi.org/10.1513/AnnalsATS.

201707-553CC.

[34] Mezidi M, Guérin C. Complete assessment of respiratory mechanics during pressure support ventilation. Intensive Care Med. 2019; 45: 557 – 8. https://doi.org/10.1007/s00134-018-5490-4.

[35] Bellani G, Grassi A, Sosio S, Gatti S, Kavanagh BP, Pesenti A, et al. Driving pressure is associated with outcome during assisted ventilation in acute respiratory distress syndrome. Anesthesiology. 2019; 131: 594 – 604. https://doi.org/10.1097/ALN.0000000000002846.

[36] Soundoulounaki S, Akoumianaki E, Kondili E, Pediaditis E, Prinianakis G, Vaporidi K, et al. Airway pressure morphology and respiratory muscle activity during end-inspiratory occlusions in pressure support ventilation. Crit Care. 2020; 24: 1 – 9. https://doi.org/10.1186/s13054-020-03169-x.

[37] Pinto EF, Santos RS, Antunes MA, Maia LA, Padilha GA, De Machado JA, et al. Static and dynamic transpulmonary driving pressures affect lung and diaphragm injury during pressure-controlled versus pressure-support ventilation in experimental mild lung injury in rats. Anesthesiology. 2020; 132: 307 – 20. https://doi.org/10.1097/ALN.0000000000003060.

[38] Pham T, Brochard LJ, Slutsky AS. Mechanical ventilation: state of the art. Mayo Clin Proc. 2017; 92: 1382 – 400. https://doi.org/10.1016/j.mayocp.2017.05.004.

[39] Blanch L, Villagra A, Sales B, Montanya J, Lucangelo U, Luján M, et al. Asynchronies during mechanical ventilation are associated with mortality. Intensive Care Med. 2015; 41: 633 – 41. https://doi.org/10.1007/s00134-015-3692-6.

[40] Thille AW, Rodriguez P, Cabello B, Lellouche F, Brochard L. Patient-ventilator asynchrony during assisted mechanical ventilation. Intensive Care Med. 2006; 32: 1515 – 22. https://doi.org/10.1007/s00134-006-0301-8.

[41] Vaporidi K, Babalis D, Chytas A, Lilitsis E, Kondili E, Amargianitakis V, et al. Clusters of ineffective efforts during mechanical ventilation: impact on outcome. Intensive Care Med. 2017; 43: 184 – 91. https://doi.org/10.1007/s00134-016-4593-z.

[42] de Haro C, Ochagavia A, López-Aguilar J, Fernandez-Gonzalo S, Navarra-Ventura G, Magrans R, et al. Patient-ventilator asynchronies during mechanical ventilation: current knowledge and research priorities. Intensive Care Med Exp. 2019; 7: 1 – 14. https://doi.org/10.1186/s40635-019-0234-5.

[43] Beitler JR, Sands SA, Loring SH, Owens RL, Malhotra A, Spragg RG, et al. Quantifying unintended exposure to high tidal volumes from breath stacking dyssynchrony in ARDS: the BREATHE criteria. Intensive Care Med. 2016; 42: 1427 – 36. https://doi.org/10.1007/s00134-016-4423-3.

[44] Yoshida T, Fujino Y, Amato MBP, Kavanagh BP. Fifty years of research in ards spontaneous breathing during mechanical ventilation risks, mechanisms, and management. Am J Respir Crit Care Med. 2017; 195: 985 – 92. https://doi.org/10.1164/rccm.201604-0748CP.

[45] Yoshida T, Torsani V, Gomes S, Santis RRD, Beraldo MA, Costa ELV, et al. Spontaneous effort causes occult pendelluft during mechanical ventilation. Am J Respir Crit Care Med. 2013; 188: 1420 – 7. https://doi.org/10.1164/rccm.201303-0539OC.

[46] Coppadoro A, Grassi A, Giovannoni C, Rabboni F, Eronia N, Bronco A, et al. Occurrence of pendelluft under pressure support ventilation in patients who failed a spontaneous breathing trial: an observational study. Ann Intensive Care. 2020; 10: 39. https://doi.org/10.1186/s13613-020-00654-y.

[47] Mauri T, Bellani G, Confalonieri A, Tagliabue P, Turella M, Coppadoro A, et al. Topographic distribution of tidal ventilation in acute respiratory distress syndrome: effects of positive end-expiratory pressure and pressure support. Crit Care Med. 2013; 41: 1664-73. https://doi.org/10.1097/CCM.0b013e318287f6e7.

[48] Tuinman PR, Jonkman AH, Dres M, Shi ZH, Goligher EC, Goffi A, et al. Respiratory muscle ultrasonography: methodology, basic and advanced principles and clinical applications in ICU and ED patients—a narrative review. Intensive Care Med. 2020; 46: 594-605. https://doi.org/10.1007/s00134-019-05892-8.

[49] Schreiber AF, Sabatini U, Vorona S, Bertoni M, Piva S, Goligher E. Measuring abdominal muscle function by abdominal muscle thickening on ultrasound: reproducibility, validity and normal range values. Eur Respir J. 2019; 54: OA5367. https://doi.org/10.1183/13993003.

7 神经调节通气辅助
Neurally Adjusted Ventilatory Assist
Hadrien Rozé

7.1 工作原理

呼吸中枢产生的冲动通过膈神经传导至膈肌,刺激膈肌收缩,启动自主呼吸。随后,气道内压力下降,使空气流入肺部。膈肌电活动(electroactivity of the diaphragm, EAdi)由运动单位动作电位时间、空间总和构成,其幅度与运动单位激发率和募集量变化相关。EAdi 信号与神经驱动同步,在强度上成比例[1]。神经调节通气辅助(neurally adjusted ventilation assist, NAVA)是基于鼻胃管上电极记录的 EAdi 来实现的,电极必须置于靠近膈脚肌纤维的食管和胃的交接处[2]。在 NAVA 模式下,呼吸机捕获并应用 EAdi 信号,实现同步且与患者呼吸驱动力匹配的呼吸支持。因此,NAVA 可以放大患者呼吸肌的努力,提供必要的支持来改善能力与需求失衡的困境[3]。

7.1.1 膈肌电活动信号

EAdi 采用按顺序排列的双极电极,利用特殊的处理技术采集信号以不受膈肌运动的影响。大部分干扰信号,如 ECG 信号和伪迹,将在信号采集过程中去除,使 $\Delta EAdi_{(t)}$ 以波形的形式与其他曲线(如 $P_{aw(t)}$、$Flow_{(t)}$ 和 $V_{T(t)}$ 等)同步显示在呼吸机的屏幕上[4]。EAdi 信号的意义已被许多临床研究所验证,其强度与跨膈压成正比,并且增加通气支持水平时,压力时间乘积与 EAdi 会成比例减少[5,6]。需要注意的是,EAdi 无法反映辅助呼吸肌的募集激活,而其激活能够减少膈肌负荷。在呼吸控制的神经反馈调节下,EAdi 信号幅度会随着吸气努力加强、镇静减少、支持水平降低或呼吸状况恶化而增加。

H. Rozé (✉)
Thoracic Intensive Care Unit, Department of Anesthesiology and Critical Care, Bordeaux University Hospital, Bordeaux, France
e-mail: hadrien.roze@chu-bordeaux.fr

© The Author(s), under exclusive license to Springer Nature Switzerland AG 2022
G. Bellani (ed.), *Mechanical Ventilation from Pathophysiology to Clinical Evidence*, https://doi.org/10.1007/978-3-030-93401-9_7

7 神经调节通气辅助

如果 EAdi 导管置于食管的适当位置上且工作正常，EAdi 为 0 μV 表示没有膈肌激活。当 EAdi 在非比例辅助通气（如压力支持通气）模式下使用时，0 μV 的 EAdi 可能是由于过度辅助造成的，也可能是由于持续镇静或膈神经损伤扰乱了呼吸控制。实际上，作为监测工具，EAdi 还可以用于除 NAVA 外的其他通气模式，以改善患者与呼吸机的相互作用[7]。

7.1.2 NAVA 模式

7.1.2.1 NAVA 下的触发

NAVA 由电触发（电压，μV），而不是气动触发（压力或流量）。如图 7.1 所示，NAVA 会根据 EAdi 波形所代表的神经驱动来启动和终止吸气。当 ΔEAdi 大于 0.5 μV 时，NAVA 会启动吸气；当 EAdi 下降到峰值的 70% 时（该参数无法更改），NAVA 会触发呼气并停止吸气。对于每个呼吸循环，NAVA 会根据 EAdi 波形来进行电触发吸气；如果基于流量的气动触发早于 EAdi，则可以由流量触发吸气，两种触发方式间的规则是先到先得。当电触发持续吸气时，则当吸气时间达到 2.5 s 时会强制切换至呼气相。

7.1.2.2 支持水平

呼吸机吸气时的压力水平与 EAdi 的变化（ΔEAdi）成正比，需乘以一个比例系数，即

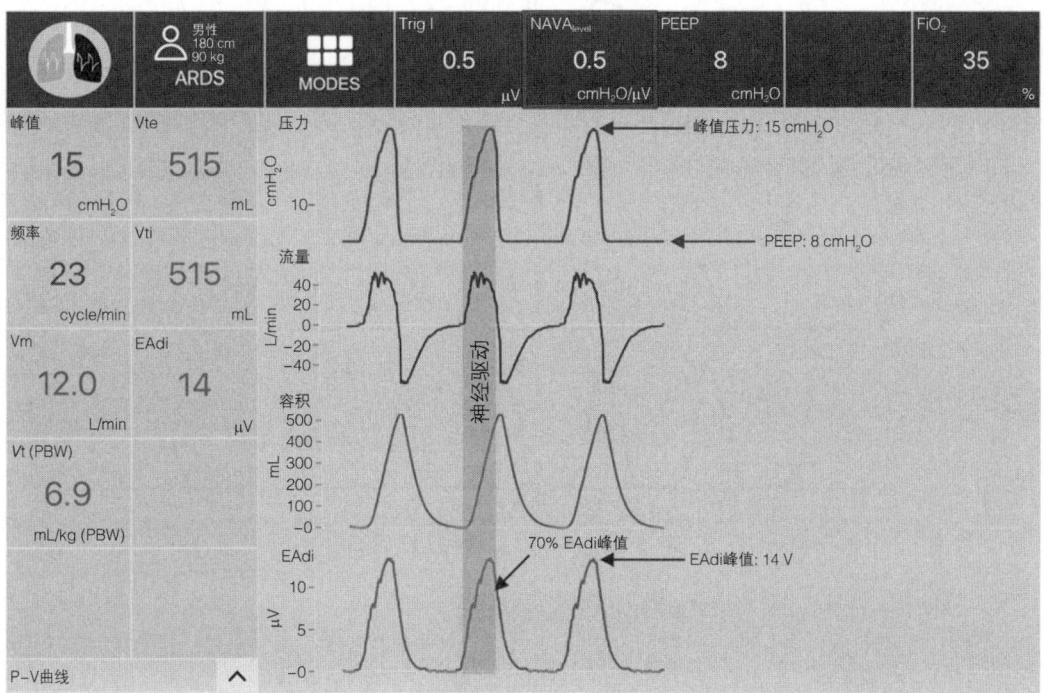

图 7.1 该图同步显示了 EAdi 和压力、流量波形，从 0.5 μV 开始吸气，到 EAdi=0.7×14=9.8 μV 时吸气停止。呼吸机提供的峰值压力水平由 EAdi 峰值（14 μV）、PEEP（8 cmH$_2$O）和 NAVA$_{level}$（0.5 cmH$_2$O/μV）决定。即峰值压力=8+0.5×14=15 cmH$_2$O。如果 NAVA$_{level}$ 增加到 1 cmH$_2$O/μV，将增加辅助的压力，峰值压力将增加为 8+1×14=22 cmH$_2$O，之后将与 EAdi 成比例变化（图片引自 iVentilate 应用，Pr Hadrien Rozé 免费提供）

$NAVA_{level}$，该系数单位为 $cmH_2O/\mu V$（见式 7.1）。

$$P_{aw(t)} = PEEP + NAVA_{level} \times \Delta EAdi_{(t)} \quad (7.1)$$

气道压力波形和 EAdi 波形的形状是相同的，两者间的比例根据 $NAVA_{level}$ 的大小增加或者减少。

$NAVA_{level}$ 人工设置范围通常为 $0.1 \sim 15\ cmH_2O/\mu V$（以 $0.1\ cmH_2O/\mu V$ 或 $0.2\ cmH_2O/\mu V$ 的幅度进行调整）。在临床实践中通常使用低于 $3\ cmH_2O/\mu V$ 的设置。$NAVA_{level}$ 对 P_{aw} 的作用取决于 $EAdi_{peak}$，如果将 $NAVA_{level}$ 加倍，在 $30\ \mu V$ 的 $EAdi_{peak}$ 下增加的压力远远多于 $5\ \mu V$ 的 $EAdi_{peak}$。为了确保患者的安全，通常需要在 NAVA 期间设置压力上限，以确保 P_{aw} 不超过气道压力报警值下 $5\ cmH_2O$ 的水平（图 7.1）。

$NAVA_{level}$ 的改变会影响与 EAdi 相关的支持水平，如图 7.2 所示。从最低水平开始，增加 $NAVA_{level}$ 会增加呼吸机输送的压力。然而，随着呼吸机支持的增加，呼吸控制的神经反馈会使 EAdi 值降低，导致传递的压力降低（图 7.2）[6,8]。

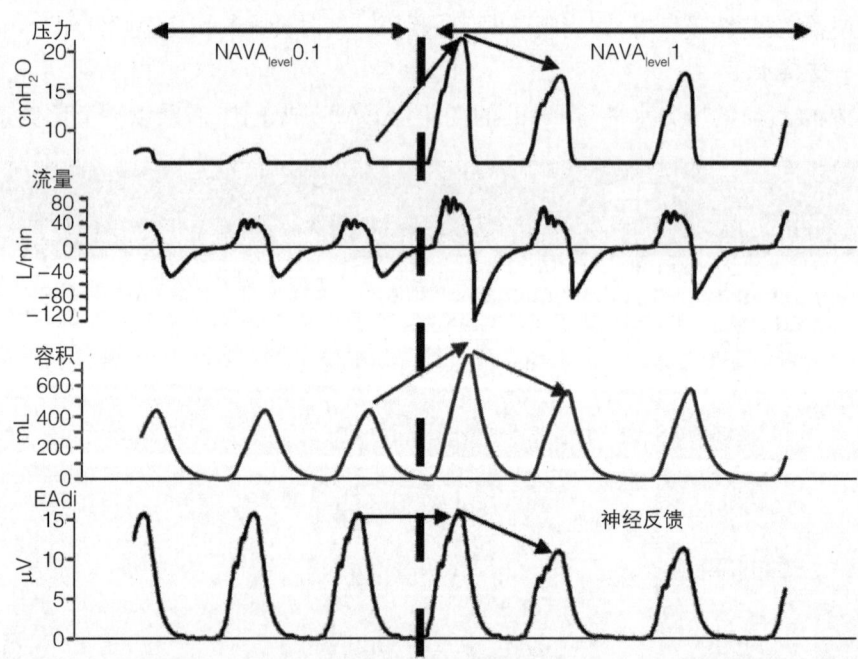

图 7.2 显示将 $NAVA_{level}$ 从 $0.1\ cmH_2O/\mu V$ 增加到 $1\ cmH_2O/\mu V$ 时对神经反馈的影响，相应的 EAdi 从 $17\ \mu V$ 降低到 $12\ \mu V$，气道压从 $22\ cmH_2O$ 降低到 $17\ cmH_2O$。（图片引自 iVentilate 应用，Pr Hadrien Rozé 免费提供）

7.2 NAVA 时如何设置辅助通气

基于对呼吸生理的不同评估方式，有不同的方法来设置 $NAVA_{level}$，利用其对呼吸力学和（或）神经反馈的作用来确定[9]。

7.2.1 气道压目标

在将主动呼吸的患者切换为 NAVA 之前,医护人员可以使用 NAVA 预览功能,该功能可以估算和显示其他通气模式(如压力支持通气模式)的患者在使用 NAVA 时输送的气道压力。可以逐步确定 $NAVA_{level}$,直到两个模式下气道峰压水平匹配,这种设定方法假定当前的辅助水平对患者最合适。由于 P_{aw} 波形的差异,气道峰压的匹配不能保证两者辅助水平近似。NAVA 压力-时间曲线不像大多数压力导向的通气模式那样是方形的,所以还有另一种设置方法,即匹配平均气道压力[10]。在 NAVA 下,呼吸间 EAdi 振幅的变异性较大,会导致压力匹配困难。最后,一旦切换到 NAVA,EAdi(P_{aw} 也是)的水平可能会因神经反馈的作用而发生变化。

7.2.2 设置不同 $NAVA_{level}$ 时潮气量的反应

如果患者在没有任何辅助的情况下出现呼吸衰竭,可以逐步增加 $NAVA_{level}$ 来评估 P_{aw} 和潮气量(V_T)的变化。通常可以观察到两个阶段的反应。

(1)第一阶段:$NAVA_{level}$ 增加会导致 P_{aw} 和 V_T 急剧增加,而在达到某个水平后,再继续增加 $NAVA_{level}$ 会使 ΔP_{aw} 减小,而 V_T 不变(第二阶段)。

(2)第二阶段:指的是存在一个"舒适区",在这个范围内辅助水平足以减轻呼吸肌的负担。神经反馈导致 EAdi 降低,进一步提高 $NAVA_{level}$ 并不会增加 V_T。最佳 $NAVA_{level}$ 是基于这两个阶段的转换点确定的,当潮气量趋于稳定时,说明已从之前的辅助不足到了患者呼吸需求得到满足的支持水平[5]。该方法的局限性在于,在确定 $NAVA_{level}$ 的过程中并不总能清晰地显示这两个阶段。

7.2.3 设置不同 $NAVA_{level}$ 时膈肌电活动的反应

NAVA 技术可以用于自主呼吸试验(spontaneous breathing trial, SBT)失败后的呼吸衰竭患者,能够监测到随着 $NAVA_{level}$ 的逐步增加,EAdi 信号下降。

首先,需要记录呼吸衰竭患者 SBT 失败时的 EAdi 值($EAdi_{maxSBT}$)。逐步滴定 $NAVA_{level}$ 使 EAdi 降低到"舒适区"。将 EAdi 振幅降至 $EAdi_{maxSBT}$ 的约 60%,对于撤机困难的患者来说已经足够了[11]。每天重复这个过程,尝试逐渐降低 $NAVA_{level}$,直到顺利通过 SBT。

另一种滴定 $NAVA_{level}$ 的方法是以 EAdi 降至在将 $NAVA_{level}$ 设置为最低值($0.1\ cmH_2O/\mu V$)时记录值($EAdi_{peak}$)的 50% 为目标。一项随机对照试验表明,与 PSV 相比,使用 NAVA 的这种流程可以显著减少机械通气持续时间[12]。

7.2.4 神经通气效率指数

神经通气效率指数(neuro-ventilatory efficiency, NVE)(V_T 与 EAdi 的比值,单位为 $mL/\mu V$)表示在没有辅助通气的情况下,呼吸肌将 EAdi 转换为潮气量的能力[13]。NVE 可以用于滴定 $NAVA_{level}$ 至不同的膈肌卸载水平,而较小的膈肌卸载与更大膈肌的活动度,以及背侧重力依赖的肺区域通气改善相关联[14]。

7.2.5 基于 NAVA 的 EAdi 衍生参数

人-机呼吸贡献(patient ventilator breath contribution,PVBC)指数被定义为无辅助时吸气 V_T 与 EAdi 变化的比值($V_{T, insp}/\Delta EAdi$)除以辅助呼吸时的比值(图 7.3)[15]。PVBC 值的范围为 0~1,其中 1 表示无辅助时患者吸气努力产生的全部潮气量。解读时必须考虑绝对的呼吸机支持,以及患者的自主呼吸努力(图 7.3)。

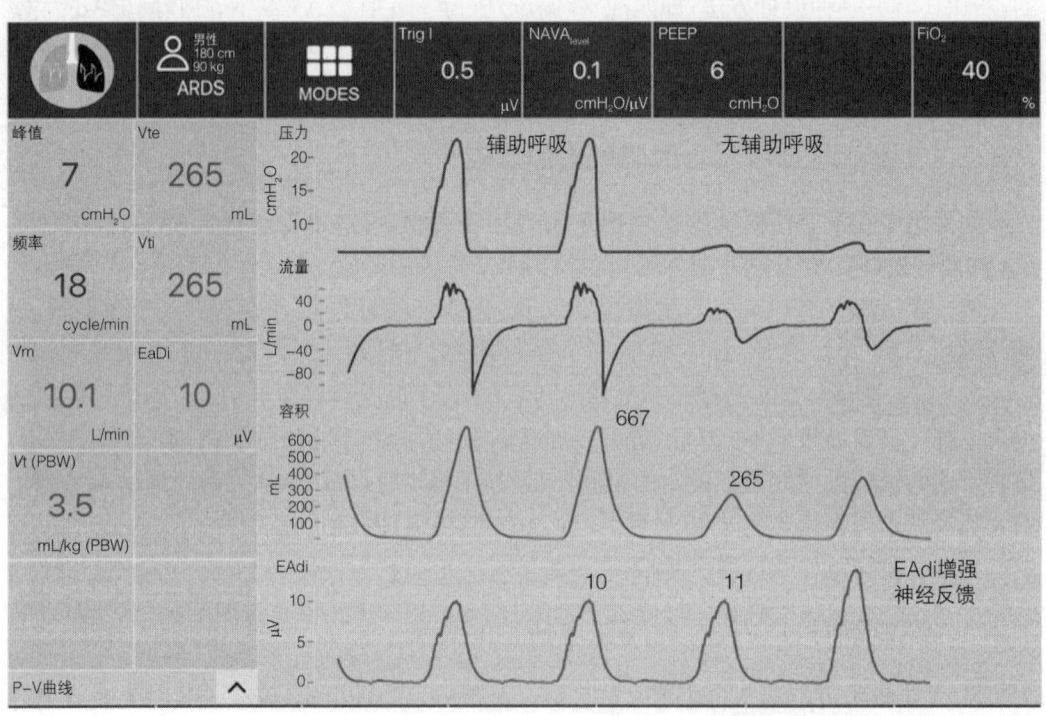

图 7.3 显示辅助呼吸($NVE_{assist} = 667/10 = 66.7$ mL/μV)与非辅助呼吸($NVE_{unassist} = 265/11 = 24$ mL/μV)之间的神经通气效率指数($NVE = V_T/EAdi$)的比较。人-机呼吸贡献指数 $= 100 \times 24/66.7 = 36\%$。(图片引自 iVentilate 应用,Pr Hadrien Rozé 免费提供)

7.3 神经调节通气辅助下如何设置呼气末正压

在 NAVA 模式下,呼气末正压(positive end-expiratory pressure,PEEP)的设置与其他模式无区别,但可能会影响呼吸肌负荷和功能,从而影响 EAdi。NVE 对 PEEP 变化的反应可用于确定一个 PEEP 水平,以得到生成相同潮气量所需的最小 EAdi(即最高的 NVE)[16]。

在 NAVA 或 PSV 模式下,EAdi 可以作为一种工具(类似于食管压),用于监测内源性 PEEP 的存在,以及施加外源性 PEEP 的效果[17]。此外,使用 NAVA 时,克服内源性 PEEP 所需的努力低于 PSV,并且不太受 PEEP 降低的影响[17]。最后,在 PSV 中,EAdi

可用于设置 PEEP,以减少内源性 PEEP 存在时的吸气触发延迟[7]。

7.4 神经调节通气辅助如何撤机

NAVA 可以与任何撤机程序相结合,从 NAVA 切换到基于 PSV、CPAP 或其他方法的 SBT。如果患者无法通过 SBT,无论采用哪种方法均可恢复使用 NAVA 模式进行机械通气,并采用与 NAVA 启动时的相同方案再次滴定 $NAVA_{level}$。研究表明,在给定的压力支持水平下,从 NAVA 开始的第一天到 SBT 成功的第一天,EAdi 可以逐日变化[13]。例如,在撤机流程的开始阶段,残留的镇静效应会降低给定辅助压力水平下的 $EAdi^{[18]}$。对给定辅助下的 EAdi 进行每日评估有助于设定 $NAVA_{level}$。如果没有残留的镇静效应,任何呼吸功能的改善都可能表现为神经驱动下降(即 EAdi 降低),并应随之降低 $NAVA_{level}$。

相较于 PSV,采用 NAVA 进行撤机可以缩短机械通气的持续时间[12]。

7.5 神经调节通气辅助的临床效果

7.5.1 对潮气量的作用

在非比例通气模式中(如 PSV),辅助水平的增加几乎总是与 V_T 的增加有关[19],患者只需尽最小的吸气努力便可轻易触发呼吸,然后被动吸气。此外,当患者停止吸气努力时,呼吸机仍然可能会继续送气而不是切换到呼气相。与此相反,在 NAVA 模式下,尽管增加了 $NAVA_{level}$,V_T 往往还能保持稳定,这表明 NAVA 能够防止过度辅助和肺过度膨胀。此外,在 NAVA 中,当呼吸中枢对膈肌输出的信号结束时,吸气就停止了。

$NAVA_{level}$ 的提高会降低 EAdi,从而自动限制肺膨胀压力和容积的增加[6,8,20]。Hering-Breuer 反射可能在潮气量的控制中起作用[21],但是人类的迷走神经抑制作用较弱,不足以改变呼吸模式。在非插管患者中,控制潮气量的其他非化学机制包括上气道传入神经、胸壁和膈肌的牵拉刺激。这可以解释为什么 NAVA 在双侧迷走神经切断的肺移植患者中仍然成功达到了保护性潮气量[22]。此外,与传统的 PSV 相比,NAVA 允许更大的呼吸模式变异度[20]。

7.5.2 对人-机不同步的作用

与 PSV 相比,NAVA 尤其可以通过减少吸气触发延迟、呼气时间过长和不同步事件的总数量来改善人-机同步性和总体人-机交互作用[23,24]。采用 NAVA 后,无效努力或延迟呼气可能会完全消失,这对于阻塞性肺疾病来说尤为重要[24,25]。

在重度肺扩张受限和低顺应性患者中,即使在 PSV 期间优化了呼气触发,使用 NAVA 仍能够显著减少 PSV 下过早切换和双重触发的不同步次数[26]。

针对支气管瘘和机械通气时严重漏气的患者,NAVA 的神经触发也适用。在这种情况下,降低气动触发的灵敏度以保证只进行神经触发,就能避免自动触发[27]。

7.5.3 无创通气或气管切开术中的神经调节通气辅助

此外,在无创通气(non-invasive ventilation,NIV)期间,相较于 PSV,NAVA 通过减少吸气触发延迟和严重不同步,降低 NAVA 无效努力、过早或延迟切换,从而改善了患者与呼吸机的同步性[28]。研究发现,使用 NAVA-NIV 代替 PSV 可以改善患者与呼吸机的交互作用,尽管其中一些研究没有使用特定的 NIV 功能进行漏气补偿。此外,相较于在 PSV 期间激活特定的 NIV 算法,NAVA 能够更好地改善人-机交互;而将 NAVA 与特定的 NIV 算法结合能提供良好同步性和低水平泄漏间的最佳平衡方案[29]。

NIV-NAVA 接入头罩使用可能更有意义。由于头罩的可压缩容积较大,患者与呼吸机的交互可能会有困难,而 NIV-NAVA 可改善其同步性[30]。

7.6 神经调节通气辅助的局限性

很明显,NAVA 无法在没有呼吸驱动的情况下使用,过度镇静会显著降低 EAdi。

存在过度呼吸驱动的情况下,应谨慎使用 NAVA,因为 NAVA 可能会放大这个问题。高呼吸驱动时使用 NAVA 比例辅助模式会增加患者自戕性肺损伤的风险。此外,选择正确的方法来设置 $NAVA_{level}$ 也十分关键,因为过高的 $NAVA_{level}$ 可能会导致不规则的呼吸模式[20]。使用 NAVA 需要插入鼻胃管,这可能存在禁忌证。最后,EAdi 信号质量差也可能会影响 NAVA 的使用。

7.7 总结

NAVA 和 EAdi 监测能够改善患者与呼吸机的交互作用,将患者的呼吸驱动考虑在内,实现更个性化的治疗。使用 NAVA 可以提高患者与呼吸机的匹配度,为实现肺和膈肌保护性通气提供可能。研究数据表明,通过基于个体神经反馈的适当设置方法,使用 NAVA 可能缩短机械通气的使用时间。

(赵立娜,肇寅辉,宫晔 译)

参考文献

[1] Sinderby C, Navalesi P, Beck J, et al. Neural control of mechanical ventilation in respiratory failure. Nat Med. 1999;5:1433-6.

[2] Barwing J, Ambold M, Linden N, Quintel M, Moerer O. Evaluation of the catheter positioning for neurally adjusted ventilatory assist. Intensive Care Med. 2009;35:1809-14.

[3] Jonkman AH, de Vries HJ, Heunks LMA. Physiology of the respiratory drive in ICU patients: implications for diagnosis and treatment. Crit Care. 2020;24:104.

[4] Sinderby CA, Beck JC, Lindström LH, Grassino AE. Enhancement of signal quality in

[5] Brander L, Leong-Poi H, Beck J, et al. Titration and implementation of neurally adjusted ventilatory assist in critically ill patients. Chest. 2009; 135: 695-703.

[6] Carteaux G, Córdoba-Izquierdo A, Lyazidi A, Heunks L, Thille AW, Brochard L. Comparison between Neurally adjusted Ventilatory assist and pressure support ventilation levels in terms of respiratory effort. Crit Care Med. 2016; 44: 503-11.

[7] Beloncle F, Piquilloud L, Rittayamai N, Sinderby C, Rozé H, Brochard L. A diaphragmatic electrical activity-based optimization strategy during pressure support ventilation improves synchronization but does not impact work of breathing. Crit Care. 2017; 21: 21.

[8] Colombo D, Cammarota G, Bergamaschi V, De Lucia M, Corte FD, Navalesi P. Physiologic response to varying levels of pressure support and neurally adjusted ventilatory assist in patients with acute respiratory failure. Intensive Care Med. 2008; 34: 2010-8.

[9] Jonkman AH, Rauseo M, Carteaux G, et al. Proportional modes of ventilation: technology to assist physiology. Intensive Care Med. 2020; 46: 2301-13.

[10] Cecchini J, Schmidt M, Demoule A, Similowski T. Increased diaphragmatic contribution to inspiratory effort during neurally adjusted ventilatory assistance versus pressure support: an electromyographic study. Anesthesiology. 2014; 121: 1028-36.

[11] Rozé H, Lafrikh A, Perrier V, et al. Daily titration of neurally adjusted ventilatory assist using the diaphragm electrical activity. Intensive Care Med. 2011; 37: 1087-94.

[12] Kacmarek RM, Villar J, Parrilla D, et al. Neurally adjusted ventilatory assist in acute respiratory failure: a randomized controlled trial. Intensive Care Med. 2020; 46: 2327-37.

[13] Rozé H, Repusseau B, Perrier V, et al. Neuro-ventilatory efficiency during weaning from mechanical ventilation using neurally adjusted ventilatory assist. Br J Anaesth. 2013; 111: 955-60.

[14] Campoccia Jalde F, Jalde F, Wallin MKEB, et al. Standardized unloading of respiratory muscles during neurally adjusted ventilatory assist: a randomized crossover pilot study. Anesthesiology. 2018; 129: 769-77.

[15] Grasselli G, Beck J, Mirabella L, Pesenti A, Slutsky AS, Sinderby C. Assessment of patient-ventilator breath contribution during neurally adjusted ventilatory assist. Intensive Care Med. 2012; 38: 1224-32.

[16] Passath C, Takala J, Tuchscherer D, Jakob SM, Sinderby C, Brander L. Physiologic response to changing positive end-expiratory pressure during neurally adjusted ventilatory assist in sedated, critically ill adults. Chest. 2010; 138: 578-87.

[17] Bellani G, Coppadoro A, Patroniti N, et al. Clinical assessment of auto-positive end-expiratory pressure by diaphragmatic electrical activity during pressure support and neurally adjusted ventilatory assist. Anesthesiology. 2014; 121: 563-71.

[18] Rozé H, Germain A, Perrier V, et al. Effect of flumazenil on diaphragm electrical activation during weaning from mechanical ventilation after acute respiratory distress syndrome. Br J Anaesth. 2015; 114: 269-75.

[19] Nava S, Bruschi C, Rubini F, Palo A, Iotti G, Braschi A. Respiratory response and inspiratory effort during pressure support ventilation in COPD patients. Intensive Care Med. 1995; 21: 871-9.

[20] Patroniti N, Bellani G, Saccavino E, et al. Respiratory pattern during neurally adjusted ventilatory assist in acute respiratory failure patients. Intensive Care Med. 2012; 38: 230-9.

[21] Leiter JC, Manning HL. The Hering-Breuer reflex, feedback control, and mechanical ventilation: the promise of neurally adjusted ventilatory assist. Crit Care Med. 2010; 38: 1915 - 6.

[22] Rozé H, Piquilloud L, Richard JCM, et al. Tidal volume during assisted ventilation after double-lung transplantation. Am J Respir Crit Care Med. 2015; 192: 637 - 9.

[23] Terzi N, Pelieu I, Guittet L, et al. Neurally adjusted ventilatory assist in patients recovering spontaneous breathing after acute respiratory distress syndrome: physiological evaluation. Crit Care Med. 2010; 38: 1830 - 7.

[24] Piquilloud L, Vignaux L, Bialais E, et al. Neurally adjusted ventilatory assist improves patient-ventilator interaction. Intensive Care Med. 2011; 37: 263 - 71.

[25] Spahija J, de Marchie M, Albert M, et al. Patient-ventilator interaction during pressure support ventilation and neurally adjusted ventilatory assist. Crit Care Med. 2010; 38: 518 - 26.

[26] Mauri T, Bellani G, Foti G, Grasselli G, Pesenti A. Successful use of neurally adjusted ventilatory assist in a patient with extremely low respiratory system compliance undergoing ECMO. Intensive Care Med. 2011; 37: 166 - 7.

[27] Rozé H, Ouattara A. Use of neural trigger during neurally adjusted ventilatory assist in a patient with a large broncho-pleural fistula and air leakage. Intensive Care Med. 2012; 38: 922 - 3.

[28] Piquilloud L, Tassaux D, Bialais E, et al. Neurally adjusted ventilatory assist (NAVA) improves patient-ventilator interaction during non-invasive ventilation delivered by face mask. Intensive Care Med. 2012; 38: 1624 - 31.

[29] Schmidt M, Dres M, Raux M, et al. Neurally adjusted ventilatory assist improves patient-ventilator interaction during postextubation prophylactic noninvasive ventilation. Crit Care Med. 2012; 40: 1738 - 44.

[30] Moerer O, Beck J, Brander L, et al. Subject-ventilator synchrony during neural versus pneumatically triggered non-invasive helmet ventilation. Intensive Care Med. 2008; 34: 1615 - 23.

8 成比例辅助通气
Proportional Assist Ventilation
Eumorfia Kondili, Evangelia Akoumianaki

8.1 引言

成比例辅助通气(proportional assist ventilation，PAV)是由 Magdy Younes 于 1992 年提出的一种辅助通气支持模式。在使用 PAV 时，呼吸机根据患者的通气需求按设定比例将压力(P_{aw})输送到气道内。目前，PAV 的更新版本 PAV+(比例辅助通气+可调增益参数)已可用于临床实践。使用 PAV+ 时，软件可以半连续测量呼吸系统力学，并自动调整呼吸机参数[2-4]。本章主要介绍 PAV 和 PAV+ 的基本操作原理、支持该模式有效性的临床证据，以及辅助通气的滴定方法。

8.2 工作原理

PAV 时，呼吸机一旦触发，所提供的压力(P_{aw})总是与瞬时流量(V')和容积(V)成正比，从而也与吸气肌压力(P_{mus})成正比[1]。呼吸机通过监测 V' 和 V 产生压力，该压力由在吸气过程的任何时刻 V' 和 V 的总和乘以预设的增益参数[辅助百分比(%assist)]计算而来：

$$P_{aw} = \%assist(V' \times R_{rs} + V_T \times E_{rs}) \tag{8.1}$$

其中，R_{rs} 和 E_{rs} 分别为呼吸系统的阻力和弹性。

临床医师将增益设定为 R_{rs} 和 E_{rs} 的百分比(最大 95%)。通过设定的辅助比例降低

E. Kondili (✉) · E. Akoumianaki
Department of Intensive Care Medicine, University Hospital of Heraklion, Medical School, University of Crete, Heraklion, Crete, Greece
e-mail: kondylie@uoc.gr

© The Author(s), under exclusive license to Springer Nature Switzerland AG 2022
G. Bellani (ed.), *Mechanical Ventilation from Pathophysiology to Clinical Evidence*, https://doi.org/10.1007/978-3-030-93401-9_8

了吸气肌必须产生的压力（P_{mus}）。因此，在使用 PAV 时，呼吸机可放大患者的吸气努力，而不对流量、容积或 P_{aw} 设定任何目标。

需要定期、准确的呼吸系统力学评估以确保 PAV 的正常功能，这在辅助通气中困难且耗时，限制了其在临床上的广泛应用。

PAV＋作为 PAV 的更新版本，内置了可以半连续无创测算呼吸力学指标的软件，以 R_{rs} 和 E_{rs} 的测量值的恒定分数为基准自动调节流量和容积进行通气辅助[2-5]。

对 R_{rs} 和 E_{rs} 的计算基于 PAV 特征：机器辅助与自主呼吸的紧密联系[2-4]。因此，在吸气结束时，假定 P_{mus} 处于下降阶段（或者已经为零）。此时进行吸气阻断，P_{aw} 相当于呼吸系统在一定容积（V_T）下的弹性回缩力[3]。基于这一原理，呼吸机自动计算 PAV＋的呼吸力学，即每隔 4~7 次呼吸后随机进行 300 ms 的吸气末阻断（图 8.1a）。

测量吸气末阻断时的气道压（$P_{aw_{occlusion}}$），并计算 E_{rs} 和顺应性（$C_{rs}=1/E_{rs}$），公式如下：

$$E_{rs}=(P_{aw_{occlusion}}-\text{PEEP})/V_T \tag{8.2}$$

以及

$$C_{rs}=V_T/(P_{aw_{occlusion}}-\text{PEEP}) \tag{8.3}$$

其中，PEEP 为呼气末正压[3]。当内源性 PEEP 存在时，得到的 E_{rs} 会高估呼吸系统的弹性，得到的 C_{rs} 则会低估呼吸系统的顺应性。

在吸气末阻断后的呼气相，可以测量 R_{rs}（图 8.1b）。基于呼气早期的呼气流量由弹性回缩力［即肺泡压（P_{alv}）］驱动，软件可以记录呼气相流量-时间曲线上的 3 个点，即呼气的流量峰值点及其后 5 ms 和 10 ms 处。通过这些点，可以计算 P_{alv} 和总呼气阻力（R_{TOT}），公式如下：

$$P_{alv}=P_{aw_{occlusion}}-\Delta V \times E_{rs} \tag{8.4}$$

以及

$$R_{TOT}=(P_{alv}-P_{aw})/V' \tag{8.5}$$

其中 ΔV 是截至关注点的呼出气体容积，V' 和 P_{aw} 分别为相应的呼气流量和气道压[4]。

取这些点 R_{TOT} 的平均值，得到估算的 R_{TOT}，即气流通过气管插管或气管切开套管产生的阻力（R_{tube}）和呼吸系统阻力（$R_{rs(PAV)}$）之和。计算公式如下：

$$R_{tube}=a+bV' \tag{8.6}$$

其中 a 和 b 为常数，分别取决于导管的长度和直径。R_{TOT} 减去 R_{tube} 得到 $R_{rs(PAV)}$[4]。

在启动 PAV＋通气时，正确设置导管的类型（气管导管或气管切开套管）和直径非常重要，不然得出的 R_{TOT} 将会不准确，可能会导致通气辅助不足或辅助过度。

需要注意的是，这种方法实际测量的是呼气阻力，而 PAV＋中基于吸气阻力（假设两

8 成比例辅助通气

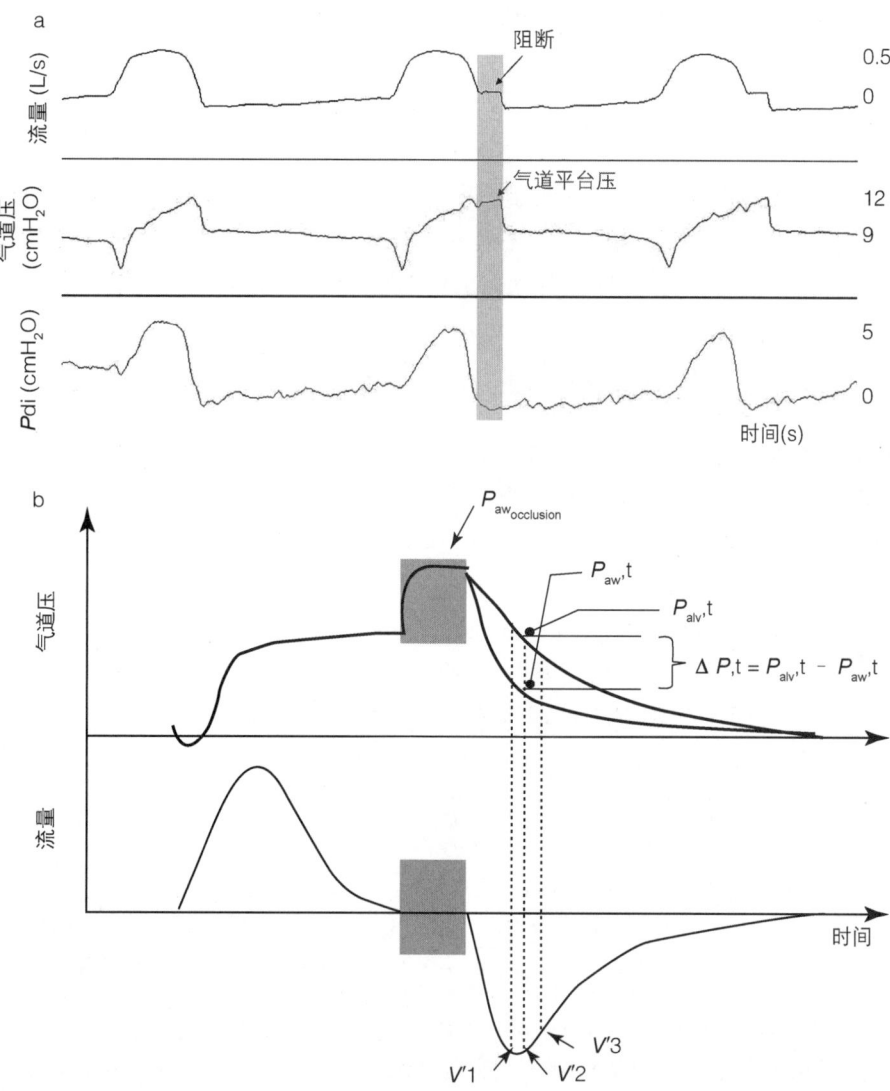

图 8.1 a. 流量、气道压(P_{aw})和跨膈压(PAV+时的Pdi-时间曲线)。在第二次呼吸中进行了吸气末阻断(阴影部分)。阻断操作在Pdi下降到0,自主吸气快结束时进行,也就是阻断时不存在患者的吸气努力。阻断操作完成时测量的P_{aw}就是$P_{aw_{occlusion}}$,可以用来计算呼吸系统的弹性。b. 呼吸系统阻力的测算:阴影区域代表吸气末阻断的时间,然后在呼气相计算呼吸系统阻力。箭头表示计算阻力的三个时间点:最大呼气流量($V'1$)点及其后 5 ms($V'2$)和 10 ms($V'3$)两个点。在这些时间点上测量气道压(P_{aw},t)、呼气潮气量(ΔV_T,t)和流量(V')。弹性($E_{rs(PAV)}$)已在吸气末阻断时计算出。各时间点的肺泡压(P_{alv},t)按照公式 P_{alv},t$=P_{aw_{occlusion}} - \Delta V_T$,t$\times E_{rs(PAV)}$ 来计算。P_{alv},t$-P_{aw}$,t的差值除以流量(V')即为各时间点的R_{TOT}。Pdi,跨膈压

者间的差异可以忽略不计)计算。然而,如果吸气阻力与呼气阻力间的差异很大(如在慢性阻塞性肺疾病中),计算出的 R_{rs} 是不准确的,使得辅助水平不足。此外,在存在内源性 PEEP(PEEPi)的情况下,R_{TOT} 的计算值会低于实际值。

8.3 PAV+ 的优势

PAV+与常规的辅助模式[如压力支持通气(PSV)、辅助容量控制(AVC)]的主要区别在于其依靠患者的吸气努力来驱动呼吸机的辅助[1,2]。这个特点及 PAV+能更好地匹配呼吸机和患者自主吸气的时间,对优化辅助水平、人-机同步性和呼吸模式等方面都有积极的作用。

8.3.1 防止支持过度或支持不足

在设置辅助机械通气时,辅助通气的目标是防止辅助过少或过多导致并发症。在 AVC 模式中,输送的 V_T 是固定的,与 P_{mus} 无关。而在 PSV 模式中,对 P_{mus} 预设定了压力支持水平,导致无辅助时的 $P_{mus}-V_T$ 曲线平行上移。在这两种模式下,呼吸机一旦被触发,就会根据呼吸力学和设定的辅助水平输送最小的 V_T。而 PAV+的主要优势在于:提供的 V_T 与吸气 P_{mus} 成正比,当改变辅助百分比时,$P_{mus}-V_T$ 关系的斜率也会随之改变(图 8.2)。如果没有 P_{mus},则不会输送 V_T。当辅助水平较高时,激活的负反馈(如 Hering-Breuer 反射和迷走神经反射)及不佳的膈肌长度-张力关系会减少 V_T,从而保护肺和膈肌免受过度辅助的影响[2]。实际上,研究表明,在使用 PAV 模式的大多数患者中,平台压和驱动压都维持在"安全"范围内[6,7]。由于 PAV 的辅助压力可以根据呼吸需求动态调整,因此与 PSV 相比,在活动或呼吸力学改变时,PAV 可以使呼吸肌做功和耗氧量的增加更小[5,8]。

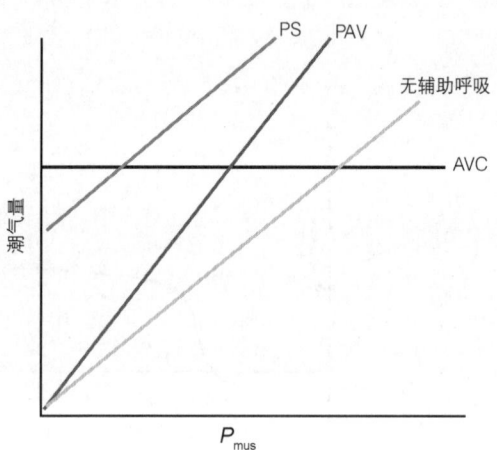

图 8.2 患者吸气努力(P_{mus})与潮气量(V_T)的关系。无辅助呼吸(浅蓝色线)、PS(橙色线)、AVC(棕色线)和 PAV+(蓝色线)。无辅助呼吸时,P_{mus} 增加将导致 V_T 呈线性增加。在 AVC 中,输送的预设 V_T 与患者的吸气努力无关,且 $P_{mus_{peak}}-V_T$ 的斜率始终为零。在 PS 中,触发后,呼吸系统会承受预先设置的压力(无论 $P_{mus_{peak}}$ 是多少),从而导致相较于无辅助的 $P_{mus}-V_T$ 曲线平行上移。而在 PAV+情况下,V_T 与 P_{mus} 呈正比,因为当改变辅助百分比时,$P_{mus}-V_T$ 关系的斜率也会随之改变。在 PS 和 AVC(而非 PAV+)中,即便在 $P_{mus_{peak}}$ 非常低的情况下,仍有可能产生较高的 V_T。(见彩色插图)

8.3.2 呼吸模式与人-机交互

与传统的辅助模式不同,在这些模式中,V_T 的变化要么完全丧失(AVC)要么被显著抑制(PS),PAV 则会提供大范围的辅助区间,以维持生理性的呼吸模式变化。PAV 时的呼吸模式更多受到患者自身呼吸需求的影响,而非辅助水平[5,9,10]。

人-机不同步(更多见于传统辅助模式)可能会损伤呼吸肌和膈肌,增加呼吸做功,导致动态肺过度充气的发生或恶化,并最终影响患者的预后[11]。相关研究表明,PAV可以明显改善患者与呼吸机的相互作用,减少无效触发、呼气触发延迟和其他人-机不同步事件的发生[5,6,9,10,12],这主要得益于PAV能够避免过度的辅助;其次,PAV还能够改善呼气不同步。

8.3.3 临床结局

一项比较PS和PAV+的随机试验探讨了PAV+的优势是否能够转化为患者临床结局的改善。研究结果表明,在PS组中,辅助通气失败及需要切回控制通气的患者比例是PAV+组的2倍。最近的一项荟萃分析也表明,与PS相比,PAV与降低撤机失败的发生率、缩短机械通气时间相关[12]。到目前为止,没有证据表明PAV+和PS在ICU和住院病死率、ICU住院时间上存在差异[6,12]。

8.4 PAV/PAV+ 应用的局限

PAV/PAV+可能导致不适当的呼吸辅助,在以下情况应谨慎使用。

(1) 低呼吸驱动的患者:需要吸气努力来驱动呼吸机,因此存在低通气风险。

(2) 动态肺过度充气:部分吸气努力未触发辅助(即呼吸机的无效触发)[5]。

(3) 高估 E_{rs} 和 R_{rs}:根据 PAV 的工作原理,存在过度辅助(压力或容量过大)的风险,这一现象称为"失控"。当流量和容量辅助设置值高于实际 R_{rs} 和 E_{rs} 值时,就会发生失控。结果是,在吸气期间呼吸机提供的压力可能超过弹性和阻力之和,并且呼吸机会在吸气努力结束后继续输送气体。需要注意的是,失控是 PAV 中应关注的问题,但在 PAV+中很少发生(仅在增益接近90%时才会出现)。

(4) 过多的吸气泄露:类似于呼吸力学指标的高估(见上文)。吸气泄露(如无创 PAV、管路漏气、支气管胸膜瘘等)可能与失控有关。呼吸机错误地将气流泄漏解释为患者的持续努力,并在患者的吸气努力结束后延长辅助支持时间。

8.5 PAV+ 吸气辅助的滴定

虽然 PAV+具有优势,但在临床实践中的推广受到限制,主要原因是不熟悉增益的设定。为解决这一问题,Carteaux 等提出根据测量的吸气努力($P_{mus_{peak}}$)来设定 PAV+增益[13]。因为 PAV+输送与 P_{mus} 成正比的 P_{aw},然后就可以计算 P_{mus},公式如下:

$$P_{mus_{peak}} = (P_{aw_{peak}} - PEEP) \times [(100 - \%assist)/\%assist] \qquad (8.7)$$

增益百分比的设定目标是使 P_{mus} 为 5~10 cmH$_2$O,相应的 P_{mus}-时间乘积为 50~150 cmH$_2$O·s/min。尽管具备可行的方法,但计算 $P_{mus_{peak}}$ 来预测实际吸气努力的准确性是存疑的,可能导致近50%的患者出现辅助过度或不足的情况[14]。此外,存在PEEPi时,$P_{mus_{peak}}$同样会被低估[14,15]。

另一种临床设置的方法是在PAV+的初始阶段设置较高的增益水平(如70%~80%),然后逐步以5%~10%的幅度降低增益百分比,直至达到不会出现高碳酸血症或呼吸窘迫的最低支持水平。对于PEEP,可以使用PAV+的顺应性测量来设置最佳PEEP;增加PEEP后,肺泡复张会改善顺应性。此外,通过连续计算V_T与C_{rs}(利用短暂阻断测量)的比值,可以监测呼吸系统的驱动压,以评估肺损伤的风险。如果在优化PEEP和辅助水平后驱动压仍然较高[如重度ARDS和(或)高呼吸驱动情况下],则可能需要使用镇静和控制通气。

8.6 总结

PAV/PAV+是一种比例辅助通气模式,其中呼吸机输送的压力总是与患者自主产生的流量和容量成比例,因此也和患者的吸气需求成比例。临床研究表明,相较于传统的辅助通气模式,PAV/PAV+与更好的人-机同步、更低的呼吸机辅助不足或过度的风险,以及降低撤机失败率相关。

(赵立娜,肇寅辉 译)

参考文献

[1] Younes M. Proportional assist ventilation, a new approach to ventilatory support. Theor Am Rev Respir Dis. 1992;145:114-20.

[2] Akoumianaki E, Kondili E, Georgopoulos D. Proportional assist ventilation. In: Ferrer M, Pelosi P, editors. ERS monographs: new developments in mechanical ventilation; 2012. p. 97-115.

[3] Younes M, Webster K, Kun J, Roberts D, Masiowski B. A method for measuring passive elastance during proportional assist ventilation. Am J Respir Crit Care Med. 2001;164:50-60.

[4] Younes M, Kun J, Masiowski B, Webster K, Roberts D. A method for non-invasive determination of inspiratory resistance during proportional assist ventilation. Am J Respir Crit Care Med. 2001;163:829-39.

[5] Kondili E, Prinianakis G, Alexopoulou C, Vakouti E, Klimathianaki M, Georgopoulos D. Respiratory load compensation during mechanical ventilation—proportional assist ventilation with load-adjustable gain factors versus pressure support. Intensive Care Med. 2006;32:692-9.

[6] Xirouchaki N, Kondili E, Vaporidi K, Xirouchakis G, Klimathianaki M, Gavriilidis G, et al. Proportional assist ventilation with load-adjustable gain factors in critically ill patients: comparison with pressure support. Intensive Care Med 2008;34:2026-2034.

[7] Vaporidi K, Psarologakis C, Proklou A, Pediaditis E, Akoumianaki E, Koutsiana E, et al. Driving pressure during proportional assist ventilation: an observational study. Ann Intensive Care. 2019;9:1.

[8] Akoumianaki E, Dousse N, Lyazidi A, Lefebvre J-C, Graf S, Cordioli RL, et al. Can proportional ventilation modes facilitate exercise in critically ill patients? A physiological cross-

over study: pressure support versus proportional ventilation during lower limb exercise in ventilated critically ill patients. Ann Intensive Care. 2017; 7: 64.

[9] Giannouli E, Webster K, Roberts D, Younes M. Response of ventilator-dependent patients to different levels of pressure support and proportional assist. Am J Respir Crit Care Med. 1999; 159: 1716 - 25.

[10] Akoumianaki E, Prinianakis G, Kondili E, Malliotakis P, Georgopoulos D. Physiologic comparison of neurally adjusted ventilator assist, proportional assist and pressure support ventilation in critically ill patients. Respir Physiol Neurobiol. 2014; 203: 82 - 9.

[11] Thille AW, Rodriguez P, Cabello B, Lellouche F, Brochard L. Patient-ventilator asynchrony during assisted mechanical ventilation. Intensive Care Med. 2006; 32: 1515 - 22.

[12] Kataoka J, Kuriyama A, Norisue Y, Fujitani S. Proportional modes versus pressure support ventilation: a systematic review and meta-analysis. Ann Intensive Care. 2018; 8: 123.

[13] Carteaux G, Mancebo J, Mercat A, Dellamonica J, Richard J-CM, Aguirre-Bermeo H, et al. Bedside adjustment of proportional assist ventilation to target a predefined range of respiratory effort. Crit Care Med. 2013; 41: 2125 - 32.

[14] Amargiannitakis V, Gialamas I, Pediaditis E, Soundoulounaki S, Prinianakis G, Vaporidi K, et al. Validation of a proposed algorithm for assistance titration during proportional assist ventilation with load-adjustable gain factors. Respir Care. 2020; 65: 36 - 44.

[15] Beloncle F, Akoumianaki E, Rittayamai N, Lyazidi A, Brochard L. Accuracy of delivered airway pressure and work of breathing estimation during proportional assist ventilation: a bench study. Ann Intensive Care. 2016; 6: 30.

9 无创通气：适应证和注意事项
Non-Invasive Ventilation: Indications and Caveats

Oriol Roca, Domenico Luca Grieco, Laveena Munshi

9.1 引言

在过去几十年中，无创通气（non-invasive ventilation，NIV）在急性呼吸衰竭患者中的适应证日益增加。相比于有创机械通气，NIV 的使用更简单，在适当的专业知识掌握和监测下，甚至可以在 ICU 外（如急诊室、高依赖病房）应用。需要注意的是，这些装置主要用于支持患者度过呼吸衰竭，等待基础药物治疗产生效果。NIV 可以使用不同的患者接口和通气模式，产生不同的生理效应。

9.2 无创通气的接口

NIV 可以通过不同的接口进行支持（图 9.1），常用的接口是面罩（包括口鼻面罩和全脸面罩）。两者主要区别在于内部无效腔大小和提供有效呼气末正压（positive end-expiratory pressure，PEEP)的能力。然而，接口间的差异在动脉二氧化碳分压、每分钟通气量或患者的吸气努力方面并不会产生显著的无效腔效应[2]。同样，这两种面罩的有效无效腔与面罩内气体容积无关。这些研究结果表明，仅考虑无效腔和二氧化碳，口鼻面罩和全脸面罩是可互换的。全脸面罩的密封性更好，能够更有效地提供PEEP，因此它可能比口鼻面罩更具有优势。

在重症患者的治疗中，另一个越来越受欢迎的接口是头罩。它是一个透明的罩子，覆

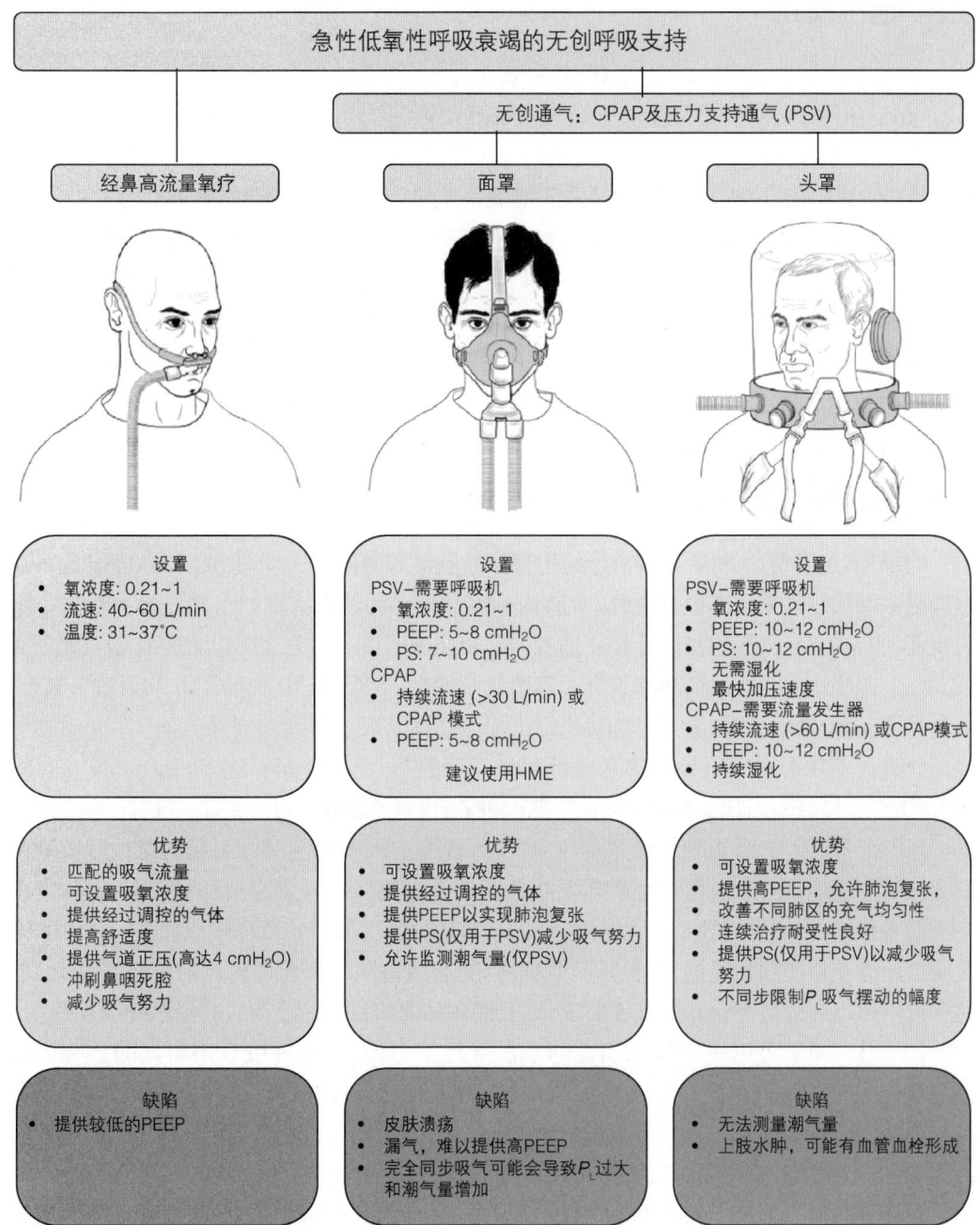

图9.1 无创呼吸支持的模式和连接接口

盖患者的整个头部。头罩由一个柔软的领口在颈部密封。与面罩相比,头罩的优势在于更好的密封性,能够更有效地提供 PEEP 而不会出现明显漏气。此外,良好的耐受性可以延长 NIV 治疗的持续时间。最重要的是,头罩需要较高的新鲜气体流量(通常高于 40 L/min),以尽量减少二氧化碳重复吸入的风险[3]。

9.3　通气模式

在临床实践中,NIV 的主要模式为双水平气道正压通气(bilevel positive airway pressure,BiPAP)或持续气道正压通气(continuous positive airway pressure,CPAP)。BiPAP 也被称为压力支持通气(NIV-PS),其特点是使用两个水平的压力:压力支持和 PEEP。与 BiPAP 不同,CPAP 不提供任何吸气支持[4]。虽然 ICU 的有创呼吸机也可提供 CPAP-NIV 模式,但为了充分满足患者对气体流量的需求,并在整个呼吸周期中维持设定压力的稳定,因此在使用头罩 CPAP 时使用空氧混合器或文丘里系统持续提供高气流是必要的。在选择口鼻和全脸面罩时,也同样建议使用。

使用比例通气模式(如 PAV 和 NAVA)进行 NIV 目前仍在评估其优化人-机交互和耐受性的效果阶段[5,6]。这些模式在临床实践中尚未被广泛应用。

9.4　无创通气的生理学效应

对 ARF 患者使用 NIV 支持治疗的生理益处已被充分阐述[7]。CPAP 和 BiPAP 均可通过肺复张增加呼气末肺容积(从而减少肺内分流和潜在的动态应变)[8],并通过减少左心室后负荷和右心室前负荷改善伴有心衰患者的心功能(见"19　心力衰竭患者的有创与无创通气")[9]。这些效应能够改善动脉氧合。需要注意的是,尽管 CPAP 和 BiPAP 均可改善氧合,但它们具有不同的生理效应。与 BiPAP 相比,仅使用 CPAP 并不能降低吸气努力[8]。这也可能部分解释了在不同病因导致的急性低氧性呼吸衰竭(acute hypoxemic respiratory failure,AHRF)患者人群中,为什么 CPAP 只能短暂改善氧合和呼吸困难,而对插管率没有影响[10]。

BiPAP 和 CPAP 各自独特的生理效应,使其成为适用于不同病因引起的急性呼吸衰竭的支持治疗措施。对于慢性阻塞性肺疾病急性加重出现高碳酸血症型呼吸衰竭的患者,由于支气管狭窄,他们的呼吸系统无法进行有效的肺泡通气,最终导致呼吸肌疲劳。BiPAP 通过吸气压力支持增加潮气量、减轻呼吸肌疲劳,更有效清除二氧化碳的同时降低呼吸做功。这一策略可以在针对炎症和支气管狭窄,以及潜在病因的目标治疗起效时提供呼吸支持。

CPAP-NIV 可以在高静水压性肺水肿导致的急性、严重呼吸衰竭时同时改善心血管和呼吸系统的生理功能。通过增加胸内压,能降低左心室的后负荷和左、右心室的前负荷。此外,在伴有呼吸窘迫、低氧和高碳酸血症的严重急性呼吸衰竭中,在治疗充血性心力衰竭的药物生效的同时,增加吸气时的气道正压辅助潮气量有助于减少呼吸做功。

对于原发性 AHRF 患者,通过 NIV 应用 CPAP/PEEP 可促进远端气道和肺泡的开放,促进肺复张,减少分流,改善呼吸力学和功能残气量。此外,在呼吸肌疲劳的情况下,可以使用 BiPAP 模式中的额外吸气支持降低呼吸做功,也可以应用 CPAP 模式促进肺复张来部分缓解。

9.5 无创通气的指征

当前指南对于在不同临床情境中使用 NIV 的推荐总结在图 9.2 中。

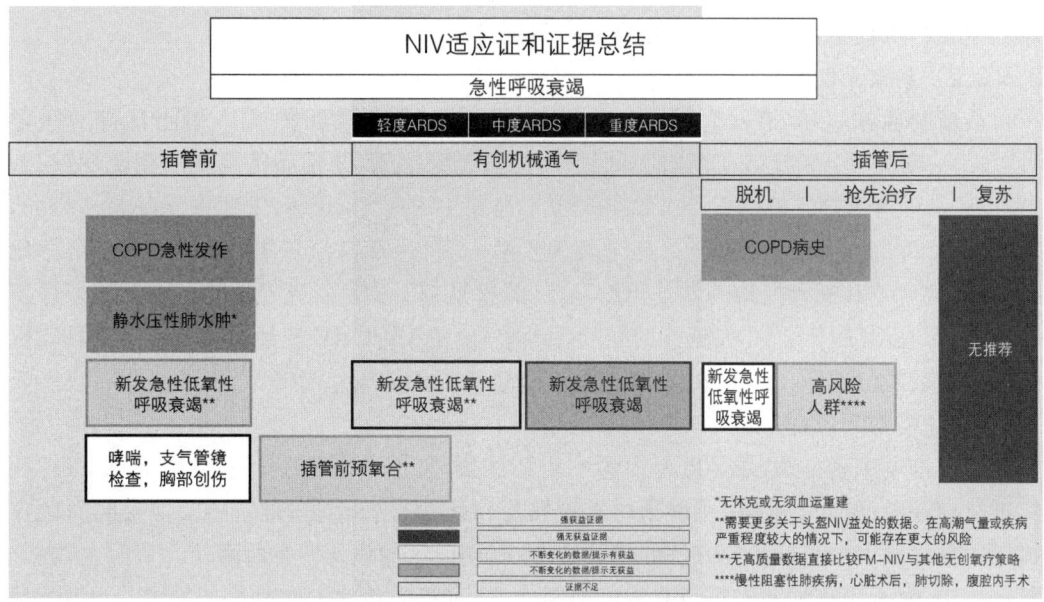

图 9.2 当前指南中在不同临床情况下使用 NIV 的推荐(见彩色插图)

9.5.1 高静水压性肺水肿

使用 NIV,特别是采用 CPAP 模式的 NIV,治疗心源性肺水肿已被广泛研究。许多临床实践指南推荐,在没有急性休克或需要行急性血运重建治疗的情况下,除了药物干预外,将 NIV 作为心源性肺水肿患者的首选支持治疗方法[11]。

9.5.2 高碳酸血症型呼吸衰竭:慢性阻塞性肺疾病急性加重

大量随机对照试验表明,在 COPD 急性加重患者中,使用面罩 NIV(尤其是 BiPAP)比使用标准氧疗更具优势。现有证据表明,NIV 预防插管和降低病死率的成功率高,因此多个共识和临床实践指南都强烈推荐使用 NIV[11,12]。

9.5.3 新发急性低氧性呼吸衰竭

9.5.3.1 面罩无创通气

与其他无创策略相比,使用预防性面罩 NIV 来避免插管的研究数据相互矛盾,一些研究数据支持使用面罩NIV能获益[13]，另一些研究则提示无差异[14]，还有一些研究甚至提示可能有害[15]。最近，一项荟萃分析比较了所有无创氧疗模式，结果显示相较于常规氧疗，使用面罩NIV具有明显更低的气管插管率（$RR=0.76$，95%CI为0.62～0.90）和病死率（$RR=0.83$，95%CI为0.68～0.99）[16]。这一数据表明，使用面罩NIV可能对预防气管插管或早期AHRF管理起着一定的作用。然而，面罩NIV的使用也不可能无风险。实际上，相比于成功使用NIV避免气管插管或早期采用有创机械通气，面罩NIV失败导致更高的病死率更令人担忧[17]。另外，在上述荟萃分析中，面罩NIV所带来的病死率获益在严重程度更高的急性呼吸衰竭中不再显现[16]。

9.5.3.2 头罩无创通气

最新的数据显示，在AHRF患者中，使用头罩NIV与面罩NIV相比具有潜在益处[18]。一项荟萃分析比较了所有无创氧疗方式，结果表明，与使用常规氧疗相比，使用头罩NIV与插管风险下降（$RR=0.26$，95%CI为0.14～0.45）和病死率降低（$RR=0.40$，95%CI为0.24～0.63）相关[15]。在与其他给氧方式（经鼻高流量氧疗和面罩NIV）相比时，降低病死率和插管风险的益处仍然存在，但这是基于少量研究得出的结论。此外最新数据显示，在COVID-19大流行期间的患者中，使用头罩NIV比经鼻高流量氧疗具有更低的插管风险（见"23 COVID-19相关呼吸衰竭的无创氧疗策略"）[19]。

9.5.4 免疫抑制患者

免疫抑制患者是AHRF患者中的一个特殊群体。一些研究表明，使用面罩NIV比标准氧疗在免疫抑制群体中更能预防气管插管和死亡[20]。但是，随着感染性疾病和免疫抑制危重症患者的支持治疗方法的显著改变，有创通气的病死率有所降低。实际上，在荟萃分析中，对于免疫抑制人群与非免疫抑制人群，有效的治疗方向是相似的[16]。因此，目前的数据并不支持在这个人群中采用不同的呼吸支持策略。

9.5.5 预充氧

早期数据显示，相较于球囊面罩通气，采用面罩NIV作为气管插管前的预氧合策略可能获益[21]，可以降低插管过程中氧合下降的发生频率和程度。有趣的是，在AHRF的气管插管过程中，评估采用NIV和HFNO组合进行预充氧的效果，发现持续使用经鼻高流量氧疗有额外的优势，能有效地减少氧合下降的风险[22]。

9.5.6 有创机械通气后的应用

9.5.6.1 早期撤机

已经有大量的研究将NIV应用于撤机策略，在特定患者（尤其是COPD患者）中，基于NIV的撤机策略能够减少有创通气的时间[23]，但这些研究并未证明其对ICU住院时间或病死率方面有改善[24]。

9.5.6.2 抢先策略

在符合撤机标准并通过自主呼吸试验的患者中，仍有10%～20%的患者拔管失败。对于拔管失败的高风险患者，拔管后接续面罩NIV经过证实是有效的预防策略，对于

COPD 患者、老年患者,以及伴有心脏或呼吸系统并发症的患者尤其有效。多项研究评估了 NIV 在某些特定手术后的抢先应用,如心脏手术、腹部手术和肺切除术等,结果发现与标准氧疗相比,抢先应用 NIV 能够降低插管率[25]。

9.5.6.3 拔管后急性呼吸衰竭的抢救

NIV 作为一种"预防"再插管的挽救手段,尚未被证明能获益(也许除了明显的急性肺水肿外)。事实上,它已经被证实会导致再插管延迟、增加病死率[26]。因为拔管失败的根本原因可能是基础疾病或蓄积的呼吸肌无力,短期使用 NIV 可能无法逆转这些原因。

9.5.7 不充分的数据

在哮喘急性发作、胸部创伤和支气管镜检查等情况下,NIV 的应用尚缺乏高质量的数据支持。

9.6 无创通气患者监测的重要性

9.6.1 无创通气患者的监测

使用任何类型的 NIV 呼吸支持治疗均可以掩盖呼吸功能恶化的表现,导致插管延迟。而延迟插管可能会引起严重的患者自戕性肺损伤(patient self-inflicted lung injury,P-SILI)、插管前后低氧血症,并可能会导致更差的预后[27]。考虑到病情可能会随时迅速恶化,并且需要足够的专业技能来识别这种情况,因此使用 NIV 时必须对患者进行严密监测。必须具备调节设备、认识通气不足、识别有害潮气量或呼吸疲劳预兆的专业技能,以准确评估必须切换到插管的时机。

P-SILI 是最近用于描述自主呼吸可能会加重肺损伤现象的术语,被认为是在肺损伤患者伴有强烈的呼吸驱动时,由自身的吸气努力所引发。强烈的吸气努力会产生剧烈的跨肺压波动,从而导致肺整体或区域的压力与容积变化,进一步加剧已经存在的肺损伤[28]。持续的强大胸腔负压同样会导致血管跨壁压和血管通透性增加,进而促进肺泡渗出[29]。此外,如果 PEEP 设置不足[可见于使用面罩 NIV 或 HFNO($2\sim7$ cmH$_2$O)期间],患者可能会经历周期性肺泡塌陷和开放,导致所谓的肺萎陷伤。最近的研究发现,在有自主吸气的 ARDS 患者中,在吸气相的初始阶段(此时呼吸机尚未开始送气),由于膈肌收缩力在肺内传输的差异,肺内的气体会从非重力依赖区向重力依赖区转移[30]。这种呼吸摆动现象会导致重力依赖区肺组织应力过大,而这与设置的吸入潮气量大小无关。最近的研究表明,呼吸摆动会加重自主呼吸时的肺损伤,该现象可以见于任何自主呼吸的患者,包括那些使用 NIV 的患者。目前还没有明确定义的最佳方案来识别自主呼吸何时可能有害,何时应该升级为有创机械通气(以及何时使用镇静/肌松剂以消除自主呼吸)。

9.6.1.1 在新发急性低氧性呼吸衰竭情况下预测无创通气失败

中到重度低氧血症(即 PaO$_2$/FiO$_2$<150 mmHg)已被反复证实与新发 AHRF 患者的 NIV 高失败风险和较差的预后相关[1,31]。近期开发了一种能够预测 NIV 失败的临床

评分量表[27]，它采用易于在床边测量的变量进行计算，包括心率、酸中毒、意识水平、氧合（PaO_2/FiO_2）和呼吸频率（HACOR 评分）（表 9.1）。该评分系统可以动态监测 NIV 期间的气管插管风险，那些 HACOR 评分大于 5 分的患者 NIV 失败风险更高。

表 9.1 预测 NIV 失败的 HACOR 评分

参　数	范　围	分　值
心率(次/分)	≤120	0
	≥121	1
pH	≥7.35	0
	7.30～7.34	2
	7.25～7.29	3
	<7.25	4
GCS	15	0
	13～14	2
	11～12	5
	≤10	10
PaO_2/F_IO_2	≥201	0
	176～200	2
	151～175	3
	126～150	4
	101～125	5
	≤100	6
呼吸频率(次/分)	≤30	0
	31～35	1
	36～40	2
	41～45	3
	≥46	4

启用 NIV 后，吸气努力没有减少，这与 NIV 治疗失败和病死率的增加相关。过强的吸气努力可能会产生过大的潮气量，导致上述 P-SILI 的发生[31,32]。因此，在面罩 NIV 治疗中，要尽早评估患者的潮气量是否低于 9 mL/kg（理想体重），同时注意使用头罩时潮

气量的测量是不可靠的。吸气努力的变化（ΔP_{es}<10 cmH$_2$O）也同样可以用于监测 NIV 的效果。最后，近期的生理学研究发现，膈肌增厚分数（diaphragmatic thickening fraction，DTF）<36%和呼吸频率与 DTF 的比值<0.6 也可以用来预测 NIV 的结局[33]。

9.6.1.2 高碳酸血症型急性呼吸衰竭无创通气治疗失败的预测

在高碳酸血症的患者中，NIV 治疗失败的病理生理机制可能不同。这些患者动脉血 pH 和 PaCO$_2$ 的变化与 NIV 失败相关[34]。因此，HACOR 评分同样可以用于评估这一人群，可以作为识别高碳酸血症患者高失败风险的工具[35]。最后，PEEPi 或呼吸肌无力导致吸气努力不足，以及人-机不同步的出现，也可能是 NIV 失败的预测因素。

9.7 总结

BiPAP 和 CPAP 具有不同的生理效应，适用于不同的临床情况。这些支持治疗设备的生理效应特性可以降低某些患者群体的插管需求和病死率，但必须密切监测，尤其是要避免延迟气管插管。还需要更多研究工作来深入地理解呼吸衰竭的不同表型，了解哪些表型能从 NIV 中获益、哪些表型 P-SILI 风险更高，以及不同表型对面罩 NIV、HFNO 或头罩反应的差异。未来研究还需要确定哪些患者从每种无创设备中获益最大，并确定切换到有创机械通气的阈值。

（赵立娜，肇寅辉　译）

参考文献

[1] Bellani G, Laffey JG, Pham T, Madotto F, Fan E, Brochard L, et al. Noninvasive ventilation of patients with acute respiratory distress syndrome. Insights from the LUNG SAFE study. Am J Respir Crit Care Med. 2017; 195(1): 67-77.

[2] Fraticelli AT, Lellouche F, L'Her E, Taillé S, Mancebo J, Brochard L. Physiological effects of different interfaces during noninvasive ventilation for acute respiratory failure. Crit Care Med. 2009; 37(3): 939-45.

[3] Taccone P, Hess D, Caironi P, Bigatello LM. Continuous positive airway pressure delivered with a "helmet": effects on carbon dioxide rebreathing. Crit Care Med. 2004; 32(10): 2090-6.

[4] Grieco DL, Maggiore SM, Roca O, Spinelli E, Patel BK, Thille AW, et al. Non-invasive ventilatory support and high-flow nasal oxygen as first-line treatment of acute hypoxemic respiratory failure and ARDS. Intensive Care Med. 2021; 47(8): 851-66.

[5] Cammarota G, Olivieri C, Costa R, Vaschetto R, Colombo D, Turucz E, et al. Noninvasive ventilation through a helmet in postextubation hypoxemic patients: physiologic comparison between neurally adjusted ventilatory assist and pressure support ventilation. Intensive Care Med. 2011; 37(12): 1943-50.

[6] Wysocki M, Richard JC, Meshaka P. Noninvasive proportional assist ventilation compared with noninvasive pressure support ventilation in hypercapnic acute respiratory failure. Crit Care Med. 2002; 30(2): 323-9.

[7] García-de-Acilu M, Patel BK, Roca O. Noninvasive approach for de novo acute hypoxemic

respiratory failure: noninvasive ventilation, high-flow nasal cannula, both or none? Curr Opin Crit Care. 2019; 25(1): 54-62.

[8] L'Her E, Deye N, Lellouche F, Taille S, Demoule A, Fraticelli A, et al. Physiologic effects of noninvasive ventilation during acute lung injury. Am J Respir Crit Care Med. 2005; 172(9): 1112-8.

[9] Luce JM. The cardiovascular effects of mechanical ventilation and positive end-expiratory pressure. JAMA. 1984; 252(6): 807-11.

[10] Delclaux C, L'Her E, Alberti C, Mancebo J, Abroug F, Conti G, et al. Treatment of acute hypoxemic nonhypercapnic respiratory insufficiency with continuous positive airway pressure delivered by a face mask: a randomized controlled trial. JAMA. 2000; 284(18): 2352-60.

[11] Rochwerg B, Brochard L, Elliott MW, Hess D, Hill NS, Nava S, et al. Official ERS/ATS clinical practice guidelines: noninvasive ventilation for acute respiratory failure. Eur Respir J. 2017; 50(2): 1602426.

[12] Vestbo J, Hurd SS, Agustí AG, Jones PW, Vogelmeier C, Anzueto A, et al. Global strategy for the diagnosis, management, and prevention of chronic obstructive pulmonary disease: GOLD executive summary. Am J Respir Crit Care Med. 2013; 187(4): 347-65.

[13] Perkins GD, Ji C, Connolly BA, Couper K, Lall R, Baillie JK, et al. An adaptive randomized controlled trial of non-invasive respiratory strategies in acute respiratory failure patients with COVID-19. medRxiv. 2021: 2021.08.02.21261379.

[14] Lemiale V, Mokart D, Resche-Rigon M, Pène F, Mayaux J, Faucher E, et al. Effect of noninvasive ventilation vs oxygen therapy on mortality among immunocompromised patients with acute respiratory failure: a randomized clinical trial. JAMA. 2015; 314(16): 1711-9.

[15] Frat JP, Thille AW, Mercat A, Girault C, Ragot S, Perbet S, et al. High-flow oxygen through nasal cannula in acute hypoxemic respiratory failure. N Engl J Med. 2015; 372(23): 2185-96.

[16] Ferreyro BL, Angriman F, Munshi L, Del Sorbo L, Ferguson ND, Rochwerg B, et al. Association of noninvasive oxygenation strategies with all-cause mortality in adults with acute hypoxemic respiratory failure: a systematic review and meta-analysis. JAMA. 2020; 324(1): 57-67.

[17] Rathi NK, Haque SA, Nates R, Kosturakis A, Wang H, Dong W, et al. Noninvasive positive pressure ventilation vs invasive mechanical ventilation as first-line therapy for acute hypoxemic respiratory failure in cancer patients. J Crit Care. 2017; 39: 56-61.

[18] Patel BK, Wolfe KS, Pohlman AS, Hall JB, Kress JP. Effect of noninvasive ventilation delivered by helmet vs face mask on the rate of endotracheal intubation in patients with acute respiratory distress syndrome: a randomized clinical trial. JAMA. 2016; 315(22): 2435-41.

[19] Grieco DL, Menga LS, Cesarano M, Rosà T, Spadaro S, Bitondo MM, et al. Effect of helmet noninvasive ventilation vs high-flow nasal oxygen on days free of respiratory support in patients with COVID-19 and moderate to severe hypoxemic respiratory failure: the HENIVOT randomized clinical trial. JAMA. 2021; 325(17): 1731-43.

[20] Hilbert G, Gruson D, Vargas F, Valentino R, Gbikpi-Benissan G, Dupon M, et al. Noninvasive ventilation in immunosuppressed patients with pulmonary infiltrates, fever, and acute respiratory failure. N Engl J Med. 2001; 344(7): 481-7.

[21] Weingart SD, Levitan RM. Preoxygenation and prevention of desaturation during emergency airway management. Ann Emerg Med. 2012; 59(3): 165-75. e1.

[22] Jaber S, Monnin M, Girard M, Conseil M, Cisse M, Carr J, et al. Apnoeic oxygenation via high-

flow nasal cannula oxygen combined with non-invasive ventilation preoxygenation for intubation in hypoxaemic patients in the intensive care unit: the single-centre, blinded, randomised controlled OPTINIV trial. Intensive Care Med. 2016; 42(12): 1877-87.

[23] Nava S, Ambrosino N, Clini E, Prato M, Orlando G, Vitacca M, et al. Noninvasive mechanical ventilation in the weaning of patients with respiratory failure due to chronic obstructive pulmonary disease. A randomized, controlled trial. Ann Intern Med. 1998; 128(9): 721-8.

[24] Girault C, Bubenheim M, Abroug F, Diehl JL, Elatrous S, Beuret P, et al. Noninvasive ventilation and weaning in patients with chronic hypercapnic respiratory failure: a randomized multicenter trial. Am J Respir Crit Care Med. 2011; 184(6): 672-9.

[25] Auriant I, Jallot A, Hervé P, Cerrina J, Le Roy L, Fournier JL, et al. Noninvasive ventilation reduces mortality in acute respiratory failure following lung resection. Am J Respir Crit Care Med. 2001; 164(7): 1231-5.

[26] Esteban A, Frutos-Vivar F, Ferguson ND, Arabi Y, Apezteguía C, González M, et al. Noninvasive positive-pressure ventilation for respiratory failure after extubation. N Engl J Med. 2004; 350(24): 2452-60.

[27] Duan J, Han X, Bai L, Zhou L, Huang S. Assessment of heart rate, acidosis, consciousness, oxygenation, and respiratory rate to predict noninvasive ventilation failure in hypoxemic patients. Intensive Care Med. 2017; 43(2): 192-9.

[28] Brochard L, Slutsky A, Pesenti A. Mechanical ventilation to minimize progression of lung injury in acute respiratory failure. Am J Respir Crit Care Med. 2017; 195(4): 438-42.

[29] Bhattacharya M, Kallet RH, Ware LB, Matthay MA. Negative-pressure pulmonary edema. Chest. 2016; 150(4): 927-33.

[30] Yoshida T, Torsani V, Gomes S, De Santis RR, Beraldo MA, Costa EL, et al. Spontaneous effort causes occult pendelluft during mechanical ventilation. Am J Respir Crit Care Med. 2013; 188(12): 1420-7.

[31] Frat JP, Ragot S, Coudroy R, Constantin JM, Girault C, Prat G, et al. Predictors of intubation in patients with acute hypoxemic respiratory failure treated with a noninvasive oxygenation strategy. Crit Care Med. 2018; 46(2): 208-15.

[32] Tonelli R, Fantini R, Tabbì L, Castaniere I, Pisani L, Pellegrino MR, et al. Early inspiratory effort assessment by esophageal manometry predicts noninvasive ventilation outcome in de novo respiratory failure. A pilot study. Am J Respir Crit Care Med. 2020; 202(4): 558-67.

[33] Mercurio G, D'Arrigo S, Moroni R, Grieco DL, Menga LS, Romano A, et al. Diaphragm thickening fraction predicts noninvasive ventilation outcome: a preliminary physiological study. Crit Care. 2021; 25(1): 219.

[34] Brochard L, Mancebo J, Wysocki M, Lofaso F, Conti G, Rauss A, et al. Noninvasive ventilation for acute exacerbations of chronic obstructive pulmonary disease. N Engl J Med. 1995; 333(13): 817-22.

[35] Duan J, Wang S, Liu P, Han X, Tian Y, Gao F, et al. Early prediction of noninvasive ventilation failure in COPD patients: derivation, internal validation, and external validation of a simple risk score. Ann Intensive Care. 2019; 9(1): 108.

10 经鼻高流量氧疗：从生理学到临床实践
High Flow Nasal Oxygen：From Physiology to Clinical Practice

Sharon Einav, Marta Velia Antonini

10.1 引言

将氧气加温、加湿后通过宽径鼻导管输氧最初是设计用来提高赛马成绩的。将这种方法巧妙运用于人类是从在新生儿中实施开始的。既往在新生儿使用经鼻持续正压通气（continuous positive airway pressure，CPAP）的实践中已经证实，使用直径与新生儿鼻孔直径相匹配的鼻导管可以有效地控制漏气。由于新生儿胸壁具有相对较高的顺应性，经鼻输送高速气流，与给定压力相比，似乎能提供近似的呼吸支持水平，且气压伤和鼻腔结构损伤的风险更低[1,2]。事实上，目前儿科研究正关注基于呼吸做功来调整流速，以提高新生儿氧疗的精确性[3]。也有人认为，在有呼吸暂停倾向的人群中，高流速可能触发自主呼吸，但这一假设尚未得到证实。

经鼻高流量氧疗（high flow nasal oxygen，HFNO）在新生儿中的使用经验是一种典型的模式转变，使得这种设备从马转移到人类中应用。但是，正常成人的生理和病理与新生儿或者儿童存在极大的差异，因此将新生儿或儿童的 HFNO 的使用经验和设备研究直接推广至成人中使用是错误的。这些高流量氧疗设备操作简单、使用方便，现如今已普遍应用于危重成人患者[4]。因此，本章将重点讨论成人经鼻高流量氧疗的生理效应及其对治疗和未来研究的影响。

S. Einav (✉)
Surgical Intensive Care, Intensive Care Unit, Shaare Zedek Medical Center, Jerusalem, Israel
Anesthesiology and Intensive Care, Hebrew University Faculty of Medicine, Jerusalem, Israel
e-mail: einav_s@szmc.org.il

M. V. Antonini
Department of Biomedical, Metabolic and Neural Sciences, University of Modena and Reggio Emilia, Modena, Italy

© The Author(s), under exclusive license to Springer Nature Switzerland AG 2022
G. Bellani (ed.), *Mechanical Ventilation from Pathophysiology to Clinical Evidence*, https://doi.org/10.1007/978-3-030-93401-9_10

10.2 无效腔,气体混合和冲刷

在健康的成年人中,解剖无效腔等于生理无效腔,通常接近 2 mL/kg(体重)。因此,一个正常的成年人,约三分之一的潮气量(每次)属于无效通气。病理进程可能显著增加生理无效腔,这种变化已被认为与病死率相关。当解剖无效腔增加时,通过减少无效通气从而减少生理无效腔可能是至关重要的。

在吸气开始之前,用含氧量高的气体冲刷呼吸道已经被长期用于增加吸入氧浓度(inspired oxygen,FiO_2)。这种方法的主要限制是无法匹配高吸气流速,在呼吸困难患者中吸气流速可能超过 50 L/min[5],而且这样的流速在开放吸气时引起严重的不适[6]。如果患者的吸气峰流速与设定的流速不匹配,则会吸入环境空气,降低吸入气体的 FiO_2。

经鼻高流量氧疗系统可以在高达 60 L/min 的吸气流速下维持气体湿度[7]。实验室研究[8]、人体志愿者研究[9]及气道疾病患者研究[10,11]表明,气道湿化可以改善气道黏膜纤毛清除分泌物的能力,并防止冷气流引起的气道阻力增加。一些设备还可以根据患者的喜好调节吸入气流的温度,增加患者耐受性[12](表 10.1)。

表 10.1 独立的经鼻高流量氧疗设备的特点

设 备	流量(L/min)	相对湿度(%)	气体温度℃(℉)
Vapotherm	5~40	95~100	33~43(91.4~109.4)
Optiflow	1~60	100	37(98.6)
Airvo	2~60(成人) 2~25(青少年)	95(在 10~30℃间)	37(98.6),34(93),31(88)

通过经鼻高流量氧疗系统可以提供稳定的 FiO_2。使用超过患者所需的流速可以防止空气混入(导致 FiO_2 下降),并用新鲜气体替换上呼吸道解剖无效腔中呼出的气体。高氧流的冲刷效应已在模拟模型和人体研究中得到描述,并且可能在张开嘴巴时更有效[13,14]。

10.2.1 应用前景

部分呼吸机已经配备了 HFNO 模块,可以提供恒定的流速和 FiO_2,性能与独立的 HFNO 设备相当[15],这为 HFNO 与其他通气模式相结合提供了可能性。Grofalo 等最近描述了健康志愿者同时接受头罩 CPAP(5 cmH_2O 和 10 cmH_2O)和 HFNO(30 L/min、40 L/min 和 50 L/min 流量)的治疗。任何时候都没有头罩起雾或不适的问题,并且在所有流速下,联合使用 CPAP 和 HFNO 的呼吸频率均略低于仅使用 HFNO 的情况,但差异是显著的[16]。

10.3 呼气末正压的产生(或无)

描述新生儿和儿科人群使用 HFNO 产生高 PEEP 的研究层出不穷。这些研究可能导致了一种错误的观念,即这种效应在成人患者中也是相同的。事实上,成人患者中 HFNO 和 PEEP 之间的关系似乎比儿童中观察到的更为复杂。

早期的研究表明,在健康的成年志愿者和计划进行心脏手术的患者中,喉部压力几乎与输送气体的流速同步上升,但即使在 50 L/min 的气流下,闭合口腔时的喉部压力也很少超过 7~8 cm H_2O[17,18]。气体泄漏似乎只影响初始压力,而不影响由增加的气流产生的压力增量[18,19]。由于压力通常在气道中保持一致,喉部压力的上升反映了肺泡压某种程度的上升。PEEP 的产生量主要取决于设定的气流速率,但也与峰值吸气流速和潮气量有关,这两者都由患者决定并可能随时间而变化(图 10.1)。

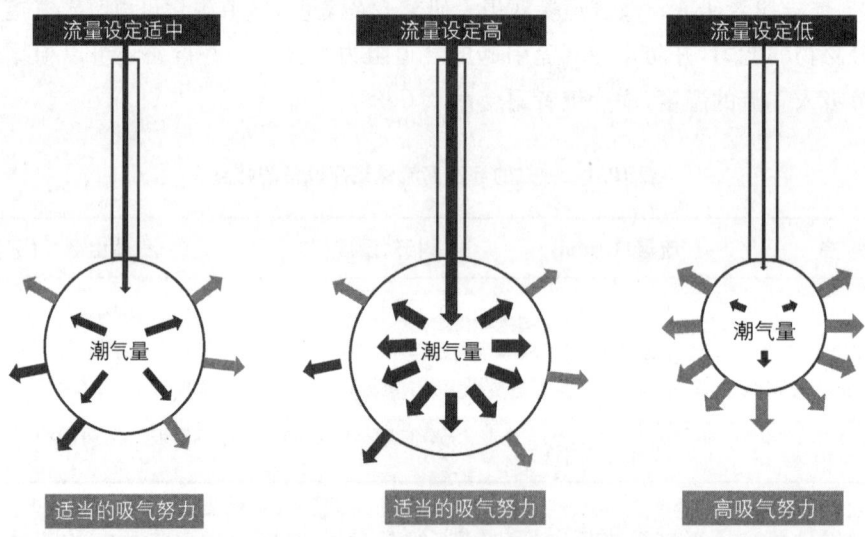

图 10.1 设定流速、吸气努力产生的负压、潮气量与呼气末正压的关系。较高的设定流速和较高的自发潮气量增加了 HFNO 产生的 PEEP,而吸气努力产生的负压增加降低了 HFNO 产生的 PEEP(引自 Sun YH et al. Clin Respir J. 2019 Dec;13(12):758-764. doi:https://doi.org/10.1111/crj.13087. Epub 2019 Sep 8. PMID:31465634 and Okuda M et al. BMJ Open Respir Res. 2017 July 20;4(1):e000200. doi:https://doi.org/10.1136/bmjresp-2017-000200. PMID:29071075;PMCID:PMC5647476)

10.3.1 应用前景

对于拔管后的患者,电阻抗断层扫描(electrical impedance tomography, EIT)显示,呼气末总肺阻抗、区域肺复张和过度膨胀随着 HFNO 流速的增加而同步增加。然而,腹侧区域肺复张的程度比背侧区域更大,似乎取决于基线未复张区域的占比[20]。实际上,提高 HFNO 流速并不总是会产生预测的呼气末肺容积增量,尤其是在肺的重力依赖区[21]。

尽管如此,那么如何改善肺通气呢? 油酸诱导猪肺损伤 4 小时后,通过经鼻高流量氧疗系统给予猪高氧气体和氦氧混合气可改善通气效率和通气分布(主要是氦氧混合气),并减少呼吸做功(包括高氧气体和氦氧混合气)[22]。

另外,未来可能受益于 HFNO 的患者或将被提前识别。肺可复张性,通过 CT 定量非通气肺组织来评估,似乎与 HFNO 治疗失败有关,而与 NIV 治疗无关[23]。HFNO 的个体化治疗可能需要在治疗开始前测量肺可复张性。

10.4 呼吸做功

一些研究表明,HFNO 最重要的作用可能是降低了呼吸做功(work of breathing,WOB)。

10.4.1 正常成人和低氧性呼吸衰竭的呼吸做功

Takashima 等使用超声测量来研究在有和没有使用 HFNO 时成年危重症患者的膈肌增厚分数。无膈肌功能障碍的患者在停用 HFNO 后膈肌增厚分数增加,但在膈肌收缩减少的患者中未观察到这种现象。HFNO 还降低了膈肌矛盾收缩[24]。

肺阻抗的研究也显示,使用 HFNO 可降低 WOB。Longhini 等将正在接受支气管镜检查的患者随机分为 HFNO 组或常规面罩氧疗组。在操作过程中 HFNO 组患者 PaO_2 更稳定,呼气末肺容积(通过电阻抗测量)和膈肌缩短分数保持不变,但常规氧疗组肺容积减少,膈肌增厚分数增加[25]。Pérez-Terán 等研究了健康志愿者在无创通气(NIV)或 HFNO 呼吸支持 30 min 前后的肺阻抗变化并通过超声评估了膈肌运动。两组患者的呼吸频率均下降,呼气末肺阻抗均升高,但 NIV 组呼气末肺阻抗的变异度均高于 HFNO 组[26]。Vargas 等治疗因急性低氧性呼吸衰竭收治于 ICU 的患者时,通过高吸氧浓度非重复呼吸面罩、HFNO 和 CPAP 交替给氧 20 分钟。与面罩相比,HFNO 和 CPAP 均显著降低了吸气努力(通过食管评估),但 CPAP 对 PaO_2/FiO_2 有更大的改善[27]。Mauri 等使用电阻抗成像技术(electrical impedance tomography,EIT)研究了在恒定的 FiO_2 条件下应用传统氧疗和 HFNO 的两组急性低氧性呼吸衰竭患者,发现增加的流速显著降低了吸气努力、改善了肺通气(呼气末肺容积)及动态肺顺应性(潮气量与食管压的比值)[21]。

10.4.2 失代偿性慢性阻塞性肺疾病患者的呼吸做功

目前,临床实践指南不建议对 COPD 急性加重的患者使用 HFNO。然而,最近的一些研究表明,这种方法在未来可能需要被重新审视。Di Mussi 等研究了因高碳酸血症型呼吸衰竭而接受插管治疗的 COPD 患者,在拔管后,给予预设的常规氧疗与 HFNO 交替使用。当常规氧疗切换为 HFNO 时,中枢呼吸驱动(通过膈肌电活动的减少来评估)和呼吸做功(通过吸气时跨膈压-时间乘积来评估)均有改善。当从 HFNO 改回常规氧疗时,这种改善将被逆转。由于在整个研究期间,均滴定 FiO_2 以达到 88%~92% 的稳定的动脉血氧饱和度目标,因此这种(中枢呼吸驱动和呼吸做功的)变化被归因于 HFNO 的使用[28]。接受 HFNO 治疗 COPD 患者的运动表现的研究还显示,CO_2 产生显著减少,运动持续时间增加,肌肉组织中的脱氧血红蛋白减少[29,30]。将这些研究结果外推至急性加重的 COPD 患者则提示 HFNO 可增加患者的耐力,降低疲劳和插管的可能性。

10.4.3 应用前景

最近的一项研究将插管患者在自主呼吸试验期间产生的平均吸气流速与拔管后患者描述为最舒适的 HFNO 设置流速(每次增加 10 L/min,从 20 L/min 到 60 L/min 进行测试)进行了比较。其间滴定 FiO_2 以维持动脉血氧饱和度为 92%～97%。拔管前的平均吸气流速与患者认为最舒适的 HFNO 吸气流速相关[31]。这个发现的重要性可能远远不止于患者舒适度方面,实时监测呼吸做功并自动调节流速可能是在 HFNO 治疗过程中改善呼吸同步性和维持氧合稳定的一种方法[3]。迄今为止,在使用 HFNO 治疗期间无创评估呼吸做功一直受到单向气流的影响而无法准确监测。然而,Montecchia 等最近描述了使用两个呼吸流量记录仪并结合了一种漏气校正的算法。对一个肺模型和两名健康成年志愿者的测量结果显示该方法提供了可靠的呼吸流速和容积测算(计算呼吸做功所需),相对误差<1%[32]。

10.5 注意事项

HFNO 的使用存在三个主要安全问题：缺乏设备报警、治疗期间的呼吸肌疲劳和 P-SILI。

对于没有使用镇静剂和能够说话的患者来说,缺乏设备警报似乎不是一个主要问题。然而,呼吸肌疲劳已经被一些研究强调为一个主要的问题,在 ICU 使用无创呼吸支持时发生呼吸肌疲劳会导致病死率升高,即使使用带有报警的设备也是如此。Frizola 等对猪模型的研究发现气管压力以流量依赖的方式增加,而通过两个鼻孔给予相似的流量时,增加的压力比单一鼻孔给氧更大[19]。虽然这一结论可能看起来微不足道,但立刻让人想到对于神志欠清或躁动的患者发生鼻导管移位时的临床意义。事实上,鼻导管的意外受压或堵塞已在文献中被广泛报道[15]。此外,患者可能在治疗期间睡着和(或)可能因无法产生足够的气流来寻求帮助。无论使用何种 HFNO 设备,低氧血症患者都应该被安置在充分监护的环境中。

最后,P-SILI 被认为是在新生儿中使用 HFNO 的一个重要问题。因此,在其他 P-SILI 高危人群中使用 HFNO 时,无法监测压力或容量是令人担忧的问题[14]。

10.6 总结

由于这些单一设备使用简单且高效,使 HFNO 得到了普遍应用。HFNO 提供了些许明显的生理优势,包括氧合气体冲刷气道无效腔、减少无效呼吸、即便速度高也维持气道湿度、根据舒适水平调整温度并在吸气流速变化的情况下提供稳定的 FiO_2。成人产生的 PEEP 相对较低,不仅取决于设定流速,还取决于患者相关变量(闭口、吸气峰流速、潮气量和肺顺应性)。HFNO 的主要作用似乎与减少呼吸做功和减少呼吸肌疲劳有关。HFNO 对通气的影响需要进一步阐明,很可能取决于其他因素而不只是设定流速。虽然指南不建议对 COPD 急性加重的患者使用 HFNO,但有初步数据表明,使用 HFNO 可能会在这些患者吸气开始时减少吸气肌的负荷,从而增加呼吸耐力。展望未来,发展方向可能包括使 HFNO 与其他通气模式相结合,通过高流量设备给予混合气体(如高氧气体和氦氧混合气),个体化评估肺可复张性和通气模式以选择适合 HFNO 的患者,以及设置设备以匹配患者的吸气流速和呼吸做功。无论其使用的适应证如何,HFNO 都应始终在监护环境中使用,以确保患者的安全。

(陈珵,金珊珊 译)

参考文献

[1] Wilkinson D, Andersen C, O'Donnell CP, De Paoli AG, Manley BJ. High flow nasal cannula for respiratory support in preterm infants. Cochrane Database Syst Rev. 2016; 2: CD006405. https://doi.org/10.1002/14651858.CD006405.pub3.

[2] Hong H, Li XX, Li J, Zhang ZQ. High-flow nasal cannula versus nasal continuous positive airway pressure for respiratory support in preterm infants: a meta-analysis of randomized controlled trials. J Matern Fetal Neonatal Med. 2021; 34(2): 259-66. https://doi.org/10.1080/14767058.2019.1606193.

[3] Kovatis KZ, Locke RG, Mackley AB, Subedi K, Shaffer TH. Adjustment of high flow nasal cannula rates using real-time work of breathing indices in premature infants with respiratory insufficiency. J Perinatol. 2021; 41(7): 1711-7. https://doi.org/10.1038/s41372-021-00977-z.

[4] Gershengorn HB, Hu Y, Chen JT, Hsieh SJ, Dong J, Gong MN, Chan CW. The impact of high-flow nasal cannula use on patient mortality and the availability of mechanical ventilators in COVID-19. Ann Am Thorac Soc. 2021; 18(4): 623-31. https://doi.org/10.1513/AnnalsATS.202007-803OC.

[5] Chiumello D, Pelosi P, Croci M, Bigatello LM, Gattinoni L. The effects of pressurization rate on breathing pattern, work of breathing, gas exchange and patient comfort in pressure support ventilation. Eur Respir J. 2001; 18(1): 107-14. https://doi.org/10.1183/09031936.01.00083901.

[6] Chanques G, Constantin JM, Sauter M, Jung B, Sebbane M, Verzilli D, et al. Discomfort associated with underhumidified highflow oxygen therapy in critically ill patients. Intensive Care Med. 2009; 35(6): 996-1003.

[7] Chikata Y, Izawa M, Okuda N, Itagaki T, Nakataki E, Onodera M, Imanaka H, Nishimura M. Humidification performance of two high-flow nasal cannula devices: a bench study. Respir Care. 2014; 59(8): 1186-90. https://doi.org/10.4187/respcare.02932.

[8] Kilgour E, Rankin N, Ryan S, Pack R. Mucociliary function deteriorates in the clinical range of inspired air temperature and humidity. Intensive Care Med. 2004; 30(7): 1491-4. https://doi.org/10.1007/s00134-004-2235-3.

[9] Salah B, Dinh Xuan AT, Fouilladieu JL, Lockhart A, Regnard J. Nasal mucociliary transport in

healthy subjects is slower when breathing dry air. Eur Respir J. 1988; 1(9): 852-5.

[10] Hasani A, Chapman TH, McCool D, Smith RE, Dilworth JP, Agnew JE. Domiciliary humidification improves lung mucociliary clearance in patients with bronchiectasis. Chron Respir Dis. 2008; 5(2): 81-6. https://doi.org/10.1177/1479972307087190.

[11] Fontanari P, Zattara-Hartmann MC, Burnet H, Jammes Y. Nasal eupnoeic inhalation of cold, dry air increases airway resistance in asthmatic patients. Eur Respir J. 1997; 10(10): 2250-4. https://doi.org/10.1183/09031936.97.10102250.

[12] Mauri T, Galazzi A, Binda F, Masciopinto L, Corcione N, Carlesso E, Lazzeri M, Spinelli E, Tubiolo D, Volta CA, Adamini I, Pesenti A, Grasselli G. Impact of flow and temperature on patient comfort during respiratory support by high-flow nasal cannula. Crit Care. 2018; 22(1): 120. https://doi.org/10.1186/s13054-018-2039-4.

[13] Onodera Y, Akimoto R, Suzuki H, Okada M, Nakane M, Kawamae K. A high-flow nasal cannula system with relatively low flow effectively washes out CO_2 from the anatomical dead space in a sophisticated respiratory model made by a 3D printer. Intensive Care Med Exp. 2018; 6(1): 7. https://doi.org/10.1186/s40635-018-0172-7.

[14] Sivieri EM, Foglia EE, Abbasi S. Carbon dioxide washout during high flow nasal cannula versus nasal CPAP support: an in vitro study. Pediatr Pulmonol. 2017; 52(6): 792-8. https://doi.org/10.1002/ppul.23664.

[15] Zhou Y, Ni Z, Ni Y, Liang B, Liang Z. Comparison of actual performance in the flow and fraction of inspired O_2 among different high-flow nasal cannula devices: a bench study. Can Respir J. 2021; 2021: 6638048. https://doi.org/10.1155/2021/6638048.

[16] Garofalo E, Bruni A, Pelaia C, Cammarota G, Murabito P, Biamonte E, Abdalla K, Longhini F, Navalesi P. Evaluation of a new interface combining high-flow nasal cannula and CPAP. Respir Care. 2019; 64(10): 1231-9. https://doi.org/10.4187/respcare.06871.

[17] Groves N, Tobin A. High flow nasal oxygen generates positive airway pressure in adult volunteers. Aust Crit Care. 2007; 20(4): 126-31. https://doi.org/10.1016/j.aucc.2007.08.001.

[18] Parke RL, McGuinness SP. Pressures delivered by nasal high flow oxygen during all phases of the respiratory cycle. Respir Care. 2013; 58(10): 1621-4. https://doi.org/10.4187/respcare.02358.

[19] Frizzola M, Miller TL, Rodriguez ME, Zhu Y, Rojas J, Hesek A, Stump A, Shaffer TH, Dysart K. High-flow nasal cannula: impact on oxygenation and ventilation in an acute lung injury model. Pediatr Pulmonol. 2011; 46(1): 67-74. https://doi.org/10.1002/ppul.21326.

[20] Zhang R, He H, Yun L, Zhou X, Wang X, Chi Y, Yuan S, Zhao Z. Effect of postextubation high-flow nasal cannula therapy on lung recruitment and overdistension in high-risk patient. Crit Care. 2020; 24(1): 82. https://doi.org/10.1186/s13054-020-2809-7.

[21] Mauri T, Alban L, Turrini C, Cambiaghi B, Carlesso E, Taccone P, Bottino N, Lissoni A, Spadaro S, Volta CA, Gattinoni L, Pesenti A, Grasselli G. Optimum support by high-flow nasal cannula in acute hypoxemic respiratory failure: effects of increasing flow rates. Intensive Care Med. 2017; 43(10): 1453-63. https://doi.org/10.1007/s00134-017-4890-1.

[22] Jassar RK, Vellanki H, Zhu Y, Hesek AM, Wang J, Rodriguez E, Wolfson MR, Shaffer TH. High flow nasal heliox improves work of breathing and attenuates lung injury in a newborn porcine lung injury model. J Neonatal Perinatal Med. 2015; 8(4): 323-31. https://doi.org/10.3233/NPM-15915039.

[23] Koga Y, Kaneda K, Fujii N, Tanaka R, Miyauchi T, Fujita M, Hidaka K, Tsuruta R. Association between increased nonaerated lung weight and treatment failure in patients with de novo acute respiratory failure: difference between high-flow nasal oxygen therapy and noninvasive ventilation in a multicenter retrospective study. J Crit Care. 2021; 9(65): 221-5. https://doi.org/10.1016/j.jcrc.2021.06.025.

[24] Takashima T, Nakanishi N, Arai Y, Oto J. The effect of high-flow nasal cannula on diaphragm dysfunction including paradoxical diaphragmatic contraction in the intensive care unit. J Med Investig. 2021; 68(1.2): 159-64. https://doi.org/10.2152/jmi.68.159.

[25] Longhini F, Pelaia C, Garofalo E, Bruni A, Placida R, Iaquinta C, Arrighi E, Perri G, Procopio G, Cancelliere A, Rovida S, Marrazzo G, Pelaia G, Navalesi P. High-flow nasal cannula oxygen therapy for outpatients undergoing flexible bronchoscopy: a randomised controlled trial. Thorax. 2021; 77(1): 58-64. https://doi.org/10.1136/thoraxjnl-2021-217116.

[26] Pérez-Terán P, Marin-Corral J, Dot I, Sans S, Muñoz-Bermúdez R, Bosch R, Vila C, Masclans JR. Aeration changes induced by high flow nasal cannula are more homogeneous than those generated by non-invasive ventilation in healthy subjects. J Crit Care. 2019; 53: 186-92. https://doi.org/10.1016/j.jcrc.2019.06.009.

[27] Vargas F, Saint-Leger M, Boyer A, Bui NH, Hilbert G. Physiologic effects of high-flow nasal cannula oxygen in critical care subjects. Respir Care. 2015; 60(10): 1369-76. https://doi.org/10.4187/respcare.03814.

[28] Di Mussi R, Spadaro S, Stripoli T, Volta CA, Trerotoli P, Pierucci P, Staffieri F, Bruno F, Camporota L, Grasso S. High-flow nasal cannula oxygen therapy decreases postextubation neuroventilatory drive and work of breathing in patients with chronic obstructive pulmonary disease. Crit Care. 2018; 22(1): 180. https://doi.org/10.1186/s13054-018-2107-9.

[29] Chen YH, Huang CC, Lin HL, Cheng SL, Wu HP. Effects of high flow nasal cannula on exercise endurance in patients with chronic obstructive pulmonary disease. J Formos Med Assoc. 2021; https://doi.org/10.1016/j.jfma.2021.05.018.

[30] Cirio S, Piran M, Vitacca M, Piaggi G, Ceriana P, Prazzoli M, Paneroni M, Carlucci A. Effects of heated and humidified high flow gases during high-intensity constant-load exercise on severe COPD patients with ventilatory limitation. Respir Med. 2016 Sep; 118: 128-32. https://doi.org/10.1016/j.rmed.2016.08.004.

[31] Butt S, Pistidda L, Floris L, Liperi C, Vasques F, Glover G, Barrett NA, Sanderson B, Grasso S, Shankar-Hari M, Camporotaa L. Initial setting of high-flow nasal oxygen post extubation based on mean inspiratory flow during a spontaneous breathing trial. J Crit Care. 2021; 63: 40-4. https://doi.org/10.1016/j.jcrc.2020.12.022.

[32] Montecchia F, Midulla F, Papoff P. A flow-leak correction algorithm for pneumotachographic work-of-breathing measurement during high-flow nasal cannula oxygen therapy. Med Eng Phys. 2018; 54: 32-43. https://doi.org/10.1016/j.medengphy.2018.02.004.

11 机械通气和体外膜肺氧合患者的护理

Nursing of Mechanically Ventilated and ECMO Patient

Marta Velia Antonini, Johannes Mellinghoff

ICU 收治的急性呼吸衰竭（acute respiratory failure，ARF）或急性呼吸窘迫综合征（acute respiratory distress syndrome，ARDS）患者具有复杂的临床需求，比如从严格的呼吸机管理来看，要提供氧合和二氧化碳清除，防止对肺部造成额外的损伤[1]。这些危重症患者常常不稳定，可能需要除了机械通气外的额外措施，如俯卧位和体外生命支持[1]。为确保这些治疗的耐受性，他们通常需要长时间的深度镇静，可能还需要肌肉松弛[1,2]，这会影响康复工作并可能导致心理障碍。

本章旨在介绍需要机械通气、俯卧位和（或）体外支持的 ICU 患者护理的主要特点和挑战。

11.1 机械通气

护士是多学科医疗团队的重要成员，在实施基于循证的医疗决策过程中起着关键作用，如 ABCDEF 集束化策略[3,4]，旨在解除重症患者因治疗造成的医源性不良后果，包括疼痛、焦虑/镇静、谵妄、固定不动和睡眠紊乱。为了最大程度地促进康复、减少 ICU 停留时间和重症监护后综合征（PICS 综合征，见"26 患者的长期随访"），这些策略对于最小化重症监护治疗的长期影响并改善认知和身体康复至关重要[5]。

护士更具体地参与以下集束化策略项目的实施。

M. V. Antonini (✉)
ECMO Team — AUSL della Romagna, Cesena, Italy
Department of Biomedical, Metabolic and Neural Sciences, University of Modena and Reggio Emilia, Modena, Italy
e-mail: velian@unimore.it

J. Mellinghoff
University of Brighton, School of Sport and Health Sciences, Brighton, UK

© The Author(s), under exclusive license to Springer Nature Switzerland AG 2022
G. Bellani (ed.), *Mechanical Ventilation from Pathophysiology to Clinical Evidence*, https://doi.org/10.1007/978-3-030-93401-9_11

(1) A 和 C：评估、预防和管理疼痛，选择镇痛和镇静剂。这两项聚焦于疼痛评估和管理，包括镇痛和镇静药物的选择。此外，根据镇静目标调整这些药物有利于轻度镇静那些更清醒、警觉的患者，可以减少机械通气的时间并防止谵妄（图 11.1）。护士实施和导向的操作方案/流程能够系统地评估和管理疼痛和焦虑，对预后产生积极影响[4,6]。

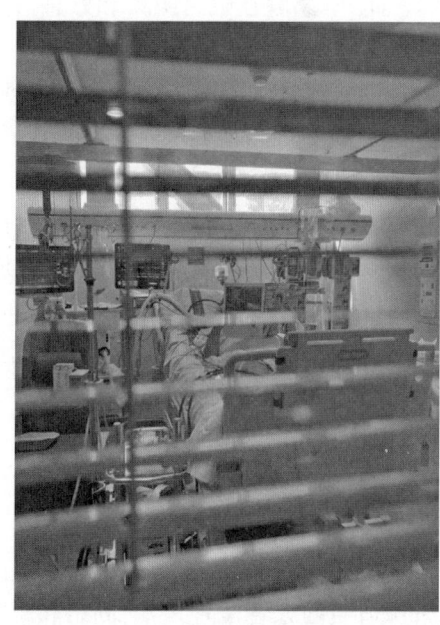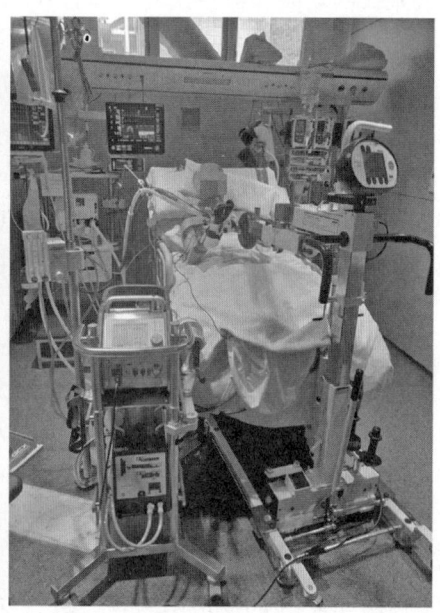

图 11.1　ECMO 支持下的康复治疗。由 Jordi Riera MD PhD 提供，并获得了患者的许可（见彩色插图）

(2) B：包括自发觉醒试验（spontaneous awakening trials，SAT）和自主呼吸试验（spontaneous breathing trials，SBT）。基于机构/国家角色职责的要求，SAT 与 SBT 的联合应用有利于促进团队成员间的沟通和协调[4,6]。床旁患者监测作为重要的护理干预手段，可观察患者自发/辅助呼吸时的呼吸努力，这对于可能出现的人-机不同步的检测和管理非常关键。将"R"加入 ABCDEF 集束化策略中用于控制呼吸驱动，可以使操作人员根据患者特定情况调整机械通气设置，并应尽快促进恢复自主呼吸[2]。

(3) D：谵妄。推荐使用经过验证和可靠的监测工具，如 ICU 谵妄评估量表（CAM-ICU）[7]，以评估和预防谵妄，是 ICU 床旁护理的基础[4]。谵妄经常发生在危重症患者中，其作为短期和长期不良预后的预测因素，包括更高的病死率、延长机械通气时间、延长 ICU 和住院时间，以及使存活患者发展为 PICS，被越来越多人所认识[5]。

(4) E：早期活动与锻炼以预防和管理 ICU 获得性虚弱，这种活动性虚弱会延长机械通气/住院时间并增加病死率，是 ICU 护理实践的另一个方面。卧床休息与神经肌肉功能障碍和身体受损密切相关。因此，重症患者的早期康复治疗是一种安全、可行的干预措施[8]：在适当的安全考虑下，机械通气的成年人活动是可行的，可提高认知/身体恢复，同时将不良事件的风险降至最低（图 11.1）[8]。目前，康复实施的主要障碍是结构/环境问题和流程/文化因素，而不是患者本身相关问题。

（5）F：家庭参与和进入ICU的许可主要由护理人员来协调。自COVID-19大流行以来，ICU限制探视政策对家庭和医疗工作人员都产生了负面影响，导致两个群体的压力强度均有所增加[9]。具体来说，床边缺乏家人的陪伴是发生谵妄的危险因素[10]。家人是重症监护环境的一个组成部分，是康复的关键决定因素，还对ICU幸存者如何应对PICS及长期或永久的功能和神经认知障碍产生影响。此外，家庭在临终决策和姑息治疗中也扮演着重要角色[10]。

统筹患者及其亲属和临床团队之间的联系是以家庭为中心的护理理念的体现，是一种跨职业的策略（和文化）。ICU护士在此发挥重要作用，因为他们一直在床边，与家人建立特殊关系，并且是识别和满足家庭需求、提供必要支持和护理的关键专业人士[11]。

ABCDEF(R)并不是唯一的集束化护理策略。ICU护士有责任促进或实施基于循证策略的护理干预措施，如旨在减少可预防感染发生率的护理流程[12]，特别是以下几点。

（1）呼吸机相关性肺炎（ventilator associated pneumonia，VAP）预防策略，包括对患者适当的体位、监测气管插管气囊压力变化、口咽/气管吸引和呼吸机管路的管理。此外，良好的口腔护理是ICU患者的基本卫生需要，可以预防不适和局部或全身并发症。

（2）导管相关的血流感染的预防，包括置管前备皮、确保无菌技术的实施、提供可靠的固定、伤口敷料覆盖及换药、定期观察穿刺部位、适当的导管管理，以及使用一次性传感器和输液器[13]。

（3）预防导管相关尿路感染的措施，包括采用适当的尿管留置技术、固定和管理方案（包括会阴护理）[14]。

（4）护士主导的肠内营养方案可以优化ICU患者的热卡、蛋白质和其他营养素的摄入目标，从而预防这类高危患者发生营养不足[15]。同时，根据护理流程进行血糖监测和胰岛素管理可以实现安全有效的血糖控制。

11.2 俯卧位

俯卧位（prone position，PP）是一种对于需要机械通气的重症ARDS患者有益的治疗方法（见"29 俯卧位通气"）[16]。虽然PP被认为是一种无创且相对廉价的干预措施，但该操作过程本身很复杂，显著增加工作量，需要多学科协作[17,18]，同时还需要全面了解相关的并发症和不良事件[19]。

文献中描述了三种不同类别的翻转操作方法：手动、机械升降辅助和使用专用的俯卧床。手动是最广泛使用的策略，可以使用搬动和减少摩擦的工具，如滑动床单或翻身板。它需要一个至少4~5名经验丰富成员的工作小组（理想情况下每侧2名成员），1名小组长在头部负责气道固定/管理，同时指挥团队保持协同[17,18]。此外，可能需要专门的团队成员负责移动诸如胸腔引流管[19]或体外膜肺氧合（ECMO）导管之类的设备。上面是理想配置，如果需要在人力有限时执行PP，则应该至少由3名医疗专业人员（healthcare professionals，HCP）小心地执行。

建议制定和实施机构内的操作规范和核查清单,用于指导患者、团队和设备准备、体位翻转流程和操作后护理,标准化 PP 操作流程。因此,总体目标是确保一致性,提高不良事件的可预测性,以最小化对患者或医疗保健提供者的潜在危害[19]。教育和培训多学科团队,特别是模拟培训,以增加团队信心,使其具备相应技能以应对相关风险[19,20]。在 COVID-19 大流行期间,有报道专门的多学科团队和训练有素的 PP 小组减轻了 ICU 工作人员的心理压力并提高了操作的安全性和效率[21]。

卧床休息或长时间的俯卧位可能会导致不良事件和并发症。护士实施的保护性策略可能有助于预防这些并发症或减少其发生。面部水肿、眼睑/眶周水肿和(或)结膜水肿/渗出是常见的不良反应,但一旦回到仰卧位,通常会迅速恢复[17,19,22,23],而其他眼部并发症(由水肿恶化),如眼球损伤/角膜擦伤,仍可能持续存在。

俯卧位相关压疮是报道最多的损伤[18,22-25],是唯一与俯卧位持续时间正相关的常见并发症[25]。需要俯卧位的 ARDS 患者可能存在多种增加压力性损伤(pressure injury,PI)发生率的危险因素,如心血管不稳定引起的周围灌注不足、血管活性/正性肌力药物的使用、急性或既往器官功能障碍、长时间卧床和 ICU 住院、营养摄入不足或存在合并症(如糖尿病等)。尽管报告的 PI 多为低级别,因此不需要任何特定干预即可完全恢复[25,26],但医疗保健提供者仍应考虑采用多模式预防策略,其中包括:

(1) 细心、连续的皮肤/眼部护理和评估[19,24,27]。由于存在多种潜在机制导致损伤的高风险,需要将面部视为这类患者的重点关注区域[24]。

(2) 为了最小化剪切力、重新分配压力,以及同时吸收水分,可以在易受压的部位(表 11.1),如骨性突起处[18,19]、医疗设备接触区域下方使用预防性敷料[27]。

(3) 谨慎使用胶带/固定装置[27]。

(4) 使用专用床或床垫以及技术/定位装置来减轻受压和重新分配压力[19,24]。

(5) 优化患者的营养状况,因为营养好的患者 PI 发生率降低[22,27]。

实施长期随访(见"26 患者的长期随访")可能有助于发现在 ICU 期间可能被忽视的长时程损害,需要提高认识以改善临床实践。

虽然预防 PI 的集束化策略中通常包括让患者活动的方案[27],但由于需要长时间的 PP 和预防导管移位脱落,上述集束化策略的应用可能受限[24]。一旦患者进入 PP 状态,可以采取头高脚低位(又称反特伦德伦堡位)[19,28],并按照操作规范定期改变头部和四肢的姿势(表 11.1),以避免臂丛神经损伤和股外侧皮神经受压,这两种情况都曾在长时间 PP 后被报道过。

PI,特别是与医疗设备相关的 PI,如果存在进行中的特定治疗(如接受体外生命支持)或高剂量预防性抗凝治疗(如 COVID-19 患者),可能会与出血并发症有关[24]。

导管移位/脱落或阻塞可能导致失去血管内通路、气管插管/气管切开插管、胸腔引流管和其他维持生命治疗的通路[18,22,23,25],是令人担忧的严重并发症。为了防止这些导管设备相关的并发症,在翻身过程中建议断开非必要输液、电路和其他监测设备[19]。然而,为了保证工作状态和预防并发症,尽可能减少需要关闭的设备系统,平衡以下风险。

表 11.1 患者俯卧位前后的准备和管理(已标注易于发生与俯卧位相关伤害的高风险区域)

	俯 卧 位 之 前	俯 卧 位 之 后
核查表	制定并实施规范/核查表以明确 • 团队角色/职责分配和患者在俯卧位前、中、后的位置 • 俯卧位前患者的准备 • 设备和仪器的准备 • 俯卧位技术要点和流程 • 俯卧位后的全方位护理 • 非紧急/紧急的换位技术和程序	立即恢复完整的生命体征监测 • 将 ECG 电极放置在适应体位的合适位置 • 如果使用过程中有创动脉压监测系统被断开，请执行零点校准 • 如果留置了肺动脉导管，建议在俯卧前断开连接。应仔细评估肺动脉压力组长选择在特定案例中断开连接。应仔细评估肺动脉压力的意外阻塞，这可以通过肺动脉楔压床旁推断。如果确实发生了上述情形，应通知医生将导管退回
设备	检查/记录插管深度并牢牢固定以防意外移位 • 气管插管：调整位置（口中央），避免边界位或嘴唇压迫；保持通气管末端朝向患者，避免向外弯曲 • 监测颈内静脉导管/管监深度；必要时，操纵前增加管线以防止牵引 • 鼻饲管：暂停鼻饲喂养，检查胃剩余量（考虑俯卧位前丢弃鼻饲液），冲洗鼻饲管以防堵塞 • 胸管：仅在确定安全时清理，否则保持较低位置以便排空 • 导尿管和其他管路的引流袋和引流设备 SpO_2 和有创动脉压监测应在整个病程中持续进行；连续的 $EtCO_2$ 监测是可取的，因为它可能早期提示呼吸机回路断开或气道移位	检查气管插管(ET)的位置，与之前的深度比较。查有无堵塞。确认气管套囊的压力在指定范围内，即 20～30 cmH_2O。使用封闭式吸痰系统以便于痰液抽吸 • 如有胸腔引流管关闭了，重新打开，并在需要时恢复抽吸 • 维持静脉输液，确保在程序进行中没有关闭的导管，检查是否有流动阻塞 • 为程序重新打开任何关闭的导管，并确保没有管道在患者身体下面通过
镇静	评估镇静深度和镇痛药的需要 • 可能需要增加维持剂量和（或）给予负荷剂量 • 在镇静需要增加的情况下，根据需要考虑使用神经肌肉阻断药物(NMBA)	

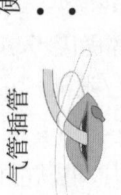

续 表

俯卧位之前	俯卧位之后
保持皮质清洁和滋润 • 检查设备下方的皮肤，确认皮肤的完整性或压疮的存在情况，记录设备相关的损伤 • 应用预防压疮的敷料 • 清洁/润滑眼睛，闭合或贴紧眼睑，确保睫毛向外 • 使用专门的床垫/床和装置来卸载压力并重新分配压力	• 在俯卧位过程中调整垫子/枕头，泡沫表面或任何装置的位置，以卸载/重新分配压力点 • 仔细评估可能的不良血流动力学效应，因为骨盆/胸部支撑的姿势。妥善放置头部/上肢的位置（游泳者可能会阻碍静脉回流，避免异常伸展或核查表、调整支撑点的位置 • 考虑使用反向特伦德伦堡体位，同时将床头抬高30°，以最小化面部水肿和减少胃内容物/管饲营养吸入风险，以确保良好的眼压 • 评估高风险区域：眼睛、耳朵（不弯曲）、下巴、手、髂嵴、腿前部和膝盖、脚背、男性生殖器；减轻明显压力；确保气管插管不对唇角/唇施加压力，也不使导管压迫颈部/面部，或管线/管道在患者身体下面穿过

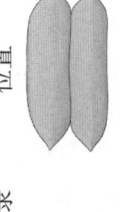

位置

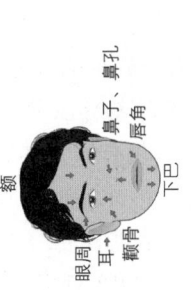

高风险区域

(1) 发生导管相关感染的机会增加。

(2) 短时间内缺失生命体征监护：至少应在整个过程中保留脉搏、血氧饱和度和有创动脉血压的持续监测[17,18]。而 $EtCO_2$ 可以提示呼吸机管路脱落或导管移位[17,18]，因此建议在整个过程中持续监测。

需要保证提供生命支持设备（如正性肌力/血管活性药物输注泵）通路的完整性。如果需要，可以增加静脉输液管的长度以防止牵拉，但密切关注输液线的长度/管径/柔韧性改变对压力监测和静脉输液带来的可能后果。

尽管罕见，但气管插管意外脱管被认为是最严重的潜在不良事件[18,23]。进行仔细的人工气道评估，包括插管深度，以确保其通畅和功能正常。在操作前后，仔细地固定所有设备对于提高患者安全至关重要（表 11.1）[19,25,29]。将呼吸机靠近患者，并将呼吸机朝向患者以防止管道过度牵拉，可避免对机械通气的不必要影响。总体而言，整个多学科团队需要随时准备好将患者紧急重新调整回仰卧位，可能需要进行困难的再插管[19,29]。

11.3 体外膜肺氧合

ECMO 技术发展至今已经成为一种确定性支持策略，可以改善传统治疗无效（包括优化机械通气和俯卧位）的重症 ARF 患者的临床预后[30,31]。

ECMO 被认为是一种安全技术，只要由有经验的团队在专业的 ECMO 中心开展[31]。对 ECLS 生理学的进一步理解和技术的进步提高了管路操作管理能力和生物相容性，从而减少和避免了相关并发症[32]。然而，ECLS 仍然是一种复杂、存在技术挑战、高风险和资源密集度高的治疗方式，具有较高的病死率和较多并发症[30,32]，且与不同的临床结局有关[33]。

制定符合体外生命支持组织（Extracorporeal Life Support Organization，ELSO）指南的操作规范/核查清单[30]，并组建一个明确角色和责任的多学科团队[30,34]是限制不良事件和改善生存率的关键。迄今为止，没有关于 ECMO 患者床旁管理的工作人员配置的国际共识，也没有针对专业人士的正式资质认证流程。考虑到这种情况，护士和 ECMO 专家的角色、职责、能力和界限需要考虑当地的政策、需求和可用的人力资源，同时遵守各国法律[32,33]。ECMO 专家被定义为从不同专业背景招募的技术专家（包括体外循环灌注师、物理治疗师和护师），具有重症监护技能，经过培训和具备经验，能够管理体外循环系统和 ECMO 患者的临床需求，在 ECMO 医生的指导和监督下工作[32,33,36]。

最近的一项调查[32]表明 1∶1 的护士-患者比为最常见的工作人员配比，由担任日常管路管理的护士担任 ECMO 专家，并由灌注师进行技术支持[32]。这种策略似乎是合理和可取的[33]，但不同的护士-患者比，如 2∶1 或 2∶3～1∶4，也被建议过或者报道过[32,35]。将 ECMO 患者分组可能可以优化管理和资源分配[37]。

无论采用何种护理模式，ECLS 都会增加护士的工作量并扩展其职责，成为提供 24 小时床旁护理的专业人员。此外，严密监测 ECMO 系统与患者及其相互作用，及时响应常规和特定要求的同时始终准备应对紧急情况和并发症，这些都强调了照顾这个患者群体的复杂性[32,38]。

对 ECMO 团队的每个成员进行持续的标准化和专业的多学科教学和培训,包括 ECMO 支持的理论和实践都是必要的[35,38,39],以获得 ECMO 床旁有效/安全护理和监测/管理 ECMO 回路所需的高级技能和知识[32,35-38,40]。

在 ECMO 患者中开展护理工作可能具有挑战性,但日常护理仍然是确保卫生、改善舒适度并预防或发现并发症,如感染、压力性损伤、出血和导管/回路相关问题的关键[41,42]。特定的规范化流程,包括安全措施和由训练有素的专业人员谨慎实施的临床路径,可以限制相关不良事件的发生[38]。

主要医学并发症包括出血、血栓形成和溶血[43]。由于需要全身系统性抗凝作为治疗基础,故例如口腔护理等基本干预措施可能会引起严重出血[42]。因此,护理操作应谨慎进行,避免不必要的操作。持续监测凝血状态/溶血参数可以预防和早期识别即将发生的并发症,通常需要进行重复和多次的检测[37,43]。无论使用哪种评估凝血功能的方式,都需要优化采血技术以确保结果的准确度,否则可能会对抗凝管理产生负面影响。

此外,在 ECMO 机器运行期间,患者可能会经历特定的 ECLS 状况,如引流障碍、回流阻塞和 V-V 配置时的再循环,以及机械性并发症,任何管理 ECMO 患者的护士都需要能够依赖团队中不同的角色与分工来识别和解决问题(表 11.2)[38]。

气体交换和(或)血流动力学稳定受损的患者往往高度依赖 ECMO 的支持,可能导致心脏停搏,在支持期间并发症的发生率更高并会降低生存率。在 ECMO 期间,既需要定期、主动检查管路及时发现问题[37,38],又需要通过及时和适当的干预/故障排除来应对紧急情况和重大并发症[38]。

在搬动 ECMO 患者使其接受护理或康复治疗、医疗操作检查流程或转运之前,应仔细固定所有导管[31,37]。导管插入部位敷料可预防感染,减少局部出血,并有助于固定导管[35,38]。

在移动期间如果可行,由 1~2 名成员[灌注师和(或)ECMO 专家]负责管路以防止并发症,包括管路断开或意外脱管,并确保整个期间引流的有效性和体外膜肺血流(extracorporeal blood flow, EBF)的稳定连续[41]。有时,通过微调患者在床上的姿势,可以防止 ECLS 带来持续损害[41]。由训练有素的多学科团队来进行这类患者的物理康复治疗和早期运动是可行和安全的,这些干预措施可能与改善预后有关[43]。

如果在优化 ECMO 支持条件下仍存在难治性低氧血症,PP 可能是一个合理、有效的选择[44,45]。尽管同时进行 PP 和 ECMO 时导管移位是最令人担忧的并发症,但据我们所知,迄今为止没有出现这种并发症的报道[45]。即使穿刺部位出血是一种普遍现象[44-46],但这可能与 PP 无关。然而,可以观察到 EBF 在 PP 过程中出现下降[44,45],需要操作者使用装置避免压迫导管、保持管路通畅。此外,如果 EBF 严重受损,可能需要迅速将 PP 恢复到仰卧位。

建议在灌注师和医师随时提供支持的情况下搬动患者、进行护理干预。可能需要调节机械通气和 EBF 设置以满足增加的氧供需求。同时,基于同样的理由,可能需要调整患者的镇静水平[41]。

表 11.2 基本 ECMO 流程，命名，监测，以及与 ECMO 支持可能相关的主要机械并发症；同时也包括与 V-V 体外循环支持的生理学和病理生理学相关的一些典型的情景

ECMO 流程及核查表 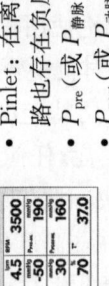	· 开发并实施标准化 ECMO 流程，并制定清晰定义团队角色/责任的流程/核查表，重点关注 · 插管和 ECMO 启动 · 直接灌注/组装，报警设置与监测 · 并发症预防，早期识别与故障康复 · 患者管理，床旁护理和插管的管理 · 出凝血管理 · 跨院内 ECMO 运输 · ECMO 紧急情况下的管路更换 · ECMO 拆机 · 临床评估主要不良事件 · ECMO 项目评估	ECMO 设置 & 监测 RPM 3500 BF 4.5 Pven -50 Part 190 SvO2 30 SaO2 160 70 37.0	· 泵速（RPM）：根据前负荷和后负荷产生 EBF，通过流量计以 LPM 读数显示 EBF · 扫气流量（SGF）或新鲜气体流量（FGF）：气体流向膜肺（ML）的流量，以 LPM 读数 · 设备氧分数（FdO₂）或扫气中的氧分数（FsO₂）：SGF 的氧分数（0.21～1），由气体/氧气混合器或气体调节器控制 · Pinlet：在离心泵入口处的负压 · 路也存在负压 · P_pre（或 P_静脉）：在 ML 入口处的正压 · P_post（或 P_动脉）：在 ML 出口处的正压，P_post < P_pre · ΔP：ML 入口/出口之间的压力梯度，计算为 ΔP = P_pre − P_post。ΔP/EBF 表示 ML 阻力 · S_pre O₂：在 ML 入口处的氧饱和度 · S_post O₂：在 ML 出口处的氧饱和度
引流不足	· 引流不足或引流失败是在血液经引流导管时，出现了血流不足与导管压力的不匹配，这可能是由于过度血管内负压（和）回流不足引起。ECMO 导管周围血流与导管开孔部分堵塞，暂时性血流阻塞，出现了血流量与 ECMO 流量的不匹配，从而出现 ECMO 导管的振动或摆动（"抖管"） 鉴别诊断 · 绝对/相对低血容量状态 · 增加的 IBP 或 CVP（张力性气胸、心包填塞，AIH） · 咳嗽，人-机对抗和躁动 · ECMO 导管的阻塞	气体进入	气体可能进入 ECMO 循环，产生微小气泡甚至气泡至导致离心泵失压的大规模气体栓塞，进而形成"气锁"。如果在循环的负压侧发生任何断开或静脉导管的开放端口，大气中的空气可能被吸入。此外，如果血液暴露于过度负压下，还可能产生气泡

续表

再循环	高度氧合的血液从回流管返回至机体[在ECMO中被称为再循环分数(RF)=再循环血流(RBF)/体外血流(EBF)]，RF升高不利于气体交换，导致体外循环的效率降低。如果旋转泵速度增加且导管道之间的距离氧减少，可使RF增高，引流导管中的血液颜色（富氧血的颜色）与回流导管中的血液颜色（较红的血液）看起来很相似	泵故障发生在离心泵(CP)无法提供EBF时：EBF的缺失导致支持丧失。CP可能因涉及泵头的并发症（脱落、血栓形成或大量空气栓塞）或涉及泵控制、驱动单元的问题（电源丧失和电池耗尽、电子/机械故障）而失败
回流受阻	由于出口端对离心泵的阻力的（如凝血）或外在的（如管路弯曲、压缩、张力性气胸或胸迫）阻力可能是内在的，增加了 $\triangle P$（膜肺内部的压差）。回流阻碍损害了 EBF 对体外生命体质(ECLS)的效率	凝血块/血栓和纤维蛋白沉积的渐进或急性形成减少了 ML 内用于体外气体交换的可用面积，损害凝血合/二氧化碳清除的效果。凝血块、血纤维蛋白可通过亮光照射膜肺发现（"手电筒测试"）。由于更高的阻力影响EBF：P_{pre} 减少而 P_{post} 增加了 $\triangle P$。此外，如果 ML 内部有广泛的血栓形成，可能会出现系统性凝血或溶血
管路断裂	管路断裂：如果发生在泵前，会导致失血。体外循环的任何组件的空气进入；如果发生在泵后，空气进入循环系统中断都需要紧急停止ECMO以防止进一步的空气进人/失血，并处理管路破裂/更换组件；否则，ECLS将会突然中断	任何影响提供FGF到ML的气体管线问题（不适当的FGF/FdO₂设置、意外断开连接、气源耗尽）都会损害ML的气体交换功能。水分可能在气体内纤维内聚集，减少体外二氧化碳清除，需要定期清除（"吹膜"）
意外脱管	ECMO插管/接头的意外移除或显著位移 • 如果是引流导管，空气会通过导管进入循环系统 • 如果是回流导管，则会导致失血性休克。两种情况下，脱离部位都会发生血液丢失，意外脱管系统将会突然中断。急停止ECMO。体外生命支持系统将会突然中断	

ECMO，体外膜肺氧合；RPM，每分钟转速；CP(s)，离心泵；EBF，体外血流；FGF，新鲜气流量；ML，膜肺（人工肺）；SGF，换气流量；LPM，L/min；ECLS，体外生命支持；IAP，腹腔压；ITP，胸腔压；PTX，气胸；IAH，腹腔高压；V-V，静脉-静脉；RF，回流分数；RBF，回流血流量；CVL，中心静脉导管（见彩色插图）；FdO₂，设备氧浓度；FsO₂，换气浓度。
注意：关于如何预防、早期发现和处理ECLS的机械并发症和病理生理的详细讨论超出了本章的范围。

11.4 总结

ICU 护士照护进行机械通气的 ARF 或 ARDS 的危重症患者时，包括可能会进行的 PP 和 ECLS 治疗时，需要了解他们复杂需求的独特性，掌握病理生理学和治疗/支持策略的广泛知识、先进的技术技能，以及温柔的关怀技能，为这个人群及其家人提供最佳护理，从而有助于改善短期和长期的功能预后。

（陈珵，金珊珊 译）

参考文献

[1] Menk M, Estenssoro E, Sahetya SK, et al. Current and evolving standards of care for patients with ARDS. Intensive Care Med. 2020; 46(12): 2157-67. https://rdcu.be/cFuIk.

[2] Chanques G, Constantin JM, Devlin JW, et al. Analgesia and sedation in patients with ARDS. Intensive Care Med. 2020; 46(12): 2342-56. https://doi.org/10.1007/s00134-020-06307-9.

[3] Pandharipande P, Banerjee A, McGrane S, Ely EW. Liberation and animation for ventilated ICU patients: the ABCDE bundle for the back-end of critical care. Crit Care. 2010; 14(3): 157. https://doi.org/10.1186/cc8999.

[4] Balas MC, Vasilevskis EE, Burke WJ, et al. Critical care nurses' role in implementing the "ABCDE bundle" into practice. Crit Care Nurse. 2012; 32(2): 35-8, 40-7; quiz 48. https://doi.org/10.4037/ccn2012229.

[5] Mart MF, Pun BT, Pandharipande P, Jackson JC, Ely EW. ICU survivorship-the relationship of delirium, sedation, dementia, and acquired weakness. Crit Care Med. 2021; 49(8): 1227-40. https://doi.org/10.1097/CCM.0000000000005125.

[6] Chanques G, Jaber S, Barbotte E, Violet S, Sebbane M, Perrigault PF, Mann C, Lefrant JY, Eledjam JJ. Impact of systematic evaluation of pain and agitation in an intensive care unit. Crit Care Med. 2006; 34(6): 1691-9. https://doi.org/10.1097/01.CCM.0000218416.62457.56.

[7] Ely EW, Inouye SK, Bernard GR, et al. Delirium in mechanically ventilated patients: validity and reliability of the confusion assessment method for the intensive care unit (CAM-ICU). JAMA. 2001; 286(21): 2703-10. https://doi.org/10.1001/jama.286.21.2703.

[8] Hodgson CL, Stiller K, Needham DM, et al. Expert consensus and recommendations on safety criteria for active mobilization of mechanically ventilated critically ill adults. Crit Care. 2014; 18(6): 658. https://doi.org/10.1186/s13054-014-0658-y.

[9] Kentish-Barnes N, Degos P, Viau C, Pochard F, Azoulay E. "It was a nightmare until I saw my wife": the importance of family presence for patients with COVID-19 hospitalized in the ICU. Intensive Care Med. 2021; 47(7): 792-4. https://doi.org/10.1007/s00134-021-06411-4.

[10] Van Rompaey B, Elseviers MM, Schuurmans MJ, Shortridge-Baggett LM, Truijen S, Bossaert L. Risk factors for delirium in intensive care patients: a prospective cohort study. Crit Care. 2009; 13(3): R77. https://doi.org/10.1186/cc7892.

[11] Naef R, Brysiewicz P, Mc Andrew NS, et al. Intensive care nurse-family engagement from a global perspective: a qualitative multi-site exploration. Intensive Crit Care Nurs. 2021 Oct; 66: 103081. https://doi.org/10.1016/j.iccn.2021.103081.

[12] Ceballos K, Waterman K, Hulett T, Makic MB. Nurse-driven quality improvement interventions to reduce hospital-acquired infection in the NICU. Adv Neonatal Care. 2013; 13(3): 154–63. ; quiz 164–5. https://doi.org/10.1097/ANC.0b013e318285fe70.

[13] Ista E, van der Hoven B, Kornelisse RF, et al. Effectiveness of insertion and maintenance bundles to prevent central-line-associated bloodstream infections in critically ill patients of all ages: a systematic review and meta-analysis. Lancet Infect Dis. 2016; 16(6): 724–34. https://doi.org/10.1016/S1473-3099(15)00409-0.

[14] Sampathkumar P. Reducing catheter-associated urinary tract infections in the ICU. Curr Opin Crit Care. 2017; 23(5): 372–7. https://doi.org/10.1097/MCC.0000000000000441.

[15] Singer P, Blaser AR, Berger MM, et al. ESPEN guideline on clinical nutrition in the intensive care unit. Clin Nutr. 2019; 38(1): 48–79. https://doi.org/10.1016/j.clnu.2018.08.037.

[16] Guérin C, Reignier J, Richard JC, et al. Prone positioning in severe acute respiratory distress syndrome. N Engl J Med. 2013; 368(23): 2159–68. https://doi.org/10.1056/NEJMoa1214103.

[17] Guérin C, Albert RK, Beitler J, et al. Prone position in ARDS patients: why, when, how and for whom. Intensive Care Med. 2020; 46(12): 2385–96.

[18] Lucchini A, Bambi S, Mattiussi E, et al. Prone position in acute respiratory distress syndrome patients: a retrospective analysis of complications. Dimens Crit Care Nurs. 2020; 39(1): 39–46.

[19] Bamford P, Denmade C, Newmarch C, et al on Behalf of the Intensive Care Society and Faculty of Intensive Care Medicine. Guidance for: prone positioning in adult critical care. 2019. Available at https://www.ics.ac.uk/ICU/Guidance/PDFs/Prone_Position_Guidance_in_Adult_Critical_Care. Accessed Aug 2021.

[20] Montanaro J. Using in situ simulation to develop a prone positioning protocol for patients with ARDS. Crit Care Nurse. 2020 Nov; 23: e1–e13.

[21] Short B, Parekh M, Ryan P, et al. Rapid implementation of a mobile prone team during the COVID-19 pandemic. J Crit Care. 2020; 60: 230–4.

[22] Jové Ponseti E, Villarrasa Millán A, Ortiz CD. Analysis of complications of prone position in acute respiratory distress syndrome: quality standard, incidence and related factors. Enferm Intensiva. 2017; 28(3): 125–34.

[23] Munshi L, Del Sorbo L, Adhikari NKJ, et al. Prone position for acute respiratory distress syndrome. A systematic review and meta-analysis. Ann Am Thorac Soc. 2017; 14(Supplement_4): S280–8.

[24] Binda F, Galazzi A, Marelli F, et al. Complications of prone positioning in patients with COVID-19: a cross-sectional study. Intensive Crit Care Nurs. 2021; 1: 103088.

[25] Rodríguez-Huerta MD, Díez-Fernández A, Rodríguez-Alonso MJ, Robles-González M, Martín-Rodríguez M, González-García A. Nursing care and prevalence of adverse events in prone position: characteristics of mechanically ventilated patients with severe SARS-CoV-2 pulmonary infection. Nurs Crit Care. 2021; https://doi.org/10.1111/nicc.12606.

[26] Douglas IS, Rosenthal CA, Swanson DD, et al. Safety and outcomes of prolonged usual care prone position mechanical ventilation to treat acute coronavirus disease 2019 hypoxemic respiratory failure. Crit Care Med. 2021; 49(3): 490–502.

[27] Alshahrani B, Sim J, Middleton R. Nursing interventions for pressure injury prevention among critically ill patients: a systematic review. J Clin Nurs. 2021; 30(15–16): 2151–68.

[28] Bruni A, Garofalo E, Grande L, et al. Nursing issues in enteral nutrition during prone position in critically ill patients: a systematic review of the literature. Intensive Crit Care Nurs. 2020;

60: 102899.

[29] Bruni A, Garofalo E, Longhini F. Avoiding complications during prone position ventilation. Intensive Crit Care Nurs. 2021; 66: 103064.

[30] Dalia AA, Ortoleva J, Fiedler A, Villavicencio M, Shelton K, Cudemus GD. Extracorporeal membrane oxygenation is a team sport: institutional survival benefits of a formalized ECMO team. J Cardiothorac Vasc Anesth. 2019; 33(4): 902-7.

[31] Combes A, Schmidt M, Hodgson CL, et al. Extracorporeal life support for adults with acute respiratory distress syndrome. Intensive Care Med. 2020; 46(12): 2464-76.

[32] Daly KJ, Camporota L, Barrett NA. An international survey: the role of specialist nurses in adult respiratory extracorporeal membrane oxygenation. Nurs Crit Care. 2017 Sep; 22(5): 305-11.

[33] ELSO. Guidelines for training and continuing education of ECMO specialists version 1.5. 2010. Available at https://www.elso.org/Resources/Guidelines.aspx. Accessed Aug 2021.

[34] Alshammari MA, Vellolikalam C, Alfeeli S. Nurses' perception of their role in extracorporeal membrane oxygenation care: a qualitative assessment. Nurs Crit Care. 2020; https://doi.org/10.1111/nicc.12538.

[35] Combes A, Brodie D, Bartlett R, et al. International ECMO Network (ECMONet). Position paper for the organization of extracorporeal membrane oxygenation programs for acute respiratory failure in adult patients. Am J Respir Crit Care Med. 2014; 190(5): 488-96.

[36] ELSO. Guidelines for ECMO centers version 1.8. 2014. Available at https://www.elso.org/Resources/Guidelines.aspx. Accessed Aug 2021.

[37] Van Kiersbilck C, Gordon E, Morris D. Ten things that nurses should know about ECMO. Intensive Care Med. 2016; 42(5): 753-5.

[38] Hamed A, Alinier G, Hassan IF. The ECMO specialist's role in troubleshooting ECMO emergencies. Egyptian J Crit Care Med. 2018; 6: 91-3.

[39] Zakhary B, Shekar K, Diaz R, et al. Extracorporeal Life Support Organization (ELSO) ECMOed Taskforce. Position paper on global extracorporeal membrane oxygenation education and educational agenda for the future: a statement from the extracorporeal life support organization ECMOed taskforce. Crit Care Med. 2020; 48(3): 406-14.

[40] Fouilloux V, Gran C, Guervilly C, Breaud J, El Louali F, Rostini P. Impact of education and training course for ECMO patients based on high-fidelity simulation: a pilot study dedicated to ICU nurses. Perfusion. 2019; 34(1): 29-34.

[41] Redaelli S, Zanella A, Milan M, Isgrò S, Lucchini A, Pesenti A, Patroniti N. Daily nursing care on patients undergoing venous-venous extracorporeal membrane oxygenation: a challenging procedure! J Artif Organs. 2016; 19(4): 343-9.

[42] Lucchini A, Bambi S, de Felippis C, et al. Oral care protocols with specialty training lead to safe oral care practices and reduce iatrogenic bleeding in extracorporeal membrane oxygenation patients. Dimens Crit Care Nurs. 2018; 37(6): 285-93.

[43] Murphy DA, Hockings LE, Andrews RK, et al. Extracorporeal membrane oxygenation-hemostatic complications. Transfus Med Rev. 2015; 29(2): 90-101.

[44] Giani M, Martucci G, Madotto F, et al. Prone positioning during venovenous extracorporeal membrane oxygenation in acute respiratory distress syndrome. A multicenter cohort study and propensity-matched analysis. Ann Am Thorac Soc. 2021; 18(3): 495-501.

[45] Abrams D, Javidfar J, Farrand E, Mongero LB, Agerstrand CL, Ryan P, Zemmel D, Galuskin K, Morrone TM, Boerem P, Bacchetta M, Brodie D. Early mobilization of patients receiving

extracorporeal membrane oxygenation: a retrospective cohort study. Crit Care. 2014; 18(1): R38.

[46] Culbreth RE, Goodfellow LT. Complications of prone positioning during extracorporeal membrane oxygenation for respiratory failure: a systematic review. Respir Care. 2016; 61(2): 249-54.

12 闭环通气模式

Closed-Loop Ventilation Modes

Jean-Michel Arnal, Dirk Schaedler, Cenk Kirakli

12.1 引言

"闭环通气模式"是指可根据一个或多个反馈信号自动调整呼吸机的某些设置的模式。常规操作原则如下：呼吸机测量患者的某些生理变量，将其与用户设置的相应目标进行比较，然后自动调整某些呼吸机设置来降低实际值与目标值之间的差异（负反馈）。输入控制器的生理变量必须是一种在所有类型的患者中均可靠、易于测量、廉价且尽可能是可通过非侵入性设备检测的变量。通常在几次呼吸中测量它们并取平均值，以避免异常值的影响。目标值可以由用户设置或由算法确定，其可以是固定值也可以根据某些条件而变化。呼吸机设置的自动调整是逐步进行的，可以逐个呼吸调整，也可以经过多次呼吸逐渐调整。使用闭环通气模式时，临床医生需设置生理目标值，而不是具体的呼吸机参数，这需要不同的知识和思维方式。闭环通气模式的监测与传统模式下是类似的，但提供了有关患者病情动态变化的额外信息。通气支持可持续适应患者的呼吸力学、自主活动和做功的变化，有潜在益处。这可能会使患者维持在最佳通气和氧合范围内的时间更多，并提供足够的通气支持，从而降低呼吸机相关肺损伤、人-机不同步，以及辅助过度或不足所带来的风险。最终，机械通气的持续时间和病死率等临床结果可能会得到改善。这种

J.-M. Arnal (✉)
Service de Réanimation, Hôpital Sainte Musse, Toulon, France
Medical Research and New Technologies, Hamilton Medical AG, Bonaduz, Switzerland
e-mail: jean-michel@arnal.org

D. Schaedler
Department of Anesthesiology and Intensive Care Medicine, University Medical Center Schleswig-Holstein, Kiel, Germany

C. Kirakli
Intensive Care Unit, Dr. Suat Seren Chest Diseases and Surgery Training and Research Center, University of Health Sciences, Izmir, Turkey

© The Author(s), under exclusive license to Springer Nature Switzerland AG 2022
G. Bellani (ed.), *Mechanical Ventilation from Pathophysiology to Clinical Evidence*, https://doi.org/10.1007/978-3-030-93401-9_12

通气模式的潜在风险在于若培训和经验不足，可导致设定的目标不恰当、监测不充分。

强制每分钟通气（mandatory minute ventilation，MMV）、自适应支持通气（adaptive support ventilation，ASV）、INTELLiVENT-ASV 和 Smartcare/PS 都是目前市面上可用的闭环通气模式，将在本章中详细解释。

12.2 强制每分钟通气

MMV 是 1977 年首次报道的闭环模式，旨在克服间歇性强制通气的某些无效特征[1]。MMV 是一种压力支持模式，可保证用户设定的目标每分钟通气量。如果患者的自主通气没有达到目标每分钟通气量，呼吸机要么增加压力支持（pressure support，PS）水平，要么增加强制性呼吸，具体取决于生产厂商的设置。相反，当患者的自主通气量超过目标每分钟通气量时，呼吸机会降低压力支持。目前仅少数呼吸机提供 MMV 且很少使用。主要风险是目标每分钟通气量可以通过非常大的潮气量（tidal volume, V_T）来实现，会带来肺损伤的风险；或者通过非常低的潮气量结合高呼吸频率（respiratory rate，RR）来实现，可能导致无效腔通气和辅助不足。到目前为止，强制每分钟通气在协助撤机方面的价值尚不清楚[2]。

12.3 Smartcare/PS

12.3.1 操作原理

Smartcare/PS 可在压力支持通气模式下控制 PS 水平。系统不会更改其他呼吸机设置。启动 Smartcare/PS 需要一些先决条件（如启用 $EtCO_2$ 监测，PEEP 在 5~20 cmH_2O 之间，开启窒息后备通气）。启动后，Smartcare/PS 会尝试将患者带入所谓的呼吸舒适区，并使其保持在该区域。这意味着 PS 水平能维持大于 300 mL 的最小潮气量，呼气末二氧化碳分压（end-tidal partial pressure of CO_2，$PetCO_2$）低于 55 mmHg，自主 RR 在每分钟 15~30 次之间。一旦患者稳定在舒适区，压力支持会逐步降低到目标 PS。目标 PS 取决于人工气道、使用的加湿系统，以及是否启用自动管道补偿。Smartcare/PS 降低 PS 的速度取决于实际的 PS 值。PS 值越高，降低速度越慢，反之亦然。如果患者在目标 PS 上仍然稳定，并且没有超过用户定义的吸入氧浓度（inspired oxygen，FiO_2）和 PEEP 的限制，Smartcare/PS 将自动进行自主呼吸试验（spontaneous breathing trial，SBT）。如果 SBT 成功完成，Smartcare/PS 会在呼吸机屏幕上显示一条消息，建议将患者与呼吸机断开[3]。

12.3.2 监测

在 Smartcare/PS 中监控撤机过程是非常重要的。根据我们的经验，我们建议在呼吸机上设置一个特殊的智能管理界面，显示撤机诊断和 PS 水平的图表。该页面可供临床医生查房时使用,以了解过去几个小时或几天撤机的整体情况(图 12.1)。此外,许多 Smartcare/PS 细节可以被传输到患者数据管理系统(patient data management system, PDMS)。在 PDMS 的一个特殊撤机页面上,可以通过整合更多的撤机变量(如镇静评分、营养、活动能力)来更容易地评估整个撤机过程。

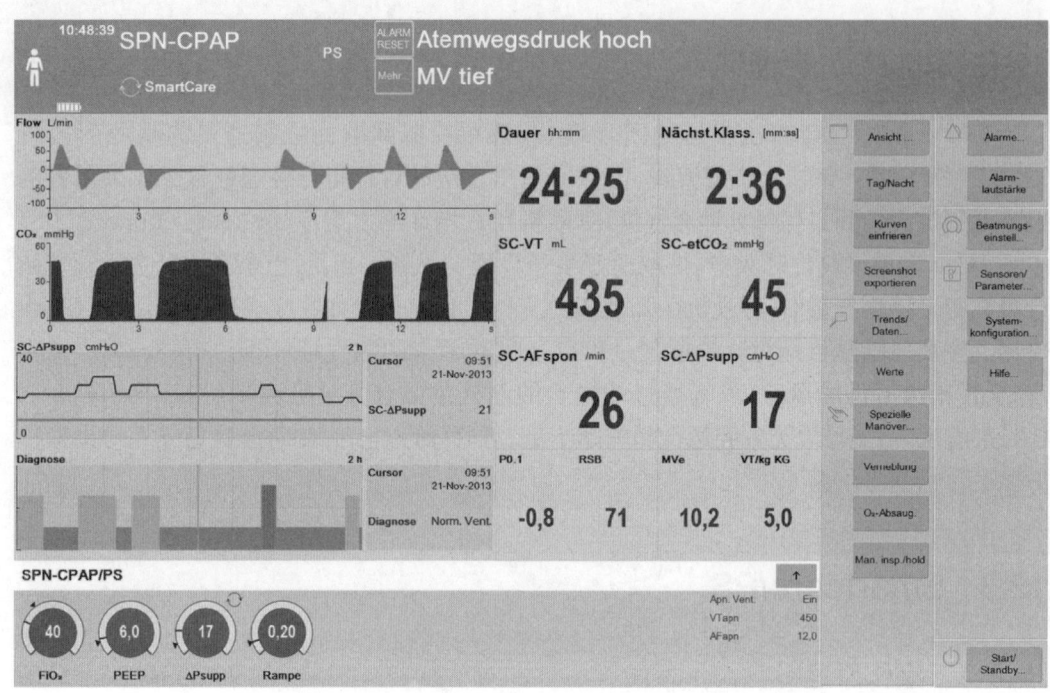

图 12.1　V500 呼吸机特殊撤机页面示例(Dräger)

12.3.3　临床证据

在一项针对 5 家欧洲大学医院的多中心随机对照试验中,Lellouche 等将 Smartcare/PS 与常规通气模式进行了比较,其中 5 家研究单位采用的常规通气模式各不相同。Smartcare/PS 组的通气时间明显低于对照组(分别为 7.5 天和 12 天,$P = 0.003$)[4]。受这一结果启发,Schädler 等进行了一项纳入 300 名患者的单中心随机对照研究。与 Lellouche 等的研究不同的是,对照组采用了标准化撤机方案。在总通气时间方面,两组之间没有发现显著差异($P = 0.178$)[5]。同样,两项较小的单中心研究[6,7]和一项多中心随机对照试验的初步结果[8]都没有检测到通气时间存在显著差异。然而,几项荟萃分析显示自动撤机对通气时间有好处(尤其是 Smartcare/PS)[9,10]。最近的一项贝叶斯网络荟萃分析明确显示,无论使用何种技术,自动撤机模式都会缩短通气时间[11]。

总之,使用 Smartcare/PS 撤机至少与标准的黄金撤机方案同样有效。进一步的发展应该改善该系统的实用性(复杂的设置,Smartcare/PS 停止后的自动重启)和技术(整合肺生理模型信息、自动控制其他呼吸机参数)。此外,自动撤机系统应与 PDMS 相结合,可更好地获取患者的医疗信息(如血气分析、影像学资料、医疗诊断),并在整个撤机过程中获得更好的支持。

12.4 自适应支持通气

自适应支持通气(ASV)是一种闭环通气模式,其结合了对被动患者实施自适应压力控制通气和对自主呼吸患者实施适应性压力支持通气。这种模式的优点是优化了患者的呼吸做功和呼吸力,减少了ICU人员的工作负荷,提高患者的安全性和舒适性。

12.4.1 操作原理

ASV算法最初基于Otis方程[12]计算的最小呼吸做功,后来根据Mead方程[13,14]进行了修改,引入了最小呼吸力。ASV通过逐次测量呼气时间常数(expiratory time constant,RCexp)来评估患者的呼吸力学,然后为由临床医生设定的任何每分钟通气目标量确定V_T-RR组合,目标是最大限度地减少呼吸做功和呼吸力(图12.2)。因此,ASV在限制性疾病中自动选择低潮气量和高呼吸频率,而在阻塞性疾病中则相反。在主动呼吸的患者中,它提供呼吸压力支持并调整PS以达到最佳V_T。所以随着患者努力的增加,PS会自动降低,为撤机做准备。

12.4.2 设置和监测

初始设置和调整(被动呼吸患者):
(1) 目标每分钟通气量,以理想体重(ideal body weight,IBW)的百分比表示(最小通气量%):设定为100%,相当于100 mL/(kg·min)。
(2) 压力限制:设定为30 cm H_2O(严重阻塞性疾病可能会增加)。
(3) PEEP和FiO_2:根据脉搏氧饱和度(SpO_2)或动脉氧分压(arterial partial pressure in oxygen,PaO_2)手动设置。
(4) 必须根据$PaCO_2$以10%为单位调整最小通气量%。

初始设置和调整(自主呼吸患者):
(1) 最小通气量%:设置为100%。
(2) 压力限制:设定为30 cmH_2O(严重阻塞性疾病可能会增加)。
(3) PEEP和FiO_2:需要根据SpO_2或PaO_2进行手动设置。
(4) 必须根据患者的呼吸做功和RR以20%为单位调整最小通气量%。

必须监测呼吸力学,如RCexp、顺应性和阻力,以了解潜在的病理进程并相应地调整通气策略。除了V_T(IBW),还必须密切监测峰压和平台压、驱动压和PS水平,以避免呼吸机相关肺损伤。

12.4.3 撤机

如果患者达到可接受的PEEP和FiO_2水平并准备撤机,则将最小通气量%设置为

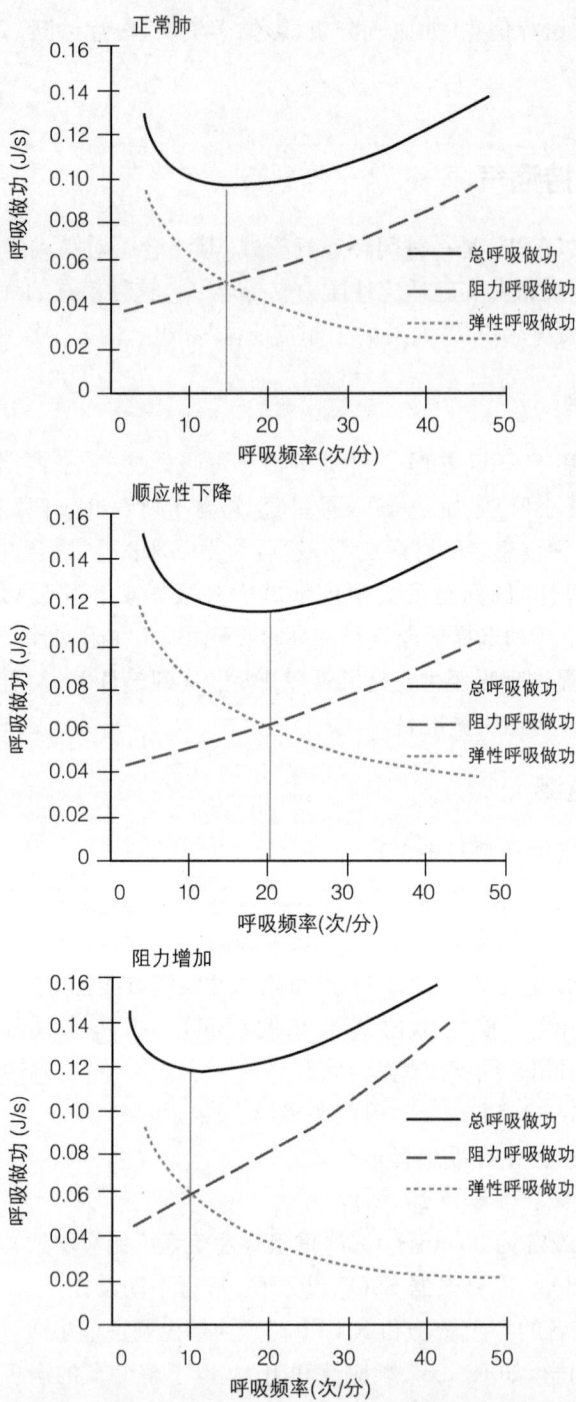

图 12.2 根据 Otis 方程，对于给定的每分钟通气量，总呼吸做功是阻力呼吸做功和弹性呼吸做功的总和，并且取决于 U 形的呼吸频率。ASV 选择与最小总呼吸做功相关的呼吸频率。与正常肺部状况相比，这种最佳呼吸频率在顺应性下降的情况下更高，在阻力增加的情况下更低

25%进行 SBT。如果试验结束时（30 分钟至 2 小时）PS 水平可接受（低于 10～12 cmH$_2$O）并且没有其他禁忌证，医生应考虑拔管。

12.4.4 临床证据

某些研究调查了 ASV 在内科、外科和神经 ICU 中被动和主动呼吸患者中相较于传统模式的优势，结果显示撤机过程或整个通气时间缩短[15-19]。还有一些证据表明，与传统通气模式相比，ASV 可以选择个体化的 V_T - RR 组合，并降低患者的代谢负荷和机械能[20-22]。目前有正在进行临床试验研究 ASV 对 ARDS 患者和儿科患者的作用（NCT03715751，NCT03930147）。

12.5 INTELLiVENT - ASV

INTELLiVENT - ASV 是基于 ASV 发展的模式，它可以全自动控制被动和自主呼吸患者的通气和氧合设置，可根据患者呼吸力学、自主活动和吸气努力以及氧合需求的变化进行调整。INTELLiVENT - ASV 同样包含自动撤机流程。

12.5.1 工作原理

在被动呼吸患者的通气支持方面，INTELLiVENT - ASV 根据测量的 PetCO$_2$ 与用户设置的目标 PetCO$_2$ 之间的差异自动设置目标每分钟通气量。对于自主呼吸患者，INTELLiVENT - ASV 根据患者的实际 RR 和 ASV 算法确定的最佳 RR 目标范围之间的差异自动设置目标每分钟通气量。一旦建定了目标每分钟通气量，ASV 控制器就选择 V_T 和 RR 的最佳组合，然后在被动呼吸患者中进行自适应压力控制通气，或在自主呼吸患者中进行自适应压力支持呼吸（图 12.3）。

在氧合支持方面，INTELLiVENT - ASV 根据测量的 SpO$_2$ 与用户设定的目标 SpO$_2$ 之间的差异自动调整 PEEP 和 FiO$_2$。氧合控制器对被动和自主呼吸的患者使用相同的规则。PEEP 和 FiO$_2$ 的调整是根据 PEEP - FiO$_2$ 表进行的，NIH 的低和高 PEEP - FiO$_2$ 表分别用于增加和减少支持水平时[23,24]。

12.5.2 设置和监测

初始设置包括激活控制器、选择患者的病情，以及设置 PetCO$_2$ 和 SpO$_2$ 目标。根据所选的患者病情（正常、急性呼吸窘迫综合征、慢性高碳酸血症或脑损伤），呼吸机建议适用于该病情的默认目标范围。当然，用户可以选择更改这些目标。用户还需要设置最大峰压、最小 FiO$_2$ 和 PEEP 的范围。最后，与任何闭环模式一样，正确设置警报至关重要，以确保在发生突发事件时向用户发出警报。

对于被动呼吸患者，监测呼吸力学（顺应性、阻力和 RCexp）有助于了解患者肺部的情况，而对 V_T(IBW)、平台压、总 PEEP 和驱动压的监测可确保所提供的通气符合保护性通气策略的要求。在氧合方面，SpO$_2$ 不能提供额外的作用，因为它是一个目标值，通常应设

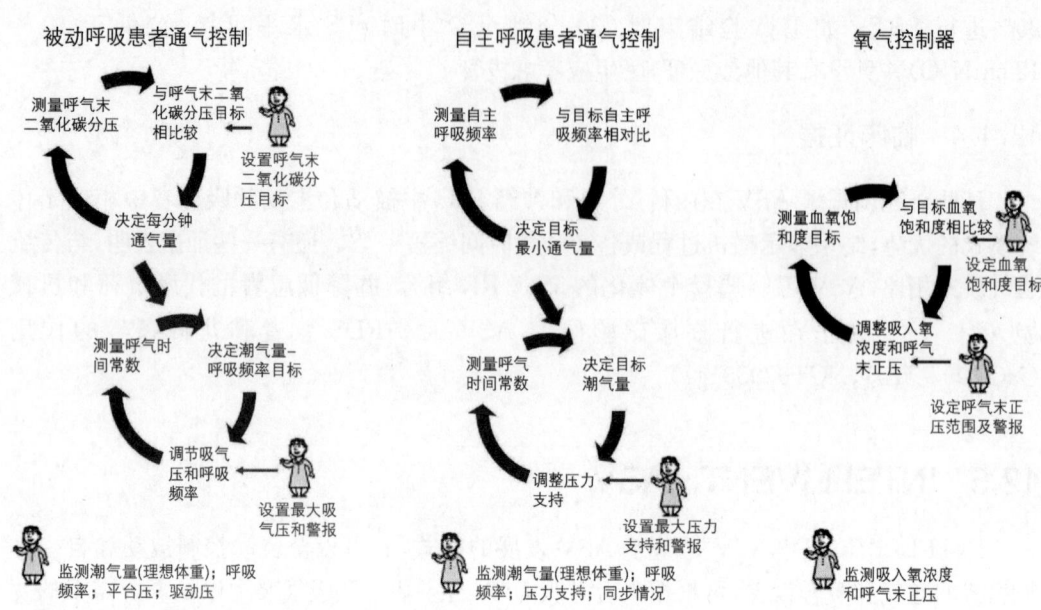

图 12.3 INTELLiVENT-ASV 的工作原理。第一个控制器确定目标每分钟通气量,然后 ASV 控制器选择吸气压力和呼吸频率

置一定的目标范围,而 FiO_2 和 PEEP 是需要监测的因变量。

12.5.3 撤机

INTELLiVENT-ASV 有一个名为快速撤机(Quick Wean)的自动撤机流程,当患者有稳定的自主呼吸时必须由操作者启动。一旦启动,呼吸机会逐渐降低 PS,并进行撤机标准的筛选。当在一定时间内达到撤机标准时,呼吸机通过减少 PEEP 和 PS 切换到自动撤机试验。撤机试验受到密切监测,如果某些变量超出目标范围,可以随时中止。相反,如果撤机试验在给定的持续时间后成功,它将自动停止,并会显示相关消息。然后由临床医生进行拔管标准筛选。撤机试验的设置、持续时间,以及开始和中止的所有标准都可以由用户自行设定。

12.5.4 临床证据

自 2010 年以来,INTELLiVENT-ASV 已应用于某些 Hamilton Medical 呼吸机。有几项研究已经在 ICU 和心脏手术后的被动和自主呼吸患者中测试了其与传统模式相比的有效性和安全性[25,29]。根据对不同时长不同通气形式呼吸的逐次分析,INTELLiVENT-ASV 维持在理想范围的时间与传统模式相同或更高,这表明其具有可靠的疗效和安全性。可行性研究表明,它可用于大多数 ICU 和心脏手术后患者且失败率极低,还可用于严重的新型冠状病毒感染 ARDS 患者[29,30]。初步数据显示,这种通气模式在缩短通气时间方面有很好的效果[28,30,31],但迄今为止还没有针对性大型随机对照试验的结果来证实,目前有一项大型多中心随机对照试验(NCT04593810)正在进行中。有研究表明,与传统通气模式相比,使用 INTELLiVENT - ASV 时可以减少手动设置呼吸机的次数,这意味着医护人员的工作负荷下降[26,27,30-32]。

12.6 总结

这几种闭环通气模式可用于 ICU 的机械通气患者。所有这些模式都是基于生理学知识的算法。重要的是,临床医生要充分理解其自动调整的"原因",以便正确设定目标,充分监测患者,并有效地使用该工具及时做出医疗决策。初步研究表明,这些模式能提供持续的肺保护性通气并有可能减少通气时间,还能最小化呼吸机相关损伤的风险,然而还需要进一步的证据来充分评估其价值。这些模式在未来可能会整合机器学习和人工智能,以进一步提高机械通气的安全性和个体化。

(陈珵,金珊珊 译)

参考文献

[1] Hewlett AM, Platt AS, Terry VG. Mandatory minute volume. Anaesthesia. 1977;32:163-9. https://doi.org/10.1111/j.1365-2044.1977.tb11588.x.

[2] Davis S, Potgieter PD, Linton DM. Mandatory minute volume weaning in patients with pulmonary pathology. Anaesth Intensive Care. 1989;17:170-4. https://doi.org/10.1177/0310057X8901700208.

[3] Dojat M, Brochard L, Lemaire F, Harf A. A knowledge-based system for assisted ventilation of patients in intensive care units. Int J Clin Monit Comput. 1992;9:239-50. https://doi.org/10.1007/BF01133619.

[4] Lellouche F, Mancebo J, Jolliet P, Roeseler J, Schortgen F, Dojat M, et al. A multicenter randomized trial of computer-driven protocolized weaning from mechanical ventilation. Am J Respir Crit Care Med. 2006;174:894-900. https://doi.org/10.1164/rccm.200511-1780OC.

[5] Schädler D, Engel C, Elke G, Pulletz S, Haake N, Frerichs I, et al. Automatic control of pressure support for ventilator weaning in surgical intensive care patients. Am J Respir Crit Care Med. 2012;185:637-44. https://doi.org/10.1164/rccm.201106-1127OC.

[6] Rose L, Presneill JJ, Johnston L, Cade JF. A randomised, controlled trial of conventional versus automated weaning from mechanical ventilation using SmartCare/PS. Intensive Care Med. 2008;34:1788-95. https://doi.org/10.1007/s00134-008-1179-4.

[7] Stahl C, Dahmen G, Ziegler A, Muhl E. Comparison of automated protocol-based versus non-protocol-based physician-directed weaning from mechanical ventilation. Intensivmed. 2009;46:441-6.

[8] Burns KE, Meade MO, Lessard MR, Hand L, Zhou Q, Keenan SP, et al. Wean earlier and automatically with new technology (the WEAN study). A multicenter, pilot randomized controlled trial. Am J Respir Crit Care Med. 2013;187:1203-11. https://doi.org/10.1164/rccm.201206-1026OC.

[9] Burns KE, Lellouche F, Nisenbaum R, Lessard MR, Friedrich JO. Automated weaning and SBT systems versus non-automated weaning strategies for weaning time in invasively ventilated

critically ill adults. Cochrane Database Syst Rev. 2014; 2014: CD008638. https://doi.org/10.1002/14651858.CD008638.pub2.

[10] Rose L, Schultz MJ, Cardwell CR, Jouvet P, McAuley DF, Blackwood B. Automated versus non-automated weaning for reducing the duration of mechanical ventilation for critically ill adults and children. Cochrane Database Syst Rev. 2014; 2014: CD009235. https://doi.org/10.1002/14651858.CD009235.pub3.

[11] Neuschwander A, Chhor V, Yavchitz A, Resche-Rigon M, Pirracchio R. Automated weaning from mechanical ventilation: results of a Bayesian network meta-analysis. J Crit Care. 2021; 61: 191-8. https://doi.org/10.1016/j.jcrc.2020.10.025.

[12] Otis AB, Fenn WO, Rahn H. Mechanics of breathing in man. J Appl Physiol. 1950; 2: 592-607. https://doi.org/10.1152/jappl.1950.2.11.592.

[13] Mead J. The control of the respiratory frequency. Ann N Y Acad Sci. 1963; 109: 724-9. https://doi.org/10.1111/j.1749-6632.1963.tb13500.x.

[14] Ceylan G, Topal S, Atakul G, Colak M, Soydan E, Sandal O, et al. Randomized crossover trial to compare driving pressures in a closed-loop and a conventional mechanical ventilation mode in pediatric patients. Pediatr Pulmonol. 2021; 56: 3035-43. https://doi.org/10.1002/ppul.25561.

[15] Kirakli C, Naz I, Ediboglu O, Tatar D, Budak A, Tellioglu E. A randomized controlled trial comparing the ventilation duration between adaptive support ventilation and pressure assist/control ventilation in medical patients in the ICU. Chest. 2015; 147: 1503-9. https://doi.org/10.1378/chest.14-2599.

[16] Kirakli C, Ozdemir I, Ucar ZZ, Cimen P, Kepil S, Ozkan SA. Adaptive support ventilation for faster weaning in COPD: a randomised controlled trial. Eur Respir J. 2011; 38: 774-80. https://doi.org/10.1183/09031936.00081510.

[17] Ghodrati M, Pournajafian A, Khatibi A, Niakan M, Hemadi MH, Zamani MM. Comparing the effect of adaptive support ventilation (ASV) and synchronized intermittent mandatory ventilation (SIMV) on respiratory parameters in neurosurgical ICU patients. Anesth Pain Med. 2016; 6: e40368. https://doi.org/10.5812/aapm.40368.

[18] Zhu F, Gomersall CD, Ng SK, Underwood MJ, Lee A. A randomized controlled trial of adaptive support ventilation mode to wean patients after fast-track cardiac valvular surgery. Anesthesiology. 2015; 122: 832-40. https://doi.org/10.1097/ALN.0000000000000589.

[19] Gruber PC, Gomersall CD, Leung P, Joynt GM, Ng SK, Ho KM, Underwood MJ. Randomized controlled trial comparing adaptive-support ventilation with pressure-regulated volume-controlled ventilation with automode in weaning patients after cardiac surgery. Anesthesiology. 2008; 109: 81-7. https://doi.org/10.1097/ALN.0b013e31817881fc.

[20] Arnal JM, Wysocki M, Nafati C, Donati S, Granier I, Corno G, et al. Automatic selection of breathing pattern using adaptive support ventilation. Intensive Care Med. 2008; 34: 75-81. https://doi.org/10.1007/s00134-007-0847-0.

[21] Chen YH, Hsiao HF, Hsu HW, Cho HY, Huang CC. Comparisons of metabolic load between adaptive support ventilation and pressure support ventilation in mechanically ventilated ICU patients. Can Respir J. 2020;2020: 2092879. https://doi.org/10.1155/2020/2092879.

[22] Buiteman-Kruizinga LA, Mkadmi HE, Schultz MJ, Tangkau PL, van der Heiden PLJ. Comparison of mechanical power during adaptive support ventilation versus nonautomated pressure-controlled ventilation-a pilot study. Crit Care Explor. 2021;3: e0335. https://doi.org/

10.1097/CCE.0000000000000335.

[23] Acute Respiratory Distress Syndrome Network, Brower RG, Matthay MA, Morris A, Schoenfeld D, Thompson BT, Wheeler A. Ventilation with lower tidal volumes as compared with traditional tidal volumes for acute lung injury and the acute respiratory distress syndrome. N Engl J Med. 2000;342: 1301-8. https://doi.org/10.1056/NEJM200005043421801.

[24] Acute Respiratory Distress Syndrome Network. Higher versus lower positive end-expiratory pressures in patients with acute respiratory distress syndrome. N Engl J Med. 2004;351: 327-36. https://doi.org/10.1056/NEJMoa032193.

[25] Arnal JM, Wysocki M, Novotni D, Demory D, Donati D, Granier I, et al. Safety and efficacy of a fully closed-loop control ventilation (IntelliVent-ASV®) in sedated ICU patients with acute respiratory failure: a prospective randomized crossover study. Intensive Care Med. 2012;38: 781-7. https://doi.org/10.1007/s00134-012-2548-6.

[26] Lellouche F, Bouchard PA, Simard S, L'Her E, Wysocki M. Evaluation of fully automated ventilation: a randomized controlled study in post-cardiac surgery patients. Intensive Care Med. 2013;39: 463-71. https://doi.org/10.1007/s00134-012-2799-2.

[27] Bialais E, Wittebole X, Vignaux L, Roeseler J, Wysocki M, Meyer J, et al. Closed-loop ventilation mode (IntelliVent®-ASV) in intensive care unit: a randomized trial. Minerva Anestesiol. 2016;82: 657-68.

[28] Wendel Garcia PD, Hofmaenner DA, Brugger SD, Acevedo CT, Bartussek J, Camen G, et al. Closed-loop versus conventional mechanical ventilation in COVID-19 ARDS. J Intensive Care Med. 2021;36(10): 1184-93. https://doi.org/10.1177/08850666211024139.

[29] Arnal JM, Garnero A, Novotni D, Demory D, Ducros L, Berric A, et al. Feasibility study on full closed-loop control ventilation (IntelliVent-ASV) in ICU patients with acute respiratory failure: a prospective observational comparative study. Crit Care. 2013;17: R196. https://doi.org/10.1186/cc12890.

[30] Beijers AJ, Roos AN, Bindels AJ. Fully automated closed-loop ventilation is safe and effective in post-cardiac surgery patients. Intensive Care Med. 2014;40: 752-3. https://doi.org/10.1007/s00134-014-3234-7.

[31] Arnal JM, Garnero A, Novotni D, Corno G, Donati SY, Demory D, et al. Closed loop ventilation mode in intensive care unit: a randomized controlled clinical trial comparing the numbers of manual ventilator setting changes. Minerva Anestesiol. 2018;84: 58-67. https://doi.org/10.23736/S0375-9393.17.11963-2.

[32] Fot EV, Izotova NN, Yudina AS, Smetkin AA, Kuzkov VV, Kirov MY. Automated weaning from mechanical ventilation after off-pump coronary artery bypass grafting. Front Med (Lausanne). 2017;4: 31. https://doi.org/10.3389/fmed.2017.00031.

13 气道压力释放通气
Airway Pressure Release Ventilation

Niklas Larsson

13.1 引言

气道压力释放通气(airway pressure release ventilation，APRV)是一种基于时间周期、压力限制性的机械通气模式。该模式下可以实现无限制的自主通气，独立于机器控制的呼吸[1]。APRV 模式利用两种不同压力水平的持续气道正压通气(continuous positive airway pressure，CPAP)来实现。正如该模式的名称所示，具有较高压力水平的长时相被较低压力水平的短时相(压力释放)分隔开。由于机器传输的气道压力是连续的，患者可以在呼吸周期的任何部分自由自主呼吸。实际上，自主呼吸仅限于在较高压力期进行，因为患者在短暂的低压期会由于气道压力梯度而呼气。

APRV 中的呼吸机控制与其他通气模式不同，两个不同的压力水平，P-high 和 P-low，是独立设置的。T-high 和 T-low 为每个呼吸周期中设置的每个压力所持续的时间。这四个参数共同决定了驱动压、呼吸频率和吸呼比。正确的设置中需要把 T-low 设得足够短，以避免完全呼气，这样能保留适当的 autoPEEP；并且实际 PEEP 和机器控制的潮气量都主要来自时间参数 T-low，而不是设定的压力值。如果设置不正确，APRV 可以提供传统的压力控制通气模式，但这样的设置更难管理(图 13.1)。

13.2 生理学

从生理角度来看，APRV 与其他类型的机械通气有着根本的不同。APRV 并非通过压力的增加来进行相对较短的吸气，而是长时间保持肺部扩张。高压期被短暂的呼气打

N. Larsson (✉)
Council of Västerbotten, Anaesthesia and Intensive Care, Umeå, Sweden
e-mail: niklas.larsson@regionvasterbotten.se

© The Author(s), under exclusive license to Springer Nature Switzerland AG 2022
G. Bellani (ed.), *Mechanical Ventilation from Pathophysiology to Clinical Evidence*, https://doi.org/10.1007/978-3-030-93401-9_13

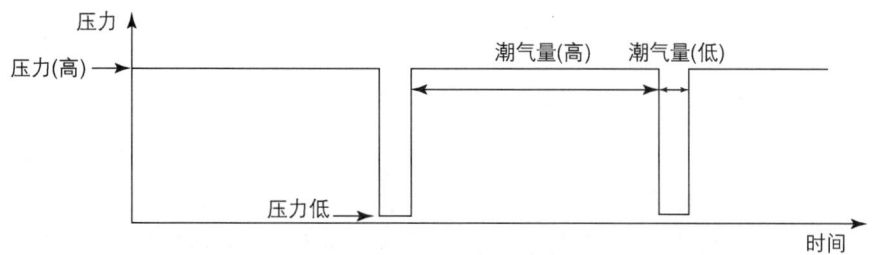

图 13.1 APRV 中的压力波形示意图。持续较长时间的高压期被短暂的压力释放期所隔断,以促进机械控制的呼吸。患者可以在整个机械呼吸周期中自由连续呼吸

断,然后随着高压水平的恢复立即吸气[2]。长时间保持肺膨胀可使不张的肺组织复张,并允许气体在无效腔和肺泡腔之间扩散[3-5]。随着扩散后有效的气体交换,优化 APRV 设置的患者由于肺泡通气改善从而可促进 CO_2 的排出[6]。这可能会起到肺保护的作用,因为较好的肺泡通气降低了呼吸机诱导肺损伤(ventilator induced lung injury,VILI)的可能性[7]。动物实验表明,APRV 可能通过减少肺的去复张和优化通气肺泡形态保持肺部结构的均一性,起到肺保护作用[8,9]。

13.3 指征

APRV 可以显著改善严重低氧血症患者的氧合[6,10,11]。APRV 对于患者预后的作用仍未得到证实[10,12]。与低潮气量通气相比,APRV 已被证实可以改善氧合并缩短 ICU 住院时间[13]。APRV 也被证明可以改善血流动力学和肺功能[11]。与系统综述相比,单中心的数据表明,在具备训练有素工作人员的医疗中心系统地应用 APRV 可能产生保护患者免受肺损伤的效果[14]。然而,目前还没有大型多中心研究将 APRV 与传统通气模式进行比较,而且还没有明确定义 APRV 的最佳通气方式。已发表文献存在临床实践和通气方案的异质性导致无法得出相应的结论[5]。

APRV 没有绝对指征。在难治性低氧血症或被认为需要肺复张的患者中,可以考虑应用 APRV。由于 APRV 允许独立于机器触发呼吸的自主呼吸,该模式可用于早期机械通气人-机不同步的患者,或即将从控制通气转换为辅助自主通气的患者。此外,APRV 可用于减少镇静和肌松剂的需求[11]。为确保在病情复杂的患者中应用 APRV 模式,APRV 可以先在其他患者中大量使用以获得经验。一般来说,与阻塞性肺疾病相比,为限制性肺疾病或健康肺患者进行 APRV 更容易设置。

13.4 设置

设置 T-high、P-high、T-low 和 P-low 时必须使它们相互关联,以实现预期的生理效果。随着参数设置的个体化调整,任何变化的结果都始终基于时间和压力间的相互作用。

13.4.1　P-high

通常情况下，P-high 应设置为实现肺复张和吸气并且在此基础上仍然可以进行舒适的自主呼吸的程度。通常该压力接近（或略低于）传统通气中的平台压（plateau pressure，P_{plat}）。对于大多数患者，包括儿童和成人，20～25 cmH_2O 之间的 P-high 是合适的。一些患者，如极度肥胖或胸壁或腹部顺应性降低者，可能需要更高的压力。P-high 的初始设置可以根据 P_{plat} 来计算。P-high 的滴定可通过密切观察患者的自主呼吸努力来调整。正确设置的 P-high 可达到最佳顺应性，患者可以安静地使用腹部肌肉来促进呼气。吸气时腹部肌肉的激活可能意味着患者试图免受过高 P-high 的伤害，如果患者需要激活辅助呼吸肌，则应考虑调整 P-high，过低的 P-high 将导致肺去复张和顺应性下降。然而，P-high 设置过高将导致肺过度膨胀，同样会导致顺应性降低。因此，呼吸困难可能是 P-high 过高或过低的表现，有时尝试增加或减少压力是识别可能问题的唯一方法。

P-high 的最佳设置应实现最大程度的肺复张而没有肺泡过度膨胀，从而优化气体交换和通气/灌注匹配。相反，缺氧和高碳酸血症都可能由 P-high 过低导致的去复张或 P-high 过高导致的过度扩张和肺泡无效腔增加引起。应密切关注 P-high 对气体交换的影响，如出现低氧或高碳酸血症问题，应立即对 P-high 进行评估。

13.4.2　T-high

通过 T-high 设定 P-high 的持续时间。在 APRV 中，T-high 期应尽可能长，因为肺复张需要时间，而太短的 P-high 不利于肺复张至最佳状态。相反，T-high 是压力释放频率的主要决定因素。T-high 设置时间过长将导致呼吸支持不足。对于大多数成年患者，T-high 初始值设置在 4～6 秒。

除了阻塞性肺疾病患者，成人 T-high 低于 4 秒与 APRV 生理效应绝对不一致，因为 P-high 的持续时间不足以达到肺泡和无效腔间气体有效扩散至稳定状态。由于吸气时间长，在 APRV 中可设定的呼吸频率非常有限。严重气道阻塞的患者可能偶尔需要较短的 T-high，因为他们延长的呼气相里包括压力的缓慢下降，并且由于 P-low 的时间较长，需要更频繁的压力释放。

一般来说，T-high 应尽可能长（通常在呼吸周期的 90% 以上），同时避免高碳酸血症或呼吸肌肉疲劳。延长 T-high 将有助于稳定肺复张，并通过增加气体扩散促进气体交换。然而，由于 T-high 的延长会降低压力释放频率，因此必须密切关注动脉 CO_2 水平和 T-high 延长时出现的肌肉疲劳迹象。$PaCO_2$ 升高时应尝试缩短 T-high，除非 T-high 接近 4 秒。在这种情况下，应考虑 T-high 是否太短，无法通过增加扩散促进气体交换来实现肺复张。

13.4.3　P-low

P-low 通常不作为目标压力，因为实际 PEEP 将由内源性 PEEP 来确定，而内源性

PEEP 是基于 T-low 的应变量,而不是设定的压力值。因此,P-low 可以常规地设置为 0 cmH$_2$O,最小化呼气气流阻力使呼气峰流速(peak expiratory flow rate,PEFR)达到最大值。过短的 T-low 会显著增加内源性 PEEP,常规测量的内源性 PEEP 的值可能与实际内源性 PEEP 值不相关,因为实际值与顺应性和气道阻力相关而存在个体化差异。

在 P-low 期存在气流是可能的,因为它本质上是低水平的 CPAP,所以自主呼吸是可能的。由于压力释放的 P-low 期很短,通常在 P-low 期没有足够的时间进行任何协调的呼吸努力。

13.4.4 T-low

T-low 是压力释放到较低压力水平的持续时间。正如模式名称所示,APRV 模式中的通气是由 T-low 期的压力释放产生的。T-low 被限制在很短的时间内,以避免去复张并限制呼出的潮气量。由于在呼气末肺内保留了大量超过功能残气量的气体,故产生了相当大的内源性 PEEP。T-low 的精确滴定在已发表的方案中有所不同,但一般来说,设定的目标为呼气流速下降至期望值。因此,T-low 被设置为允许呼气流速下降到 PEFR 的预设百分比,通常为 50%~75%。这种做法可以实现通气的自动个体化,因为呼出的潮气量将由肺容量、气流阻力和顺应性决定(图 13.2)。

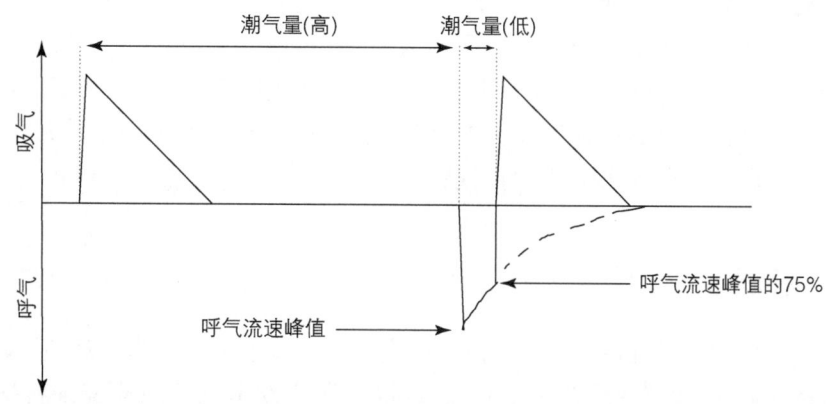

图 13.2 在没有自主呼吸的情况下,T-high 期和 T-low 期的气流量。T-low 的终点被设置为呼气流速恰好下降到其峰值的 75% 的时间点。虚线显示了理论上的持续呼气,在没有压力对抗的情况下会继续呼气

呼气流速的目标降低值可以在不同的临床场景中一致地调整潮气量以适应患者特征。呼气流速降至 PEFR 的 75% 可以作为儿科及阻塞性或限制性肺疾病成人患者的通气目标。对于阻塞性肺疾病患者,可能需要大大延长 T-low 以达到呼气流速降低的目标。

13.5 自主呼吸

在应用 APRV 模式时通常鼓励自主呼吸。由于 APRV 中的自主呼吸将有助于保留膈肌功能,减少镇静深度,并改善血流动力学,所以在前 24 小时通气内以自主呼吸产生

50%的每分钟通气量为目标[13,15,16]。如果没有自主呼吸努力,在几分钟内将相对稳定患者的 T-high 加倍,可能会使其受到短暂的挑战。由于每分钟通气量低,这会促使动脉 CO_2 迅速上升,从而刺激呼吸。如果该过程无法产生呼吸努力,建议减少镇静深度。在动脉 CO_2 低的情况下,可以将减少镇静降低和增加 T-high 联合使用,以保留更多的 CO_2。一旦恢复自主呼吸,这将有助于 P-high 的设置。

根据作者的经验,在健康肺的患者中,即使没有自主呼吸,APRV 也几乎总是会在通气开始后立即促进正常的气体交换。始终鼓励患者自主呼吸,但当 APRV 应用于严重病变的肺时,通常需要长达 24 小时才能充分排出 CO_2(允许自主呼吸时)。即便允许患者自主呼吸,最初阶段的高碳酸血症也可能非常麻烦。

在作者所在的机构中,应用 APRV 的患者几乎都允许自主呼吸,目标通常是尽快达到 50%的每分钟通气量。即使是之前接受过肌松剂治疗的患者,如果切换至 APRV 模式,也可以保留自主呼吸,尽管这类患者的过渡可能具有挑战性。

13.6 撤机

当患者病情稳定、呼吸状态改善时,在 APRV 模式可进行序贯撤机。通气支持下降的起始是通过增加 T-high 来实现的,T-high 降低了释放的频率,从而降低了呼吸支持的水平。在此阶段,根据上述原理监测和滴定 P-high、T-low 和 P-low。当达到最大 T-high 时(对于许多呼吸机来说可能是 30 秒),呼吸机模式可以切换到 CPAP,设置的 PEEP 与 P-high 相同,压力支持为 0。如果患者能耐受,则通过部分减少 CPAP 来完成进一步的撤机,直到患者被认为可以拔管。

13.7 总结

APRV 使用的设置在概念上与传统的机械通气非常不同。为了从 APRV 的理论优势中获益,必须以特定的目标来设置参数,以促使 APRV 实现其可能的特殊生理效应。事实上,尽管传统通气模式的参数设置,如潮气量和频率、内源性 PEEP、吸呼比和驱动压,都可以通过 APRV 的设置来实现,但作者强烈鼓励操作者不要以传统参数作为设置的目标。相反,应将重点放在特定的 APRV 设置上(分别为 P 和 T,高压和低压),以使该模式的生理收益最大化。然而,到目前为止,还没有明确的证据表明 APRV 对预后有益。对于最佳设置也没有达成共识。

(陈珵,金珊珊　译)

参考文献

[1]　Stock MC, Downs JB, Frolicher DA. Airway pressure release ventilation. Crit Care Med. 1987; 15(5): 462-6.

[2] Habashi NM. Other approaches to open-lung ventilation: airway pressure release ventilation. Crit Care Med. 2005; 33(3 Suppl): S228-40.

[3] Kollisch-Singule M, Emr B, Jain SV, Andrews P, Satalin J, Liu J, et al. The effects of airway pressure release ventilation on respiratory mechanics in extrapulmonary lung injury. Intensive Care Med Exp. 2015; 3(1): 35.

[4] Nieman GF, Al-Khalisy H, Kollisch-Singule M, Satalin J, Blair S, Trikha G, et al. A physiologically informed strategy to effectively open, stabilize, and protect the acutely injured lung. Front Physiol. 2020; 11: 227.

[5] Fredericks AS, Bunker MP, Gliga LA, Ebeling CG, Ringqvist JRB, Heravi H, et al. Airway pressure release ventilation: a review of the evidence, theoretical benefits, and alternative titration strategies. Clin Med Insights Circ Respir Pulm Med. 2020; 14: 1179548420903297.

[6] Maung AA, Luckianow G, Kaplan LJ. Lessons learned from airway pressure release ventilation. J Trauma Acute Care Surg. 2012; 72(3): 624-8.

[7] Roy SK, Emr B, Sadowitz B, Gatto LA, Ghosh A, Satalin JM, et al. Preemptive application of airway pressure release ventilation prevents development of acute respiratory distress syndrome in a rat traumatic hemorrhagic shock model. Shock (Augusta, Ga). 2013; 40(3): 210-6.

[8] Kollisch-Singule M, Emr B, Smith B, Roy S, Jain S, Satalin J, et al. Mechanical breath profile of airway pressure release ventilation: the effect on alveolar recruitment and microstrain in acute lung injury. JAMA Surg. 2014; 149(11): 1138-45.

[9] Kollisch-Singule M, Jain S, Andrews P, Smith BJ, Hamlington-Smith KL, Roy S, et al. Effect of airway pressure release ventilation on dynamic alveolar heterogeneity. JAMA Surg. 2016; 151(1): 64-72.

[10] Lim J, Litton E. Airway pressure release ventilation in adult patients with acute hypoxemic respiratory failure: a systematic review and meta-analysis. Crit Care Med. 2019; 47(12): 1794-9.

[11] Li J-Q, Li N, Han G-J, Pan C-G, Zhang Y-H, Shi X-Z, et al. Clinical research about airway pressure release ventilation for moderate to severe acute respiratory distress syndrome. Eur Rev Med Pharmacol Sci. 2016; 20(12): 2634-41.

[12] Carsetti A, Damiani E, Domizi R, Scorcella C, Pantanetti S, Falcetta S, et al. Airway pressure release ventilation during acute hypoxemic respiratory failure: a systematic review and meta-analysis of randomized controlled trials. Ann Intensive Care. 2019; 9(1): 44.

[13] Zhou Y, Jin X, Lv Y, Wang P, Yang Y, Liang G, et al. Early application of airway pressure release ventilation may reduce the duration of mechanical ventilation in acute respiratory distress syndrome. Intensive Care Med. 2017; 43(11): 1648-59.

[14] Andrews PL, Shiber JR, Jaruga-Killeen E, Roy S, Sadowitz B, O'Toole RV, et al. Early application of airway pressure release ventilation may reduce mortality in high-risk trauma patients: a systematic review of observational trauma ARDS literature. J Trauma Acute Care Surg. 2013; 75(4): 635-41.

[15] Kreyer S, Putensen C, Berg A, Soehle M, Muders T, Wrigge H, et al. Effects of spontaneous breathing during airway pressure release ventilation on cerebral and spinal cord perfusion in experimental acute lung injury. J Neurosurg Anesthesiol. 2010; 22(4): 323-9.

[16] Hering R, Bolten JC, Kreyer S, Berg A, Wrigge H, Zinserling J, et al. Spontaneous breathing during airway pressure release ventilation in experimental lung injury: effects on hepatic blood flow. Intensive Care Med. 2008; 34(3): 523-7.

第二部分
临床情景

14 急性低氧性呼吸衰竭和急性呼吸窘迫综合征
Acute Hypoxaemic Respiratory Failure and Acute Respiratory Distress Syndrome

Bairbre McNicholas, Emanuele Rezoagli, John G. Laffey

14.1 急性低氧性呼吸衰竭和急性呼吸窘迫综合征：定义的难题

急性呼吸窘迫综合征（acute respiratory distress syndrome，ARDS）是一种急性肺部炎症过程，可使肺泡腔渗出富含蛋白质的液体，导致非静水压性肺水肿，引起难治性低氧血症，增加肺的"僵硬度"，并使肺清除二氧化碳的能力受损（表 14.1）[8]。自 1967 年 Ashbaugh 和 Petty 正式描述 ARDS 以来，ARDS 的临床诊断标准经历了多次更新[9]。1988 年，基于胸部 X 线出现渗出的肺象限数、低氧血症的程度、PEEP 和肺顺应性，Murray 提出了一种肺损伤评分系统[10]。后来被 1994 年美国欧洲共识会议的定义所取代[11]，而目前公认的定义是"柏林定义"[7]。ARDS 柏林定义中的改变主要为纳入了无创通气、阐明"急性"的定义，以及排除心力衰竭作为病因的流程[12]。最新的定义调整了包括在资源有限的环境中使用 SpO_2 作为 ARDS 的诊断依据，以及使用肺部超声作为评估手段[13,14]。

表 14.1 基于已发表的大型临床研究中的 AHRF 特征和基于柏林定义的 ARDS 特征

特点	AHRF					ARDS
	Lewandowski AJRCCM 1995[1]	The ARF Study Group AJRCCM 1999[2]	FLORALI study group and REVA network 2015[3]	PROVENT Lancent Respir Med 2016[4]	LUNG SAFE 2016[5]/Eur Respir Journal 2021[6]	柏林定义[7]
时间	未定义	在"急性"起病	未定义	未定义	未定义	一周内急性起病的已知损伤,新发或已有呼吸道症状加重
胸部影像学	胸部 X 线检查中观察到肺实变的象限数(0~4)[b]	在 ALI/ARDS 患者胸部正位片[a]中可见双侧渗出	在 ALI/ARDS 患者中	未定义	在 CXR 或 CT 中可见单侧或双侧新发的肺实质异常[c]	双侧浸润影不能完全用积液、肺萎陷或结节解释
肺水肿的原因	未定义	肺动脉楔压<18 mmHg 或 ALI/ARDS 患者没有左心房高压[a]的临床证据	排除心源性肺水肿	未定义	未定义	不能完全用心力衰竭或液体过负荷解释的呼吸衰竭。需要客观的评估(如心脏超声)在没有危险因素的情况下排除静水压肺水肿
氧合	未定义	ALI: $PaO_2/FiO_2 \leq 300$ mmHg; ARDS: $PaO_2/FiO_2 \leq 200$ mmHg[a]	$PaO_2/FiO_2 \leq 300$ mmHg	未定义	$PaO_2/FiO_2 \leq 300$ mmHg[c]	轻度 ARDS: 200 mmHg < $PaO_2/FiO_2 \leq 300$ mmHg; 中度 ARDS: 100 mmHg < $PaO_2/FiO_2 \leq 200$ mmHg; 重度 ARDS: $PaO_2/FiO_2 \leq 100$ mmHg
呼吸支持	不管 FiO_2 水平如何,有创机械通气≥24 h	不管 FiO_2 水平如何,有创机械通气≥24 h	吸入氧流量大于等于 10 L/min 超过 15 min	有创机械通气	机械通气支持的 CPAP、EPAP 或 PEEP≥5 cmH_2O	轻度 ARDS: PEEP 或 CPAP≥5 cmH_2O; 中度 ARDS: PEEP≥5 cmH_2O; 重度 ARDS: PEEP≥5 cmH_2O

续　表

特点	AHRF					ARDS	
	Lewandowski AJRCCM 1995[1]	The ARF Study Group AJRCCM 1999[2]	FLORALI study group and REVA network NEJM 2015[3]	PROVENT Lancent Respir Med 2016[4]	LUNG SAFE JAMA 2016[5]/Eur Resp Journal 2021[6]	柏林定义[7]	
呼吸频率	未定义	未定义	>25次/分	未定义	未定义		
PaCO₂水平	未定义	未定义	PaCO₂≤45 mmHg	未定义	未定义		
危险因素	未定义	未定义	缺乏:潜在慢性呼吸衰竭病史;哮喘或慢性呼吸衰竭恶化;心源性肺水肿;严重中性粒细胞减少;血流动力学不稳定;使用血管活性药;GCS≤12;无创通气禁忌证;迫切需要气管插管;拒绝插管;不入组的决定	未定义	未定义		

AHRF,急性低氧性呼吸衰竭;ARDS,急性呼吸窘迫综合征;ALI,急性肺损伤;CXR,胸部X线片;FiO₂,吸入氧浓度;CPAP,持续气道正压;EPAP,呼气末正压;GCS,格拉斯哥昏迷评分;PaCO₂,动脉二氧化碳分压

a 来自AECC的ALI/ARDS诊断标准
b 来自Murray肺损伤评分
c 来自ARDS柏林定义

虽然 ARDS"典型"的病理改变是弥漫性肺泡损伤,但在死亡时符合 ARDS 标准的患者中只有少数在尸检时存在这种病理改变,故而目前 ARDS 的标准缺乏特异性[15]。

其他肺部因素导致的急性低氧性呼吸衰竭(acute hypoxaemic respiratory failure, AHRF)共同被归为定义不明确的类别,其特征是肺源性低氧血症急性发作伴影像学上单侧渗出[7]。鉴于 ARDS 与其他因素导致的 AHRF 之间的关键区别在于后者的胸部影像学没有双侧肺渗出,我们用单侧浸润 AHRF(unilateral-infiltrate AHRF,uAHRF)来描述它们(图 14.1)。目前尚无 uAHRF 的标准定义,相关研究中纳入了不同的呼吸支持方式(氧疗到有创通气)、氧合标准(无,$PaO_2/FiO_2 < 300$ mmHg)、影像学标准(无,新发的渗出)、持续时间(无,24 h,1 周)、是否需要呼气末正压支持(无,$PEEP \geqslant 5$ cmH_2O)[2,12](表 14.1)。缺乏一致的诊断标准是定义不明确的主要障碍。

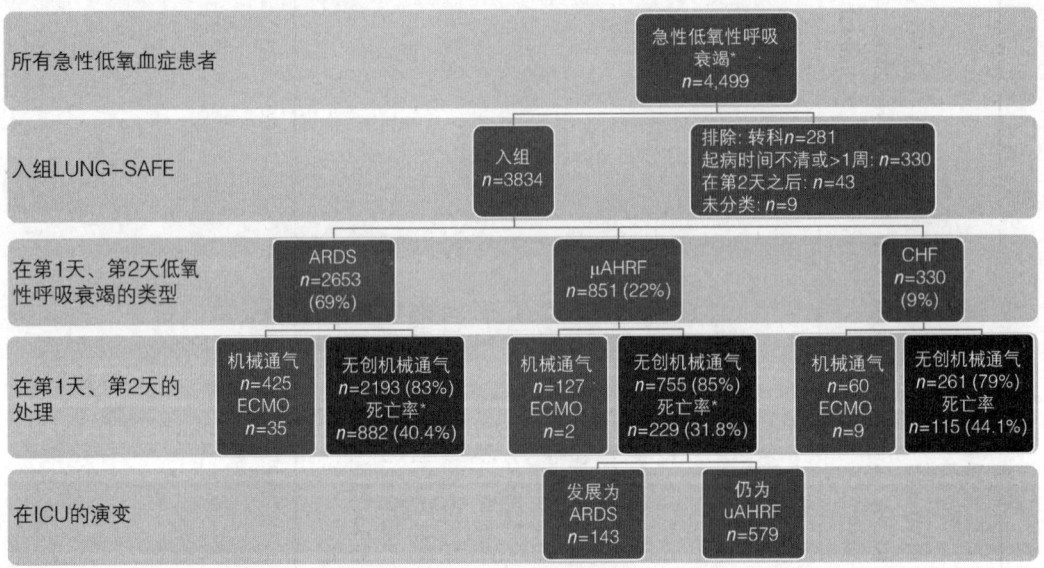

图 14.1 LUNG SAFE 队列中 AHRF 患者的分布和结局。AHRF 的定义符合以下标准:① $PaO_2/FiO_2 \leqslant 300$ mmHg;② 胸部影像学检查显示新的肺渗出灶;③ 呼吸机支持并且呼气末正压(PEEP)$\geqslant 5$ cmH_2O。患者分为 3 组:① ARDS,即完全符合柏林定义 ARDS 的所有标准;② CHF,临床医生认为呼吸衰竭完全可由心力衰竭或液体超负荷解释;③ uAHRF:符合柏林定义 ARDS 的标准,除了胸部影像学检查仅显示单侧渗出灶。uAHRF,单侧渗出性 AHRF;ARDS,急性呼吸窘迫综合征;CHF,充血性心力衰竭;ECMO,体外膜肺氧合;NIV,无创通气。经许可改编自 Pham et al. Eur Resp Journal[6]

尽管 ARDS 与 uAHRF 的定义之间存在重叠,尤其是在比较"局灶性"ARDS 与 uAHRF 时[2,6],但 uAHRF 仍然是一个独立的定义,因为事实上只有很少一部分 uAHRF 患者会演变为 ARDS[6]。考虑到当前 uAHRF 定义缺乏敏感性,以及对 ARDS 的认识不足,优化管理有单侧渗出的急性低氧血症的患者非常重要[16]。此外,在 AHRF 患者中采用"肺保护性"通气策略可能并非最佳选择,尤其是在根本的呼吸力学与 ARDS 存在显著区别的情况下[17]。

一个不满足 ARDS 及 uAHRF 定义的患者人群是快速增长的、使用经鼻高流量氧疗(high flow nasal oxygen,HFNO)的急性低氧血症患者群体,因为这种治疗所产生的 PEEP 不足 5 cmH_2O。

14.2 流行病学：已知与未知

流行病学研究大大提高了我们对 ARDS 发病率、管理和预后的认知。直到最近，这些研究仍仅限于部分地区和国家，从而导致其评估的 ARDS 和 AHRF 的发病率具有很大差异[18]。然而，最近一些大型多国协作的研究对于 ARDS/uAHFR 的发病率存在地域差异提出了质疑。LUNG SAFE（了解严重急性呼吸衰竭的全球影响的大型观察性调查）研究使用直接获得的临床信息确定了 ARDS 和 uAHRF 的发生率，而不需要医生识别 ARDS[5]。研究发现 10% 的 ICU 患者和 24% 的机械通气患者符合 ARDS 的标准，而 4% 的 ICU 患者出现严重到需要无创或有创通气的 uAHRF（图 14.1）。对 ARDS 的认识不足是主要问题，在发病第 1 天只有 30% 的 ARDS 患者被识别，在任何时间点都只有 60% 的 ARDS 能得到识别，ARDS 发病率的地理差异有限。LUNG SAFE 研究还报告了 ARDS 患者的病死率为 40%，这使得那些表明 ARDS 病死率随时间推移而降低的随机对照试验数据被质疑[18]。

与 ARDS 相比，由于缺乏公认的定义导致 uAHRF 的流行病学研究存在更大的异质性（表 14.1）[1,2,4,19-21]。最近，PRoVENT 研究对 AHRF 的流行病学进行了类似的全球评估。在机械通气开始时没有 ARDS 的患者中，30% 的患者被认为有 ARDS 的风险（肺损伤预测评分>4），但这些患者中只有 7% 在后续随访期间实际发生 ARDS；然而被认为没有 ARDS 风险的人群中实际发生 ARDS 的占 3%。与被认为没有 ARDS 风险的患者相比，有 ARDS 风险的有创机械通气患者感染、肺部并发症更多，ICU 住院时间更长。

14.3 病理生理学：见解与分歧

ARDS"经典"的病理生理学特征是由于肺泡实变和渗透性肺水肿导致重力依赖区肺萎陷而使肺泡功能广泛丧失。因此，肺顺应性通常（并非总是）严重降低，肺泡分流和无效腔增加，而气道阻力通常保持不变。这种"经典"ARDS 病理生理学的变化取决于肺渗出的分布（即局灶性还是弥漫性）等特征，不论潜在原发病在肺内还是肺外。而原发病不同常使病理学表现不同，相较于肺外病因，肺部疾病导致的 ARDS 有更明显的肺泡塌陷、纤维状渗出物、肺泡壁水肿，并且胶原蛋白含量增加[22]。电子烟成分中维生素 E 醋酸酯诱导的 ARDS 的发生和 COVID-19 大流行，增加了人们对肺泡上皮、内皮、凝血和免疫系统之间复杂相互作用的认识[23]。

最近，ARDS 患者肺部影像学和生物学的最新进展能够更好地定义 ARDS：① 肺部影像学标准（即局灶性与非局灶性或弥漫性比较）：与肺泡渗液的清除能力不同有关，且与不同预后相关[24]；② 炎性生物标志物（如高炎症表型 2 与表型 1 比较）：对应的治疗方式不同（如液体管理和 PEEP 策略），预后也不同[25]。CT 研究发现，由于肺泡实变、水肿和塌陷，顺应性差的"僵硬"肺通常是小容积肺，即"婴儿肺"[26]。此外，对俯卧位 ARDS 患者 CT 的研究发现可以将出现炎症的肺组织视为功能性海绵（与湿海绵一样随位置改变而发生变化）[27]。使用 ^{18}F-D-葡萄糖的 PET 研究表明，在无通气实变区和明显"正常"

通气区域的肺组织都可以存在炎症反应[28]。

由于 uAHRF 包含更多不同的导致急性重度缺氧和 CT 单侧肺渗出的致病条件,因此病理生理进程可能存在更大的变异性。其中可能由一种病理生理学特征占主导地位,如分流(如支气管肺炎)、气道阻力增加(如哮喘急性加重期)、弹性回缩力降低伴动态过度通气(哮喘、COPD)。重要的是,ARDS 中占主导地位的病理生理学特征(如肺顺应性降低)在 uAHRF 中较少出现,这对通气管理有重要意义。

14.4 呼吸支持方式

近年来,特别是在 COVID-19 大流行期间,HFNO 的应用大幅增加,用以改善氧合、减少呼吸做功。越来越多的证据支持其使用,并且逐渐被认为是 uAHRF 和 ARDS 患者的第一级"高级呼吸支持"模式[20,29]。无创通气(non-invasive ventilation,NIV)策略在治疗 COPD 急性加重、哮喘,以及肺炎导致的 AHRF 的疾病中具有确切的证据[12]。AHRF 的不同亚型可能会使 NIV 和 HFNO 的治疗反应存在差异,有研究发现 HFNO 在 AHRF 中优于 NIV[20],而在一项 COVID-19 导致 AHRF 的研究中使用 NIV 可以减少有创通气(invasive mechanical ventilation,IMV)的需求,而 HFNO 无效[30]。

NIV 在 ARDS 中的作用更具争议性,因为在呼吸驱动增加的情况下可能导致"自戕性肺损伤"[31]。在 LUNG SAFE 研究中,使用 NIV 治疗成功的 ARDS 患者的病死率最低[12]。然而,有超过三分之一的患者 NIV 治疗失败,该失败队列的病死率为 45%。在倾向匹配分析中,P/F<150 的 ARDS 患者接受 NIV 治疗的病死率较接受有创机械通气治疗的更高[12]。在 NIV 治疗失败的患者中,建立有创机械通气后潮气量和每分钟通气量大幅减少。由于未能在该队列患者中实施早期肺保护性通气,这引起了对治疗无反应的患者持续使用 NIV 的担忧[12]。在 AHRF 队列研究中也报告了类似的现象,在开始 NIV 后 1 小时内没有减少呼吸做功且改善氧合的患者需要有创机械通气的可能性增加了 4 倍[3]。这些结论强调,无论 AHRF 的病因如何,都需要在开始 NIV 治疗后定期评估患者对 NIV 的反应。

个性化和恰当地选择患者对于 NIV 治疗在 ARDS 和 AHRF 中能否发挥最佳疗效至关重要。预测评分(如 HACAR 或 ROX 指数)可用于识别无反应或可能治疗无效的患者[32,33]。

14.5 有创机械通气:从"保护性"到"个体化"

有创机械通气作为其他高级呼吸支持治疗失败患者的挽救措施,也可能会恶化 ARDS 的严重程度,高潮气量会增加僵硬肺部受到的剪切应力,导致容积伤、气压伤和生物伤[34]。将潮气量限制在 6~8 mL/kg(理想体重),且平台压低于 30 cmH_2O 的肺通气策略可以提高 ARDS 患者的生存率[35]。然而,优化 ARDS 患者其他通气参数设置的方法尚不清楚,如氧滴定的目标(保守与开放相比)、PEEP(较低与较高相比)和肺复张手法(开放与不开放相比)。ARDS 患者优化通气未来的进展可能包括开发在床旁个性化设置呼吸机的策略[36,37]。关于最佳 PEEP 的设置,基于氧合和(或)肺顺应性的反应,应用递增法滴定PEEP似乎是可靠的[38]。在LIVE研究中突显了ARDS中"个体化"通气的潜力，随机分配至实验组的患者基于ARDS浸润范围是局灶性还是弥漫性采用两种不同的通气策略，而对照组则接受标准化的"保护性通气"策略[17]。虽然在初步分析中没有发现结果差异，但浸润范围错误分类概率很高，重新分类后，发现个性化通气组有获益[17]。这些数据表明，需要以肺生理学为基础来调整肺通气参数，而不是采用"一刀切"的通气策略[39]。因此，近年来使用驱动压等动态指标来指导床旁潮气量的滴定得到了广泛的应用[40]。

因为现有的证据基础有限，uAHRF患者有创机械通气的最佳设置方法并不明确。虽然高潮气量通气即使在发病前正常的肺中也是有害的[4,41]，在uAHRF患者中理应避免，但对这类患者滴定潮气量的最佳方法尚不清楚。在uAHRF患者中采用极低潮气量通气可能没有额外获益，尤其是在肺顺应性保留的情况下，还需要采取相关措施以确保患者对这些策略的耐受性（如镇静）。事实上，即使在ARMA研究中，肺顺应性最高的前四分之一ARDS患者也没有从ARDSnet的肺保护策略中获得病死率相关的益处[35]。

14.6 通气支持的辅助手段

对于确诊为中至重度ARDS的有创通气患者采用俯卧位治疗有明确的证据支持[42]，已成为标准的治疗措施。尽管如此，在此类患者群体中俯卧位的使用率仍然很低[5]。COVID-19大流行期间的一项最新创新是将俯卧位拓展应用到接受无创呼吸支持的清醒患者中，一项大型荟萃分析已证明了其可以降低有创通气的需求[43]。清醒俯卧位在非COVID-19的uAHRF或ARDS患者中的作用，以及俯卧位在有创通气的uAHRF患者中的作用仍有待明确。

一些研究结论支持在中重度ARDS患者中使用神经肌肉阻滞剂[44]，但并非所有的研究都支持该结论[45]，尽管方法学上的差异可以部分解释这两种不同的结果。目前尚没有关于在uAHRF中使用肌松剂的数据。

来自观察性研究的数据表明，ARDS的辅助治疗方法多种多样，最近的SAGE研究发现，全身性类固醇（41.5% vs. 19.4%）和神经肌肉阻滞（27.4% vs. 25.6%）的使用较为频繁，但俯卧位使用率较低（5.8% vs. 7.9%）；在中重度ARDS中辅助治疗清晰地显示出了它的益处[46]。其他研究发现关键的循证治疗未得到充分使用，这表明从业者是根据经验进行个体化治疗，而非患者的需求[47,48]。

14.7 急性低氧性呼吸衰竭和急性呼吸窘迫综合征的特殊治疗

尽管已有50多年的研究和许多阴性的临床试验，但尚无治疗ARDS的特效药物[49]。治疗uAHRF的药理学策略侧重于基础疾病的管理，并且缺乏针对该人群的药理学试验。

最近一项地塞米松治疗中重度ARDS[50]的试验中，地塞米松可降低COVID-19 AHRF的病死率、延缓病情进展，表明类固醇治疗目前可能被过早地放弃[51]。需要针对特定的亚表型进行治疗的概念逐渐获得证据的支持，如那些"高炎症"反应的患者。Calfee等在对辛伐他汀治疗ARDS的HARP研究结果的再分析中发现，具有高炎症亚表型的患者似乎受益于辛伐他汀治疗[52]。这些发现强调了开发实时人群富集策略的重要性,可以在未来的临床试验中进行靶向治疗[53]。

14.8 临床结局

LUNG SAFE 的数据强调,尽管支持性治疗取得了进展,但 ARDS 患者仍有高达 40% 的住院病死率(图 14.1)[5]。最近,纳入了中重度 ARDS 患者的美国 SAGE 研究同样证实了与之类似的病死率(40.7%)。ARDS 被认为是直接导致并发症和死亡的一个实际因素[54,55]。在对两项脓毒症研究(EARLI 和 VALID)的事后分析中,报告了严重 ARDS 的归因死亡率为 16%~18%,死亡风险在 PFR 为 120 时趋于稳定。相比之下,ICU 获得性感染和谵妄的归因死亡率分别为 11% 和 7%[56]。

与 ARDS 相比,AHRF 的结局研究不足。20 世纪 90 年代斯堪的纳维亚的一项研究发现,ARDS 和非 ARDS 相关的 ARF 病死率均为 40%[2]。在 LUNG SAFE 研究中,需要有创通气的 ARDS 患者未经校正的住院病死率为 40%,而 uAHRF 为 32%[6],数据支持了 ARDS 可能带来额外死亡风险的观点[6]。然而,当将在单侧 2 个象限渗出的 uAHRF 患者与有 2 个象限渗出的 AHRF 患者进行比较时,病死率没有差异。在多因素分析中,受累肺象限的数量,而不是象限的分布(单侧 vs. 双侧)是死亡风险的关键因素(图 14.2)[6]。

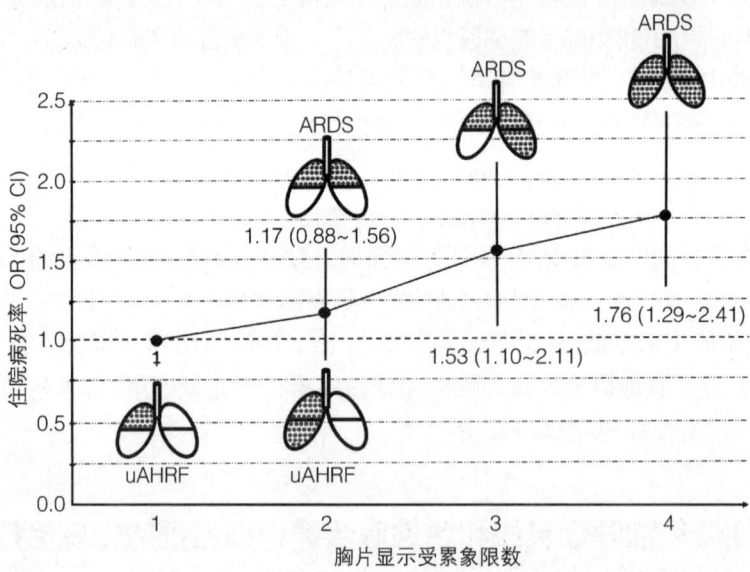

图 14.2 LUNG SAFE 队列研究中校正后的 AHRF 患者的住院死亡风险。呼吸衰竭患者可能表现为单侧浸润[AHRF(蓝点)]或双侧浸润[ARDS(红点)]。基于单侧或双侧分布,2 个象限出现浸润可分别被定义为 AHRF 或 ARDS。与仅存在一个象限浸润相比,肺浸润象限数量增加(即 2 个以上)与死亡风险逐渐增加相关。根据基线特征、合并症、是否伴随心力衰竭、ARDS 的危险因素、通气变量和地缘经济校正了 95% 置信区间的比值比(OR),比值比和 95% 置信区间用点和误差线表示,使用单象限浸润作为参照。图中数据来自 Pham et al. Eur Resp Journal[6](见彩色插图)

14.9 急性低氧性呼吸衰竭：改变范式

缺乏一套公认的诊断标准是促进理解 AHRF 和改善 AHRF 患者预后的主要障碍。迄今为止，研究工作主要集中在 ARDS 上，导致对 uAHRF 认识不足。目前迫切需要对 AHRF 进行统一的定义。根据现有的柏林定义 ARDS 标准改编而来并易于实施的标准定义可以包括以下几点：① 发病时间<1 周；② P/F<300 mmHg 的低氧血症；③ 需要高级呼吸支持(即≥40 L/min 经鼻高流量氧疗)；④ 新发肺部渗出的影像学证据；⑤ 没有心源性因素作为低氧血症的主要原因。ARDS 患者的亚群将仅根据胸部影像学检查中是否存在双侧渗出来区分。AHRF 和 ARDS 的严重程度将根据当前的 P/F 进行分级，同时还可以考虑胸部影像学受影响的象限数量。ARDS 的定义可以进一步细化，包括根据肺受累程度(肺象限数量、局灶性分布或弥漫分布)、呼吸力学特征或评估炎症和肺上皮及内皮损伤的生物标志物组来区分亚表型[52,57]。

这套新的统一诊断标准可以应用到电子病历系统中，可能会增强对 ARHF 和 ARDS 的识别，促使从业者仔细地基于基础生理学特点调整呼吸支持策略。这些定义也应构成未来研究工作的基础，应侧重于了解不同病因 AHRF 的流行病学，以充分了解 AHRF 的疾病负担和结局。干预研究可以测试不同亚型 AHRF 的呼吸支持策略，根据可治疗的特征，无论是生理性的(如 PEEP 反应性、俯卧位)还是生物学的(如类固醇反应性)对 AHRF 进行分型。

14.10 总结

AHRF 由多种临床疾病所致，当需要重症监护时，其病死率为 40%。病死率似乎更多地受到肺部受累程度的影响，这反映在受影响的肺象限数量上，而不是是否存在 ARDS 上。缺乏一套公认的 AHRF 诊断标准是推进治疗和改善预后的主要障碍，应作为紧急事项加以解决。有必要充分了解除 ARDS 外的 AHRF 的疾病负担，并为这些患者的管理和治疗策略建立证据基础。一套综合诊断标准，包括 ARDS 和其他导致 ARDS 的肺部疾病，应易于操作，并有助于早期识别这些疾病，从而实现个体化管理并减少医源性损伤。在全球层面，了解 AHRF 的负担将使政策制定者能够规划和配备适当的人员和设备，并对长期影响进行后续研究[58]。最终，这种方法应该能推动开发新的特异性疗法和个体化支持方法，从而改善 AHRF 患者的预后。

（高甜甜，周媛 译）

参考文献

[1] Lewandowski K, et al. Incidence, severity, and mortality of acute respiratory failure in Berlin, Germany. Am J Respir Crit Care Med. 1995；151(4)：1121-5.

[2] Luhr OR, et al. Incidence and mortality after acute respiratory failure and acute respiratory distress syndrome in Sweden, Denmark, and Iceland. The ARF study group. Am J Respir Crit Care Med. 1999; 159(6): 1849-61.

[3] Frat JP, et al. Predictors of intubation in patients with acute hypoxemic respiratory failure treated with a noninvasive oxygenation strategy. Crit Care Med. 2018; 46(2): 208-15.

[4] Neto AS, et al. Epidemiological characteristics, practice of ventilation, and clinical outcome in patients at risk of acute respiratory distress syndrome in intensive care units from 16 countries (PRoVENT): an international, multicentre, prospective study. Lancet Respir Med. 2016; 4(11): 882-93.

[5] Bellani G, et al. Epidemiology, patterns of care, and mortality for patients with acute respiratory distress syndrome in intensive care units in 50 countries. JAMA. 2016; 315(8): 788-800.

[6] Pham T, et al. Outcome of acute hypoxaemic respiratory failure: insights from the LUNG SAFE study. Eur Respir J. 2021; 57(6): 2003317.

[7] Ranieri VM, et al. Acute respiratory distress syndrome: the Berlin definition. JAMA. 2012; 307(23): 2526-33.

[8] Rezoagli E, Fumagalli R, Bellani G. Definition and epidemiology of acute respiratory distress syndrome. Ann Transl Med. 2017; 5(14): 282.

[9] Ashbaugh DG, et al. Acute respiratory distress in adults. Lancet. 1967; 2(7511): 319-23.

[10] Murray JF, et al. An expanded definition of the adult respiratory distress syndrome. Am Rev Respir Dis. 1988; 138(3): 720-3.

[11] Bernard GR, et al. The American-European consensus conference on ARDS. Definitions, mechanisms, relevant outcomes, and clinical trial coordination. Am J Respir Crit Care Med. 1994; 149(3 Pt 1): 818-24.

[12] Bellani G, et al. Noninvasive ventilation of patients with acute respiratory distress syndrome. Insights from the LUNG SAFE study. Am J Respir Crit Care Med. 2017; 195(1): 67-77.

[13] Riviello ED, et al. Hospital incidence and outcomes of the acute respiratory distress syndrome using the Kigali modification of the Berlin definition. Am J Respir Crit Care Med. 2016; 193(1): 52-9.

[14] Cressoni M, et al. Lung inhomogeneity in patients with acute respiratory distress syndrome. Am J Respir Crit Care Med. 2014; 189(2): 149-58.

[15] Thille AW, et al. Chronology of histological lesions in acute respiratory distress syndrome with diffuse alveolar damage: a prospective cohort study of clinical autopsies. Lancet Respir Med. 2013; 1(5): 395-401.

[16] Laffey JG, et al. Geo-economic variations in epidemiology, patterns of care, and outcomes in patients with acute respiratory distress syndrome: insights from the LUNG SAFE prospective cohort study. Lancet Respir Med. 2017; 5(8): 627-38.

[17] Constantin JM, et al. Personalised mechanical ventilation tailored to lung morphology versus low positive end-expiratory pressure for patients with acute respiratory distress syndrome in France (the LIVE study): a multicentre, single-blind, randomised controlled trial. Lancet Respir Med. 2019; 7(10): 870-80.

[18] McNicholas BA, Rooney GM, Laffey JG. Lessons to learn from epidemiologic studies in ARDS. Curr Opin Crit Care. 2018; 24(1): 41-8.

[19] Vincent JL, et al. The epidemiology of acute respiratory failure in critically ill patients(*). Chest. 2002; 121(5): 1602-9.

[20] Frat JP, et al. High-flow oxygen through nasal cannula in acute hypoxemic respiratory failure. N Engl J Med. 2015; 372(23): 2185-96.

[21] Tavernier E, et al. Awake prone positioning of hypoxaemic patients with COVID-19: protocol for a randomised controlled open-label superiority meta-trial. BMJ Open. 2020; 10(11): e041520.

[22] Negri EM, et al. Acute remodeling of parenchyma in pulmonary and extrapulmonary ARDS. An autopsy study of collagen-elastic system fibers. Pathol Res Pract. 2002; 198(5): 355-61.

[23] Meyer NJ, Gattinoni L, Calfee CS. Acute respiratory distress syndrome. Lancet. 2021; 398 (10300): 622-37.

[24] Mrozek S, et al. Elevated plasma levels of srage are associated with nonfocal CT-based lung imaging in patients with ARDS: a prospective multicenter study. Chest. 2016; 150(5): 998-1007.

[25] Famous KR, et al. Acute respiratory distress syndrome subphenotypes respond differently to randomized fluid management strategy. Am J Respir Crit Care Med. 2017; 195(3): 331-8.

[26] Gattinoni L, Pesenti A. The concept of "baby lung". Intensive Care Med. 2005; 31(6): 776-84.

[27] Gattinoni L, Pesenti A, Carlesso E. Body position changes redistribute lung computed-tomographic density in patients with acute respiratory failure: impact and clinical fallout through the following 20 years. Intensive Care Med. 2013; 39(11): 1909-15.

[28] Bellani G, et al. Lung regional metabolic activity and gas volume changes induced by tidal ventilation in patients with acute lung injury. Am J Respir Crit Care Med. 2011; 183(9): 1193-9.

[29] Azoulay E, et al. Effect of high-flow nasal oxygen vs standard oxygen on 28-day mortality in immunocompromised patients with acute respiratory failure: the high randomized clinical trial. JAMA. 2018; 320(20): 2099-107.

[30] Perkins, G. D., et al., An adaptive randomized controlled trial of non-invasive respiratory strategies in acute respiratory failure patients with COVID-19. medRxiv. 2021; https://doi.org/10.1101/2021.08.02.21261379.

[31] Grieco DL, et al. Non-invasive ventilatory support and high-flow nasal oxygen as firstline treatment of acute hypoxemic respiratory failure and ARDS. Intensive Care Med. 2021; 47(8): 851-66.

[32] Duan J, et al. Assessment of heart rate, acidosis, consciousness, oxygenation, and respiratory rate to predict noninvasive ventilation failure in hypoxemic patients. Intensive Care Med. 2017; 43(2): 192-9.

[33] Roca O, et al. An index combining respiratory rate and oxygenation to predict outcome of nasal high-flow therapy. Am J Respir Crit Care Med. 2019; 199(11): 1368-76.

[34] Imai Y, et al. Injurious mechanical ventilation and end-organ epithelial cell apoptosis and organ dysfunction in an experimental model of acute respiratory distress syndrome. JAMA. 2003; 289(16): 2104-12.

[35] Acute Respiratory Distress Syndrome Network, et al. Ventilation with lower tidal volumes as compared with traditional tidal volumes for acute lung injury and the acute respiratory distress syndrome. N Engl J Med. 2000; 342(18): 1301-8.

[36] Pelosi P, et al. Vertical gradient of regional lung inflation in adult respiratory distress syndrome. Am J Respir Crit Care Med. 1994; 149(1): 8-13.

[37] Writing Group for the Alveolar Recruitment for Acute Respiratory Distress Syndrome Trial (ART) Investigators, et al. Effect of lung recruitment and titrated positive end-expiratory

pressure (PEEP) vs low PEEP on mortality in patients with acute respiratory distress syndrome: a randomized clinical trial. JAMA. 2017; 318(14): 1335 - 45.

[38] Goligher EC, et al. Oxygenation response to positive end-expiratory pressure predicts mortality in acute respiratory distress syndrome. A secondary analysis of the LOVS and ExPress trials. Am J Respir Crit Care Med. 2014; 190(1): 70 - 6.

[39] Tobin MJ. The dethroning of 6 ml/kg as the "go-to" setting in acute respiratory distress syndrome. Am J Respir Crit Care Med. 2021; 204(7): 868 - 9.

[40] Amato MB, et al. Driving pressure and survival in the acute respiratory distress syndrome. N Engl J Med. 2015; 372(8): 747 - 55.

[41] Gajic O, et al. Ventilator settings as a risk factor for acute respiratory distress syndrome in mechanically ventilated patients. Intensive Care Med. 2005; 31(7): 922 - 6.

[42] Guerin C, et al. Prone positioning in severe acute respiratory distress syndrome. N Engl J Med. 2013; 368(23): 2159 - 68.

[43] Ehrmann S, et al. Awake prone positioning for COVID-19 acute hypoxaemic respiratory failure: a randomised, controlled, multinational, open-label meta-trial. Lancet Respir Med. 2021; 9(12): 1387 - 95.

[44] Papazian L, et al. Neuromuscular blockers in early acute respiratory distress syndrome. N Engl J Med. 2010; 363(12): 1107 - 16.

[45] National Heart L, et al. Early neuromuscular blockade in the acute respiratory distress syndrome. N Engl J Med. 2019; 380(21): 1997 - 2008.

[46] Qadir N, et al. Variation in early management practices in moderate-to-severe ARDS in the United States: the severe ARDS—generating evidence study. Chest. 2021; 160(4): 1304 - 15.

[47] Duggal A, et al. Patterns of use of adjunctive therapies in patients with early moderate to severe ARDS: insights from the LUNG SAFE study. Chest. 2020; 157(6): 1497 - 505.

[48] Gupta S, et al. Factors associated with death in critically ill patients with coronavirus disease 2019 in the US. JAMA Intern Med. 2020; 180(11): 1436 - 47.

[49] Horie S, et al. Emerging pharmacological therapies for ARDS: COVID-19 and beyond. Intensive Care Med. 2020; 46(12): 2265 - 83.

[50] Villar J, et al. Dexamethasone treatment for the acute respiratory distress syndrome: a multicentre, randomised controlled trial. Lancet Respir Med. 2020; 8(3): 267 - 76.

[51] RECOVERY Collaborative Group, et al. Dexamethasone in hospitalized patients with Covid-19. N Engl J Med. 2021; 384(8): 693 - 704.

[52] Calfee CS, et al. Acute respiratory distress syndrome subphenotypes and differential response to simvastatin: secondary analysis of a randomised controlled trial. Lancet Respir Med. 2018; 6(9): 691 - 8.

[53] Shankar-Hari M, Rubenfeld GD. Population enrichment for critical care trials: phenotypes and differential outcomes. Curr Opin Crit Care. 2019; 25(5): 489 - 97.

[54] Ketcham SW, et al. Causes and characteristics of death in patients with acute hypoxemic respiratory failure and acute respiratory distress syndrome: a retrospective cohort study. Crit Care. 2020; 24(1): 391.

[55] Prescott HC, et al. Late mortality after acute hypoxic respiratory failure. Thorax. 2018; 73(7): 618 - 25.

[56] Auriemma CL, et al. Acute respiratory distress syndrome-attributable mortality in critically ill patients with sepsis. Intensive Care Med. 2020; 46(6): 1222 - 31.

[57] Bos LD, et al. Identification and validation of distinct biological phenotypes in patients with acute respiratory distress syndrome by cluster analysis. Thorax. 2017; 72(10): 876-83.

[58] Levitt JE, et al. Identification of early acute lung injury at initial evaluation in an acute care setting prior to the onset of respiratory failure. Chest. 2009; 135(4): 936-43.

15 呼吸机诱发的肺损伤和肺保护性通气
Ventilator-Induced Lung Injury and Lung Protective Ventilation

Guillermo M. Albaiceta, Laura Amado-Rodríguez

机械通气是呼吸衰竭患者必不可少的支持性治疗：它可以改善气体交换、减少呼吸做功，并确保无法自主通气的患者得到通气。然而，高气道压力会引发呼吸系统的各种反应，在某些情况下可能是有害的，并导致肺损伤的发生或恶化，称为呼吸机诱导的肺损伤（ventilation-induced lung injury，VILI）[1]。

在现代机械通气机发明之前，正压通气就被认为是有害的。早在1744年，英国医生John Fothergill就推测，当试图挽救"明显死亡"的患者时，实施口对口人工呼吸可能比使用风箱更安全[2]。他的关注点在于，从风箱或另一个人的气道吹入气体后肺所承受的机械负荷，而前者产生的容积可能更大。

避免重症患者发生 VILI 是一个重要的治疗目标，与改善生存率相关。在本章我们将回顾机械通气可能导致肺损伤的机制，以及临床评估方法和具有证据支持的保护性肺通气策略。

G. M. Albaiceta (✉)
Unidad de Cuidados Intensivos Cardiológicos, Hospital Universitario Central de Asturias, Oviedo, Spain

Departamento de Biología Funcional, Instituto Universitario de Oncología del Principado de Asturias. Universidad de Oviedo, Oviedo, Spain

Instituto de Investigación Sanitaria del Principado de Asturias, Oviedo, Spain
Centro de Investigación Biomédica en Red-Enfermedades Respiratorias, Madrid, Spain
e-mail: guillermo.muniz@sespa.es

L. Amado-Rodríguez
Unidad de Cuidados Intensivos Cardiológicos, Hospital Universitario Central de Asturias, Oviedo, Spain

Instituto de Investigación Sanitaria del Principado de Asturias, Oviedo, Spain
Centro de Investigación Biomédica en Red-Enfermedades Respiratorias, Madrid, Spain

Departamento de Medicina, Instituto Universitario de Oncología del Principado de Asturias, Universidad de Oviedo, Oviedo, Spain

© The Author(s), under exclusive license to Springer Nature Switzerland AG 2022
G. Bellani (ed.), *Mechanical Ventilation from Pathophysiology to Clinical Evidence*, https://doi.org/10.1007/978-3-030-93401-9_15

15.1 呼吸系统的机械敏感性

大部分细胞是具有机械敏感性的，它们会感知机械刺激并产生反应。这尤其适用于承受持续或循环力的组织，如呼吸系统，其具有多种细胞机械传感器，包括质膜中的牵拉激活离子通道（如 Piezo 和 TRPV 家族）、细胞骨架或核膜本身。这些传感器的激活触发细胞重编程并诱导基因表达的变化。

在生理条件下，通气驱动响应血气或气道牵拉等多种反馈机制，以调节通气的频率、幅度和模式，从而决定施加在呼吸系统上的机械负荷[3]。呼吸系统的上皮细胞被潮汐式牵拉，激活细胞增殖/迁移及表面活性物质的分泌。这些机械依赖性通路的过度或持续激活可能导致病理反应。其中，炎症、细胞存活调节和细胞外基质重塑在 VILI 的病程中起着核心作用（图 15.1）。

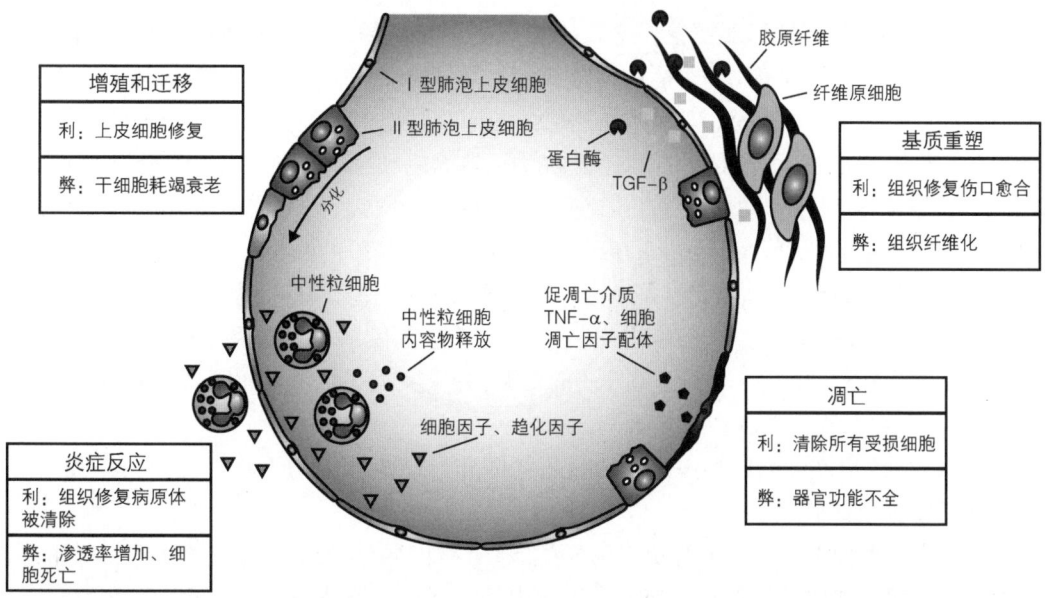

图 15.1 对呼吸机引起的肺损伤中涉及的机械牵拉的生物学反应。如图所示，这些机制都具有促进修复（PROS）和致病作用（CONS）

机械牵拉本身可能诱导肺泡上皮中促炎因子的释放。生成的趋化因子梯度从循环中招募中性粒细胞。活化的中性粒细胞在肺泡间隙和间质内释放含有蛋白酶、活性氧和炎症介质的颗粒，导致组织破坏[4]。上皮屏障完整性的丧失促进了这些介质从肺泡释放到循环中，反之亦然[5]。值得注意的是，一些释放的分子，如白细胞介素-1β 或白细胞介素-6，也是有助于组织修复的生长因子[6]。

机械刺激通过各种细胞内机制调节细胞存活。牵拉本身可以刺激细胞分裂和分化，从而促进上皮修复[7]。然而，机械受体的过度激活会引起细胞周期停滞和（或）细胞凋亡[8]。尽管细胞凋亡可以去除受损细胞而不会引起明显的炎症反应，但细胞大量损失会导致组织功能障碍。

最后,机械牵拉导致基质重塑途径的激活,包括基质合成、加工和降解[9]。几种炎症介质,如 TGF-β,能够激活胶原合成和沉积。机械牵拉促进蛋白酶(弹性蛋白酶、基质金属蛋白酶)从肺泡或募集的炎症细胞中释放,这些蛋白酶不仅可以切割细胞外基质的成分,还可以切割细胞因子和趋化因子等其他分子。在急性期,蛋白酶使肺泡破坏,抑制蛋白酶可能会防止 VILI 产生,然而越来越多的证据表明,它们通过胶原蛋白和细胞因子在后期的修复中发挥作用[10]。

所有这些致病机制是为了保持呼吸系统完整性的极端生理反应。这种对拉伸反应的双重作用(图 15.1)可能解释了大多数针对 VILI 的治疗在临床中失败的原因,因为大多数机制可能在短期内损害肺功能,但对于有效的组织修复/再生是必需的。为了有效治疗,干预不仅必须针对相关通路,而且还必须在特定时间窗内避免干扰内在的组织修复机制。

15.2 呼吸机诱发的肺损伤的病理生理学

机械敏感性是一种局部现象。这意味着只能感受到局部的拉伸或压力,而不是整体的肺容积。在健康的肺部,空气是均匀分布的。尽管肺底和非重力依赖区由于其较高的顺应性而获得较大的气体量,但气体在相邻的肺泡和腺泡中均匀分布。由于这些原因,正常通气、无损伤的肺可能对 VILI 有抵抗力。在均一的肺实质中,只有潮气量(tidal volume, V_T)高到足以令局部过度扩张,甚至在沿全肺分布后仍能增加跨肺压时,才可能造成损害。功能残气量(functional residual capacity, FRC)的测量已被提出作为可用于通气的组织量的标记[11,12],因此,只有当 V_T/FRC(呼吸系统的应变)的值增加到一定值(阈值约为 1.5)以上时,才会出现 VILI。稳定机制的效用,确保呼吸系统内力均匀分布的稳定机制的有效性,解释了其对远高于 6 mL/kg 的 V_T(大多数健康哺乳动物的正常 V_T)的耐受性(不会对正常的肺造成伤害)。

导致 VILI 出现的临床相关因素为吸入气体和(或)扩张力的不均一分布。有几个因素会使已受损伤的肺发生 VILI。

(1) 暴露于促炎环境中的肺更容易发生 VILI,因为全身炎症和损伤性通气具有协同作用[13]。然而,这种机制在没有肺损伤患者中的相关性尚不清楚。

(2) 由于组织顺应性的区域差异,吸入气体的不均匀分布可能导致局部肺泡过度扩张。当大量肺泡由于肺泡塌陷、渗出或区域顺应性极低而无法通气时,大部分气体将流入通气区("婴儿肺")。这就是提出根据肺泡可通气的量决定潮气量的原因[14]。使用不适当的大潮气量将导致局部肺泡过度扩张。在急性呼吸窘迫综合征(acute respiratory distress syndrome, ARDS)患者中,非重力依赖区和肺尖区由于没有促进塌陷的重力作用,通常能保持充气,因此会被过度拉伸[15]。

(3) 空气-组织界面的共存导致沿组织结构的力非均质分布,从而放大它们的量级。通气和非通气肺泡之间隔膜上的区域压力增加量,由肺泡容积的比值的三分之二次方决定(因此,在通气不良的区域,30 cmH_2O 的气道压力可能会局部放大至 120 cmH_2O)[16]。

(4) 异常的气体分布和保留呼气末容积的机制失效(即表面活性物质耗尽、胸壁不稳定等)可能会促进呼吸周期中肺泡大小的巨大变化(称为肺泡不稳定)和呼气末肺泡塌陷。这些肺泡通气的巨大变化增加了肺泡/气道细胞的机械负荷[16]。

所有这些机制都共同使肺泡细胞上承受的张力和压力异常增加,触发先前描述的生化反应,从而使肺持续损伤。从临床角度来看,所有这些机制都被归类为气压伤、容积伤、萎陷伤和生物伤,并且可能是混合发生的。表 15.1 定义了这些概念及其对临床管理的影响,将在后面讨论。

表 15.1 呼吸机诱导肺损伤的经典机制

名 称	定 义
气压伤	跨肺压升高引起的损伤,导致大量漏气到肺泡造成损伤
容积伤	肺泡过度扩张造成的损伤
萎陷伤	由肺泡潮汐通气造成的损伤,反复充气/塌陷循环或肺泡结构过度变形所引起
生物伤	呼吸机引起的肺损伤导致的炎症介质和其他分子释放到循环中

15.3 呼吸机诱导肺损伤的床旁评估

VILI 与其他形式的肺损伤共存,使得在临床中识别和监测 VILI 存在困难。由于 VILI 导致异质性的肺部反应,因此几乎不可能将通气造成的肺损伤与先前潜在疾病所致的肺损伤区分开来。由于这些原因,VILI 的概念已被转变为呼吸机相关肺损伤(ventilator-associated lung injury,VALI)[17]。

作为一种由过度机械负荷引起的现象,使用呼吸力学监测 VILI/VALI 非常令人感兴趣。平台压代表吸气末肺泡压,由于其易于测量,因此被广泛使用。有人建议平台压应保持在 28~30 cmH$_2$O[18]。然而,对于胸壁顺应性受损或自主呼吸的患者,平台压测量时可能会产生误差。在这些情况下,食管压力监测可以估计胸膜压力并计算跨肺压,即施加在肺实质上的真正扩张力。建议使吸气末跨肺压在 20~25 cmH$_2$O 以避免过度膨胀,使呼气末跨肺压力高于 0 cmH$_2$O 避免肺泡塌陷[11]。

驱动压(平台压减去 PEEP)反映了给定 PEEP 下所施加的 V_T 与呼吸系统顺应性之间的关系,由于其与 VILI 潜在的周期性损伤机制相关,已成为更好的衡量损伤性通气的指标。驱动压以 15 cmH$_2$O 为阈值与 ARDS 更好的预后相关[19]。呼吸系统或肺顺应性可能因不同的呼吸设置而不同。然而,在极端情况之外(由于非常高的 V_T 或 PEEP 水平导致顺应性大幅下降,提示肺过度扩张),几种现象(包括周期性复张、肺泡过度扩张或呼气末肺容量增加)的共存对 VILI 机制产生矛盾的作用,使顺应性成为持续损害的不可靠标志。同样的推论也适用于静态压力-容积曲线[20]。已在动物模型和病理生理学研究中测试了肺应变(定义为 V_T 与 FRC 的比)或 V_T 与呼气末肺容积的比(替代指标)[11,12,21],尽管这些测量可以通过调整其参数以适应通气肺泡的数量来帮助确定安全的 V_T,但尚未提供可靠的临床证据。所有这些基于呼吸力学的测量得到是反映全局的平均值。然而，如前所述，VILI 是一种因区域不均一性而增强的局部现象，因此即使"平均"呼吸力学测量值是正常的，也可能发生 VILI。

影像学检查可以提供所需的区域信息以识别暴露于不同类型机械损伤的区域。CT 已被广泛用于检查肺部对机械通气的反应。使用动态、定量的 CT 技术，能根据其放射密度识别通气和过度扩张的周期性变化。这些结果与 ARDS 患者循环中的细胞因子和无呼吸机天数相关[22]。然而，这些基于 CT 的测量很难纳入危重症患者的常规治疗中。在床旁进行的电阻抗断层扫描可以部分解决其中的问题[23]。区域顺应性，即通气变化与压力变化的比，可用于识别过度扩张(如低顺应性的通气区域)和通气的周期性变化。

最后，必须考虑使用生物标志物对 VILI 进行生物监测的可能性。目前已经提出了几种分子作为肺损伤的生物标志物，包括免疫介质(sRAGE、IL-6)、来自呼吸系统的蛋白质(表面活性蛋白、KL-6)、生长因子或在外周血中量化的基因和(或)microRNA 的复杂组合[24]。然而，这些分子中没有一个确定对 VILI 或其任何潜在发病机制(即肺泡牵拉或周期性塌陷)有特异性。

总之，由于缺乏金标准，床旁量化 VILI 十分困难，特别是在已有肺损伤的患者中。将呼吸力学和影像学技术与临床病情演变相结合，可能有助于临床医生更具保护性地调整呼吸机。

15.4　设计肺保护策略

避免产生 VILI 是当前重症治疗的主要目标。限制正压通气对肺组织施加的机械负荷是避免进一步损伤的最佳方法。保护性通气的理念就是要达到避免 VILI 发生这一目标，即使以维持较差的气体交换或需要进行进一步的侵入性支持手段(如体外气体交换)为代价。

不同的呼吸机设置对肺实质有多重影响，特别是在肺泡通气分布不均一时。大多数研究都集中在 PEEP 和 V_T，但呼吸频率或峰流速等其他设置也可能是有意义的。PEEP 通过扩张之前已通气的区域并复张未通气或塌陷区域来增加呼气末肺容积。因此，其对 VILI 机制的作用可能有所不同，从可参与通气的肺组织增加(减少应变有利于均匀通气)，到先前通气的肺泡过度扩张[21](见"17　急性呼吸窘迫综合征的呼气末正压设置")。

V_T 的调整是预防 VILI 的基石。健康的肺部中 VILI 的机制受到抑制，可以耐受中等 V_T 而不会造成明显损伤。然而，在肺损伤的实验模型中，随着 V_T 从 12 mL/kg 降至 3 mL/kg，VILI 发生率持续下降[25]。目前的共识是，对于肺损伤患者，应避免大潮气量(大致定义为 V_T 高于 8 mL/kg，或者导致平台压高于 28 cmH_2O 或驱动压超过 15 cmH_2O 的潮气量)，并且建议将按照(根据身高估算的)理想体重(而非实际体重)以 6 mL/kg 设置潮气量，作为 ARDS 患者的标准治疗[26,27]。然而，V_T 的个体化设置仍存在争议。较大潮气量应用于肺顺应性高的 ARDS 病例可能是安全的，但尚未在研究中得到验证[28]。更重要的是，目前可用的体外气体交换装备允许 CO_2 清除继而可以减少潮气量。超低 V_T 可预防吸气末过度膨胀和通气循环的肺泡巨大变化，但也可因吸气末复张不足而导致肺塌陷[29]。总体而言，尽管指南建议 ARDS 患者的 V_T 在 6 mL/kg 左右，但

V_T 的微调仍然是一个有待解决的问题,反映了目前 VILI 监测的局限性。

还可以调整其他呼吸机参数以减轻 VILI。对于给定的吸气压力,较低的呼吸频率会降低呼吸系统的机械负荷和损伤。较高的吸气流量同样与肺损伤有关,且可能与小气道损伤有关。显然,潮气量、呼吸频率和吸气流量紧密联动,不能独立设置。这种相互依赖关系的最佳解决方案尚不清楚,但实验研究表明,V_T 诱导 VILI 的关联度高于其他参数[30]。

机械通气期间保留自主呼吸也可能影响 VILI 的发展。吸气肌的收缩会在依赖区产生更高的局部跨肺压,而依赖区在肺损伤时往往通气不良。因此,自主呼吸可能有助于复张塌陷区域,使通气更加均匀,有助于减少 VILI 发生。然而,呼吸肌有时可产生非常高的跨肺压(有时不升高,甚至降低平台压和驱动压),而人-机不同步可产生非常高的 V_T(即吸气叠加)。由自主呼吸(有或没有机械通气)引发的肺损伤风险被称为"患者自戕性肺损伤"(patient self-inflicted lung injury,P‑SILI)。虽然与 P‑SILI 的相关性存在争议,但建议至少在急性肺损伤的早期阶段应监测吸气努力,避免过大的跨肺压或人-机不同步[31]。

总之,肺保护性通气策略应包括避免导致吸气末过度扩张的 V_T 和避免之前通气区在呼气末塌陷的 PEEP 水平,将呼吸频率和吸气流量调至最低水平,以确保气体交换和患者舒适度。临床上这些参数的调整必须依靠呼吸力学和影像技术,但要注意这些监测技术的局限性(图 15.2)。

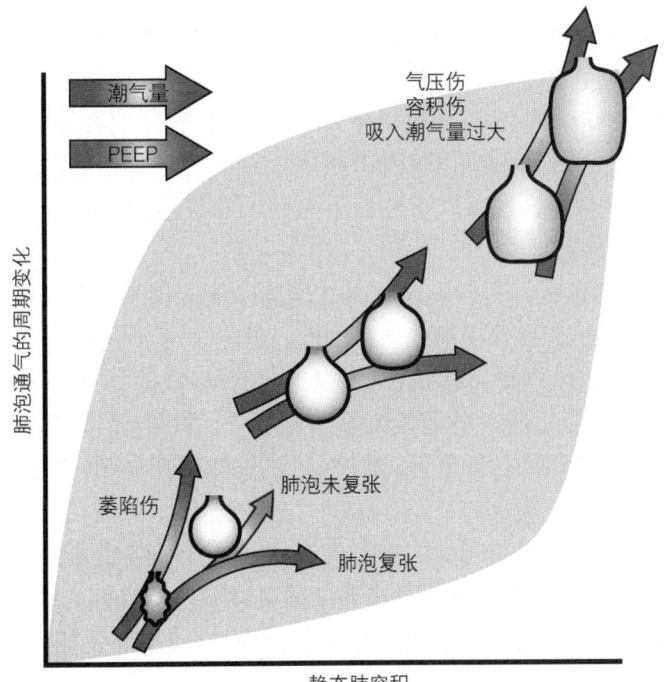

图 15.2 潮气量和 PEEP 的作用。成对的肺泡代表呼气末和吸气末肺泡充气情况。在受伤的肺中,通气设置对静态肺容积和肺泡通气周期性变化的影响取决于先前的充气情况和损伤的性质。所谓的可复张肺可能对 PEEP 有更好的反应,从而有利于静态体积的增加和通气周期肺泡变化的减少(见彩色插图)

需要有一种完全不同的策略能通过针对生物机械转导机制及其涉及肺损伤的下游途径来预防 VILI。在实验模型中,有大量的药物和生物手段可减少损伤性通气后的肺损伤。然而,这些药物均未成功转化为临床应用[32]。与实验模型相反,患者的复杂性及由牵拉触发的大多数细胞反应存在双重性质(稳态和致病性),使得确定有效的 VILI 药物治疗变得复杂。

15.5　肺保护性通气的临床证据

从 Fothergill 的预见开始,花了两个多世纪的时间才收集到足够的临床证据来支持保护性通气策略。将 V_T 从预测体重的 10 mL/kg 或 12 mL/kg 降低到 6 mL/kg 是迄今为止唯一能够降低 ARDS 患者病死率的通气策略。尽管 Amato[27]和 ARDSnet 研究人员[26]的开创性研究是重症监护管理的一个里程碑,但几年后,进一步的分析表明,生存获益与驱动压的降低有关,而非与低潮气量本身有关[19]。然而,尽管在 ARDS 患者中似乎是可行的[33],基于驱动压设置潮气量的潜在益处尚未得到证实。

对气道压力可靠性的担忧也远没有得到解决,因为胸壁弹性的改变可以在 V_T 不变的条件下形成不同的跨肺压。关于使用该参数调整 ARDS 患者通气益处的临床证据很少。使用食管压力调节 PEEP 可改善氧合和呼吸顺应性[34],但未能证明其可从患者结局中受益[35]。

在使用低 V_T 策略观察到病死率的降低之后,继续降低机械能的趋势导致了所谓的超保护性肺通气策略的应用。在临床实践中,这些策略已被证明在体外支持的情况下是安全可行的[36]。虽然一些研究表明可以减少肺部炎症[29,37],但在改善病死率方面没有任何作用[38]。因为缺乏生存获益,所以不建议应用超低潮气量通气,但不排除对特定高危人群的有潜在益处的可能性。

既往无肺部疾病的患者是否会发生 VALI 的临床证据很少。对健康的肺部,即使在手术过程中短时间通气也会导致功能残气量降低。虽然一定水平的 PEEP 可能会减轻肺应力,并使呼吸机的参数设置更具保护性,但根据研究,在没有 ARDS 的患者中,与较高的 PEEP 水平相比,基于低 PEEP 的通气策略并不差[39]。同样,无 ARDS 患者的 V_T 与不同的结果有关。一项比较该人群中低 V_T 和中 V_T 的临床研究显示,两种策略的临床结局无明显差异[39]。

总体而言,临床数据显示,潮气量的影响大于任何其他呼吸机参数,足以提高 ARDS 患者的生存率。相反,其他呼吸机参数设置尚未能证明其临床获益,表明其对 VILI 产生的影响很小或被其副作用抵消。在这种情况下,当前的挑战是寻找能够从微调这些参数或进一步优化 V_T 中受益的特定人群。

15.6　总结

VILI 可以看作是肺暴露于异常机械力的反应。VILI 中的生物学反应可以概括为肺部对损伤的标准反应(包括炎症、细胞凋亡和基质重塑)。目前,改善 VILI 的唯一方法是使用保护性通气策略,包括低 V_T(可能还有低驱动压)和适度的 PEEP 水平。由于缺乏 VILI 监测的金标准,使得临床医生调整呼吸机参数成为了一项艰巨的任务。临床试验表明,导致低驱动压的低 V_T 可降低 ARDS 患者的病死率,而它们在既往无肺损伤的患者中的作用存在争议。能够识别持续机械性肺损伤的监测技术、个体化滴定呼吸机参数,以及针对 VILI 的分子机制的新型药物治疗方法是必要的,可以改善机械通气患者的预后。

(高甜甜,周媛 译)

参考文献

[1] Dreyfuss D, Saumon G. Ventilator-induced lung injury: lessons from experimental studies. Am J Respir Crit Care Med. 1998; 157: 294 – 323.

[2] Fothergill J. Observations on a case published in the last volume of the medical essays, &c. of recovering a man dead in appearance, by distending the lungs with air. Philos Trans R Soc. 1744; 43: 275 – 81.

[3] Albaiceta GM, Brochard L, Dos Santos CC, et al. The central nervous system during lung injury and mechanical ventilation: a narrative review. Br J Anaesth. 2021; 127: 648 – 59.

[4] Williams AE, Chambers RC. The mercurial nature of neutrophils: still an enigma in ARDS? Am J Physiol Lung Cell Mol Physiol. 2014; 306: L217 – 30.

[5] Haitsma JJ, Uhlig S, Goggel R, Verbrugge SJ, Lachmann U, Lachmann B. Ventilator-induced lung injury leads to loss of alveolar and systemic compartmentalization of tumor necrosis factor-alpha. Intensive Care Med. 2000; 26: 1515 – 22.

[6] Geiser T, Jarreau PH, Atabai K, Matthay MA. Interleukin-1beta augments in vitro alveolar epithelial repair. Am J Physiol Lung Cell Mol Physiol. 2000; 279: L1184 – 90.

[7] López-Martínez C, Huidobro C, Albaiceta GM, López-Alonso I. Mechanical stretch modulates cell migration in the lungs. Ann Transl Med. 2018; 6: 28.

[8] Crosby LM, Luellen C, Zhang Z, Tague LL, Sinclair SE, Waters CM. Balance of life and death in alveolar epithelial type II cells: proliferation, apoptosis, and the effects of cyclic stretch on wound healing. Am J Physiol Lung Cell Mol Physiol. 2011; 301: L536 – 46.

[9] Pelosi P, Rocco PR. Effects of mechanical ventilation on the extracellular matrix. Intensive Care Med. 2008; 34: 631 – 9.

[10] Blazquez-Prieto J, Lopez-Alonso I, Amado-Rodriguez L, Huidobro C, Gonzalez-Lopez A, Kuebler WM, Albaiceta GM. Impaired lung repair during neutropenia can be reverted by matrix metalloproteinase-9. Thorax. 2018; 73: 321 – 30.

[11] Chiumello D, Carlesso E, Cadringher P, et al. Lung stress and strain during mechanical ventilation for acute respiratory distress syndrome. Am J Respir Crit Care Med. 2008; 178: 346 – 55.

[12] Gonzalez-Lopez A, Garcia-Prieto E, Batalla-Solis E, Amado-Rodriguez L, Avello N, Blanch L, Albaiceta GM. Lung strain and biological response in mechanically ventilated patients. Intensive Care Med. 2012; 38: 240 – 7.

[13] Smith LS, Gharib SA, Frevert CW, Martin TR. Effects of age on the synergistic interactions between lipopolysaccharide and mechanical ventilation in mice. Am J Respir Cell Mol Biol. 2010;

43: 475-86.

[14] Gattinoni L, Marini JJ, Pesenti A, Quintel M, Mancebo J, Brochard L. The "baby lung" became an adult. Intensive Care Med. 2016; 42: 663-73.

[15] Puybasset L, Gusman P, Muller JC, Cluzel P, Coriat P, Rouby JJ. Regional distribution of gas and tissue in acute respiratory distress syndrome. III. Consequences for the effects of positive end-expiratory pressure. CT Scan ARDS Study Group. Adult Respiratory Distress Syndrome. Intensive Care Med. 2000; 26: 1215-27.

[16] Mitzner W. Mechanics of the lung in the 20th century. Compr Physiol. 2011; 1: 2009-27.

[17] International consensus conferences in intensive care medicine. Ventilator-associated lung injury in ARDS. American Thoracic Society, European Society of Intensive Care Medicine, Societe de Reanimation Langue Francaise. Intensive Care Med. 1999; 25: 1444-52.

[18] Villar J, Martín-Rodríguez C, Domínguez-Berrot AM, et al. A quantile analysis of plateau and driving pressures: effects on mortality in patients with acute respiratory distress syndrome receiving lung-protective ventilation. Crit Care Med. 2017; 45: 843-50.

[19] Amato MB, Meade MO, Slutsky AS, et al. Driving pressure and survival in the acute respiratory distress syndrome. N Engl J Med. 2015; 372: 747-55.

[20] Albaiceta GM, Blanch L, Lucangelo U. Static pressure-volume curves of the respiratory system: were they just a passing fad? Curr Opin Crit Care. 2008; 14: 80-6.

[21] Garcia-Prieto E, Lopez-Aguilar J, Parra-Ruiz D, Amado-Rodriguez L, Lopez-Alonso I, Blazquez-Prieto J, Blanch L, Albaiceta GM. Impact of recruitment on static and dynamic lung strain in acute respiratory distress syndrome. Anesthesiology. 2016; 124: 443-52.

[22] Terragni PP, Rosboch G, Tealdi A, et al. Tidal hyperinflation during low tidal volume ventilation in acute respiratory distress syndrome. Am J Respir Crit Care Med. 2007; 175: 160-6.

[23] Frerichs I, Amato MBP, van Kaam AH, et al. Chest electrical impedance tomography examination, data analysis, terminology, clinical use and recommendations: consensus statement of the translational EIT development study group. Thorax. 2017; 72: 83-93.

[24] Spadaro S, Park M, Turrini C, et al. Biomarkers for Acute Respiratory Distress syndrome and prospects for personalised medicine. J Inflamm Lond Engl. 2019; 16: 1.

[25] Frank JA, Gutierrez JA, Jones KD, Allen L, Dobbs L, Matthay MA. Low tidal volume reduces epithelial and endothelial injury in acid-injured rat lungs. Am J Respir Crit Care Med. 2002; 165: 242-9.

[26] The Acute Respiratory Distress Syndrome Network. Ventilation with lower tidal volumes as compared with traditional tidal volumes for acute lung injury and the acute respiratory distress syndrome. N Engl J Med. 2000; 342: 1301-8.

[27] Amato MB, Barbas CS, Medeiros DM, et al. Effect of a protective-ventilation strategy on mortality in the acute respiratory distress syndrome. N Engl J Med. 1998; 338: 347-54.

[28] Deans KJ, Minneci PC, Cui X, Banks SM, Natanson C, Eichacker PQ. Mechanical ventilation in ARDS: one size does not fit all. Crit Care Med. 2005; 33: 1141-3.

[29] Amado-Rodríguez L, Del Busto C, López-Alonso I, et al. Biotrauma during ultra-low tidal volume ventilation and venoarterial extracorporeal membrane oxygenation in cardiogenic shock: a randomized crossover clinical trial. Ann Intensive Care. 2021; 11: 132.

[30] Cressoni M, Gotti M, Chiurazzi C, et al. Mechanical power and development of ventilator-induced lung injury. Anesthesiology. 2016; 124: 1100-8.

[31] Spinelli E, Mauri T, Beitler JR, Pesenti A, Brodie D. Respiratory drive in the acute respiratory

distress syndrome: pathophysiology, monitoring, and therapeutic interventions. Intensive Care Med. 2020; 46: 606-18.

[32] Uhlig S, Uhlig U. Pharmacological interventions in ventilator-induced lung injury. Trends Pharmacol Sci. 2004; 25: 592-600.

[33] Pereira Romano ML, Maia IS, Laranjeira LN, et al. Driving pressure-limited strategy for patients with acute respiratory distress syndrome. A pilot randomized clinical trial. Ann Am Thorac Soc. 2020; 17: 596-604.

[34] Talmor D, Sarge T, Malhotra A, O'Donnell CR, Ritz R, Lisbon A, Novack V, Loring SH. Mechanical ventilation guided by esophageal pressure in acute lung injury. N Engl J Med. 2008; 359: 2095-104.

[35] Beitler JR, Sarge T, Banner-Goodspeed VM, Gong MN, Cook D, Novack V, Loring SH, Talmor D, EPVent-2 Study Group. Effect of titrating positive end-expiratory pressure (PEEP) with an esophageal pressure-guided strategy vs an empirical high peep-fio2 strategy on death and days free from mechanical ventilation among patients with acute respiratory distress syndrome: a randomized clinical trial. JAMA. 2019; 321: 846-57.

[36] Combes A, Fanelli V, Pham T, Ranieri VM, European Society of Intensive Care Medicine Trials Group and the "Strategy of Ultra-Protective Lung Ventilation with Extracorporeal CO_2 Removal for New-Onset Moderate to Severe ARDS" (SUPERNOVA) Investigators. Feasibility and safety of extracorporeal CO_2 removal to enhance protective ventilation in acute respiratory distress syndrome: the SUPERNOVA study. Intensive Care Med. 2019; 45: 592-600.

[37] Rozencwajg S, Guihot A, Franchineau G, et al. Ultra-protective ventilation reduces biotrauma in patients on venovenous extracorporeal membrane oxygenation for severe acute respiratory distress syndrome. Crit Care Med. 2019; 47: 1505-12.

[38] McNamee JJ, Gillies MA, Barrett NA, et al. Effect of lower tidal volume ventilation facilitated by extracorporeal carbon dioxide removal vs standard care ventilation on 90-day mortality in patients with acute hypoxemic respiratory failure: the REST randomized clinical trial. JAMA. 2021; 326: 1013-23.

[39] Writing Committee and Steering Committee for the RELAx Collaborative Group, Algera AG, Pisani L, et al. Effect of a lower vs higher positive end-expiratory pressure strategy on ventilator-free days in ICU patients without ARDS: a randomized clinical trial. JAMA. 2020; 324: 2509-20.

16 健康肺的机械通气：在手术室和重症监护室中

Mechanical Ventilation in the Healthy Lung: OR and ICU

Fabienne D. Simonis, Frederique Paulus, Marcus J. Schultz

16.1 引言

在过去的三十年中，新增了很多关于 ARDS 患者机械通气的开创性观察性研究和随机临床试验[1]。从这些研究中得出的结论改变了我们为 ARDS 患者设置呼吸机的方式。这些研究的结果也被用于调整健康肺患者的呼吸机管理。

一方面，对 ARDS 患者有益的东西也可能对健康肺的患者有益。例如，在预防机械通气引起的肺损伤方面，考虑减少潮气量（V_T）的大小，可以防止肺组织过度膨胀。另一方面，某些策略可能会产生严重的副作用，在健康肺的患者中甚至可能比在 ARDS 患者中更多，PEEP 的增加可能会（也可能不会）使肺组织复张，但代价是肺泡过度膨胀和血流动力学不稳定。我们可能还需认识到机械通气对健康肺患者的危害程度可能小于 ARDS 患者，这可能会使某些通气策略对健康肺患者的效果降低，甚至根本无效。而不符合或尚未满足当前 ARDS 定义的患者仍可能存在肺损伤或之后出现肺损伤，因此我们可能需要实时调整呼吸机参数。需要重视的是 ICU 机械通气的患者，可能与手术患者，即手术室

F. D. Simonis (✉) · F. Paulus
Department of Intensive Care, Amsterdam University Medical Centers, Location AMC, Amsterdam, The Netherlands
e-mail: f.paulus@amsterdamumc.nl

M. J. Schultz
Department of Intensive Care, Amsterdam University Medical Centers, Location AMC, Amsterdam, The Netherlands

Laboratory of Experimental Intensive Care and Anesthesiology (L·E·I·C·A), Amsterdam University Medical Centers, Location AMC, Amsterdam, The Netherlands

Mahidol-Oxford Tropical Medicine Research Unit (MORU), Mahidol University, Bangkok, Thailand

Nuffield Department of Medicine, University of Oxford, Oxford, UK

© The Author(s), under exclusive license to Springer Nature Switzerland AG 2022
G. Bellani (ed.), *Mechanical Ventilation from Pathophysiology to Clinical Evidence*, https://doi.org/10.1007/978-3-030-93401-9_16

全麻手术期间机械通气的患者，在许多方面有所不同。例如，在危重症患者中通气总持续时间更长，而在麻醉中采用肌肉松弛剂的手术患者中很少出现自主呼吸活动。

在本章中，我们将讨论有关全身麻醉术中通气，以及无 ARDS 的 ICU 患者这两类健康肺机械通气的进展。我们有意将这些患者按照类别分开讨论和建议，原因已在上文解释过了。重点关注使用以患者预后为中心的研究得到的获益证据，忽略仅以生理学指标为终点的研究。我们还将讨论限制在两种主要呼吸机参数的设置：V_T 和 PEEP。

16.2 潮气量

多年来，在手术室，术中通气使用基于理想体重的高达 15 mL/kg 的高 V_T 是十分常见的。因此麻醉医师能够尽可能多地保持肺组织的扩张，这促进了气体交换，并避免了对更高吸入氧浓度（inspired oxygen，FiO_2）或 PEEP 的需求。

这种策略最初是在 ICU 采用的，以前 ICU 中的机械通气主要由麻醉医师承担。然而，一些动物实验表明较高的潮气量有害。这些临床前研究结果引发了一系列针对 ARDS 患者的随机临床试验，结果表明简单地将潮气量的大小减小到 6 mL/kg（理想体重）可显著改善结局[1]。因此，麻醉医师和 ICU 医生重新考虑了通气方法，并大规模采用了低潮气量通气，至少在 ARDS 患者中如此。

16.3 手术室中的潮气量

16.3.1 低潮气量的好处

许多观察性研究显示，术中通气使用的 V_T 大小与术后肺部并发症的发生有关[2,3]。3 项随机临床试验显示，减少 V_T 可预防术后肺部并发症的发生并改善预后[4-6]。虽然这 3 项试验也使用了较高的 PEEP 和较低的 V_T，但个体患者数据荟萃分析发现，较低的 V_T 而不是较高的 PEEP 可保护患者免于发生术后肺部并发症[2]。

16.3.2 低潮气量的挑战

术中低 V_T 通气可导致肺泡不稳定，增加肺不张和肺泡周期性开闭的风险。而且使用较低的 V_T 要求使用较高的呼吸频率（respiratory rate，RR）。然而，麻醉患者产生的 CO_2 通常较低，因此可以使用较低的 V_T 而不必大幅增加 RR，这一点很重要，因为麻醉医师倾向于使患者处于"过度通气"状态[7]。

16.3.3 随时间改变的潮气量

观察性研究显示，手术期间使用的 V_T 大小随时间发生了改变[7,8]。事实上，近年来，术中 V_T 已从高达 12 mL/kg（理想体重）下降到 8 mL/kg（理想体重）。然而，低 V_T [<8 mL/kg（理想体重）] 通气仍未得到充分利用[7]。这可能是由于缺乏个体化通气的意

识,因为有时麻醉医师仍然使用固定V_T,最常见的是 500 mL[7]。这通常会导致V_T过高,尤其是身材矮小的患者,最常见的是女性[9]。麻醉医师也倾向于对肥胖患者进行V_T过高的通气,这可能是因为他们仍然根据实际体重而不是理想体重来滴定V_T[7]。

16.3.4 当前建议

目前,建议术中将V_T设置得较低,为 6~8 mL/kg(理想体重)[10]。尽管有人认为不超过 10 mL/kg(理想体重)的"中间"V_T是有保护作用的,至少是无害的[11]。对于接受胸外科手术的患者,建议单肺通气时使用更低的V_T(另见"25 不同手术情境下的机械通气")。

16.4 重症监护室中的潮气量

16.4.1 低潮气量的优势

对非 ARDS 危重症患者的观察性研究发现,潮气量减少与较低的肺部并发症风险、较短的通气时间、较短的 ICU 监护时间和住院时间相关[12-14]。然而,最近的一项研究未能显示与中等潮气量[8~10 mL/kg(理想体重)]通气相比,低潮气量[4~6 mL/kg(理想体重)]通气更有益[15]。值得注意的是,在该研究中,患者通常在机械通气开始早期使用自主通气模式。由于自主通气模式下对V_T大小的控制远不如控制通气,因此在允许自发呼吸后不久两组V_T大小相当也就不足为奇了。此外,该研究的中等V_T组潮气量并不高,远低于开展这项随机临床试验前的那些观察性研究。

16.4.2 低潮气量的挑战

较低的潮气量可能会增加肺不张的风险,还可能增加镇静需求,从而增加谵妄的风险[16],并可能与更多的人-机不同步有关[17]。此外,代偿性吸气可能导致自戕性肺损伤[18]。而且,使用较低的V_T需要使用较高的 RR,可能会带来更差的预后[19]。不过应该指出的是,在上述研究中,这些挑战并未得到确切证实[15]。

16.4.3 随时间改变的潮气量

多年来,在危重症患者中V_T的设置逐渐减小。V_T的大小已经从>12 mL/kg(理想体重)[20]下降至<8 mL/kg(理想体重)[21,22]。然而也是在这些患者中,低V_T通气仍然在很大程度上未得到充分实施[21,22]。也可能是因为有时V_T被错误地基于实际体重滴定。此外,在 ICU 中,男女之间的V_T大小存在显著且持续的差异,无论是否患有 ARDS[23-24]。这可能是因为计算理想体重所必需的身高难以测量,而且身材矮小的患者往往存在被高估的风险[25]。

16.4.4 当前建议

目前,对于非 ARDS 的危重症患者没有严格的V_T建议。但较大的V_T[即>10 mL/

kg(理想体重)]的设置是不合适的[26]。根据目前的证据,我们建议在接受控制通气的患者中使用较低的V_T[6~8 mL/kg(理想体重)]。应根据理想体重而不是实际体重来滴定V_T,并对患者身高进行正确估算,以准确计算理想体重。

16.5 呼气末正压

肺部分塌陷或不张会对气体交换产生不良影响,还可能使相邻肺组织反复开闭,这可导致或加重肺损伤。许多临床前研究表明,PEEP可以复张这些不稳定的肺单位,但同时也会导致其他肺区域过度膨胀。在很长一段时间里,在手术室使用PEEP是非常少见的,这可能是由于PEEP与血流动力学不稳定相关,需要进行扩容并启动血管活性药物。

在ARDS患者中,PEEP可以明显改善氧合,从而降低对FiO_2的需求。三项随机临床试验对以较高PEEP(中位数15 cmH_2O)、"肺开放"为目标的通气策略可以改善ARDS患者预后的假设进行了检验[27-29]。然而这三项研究未能显示出较高PEEP的益处。而使用这三项研究中患者个体数据进行的一项荟萃分析表明,在中重度ARDS患者中,较高PEEP在病死率上有获益[30],而在轻度ARDS患者观察到有害的迹象。最近一项针对中重度ARDS患者的随机临床试验显示,使用较高PEEP加上积极的肺复张手法会造成伤害[31]。

同时,无论是在手术室还是在ICU,对健康肺患者都明显倾向于使用一定量的PEEP,有时甚至更高。

16.6 手术室呼气末正压的选择

16.6.1 高呼气末正压的优势

在不同手术人群中进行的几项随机临床试验表明,术中使用较高PEEP通气对减少术后并发症的发生有益处[4-6]。然而,在这三项研究中,两个研究组之间不仅有PEEP不同,在较高PEEP策略中V_T较低,而在较低PEEP策略中V_T较高。可以认为,同时使用较低的V_T会弱化较高PEEP的推定益处。因此,两项随机临床试验比较了术中低V_T低PEEP(<5 cmH_2O)和高PEEP(12 cmH_2O或更高)通气的疗效[32,33]。这两项研究均未能显示非肥胖患者[32]和肥胖患者[33]术后预后的改善。

16.6.2 高呼气末正压的挑战

在上述两项研究中还发现使用较高的PEEP可能会损害心功能并导致低血压。在这两项研究中将低V_T术中通气的低PEEP与高PEEP进行比较:在非肥胖患者中,接受术中血管活性药物的患者比例从51%增加到62%[32],在肥胖患者中这一比例从45%增加到50%[33]。虽然理论上较高的PEEP策略会增加气压伤的风险,但在这两项研究中都没有得到证实。

16.6.3 随时间改变的呼气末正压

PEEP 在手术室中的应用越来越多。一项研究评估了 30 年间 96 项研究中 8 万多名患者的术中呼吸机管理,结果显示 PEEP 略有升高[34]。这可能取决于动物研究中较高 PEEP 的阳性结果,以及上述比较高 PEEP/低 V_T 与低 PEEP/高 V_T 的术中通气研究结果。此外,这还可能取决于特定呼吸机制造商允许的较低 PEEP 值,其范围为 $2\sim5\ cmH_2O$。

16.6.4 当前建议

手术期间 PEEP 最佳水平尚未明确。新的研究旨在确定将 PEEP 滴定至最佳呼吸系统顺应性或驱动压是否优于标准的低 PEEP[35,36]。同时,我们建议使用尽可能低的 PEEP,只有在将较高 PEEP 作为挽救措施时使用高 PEEP,如在增加 FiO_2 难以改善的低氧血症中。也许使用 $5\ cmH_2O$ 的 PEEP 就足够了,这也是被广为接受的 PEEP 水平。对于接受微创腹部手术或机器人手术的患者,膈肌可能会出现上抬,在这些情况下是否应使用更高水平的 PEEP 尚不确定[37]。目前已计划进行几项研究。在此,如上文所述,我们仅建议在使用较高的 PEEP 作为挽救措施时,如在提高 FiO_2 难以改善的低氧血症情况下使用高 PEEP。

16.7 在重症监护室中呼气末正压的设置

16.7.1 高呼气末正压的优势

自重症医学创立以来,优化氧合和清除二氧化碳被视为机械通气的目标。值得注意的是,有些时期的氧合目标高于正常水平。使用 PEEP,乃至更高的 PEEP 非常适合,因为在呼气结束时使用更高的压力可以大大改善肺泡通气,并防止部分肺塌陷。PEEP,特别是高水平的 PEEP 的使用,是由"肺开放"策略可以预防肺损伤的概念推动的,这一点在几项利用动物模型模拟危重疾病场景的临床前研究中得到了证实。

一项荟萃分析纳入了非 ARDS 的危重症患者,比较低 PEEP 与无 PEEP 的效果,结果显示使用 PEEP 无获益[38]。应该指出的是,分析中纳入的研究规模小、质量差,其中大多数都早于明确 ARDS 的定义之前。最近发表的一项针对有 ARDS 风险患者的随机临床试验比较了高 PEEP($8\ cmH_2O$)与低 PEEP($0\sim5\ cmH_2O$)通气[39]。在这项非劣效性研究中,与高 PEEP 相比,低 PEEP 通气在通气时长方面并不逊色。这项研究确实表明了高 PEEP 的通气策略可以有更好的氧合,并且作为挽救疗法在低氧血症中的使用也有所增加,不过没有统计学意义。同样,在加入这项研究后的荟萃分析的结果中也得到了证实[40]。

16.7.2 高呼气末正压的挑战

非 ARDS 的患者肺塌陷部分远小于 ARDS 患者。至少在理论上与 ARDS 患者相比,健康肺患者可能需要相对较高的 PEEP 来复张相似数量的肺组织。由于健康肺患者的肺组织顺应性更高,因此相同的 PEEP 下,与 ARDS 患者相比,健康肺患者肺容量和胸内压变化更大。因此,较高 PEEP 产生的血流动力学效应可能在健康肺的危重症患者中更明显[41]。此外,使用较高的 PEEP 可能会导致延迟拔管,因为通常是在低 PEEP 条件下拔管[42]。

16.7.3 呼气末正压随时间的变化

与手术室患者类似,较高的 PEEP 越来越多地用于 ICU 的危重症患者,包括非 ARDS 的患者[34]。连续几篇以呼吸机管理为重点的全球范围综述也表明了这一点[43-45]。到目前为止,超过半数肺健康的危重症患者接受了 PEEP>5 cmH_2O 的通气,但结果存在地域差异[46]。

16.7.4 当前建议

目前缺乏关于健康肺患者 PEEP 的推荐意见。我们的建议是避免在这些患者中常规使用较高的 PEEP。较低 PEEP(<5 cmH_2O)的通气可能与较高 PEEP 的通气效果一样。

16.8 总结

我们总结了目前手术室患者以及 ICU 中对健康肺的危重症患者使用低 V_T 和高 PEEP 的证据。我们建议使用较低的 V_T,因为更大的通气量会使肺组织过度膨胀而对肺组织造成伤害,并且很有可能损害脆弱的肺结构。这比低 V_T 通气可能导致氧合变差更严重。使用较高的 PEEP 是吸引人的,因为可以想象高 PEEP 会复张更多的肺组织,并防止肺泡单元的反复打开和关闭。然而,高 PEEP 在健康肺的患者中未见获益,并且高 PEEP 通气存在血流动力学不稳定的副作用,所以我们不赞成使用这种通气策略。未来针对特定患者群体的研究可能会显示出高 PEEP 的益处。

(高甜甜,周媛 译)

参考文献

[1] Acute Respiratory Distress Syndrome Network. Ventilation with lower tidal volumes as compared with traditional tidal volumes for acute lung injury and the acute respiratory distress syndrome. The Acute Respiratory Distress Syndrome Network. N Engl J Med. 2000;342(18):1301-8.

[2] Serpa Neto A, Hemmes SNT, Barbas CSV, Beiderlinden M, Biehl M, Binnekade JM, et al. Protective versus conventional ventilation for surgery. Anesthesiology. 2015;123(1):66-78.

[3] Nguyen D-N, Guay J, Ochroch EA. Intraoperative use of low volume ventilation to decrease postoperative mortality, mechanical ventilation, lengths of stay and lung injury in patients without acute lung injury. In: Guay J, editor. Cochrane database of systematic reviews. Wiley: Chichester; 2014.

[4] Futier E, Constantin J-M, Paugam-Burtz C, Pascal J, Eurin M, Neuschwander A, et al. A trial

of intraoperative low-tidal-volume ventilation in abdominal surgery. N Engl J Med. 2013; 369(5): 428 – 37.

[5] Severgnini P, Selmo G, Lanza C, Chiesa A, Frigerio A, Bacuzzi A, et al. Protective mechanical ventilation during general anesthesia for open abdominal surgery improves postoperative pulmonary function. Anesthesiology. 2013; 118(6): 1307 – 21.

[6] Ge Y, Yuan L, Jiang X, Wang X, Xu R, Ma W. [Effect of lung protection mechanical ventilation on respiratory function in the elderly undergoing spinal fusion]. Zhong Nan Da Xue Xue Bao Yi Xue Ban. 2013; 38(1): 81 – 5.

[7] LAS VEGAS Investigators. Epidemiology, practice of ventilation and outcome for patients at increased risk of postoperative pulmonary complications: LAS VEGAS - an observational study in 29 countries. Eur J Anaesthesiol. 2017; 34(8): 492 – 507.

[8] Fernandez-Bustamante A, Frendl G, Sprung J, Kor DJ, Subramaniam B, Ruiz RM, et al. Postoperative pulmonary complications, early mortality, and hospital stay following noncardiothoracic surgery: a multicenter study by the perioperative research network investigators. JAMA Surg. 2017; 152(2): 157 – 66.

[9] Nijbroek SG, Hol L, Swart P, Hemmes SNT, Serpa Neto A, Binnekade JM, et al. Sex difference and intra-operative tidal volume: insights from the LAS VEGAS study. Eur J Anaesthesiol. 2021; 38(10): 1034.

[10] Young CC, Harris EM, Vacchiano C, Bodnar S, Bukowy B, Elliott RRD, et al. Lung-protective ventilation for the surgical patient: international expert panel-based consensus recommendations. Br J Anaesth. 2019; 123(6): 898 – 913.

[11] Karalapillai D, Weinberg L, Peyton P, Ellard L, Hu R, Pearce B, et al. Effect of intraoperative low tidal volume vs conventional tidal volume on postoperative pulmonary complications in patients undergoing major surgery: a randomized clinical trial. JAMA. 2020; 324(9): 848 – 58.

[12] Serpa Neto A, Simonis FD, Barbas CSV, Biehl M, Determann RM, Elmer J, et al. Association between tidal volume size, duration of ventilation, and sedation needs in patients without acute respiratory distress syndrome: an individual patient data meta-analysis. Intensive Care Med. 2014; 40(7): 950 – 7.

[13] Serpa Neto A, Simonis FD, Barbas CSV, Biehl M, Determann RM, Elmer J, et al. Lung-protective ventilation with low tidal volumes and the occurrence of pulmonary complications in patients without acute respiratory distress syndrome. Crit Care Med. 2015; 43(10): 2155 – 63.

[14] Serpa Neto A, Cardoso SO, Manetta JA, Pereira VGM, Espósito DC, de Oliveira Prado Pasqualucci M, et al. Association between use of lung-protective ventilation with lower tidal volumes and clinical outcomes among patients without acute respiratory distress syndrome: a meta-analysis. JAMA. 2012; 308(16): 1651 – 9.

[15] Simonis FD, Serpa Neto A, Binnekade JM, Braber A, Bruin KCM, Determann RM, et al. Effect of a low vs intermediate tidal volume strategy on ventilator-free days in intensive care unit patients without ARDS: a randomized clinical trial. JAMA. 2018; 320(18): 1872 – 80.

[16] Ferguson ND. Low tidal volumes for all? JAMA. 2012; 308(16): 1689 – 90.

[17] Kallet RH, Campbell AR, Dicker R, a., Katz J a., Mackersie RC. Effects of tidal volume on work of breathing during lung-protective ventilation in patients with acute lung injury and acute respiratory distress syndrome. Crit Care Med. 2006; 34(1): 8 – 14.

[18] Brochard L, Slutsky A, Pesenti A. Mechanical ventilation to minimize progression of lung injury in acute respiratory failure. Am J Respir Crit Care Med. 2017; 195(4): 438 – 42.

[19] Akoumianaki E, Vaporidi K, Georgopoulos D. The injurious effects of elevated or non-elevated respiratory rate during mechanical ventilation. Am J Respir Crit Care Med. 2019; 199(2): 149-57.

[20] Checkley W, Brower R, Korpak A, Thompson BT. Effects of a clinical trial on mechanical ventilation practices in patients with acute lung injury. Am J Respir Crit Care Med. 2008; 177(11): 1215-22.

[21] Serpa Neto A, Barbas CSV, Simonis FD, Artigas-Raventós A, Canet J, Determann RM, et al. Epidemiological characteristics, practice of ventilation, and clinical outcome in patients at risk of acute respiratory distress syndrome in intensive care units from 16 countries (PRoVENT): an international, multicentre, prospective study. Lancet Respir Med. 2016; 4(11): 882-93.

[22] Pisani L, Algera AG, Neto AS, Ahsan A, Beane A, Chittawatanarat K, et al. Epidemiological characteristics, ventilator management, and clinical outcome in patients receiving invasive ventilation in intensive care units from 10 Asian middle-income countries (PRoVENT-iMiC): An international, multicenter, prospective study. Am J Trop Med Hyg. 2021; 104(3): 1022-33.

[23] McNicholas BA, Madotto F, Pham T, Rezoagli E, Masterson CH, Horie S, et al. Demographics, management and outcome of females and males with acute respiratory distress syndrome in the LUNG SAFE prospective cohort study. Eur Respir J. 2019; 54(4): 1900609.

[24] Swart P, Deliberato RO, Johnson AEW, Pollard TJ, Bulgarelli L, Pelosi P, et al. Impact of sex on use of low tidal volume ventilation in invasively ventilated ICU patients-a mediation analysis using two observational cohorts. PLoS One. 2021; 16(7): e0253933.

[25] Schultz MJ, Karagiannidis C. Is gender inequity in ventilator management a "women's issue"? Eur Respir J. 2019; 54: 1901588.

[26] Rose L, Kenny L, Tait G, Mehta S. Ventilator settings and monitoring parameter targets for initiation of continuous mandatory ventilation: a questionnaire study. J Crit Care. 2014; 29(1): 123-7.

[27] Brower RG, Lanken PN, MacIntyre N, Matthay MA, Morris A, Ancukiewicz M, et al. Higher versus lower positive end-expiratory pressures in patients with the acute respiratory distress syndrome. N Engl J Med. 2004; 351(4): 327-36.

[28] Meade MO, Cook DJ, Guyatt GH, Slutsky AS, Arabi YM, Cooper DJ, et al. Ventilation strategy using low tidal volumes, recruitment maneuvers, and high positive end-expiratory pressure for acute lung injury and acute respiratory distress syndrome. JAMA. 2008; 299(6): 637.

[29] Mercat A, Richard JM, Vielle B, Jaber S, Osman D, Diehl J-L, et al. Positive end-expiratory pressure setting in adults with acute lung injury and acute respiratory distress syndrome: a randomized controlled trial. JAMA. 2008; 299(6): 646-55.

[30] Briel M, Meade M, Mercat A, Brower RG, Talmor D, Walter SD, et al. Higher vs lower positive end-expiratory pressure in patients with acute lung injury and acute respiratory distress syndrome: systematic review and meta-analysis. JAMA. 2010; 303(9): 865-73.

[31] Cavalcanti AB, Suzumura ÉA, Laranjeira LN, de Moraes Paisani D, Damiani LP, Guimarães HP, et al. Effect of lung recruitment and titrated positive end-expiratory pressure (PEEP) vs low PEEP on mortality in patients with acute respiratory distress syndrome. JAMA. 2017; 318(14): 1335.

[32] PROVE Network Investigators for the Clinical Trial Network of the European Society of Anaesthesiology, SNT H, Gama de Abreu M, Pelosi P, Schultz MJ. High versus low positive

[33] end-expiratory pressure during general anaesthesia for open abdominal surgery (PROVHILO trial): a multicentre randomised controlled trial. Lancet. 2014; 384(9942): 495 - 503.

[33] Bluth T, Serpa Neto A, Schultz MJ, Pelosi P, Gama de Abreu M. Effect of intraoperative high positive end-expiratory pressure (PEEP) with recruitment maneuvers vs low PEEP on post-operative pulmonary complications in obese patients. JAMA. 2019; 321(23): 2292.

[34] Schaefer MS, Serpa Neto A, Pelosi P, Gama De Abreu M, Kienbaum P, Schultz MJ, et al. Temporal changes in ventilator settings in patients with uninjured lungs: a systematic review. Anesth Analg. 2019; 129: 129.

[35] Ferrando C, Soro M, Unzueta C, Suarez-Sipmann F, Canet J, Librero J, et al. Individualised perioperative open-lung approach versus standard protective ventilation in abdominal surgery (iPROVE): a randomised controlled trial. Lancet Respir Med. 2018; 6(3): 193.

[36] Hol L, Nijbroek SGLH, Neto AS, De Abreu MG, Pelosi P, Hemmes SNT, et al. Driving pressure during general anesthesia for open abdominal surgery (DESIGNATION): study protocol of a randomized clinical trial. Trials. 2020; 21(1): 198.

[37] Mazzinari G, Serpa Neto A, Hemmes SNT, Hedenstierna G, Jaber S, Hiesmayr M, et al. The Association of Intraoperative driving pressure with postoperative pulmonary complications in open versus closed abdominal surgery patients - a posthoc propensity score - weighted cohort analysis of the LAS VEGAS study. BMC Anesthesiol. 2021; 21(1): 84.

[38] Serpa Neto A, Filho RR, Cherpanath T, Determann R, Dongelmans DA, Paulus F, et al. Associations between positive end-expiratory pressure and outcome of patients without ARDS at onset of ventilation: a systematic review and meta-analysis of randomized controlled trials. Ann Intensive Care. 2016; 6(1): 109.

[39] Algera AG, Pisani L, Serpa Neto A, den Boer SS, Bosch FFH, Bruin K, et al. Effect of a lower vs higher positive end-expiratory pressure strategy on ventilator-free days in ICU patients without ARDS: a randomized clinical trial. JAMA. 2020; 324(24): 2509.

[40] Pettenuzzo T, Boscolo A, De Cassai A, Sella N, Zarantonello F, Persona P, et al. Higher versus lower positive end-expiratory pressure in patients without acute respiratory distress syndrome: a meta-analysis of randomized controlled trials. Crit Care. 2021; 25(1): 247.

[41] Luecke T, Pelosi P. Clinical review: positive end-expiratory pressure and cardiac output. Crit Care. 2005; 9: 607.

[42] Blackwood B, Alderdice F, Burns K, Lavery G. Use of weaning protocols for reducing duration of mechanical ventilation in critically ill adult patients. Cochrane systematic review and meta-analysis. BMJ. 2011; 342: c7237.

[43] Esteban A, Anzueto A, Frutos F, Alia I, Brochard L, Stewart TE, et al. Characteristics and outcomes in adult patients receiving mechanical ventilation. JAMA. 2002; 287(3): 345 - 55.

[44] Esteban A, Ferguson ND, Meade MO, Frutos-Vivar F, Apezteguia C, Brochard L, et al. Evolution of mechanical ventilation in response to clinical research. Am J Respir Crit Care Med. 2008; 177(2): 170 - 7.

[45] Esteban A, Frutos-Vivar F, Muriel A, Ferguson ND, Peñuelas O, Abraira V, et al. Evolution of mortality over time in patients receiving mechanical ventilation. Am J Respir Crit Care Med. 2013; 188(2): 220 - 30.

[46] Van IJzendoorn M, Koopmans M, Strauch U, Heines S, Den Boer S, Kors B, et al. Ventilator settings in ICUs: comparing a Dutch with a global cohort. Neth J Med. 2014; 72(9): 473 - 80.

17 急性呼吸窘迫综合征的呼气末正压设置
PEEP Setting in ARDS

Emanuele Rezoagli, Giacomo Bellani

17.1 引言

呼气末正压（positive end-expiratory pressure，PEEP）是机械通气的控制或支持通气模式中在呼气时施加的正压：它确保呼气末肺泡压力高于大气压力，主要目的是防止肺泡塌陷。

在本章中，我们讨论的是"外源性 PEEP"，即呼吸机上设置的 PEEP 水平。不应将其与内源性 PEEP 混淆，后者是由于气流阻塞或流量限制而导致的不完全呼气结束时的肺泡压力。

PEEP 是危重症患者急性呼吸窘迫综合征（acute respiratory distress syndrome, ARDS）治疗的关键通气治疗手段。Ashbaugh 及其同事于 1967 年报道中首次描述了 PEEP 在逆转 ARDS 低氧血症方面的有益作用[1]。

总体而言，PEEP 增加了胸内压，胸内压根据肺和胸壁各自的顺应性而可变地分布。

在本章中我们将首先描述 PEEP 在 ARDS 中的病理生理效应。随后，我们将讨论如何根据不同的目标和不同方法所获得的主要临床结果来设置 PEEP。

17.2 病理生理：呼气末正压的益处

在 ARDS 中，PEEP 可以通过抵消由表面活性物质受损引起的表面张力升高、肺重量增加和胸壁弹性回缩力引起的叠加压力来防止部分肺泡塌陷。

这些作用可避免呼气时肺泡过度排空,从而减少肺内分流。严格说来,PEEP 的作用是预防肺泡不张[2],而肺复张是一种"吸气现象"。同时,由于 PEEP 增加通常与吸气压增加有关,因此复张和避免塌陷通常是同时进行的。另外,基于打开肺泡所需的压力高于避免萎陷的压力(滞后现象),肺复张手法(recruitment maneuvers,RM)可以与 PEEP 滴定法结合使用。

当应用 PEEP 时,一些肺泡得以重新参与气体交换,呼气末肺容积(end-expiratory lung volume,EELV)增加。这通常会导致肺应变的降低和呼吸系统顺应性的改善。反过来,产生相同潮气量所需的驱动压力会降低,这正是所期望的,因为较低的驱动压与较高的存活率之间存在很强的关联[3]。

此外,PEEP 可以通过减少萎陷伤(即通气期间肺泡的循环打开和关闭)以及减少肺的不均一性和应力,以最大限度地减少呼吸机诱导的肺损伤(ventilator induced lung injury,VILI),从而获得更均匀的通气,更少的局部高应力,这些局部高应力位于不同弹性肺单位的交界区域。

17.3　病理生理学：呼气末正压的危害

PEEP 如果设置不当,会对呼吸系统和心血管系统都产生有害影响。

高水平的 PEEP 可显著增加右心房压从而降低静脉回流的压力梯度,导致右心前负荷降低,继而导致左心前负荷降低,最终减少心输出量。

与任何其他压力一样,PEEP 倾向于影响更高顺应性的肺部区域。通常在 ARDS 中,无论 PEEP 设置得多高,塌陷区域都难以重新开放,非重力依赖区域可以被打开,而通气良好区域容易过度膨胀,会促进肺泡炎症和损伤。此外,根据肺复张和过度膨胀间的平衡,PEEP 可能会增加肺血管阻力,从而增加右心后负荷,增加发生肺源性心脏病的风险。最后,如果肺泡压力高于毛细血管压力,则可能会由于毛细血管闭塞增加肺泡无效腔通气,导致二氧化碳清除障碍。

17.4　急性呼吸窘迫综合征中呼气末正压设置的建议

目前的指南中没有建议 ARDS 中 PEEP 设置的具体水平或阈值。然而,Briel 等的个体患者数据荟萃分析表明,对中重度 ARDS 患者应有条件地推荐较高而非较低的 PEEP 水平[4]。在此研究中,高 PEEP 组和低 PEEP 组第 1 天的平均 PEEP 水平分别为(15.3 ± 3.4)cmH_2O 和(9.0 ± 3.1)cmH_2O[5]。尽管有这些建议,但 ARDS 中常规设定的 PEEP 水平仍低得令人担忧。在 LUNG SAFE 研究中,中度和重度 ARDS 患者 PEEP 的中位水平分别为 $8.3 cmH_2O$ 和 $10.1 cmH_2O$[6]。相似地,近期发表的 SAGE 研究证实,在美国 $PaO_2/FiO_2 \leqslant 150$ mmHg 的 ARDS 患者中,PEEP 的平均水平较低[7]。

遗憾的是,目前仍缺乏关于如何设置 PEEP 方法的推荐意见,并且不同技术之间哪种更优尚不清楚,这仍然是一个有很大争议的话题,我们将在本章的剩余部分集中讨论。

17.5 床旁滴定呼气末正压的策略

17.5.1 NIH 的 PEEP-FiO_2 表

根据美国国立卫生研究院（National Institutes of Health，NIH）ARDS 网络研究组织在潮气量研究中提出的一种根据 ARDS 严重程度设定 PEEP 的方法。以正常血氧为目标，分步增加 PEEP（最高至 18～24cmH_2O）的同时，在 0.3～1.0 的范围内（也是逐步地）增加 FiO_2。

随后，相同的研究人员提出了一个较高的 PEEP-FiO_2 表，与第一个组合表（标记为"较低"）相对比。为了测试 PEEP 对 VILI（即容积伤、萎陷伤、气压伤和生物伤）是否有保护作用，在两项随机对照试验中对两个组合表进行了比较[8,9]。与低 PEEP 组相比，接受较高水平 PEEP 的患者动脉氧合情况有所改善，这表明高 PEEP 使更多的肺复张；但病死率无差异。

使用 PEEP-FiO_2 组合表的一个前提是承认改善氧合与肺复张之间的关系，但实际上这种关系是相当微弱的。一方面，如果 PEEP 增加导致 EELV 增加，则部分肺灌注被引导到现在恢复通气的区域，这使右向左分流减少，从而产生更好的动脉氧合。另一方面，PEEP 可能会引起肺血管阻力（pulmonary vascular resistance，PVR）增加和肺泡过度膨胀而降低氧合。这可能使血液流向塌陷的肺单位，增加右向左分流。事实上，在增加 PEEP 后，并非所有患者的氧合都可以改善。然而，使用 PEEP-FiO_2 组合表要求 PEEP 与 FiO_2 一起增加，忽略了患者（在氧合和呼吸力学两个方面）的个体反应[10]。另一方面，该表降低了不当增加与 PEEP 不匹配的 FiO_2 的风险。

两项大型临床试验的二次分析提供了证据支持，表明 PEEP 增加导致的氧合改善与生存率提高相关[11]。

在评估气体交换时，不应忘记 $PaCO_2$ 和无效腔，因为它们对通气/灌注不匹配很敏感。Suter 等在 1975 年提出，无效腔占比的降低与氧传输的增加和静态顺应性的增加有关[12]。事实上，在恒定的每分钟通气量下，$PaCO_2$ 随 PEEP 升高表明无效腔增大，这可能是由肺泡灌注减少和过度膨胀引起的。

17.5.2 呼吸力学：呼吸系统的顺应性和驱动压

自 1975 年以来，呼吸系统的顺应性（compliance of the respiratory system，Cplrs）就已被提议作为 PEEP 滴定的目标。在两项独立的研究中，Suter 和 Falke 报道 PEEP 的增加与 FRC、Cplrs 和氧合的增加有关[12,13]。然而，使用 Cplrs 作为优化 PEEP 设置的目标是基于以下假设：Cplrs 的增加反映了肺复张导致的肺容积增加，而肺过度膨胀则会导致顺应性丧失。这主要取决于肺可复张容积的大小，以及充气不佳和未充气肺区域的开放压。此外，还有一个假设是胸壁和腹部力学不受 PEEP 的影响。此外，另一个潜在的误导性因素是潮气量相关的肺泡打开和关闭，可能导致高估 PEEP 对 Cplrs 增加的贡献。

最近，有人提出了一种基于驱动压力（driving pressure，DP）的 PEEP 优化方法，DP 为潮气量与 Cplrs 的比。Cplrs 与 EELV 成正比，因此与"婴儿肺"的大小成正比。综上所述，DP 反应的是可充气肺承受的潮气量，与病死率独立相关[3]。此外，在最近对 ALVEOLI 和 ExPress 试验的重新分析中，Yehya 等比较了按流程调整呼吸机设置后病死率与 PaO_2/FiO_2 和 DP 变化之间的关联。研究者观察到，与氧合变化相比，DP 变化与病死率的相关性更强，提示 DP 与病死率存在主要的关联[14]。

寻找较低的 DP（或更高的顺应性）作为设定 PEEP 的目标的概念，最近似乎受到 ART 试验结果的挑战[15]。据报道，在 RM 后以 Cplrs 为目标进行递减法设置 PEEP[16] 导致病死率增加。我们认为，这项研究并不意味着使用较高的 PEEP 或以更低的 DP 为目标的策略应被废除。在 ART 试验中，可能由其他因素导致了更高的病死率，如使用 60 cmH_2O 的激进性 RM（后来降低至 50 cmH_2O），共持续数分钟，需要神经肌肉阻滞剂、重要的液体扩张，且在 PEEP 滴定后需再次进行 RM。此外，PEEP 设定为比最低 DP（或最佳 Cplrs）值高 2 cmH_2O 的水平，可能导致非重力依赖区肺组织的过度膨胀[10,15]。

17.5.3 压力-容积曲线和肺容积测定

一些研究者建议使用压力-容积曲线的下拐点作为阈值，PEEP 应设置在该阈值之上。这应该可以最大限度地减少肺萎陷伤[17]。该策略的主要局限性是需要深度镇静和（可能的）肌肉松弛、某些患者拐点识别的不确定性，以及认为维持肺泡开放的压力位于 P-V 曲线的整个吸气支。由于肺泡闭合压力低于开放压力[18]，P-V 曲线显示出相关的滞后现象，这为在增加 PEEP 前应用肺复张手法提供了理论依据[10]。其他研究者建议使用呼气支滴定 PEEP。与使用吸气支相比，这在生理上更合理。然而，在重力梯度作用下（即从依赖区到非依赖区），ARDS 患者的肺在高压水平下开始塌陷。

PEEP 滴定期间肺容积的变化（另见"35 肺容积和容积二氧化碳图"）也可用于评估 PEEP 改变后充气肺容量的增加。气体稀释法（包括氦气或氮气洗出）已被用于测量 EELV。当 PEEP 增加时，EELV 必然会增加（即使没有任何复张）且与顺应性成比例。如果 EELV 的增加超过预测值（顺应性与 PEEP 变化的乘积），则认为额外增加的容积反映了重新开放肺单位的通气量[19]。最近，Chen 提出了一种 PEEP 从 15 cmH_2O 突然降低到 5 cmH_2O 的方法。如果增加的呼气量高于基于顺应性的预测值，则该差异对应"PEEP 的复张容积"。计算出复张容积的顺应性与低 PEEP 时的顺应性间的比值，称为"复张充气比"，是床旁评估肺可复张性的工具[20]。

17.5.4 肺牵张指数

肺牵张指数（stress index，SI）是用于描述容量控制通气（具有方形吸气流速波形）期间压力-时间曲线斜率的量；在 $P_{aw}=a \times t^b + c$ 公式中，为指数 b。在某些呼吸机上可以计算出 SI，而其他情况下必须"视觉评估"。SI<1 表示顺应性在吸气期间逐渐增加（吸气时复张），而 SI>1 表示过度膨胀。因此，SI 的最佳值被认为是 1[21]。与低 PEEP-FiO_2 表相比，Grasso 等将 SI 作为 PEEP 滴定的目标时，Cplrs 较高而炎症生物标志物水平较低[22]。

17.5.5 跨肺压

使用跨肺压滴定 PEEP 的想法源于：当部分压力扩张肺部时，它也以不同的比例扩张了胸壁。在 P-V 曲线右移（如肥胖）或胸壁顺应性低（如腹胀、胸腔积液或烧伤）的情况下，增加的气道压力使胸壁扩张，导致用于扩张肺泡的压力降低。因此，食管压（作为胸膜压的替代指标）已被用于分析胸壁和肺对整体气道压力消耗的贡献。估算跨肺压主要有两种方法：一种基于绝对压力值，另一种则基于吸气引起的压力摆动[23]。

在 EPVent 试验中，Talmor 等证明，与使用低 PEEP-FiO_2 表相比，根据食管压调整 PEEP 使呼气末跨肺压达到 $0\sim10$ cmH_2O（基于 FiO_2，改善氧合和 Cplrs），导致无显著性差异的 28 天病死率降低（17% vs. 39%，$P=0.055$）[24]。鉴于干预组 PEEP 的绝对值明显较高，在随后的 EPVent-2 试验中，作者比较了基于食管压调整 PEEP 与使用高 PEEP-FiO_2 表的效果。在任何结局终点上，两组之间均未观察到差异[25]。有趣的是，一项辅助分析显示，治疗对 60 日病死率的影响受基线多器官功能障碍严重程度的影响，在 APACHE-II 评分较低的情况下，基于食管压调整 PEEP 组的病死率较低[26]。

17.5.6 肺部影像学

本书有章节专门介绍下面总结的成像技术。CT 推动了对 ARDS 患者肺部气体区域分布的研究。不同研究小组利用 CT 更好地了解到肺力学、机械通气，以及肺充气和塌陷的分布之间的关系[27,28]。鉴于患者转移和放射暴露的要求，以肺部 CT 分析设置 PEEP 只可用于特定病例和为了研究的目的，因为它不适合临床常规使用。

Constantin 等基于放射成像技术区分了局灶性和弥漫性 ARDS，并在弥漫性疾病患者中设置了较高的 PEEP。这并没有使整体病死率降低，但这一结果被错误分类患者的高病死率所影响[29]。

肺超声近期被用于 PEEP 滴定，因为它是评估肺复张的可靠技术，然而它并不能提供关于过度膨胀的可靠信息[30]。

最近电阻抗成像技术（electrical impedance tomography，EIT）被推荐用于滴定 PEEP（另见"33 电阻抗体断层成像技术"），因为其具有区分区域性肺不张和过度膨胀的潜力。EIT 无辐射，可在床旁进行。此外，EIT 可以提供呼吸通气区域分布的动态信息，并可以推断 PEEP 变化后 EELV 的变化[31]。有一种方法基于递减 PEEP 法观察区域顺应性的变化[32,33]，但我们提出了一种基于递增 PEEP 的方法，在每次 PEEP 增加之前使用"诊断性"RM（图 17.1），目的是在通气期间获得稳定的 EELI 信号[34]。

新的数据表明，EIT 可以对肺灌注分布进行成像，这可能允许基于通气/灌注不匹配的评估下进行 PEEP 的优化[35]。

17.5.7 呼气末正压：急性呼吸窘迫综合征表型的作用

近年来，对 ARDS 生理学和影像学表现有了更深入的理解，可以描述同一综合征中的不同表型。

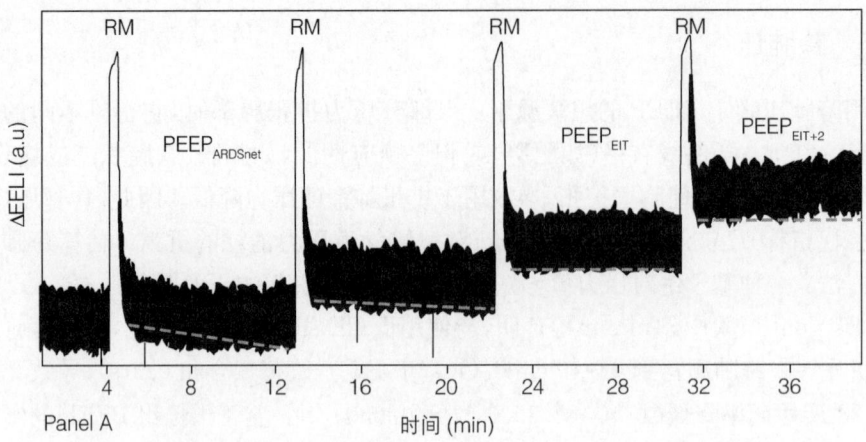

图 17.1 该图显示了 EIT 监测下呼气末正压(PEEP)变化中穿插"诊断性"肺复张手法(RM)时肺容量的变化。PEEP 水平保持不变后的第一次 RM,通过增加的呼气末肺容积(EELV),提示存在肺泡复张。然而,该 PEEP 水平不能阻止肺泡塌陷,故 EELV 又回到了基线水平。增加(2+2)cmH$_2$O 的 PEEP 可以保持肺复张后肺泡的稳定性(根据知识共享许可协议改编自参考文献[34])(见彩色插图)

　　Calfee 等的研究表明,根据临床和实验室数据,存在两种不同的 ARDS 表型。研究者观察到,只有高炎症组的患者使用较高水平的 PEEP 可降低病死率[36]。最近,在对 ARDS 随机临床试验和 LUNG SAFE 真实数据集的重新分析中证实了这些发现[37]。

17.6 总结

　　PEEP 是 ARDS 机械通气的关键参数。PEEP 可增加通气肺容积,并可避免肺不张。然而,PEEP 可导致肺泡过度膨胀和血流动力学不稳定。目前的指南建议予以中重度 ARDS 患者较高水平的 PEEP。滴定 PEEP 的不同策略包括 NIH 的 PEEP - FiO$_2$ 组合表、PEEP 递增或递减方案、食管压导管或先进的肺部成像技术(如 EIT)。

　　PEEP 滴定的主要目标包括氧合、呼吸力学,以及最近的利用影像识别肺复张与肺不张以使两者达到平衡。

　　对 ARDS 的生理学和影像学理解的进步有助于对 ARDS 的定义和管理进行更具针对性的描述,识别出哪些 ARDS 表型可以从较高和较低的 PEEP 水平中获益最大。

(高甜甜,周媛　译)

参考文献

[1] Rezoagli E, Fumagalli R, Bellani G. Definition and epidemiology of acute respiratory distress syndrome. Ann Transl Med. 2017; 5(14): 282. https://doi.org/10.21037/atm.2017.06.62.

[2] Gattinoni L, Collino F, Maiolo G, Rapetti F, Romitti F, Tonetti T, Vasques F, Quintel M. Positive end-expiratory pressure: how to set it at the individual level. Ann Transl Med. 2017; 5(14): 288. https://doi.org/10.21037/atm.2017.06.64.

[3] Amato MB, Meade MO, Slutsky AS, Brochard L, Costa EL, Schoenfeld DA, Stewart TE, Briel M, Talmor D, Mercat A, Richard JC, Carvalho CR, Brower RG. Driving pressure and survival in the acute respiratory distress syndrome. N Engl J Med. 2015; 372(8): 747-55. https://doi.org/10.1056/NEJMsa1410639.

[4] Briel M, Meade M, Mercat A, Brower RG, Talmor D, Walter SD, Slutsky AS, Pullenayegum E, Zhou Q, Cook D, Brochard L, Richard JC, Lamontagne F, Bhatnagar N, Stewart TE, Guyatt G. Higher vs lower positive end-expiratory pressure in patients with acute lung injury and acute respiratory distress syndrome: systematic review and meta-analysis. JAMA. 2010; 303(9): 865-73. https://doi.org/10.1001/jama.2010.218.

[5] Fan E, Del Sorbo L, Goligher EC, Hodgson CL, Munshi L, Walkey AJ, Adhikari NKJ, Amato MBP, Branson R, Brower RG, Ferguson ND, Gajic O, Gattinoni L, Hess D, Mancebo J, Meade MO, McAuley DF, Pesenti A, Ranieri VM, Rubenfeld GD, Rubin E, Seckel M, Slutsky AS, Talmor D, Thompson BT, Wunsch H, Uleryk E, Brozek J, Brochard LJ, American Thoracic Society, European Society of Intensive Care Medicine, and Society of Critical Care Medicine. An Official American Thoracic Society/European Society of Intensive Care Medicine/Society of Critical Care Medicine clinical practice guideline: mechanical ventilation in adult patients with acute respiratory distress syndrome. Am J Respir Crit Care Med. 2017; 195(9): 1253-63. https://doi.org/10.1164/rccm.201703-0548ST.

[6] Bellani G, Laffey JG, Pham T, Fan E, Brochard L, Esteban A, Gattinoni L, van Haren F, Larsson A, McAuley DF, Ranieri M, Rubenfeld G, Thompson BT, Wrigge H, Slutsky AS, Pesenti A, LUNG SAFE Investigators; ESICM Trials Group. Epidemiology, patterns of care, and mortality for patients with acute respiratory distress syndrome in intensive care units in 50 countries. JAMA. 2016; 315(8): 788-800. https://doi.org/10.1001/jama.2016.0291.

[7] Rezoagli E, Bellani G. The severe ARDS Generating Evidence (SAGE) study: a call for action in the daily clinical practice. Chest. 2021; 160(4): 1167-8. https://doi.org/10.1016/j.chest.2021.07.2158.

[8] Brower RG, Lanken PN, MacIntyre N, Matthay MA, Morris A, Ancukiewicz M, Schoenfeld D, Thompson BT, National Heart, Lung, and Blood Institute ARDS Clinical Trials Network. Higher versus lower positive end-expiratory pressures in patients with the acute respiratory distress syndrome. N Engl J Med. 2004; 351: 327-36. https://doi.org/10.1056/NEJMoa032193.

[9] Meade MO, Cook DJ, Guyatt GH, Slutsky AS, Arabi YM, Cooper DJ, Davies AR, Hand LE, Zhou Q, Thabane L, et al., Lung Open Ventilation Study Investigators. Ventilation strategy using low tidal volumes, recruitment maneuvers, and high positive end-expiratory pressure for acute lung injury and acute respiratory distress syndrome: a randomized controlled trial. JAMA 2008; 299: 637-645. https://doi.org/10.1001/jama.299.6.637.

[10] Rezoagli E, Bellani G. How I set up positive end-expiratory pressure: evidence- and physiology-based! Crit Care. 2019; 23(1): 412. https://doi.org/10.1186/s13054-019-2695-z.

[11] Goligher EC, Kavanagh BP, Rubenfeld GD, Adhikari NK, Pinto R, Fan E, Brochard LJ, Granton JT, Mercat A, Marie Richard JC, Chretien JM, Jones GL, Cook DJ, Stewart TE, Slutsky AS, Meade MO, Ferguson ND. Oxygenation response to positive end-expiratory pressure predicts mortality in acute respiratory distress syndrome. A secondary analysis of the LOVS and ExPress trials. Am J Respir Crit Care Med. 2014; 190(1): 70-6. https://doi.org/10.1164/rccm.201404-0688OC.

[12] Suter PM, Fairley B, Isenberg MD. Optimum end-expiratory airway pressure in patients with

acute pulmonary failure. N Engl J Med. 1975; 292(6): 284 - 9. https://doi.org/10.1056/NEJM197502062920604.

[13] Falke KJ, Pontoppidan H, Kumar A, Leith DE, Geffin B, Laver MB. Ventilation with end-expiratory pressure in acute lung disease. J Clin Invest. 1972; 51(9): 2315 - 23.

[14] Yehya N, Hodgson CL, Amato MBP, Richard JC, Brochard LJ, Mercat A, Goligher EC. Response to ventilator adjustments for predicting acute respiratory distress syndrome mortality. driving pressure versus oxygenation. Ann Am Thorac Soc. 2021; 18(5): 857 - 64. https://doi.org/10.1513/AnnalsATS.202007-862OC.

[15] Writing Group for the Alveolar Recruitment for Acute Respiratory Distress Syndrome Trial (ART) Investigators, Cavalcanti AB, Suzumura ÉA, Laranjeira LN, Paisani DM, Damiani LP, Guimarães HP, Romano ER, Regenga MM, Taniguchi LNT, Teixeira C, Pinheiro de Oliveira R, Machado FR, Diaz-Quijano FA, Filho MSA, Maia IS, Caser EB, Filho WO, Borges MC, Martins PA, Matsui M, Ospina-Tascón GA, Giancursi TS, Giraldo-Ramirez ND, Vieira SRR, Assef MDGPL, Hasan MS, Szczeklik W, Rios F, Amato MBP, Berwanger O, Ribeiro de Carvalho CR. Effect of lung recruitment and titrated positive end-expiratory pressure (PEEP) vs low PEEP on mortality in patients with acute respiratory distress syndrome: a randomized clinical trial. JAMA. 2017; 318(14): 1335 - 45. https://doi.org/10.1001/jama.2017.14171.

[16] Hickling KG. Best compliance during a decremental, but not incremental, positive end-expiratory pressure trial is related to open-lung positive end-expiratory pressure: a math-ematical model of acute respiratory distress syndrome lungs. Am J Respir Crit Care Med. 2001; 163(1): 69 - 78. https://doi.org/10.1164/ajrccm.163.1.9905084.

[17] Amato MB, Barbas CS, Medeiros DM, Schettino Gde P, Lorenzi Filho G, Kairalla RA, Deheinzelin D, Morais C, Fernandes Ede O, Takagaki TY, et al. Beneficial effects of the "open lung approach" with low distending pressures in acute respiratory distress syndrome. A prospective randomized study on mechanical ventilation. Am J Respir Crit Care Med. 1995; 152(6 Pt 1): 1835 - 46. https://doi.org/10.1164/ajrccm.152.6.8520744.

[18] Crotti S, Mascheroni D, Caironi P, Pelosi P, Ronzoni G, Mondino M, Marini JJ, Gattinoni L. Recruitment and derecruitment during acute respiratory failure: a clinical study. Am J Respir Crit Care Med. 2001; 164(1): 131 - 40. https://doi.org/10.1164/ajrccm.164.1.2007011.

[19] Ibañez J, Raurich JM, Moris SG. Measurement of functional residual capacity during mechanical ventilation. Comparison of a computerized open nitrogen washout method with a closed helium dilution method. Intensive Care Med. 1983; 9(2): 91 - 3. https://doi.org/10.1007/BF01699264.

[20] Chen L, Del Sorbo L, Grieco DL, Junhasavasdikul D, Rittayamai N, Soliman I, Sklar MC, Rauseo M, Ferguson ND, Fan E, Richard JM, Brochard L. Potential for lung recruitment estimated by the recruitment-to-inflation ratio in acute respiratory distress syndrome. A clinical trial. Am J Respir Crit Care Med. 2020; 201(2): 178 - 87. https://doi.org/10.1164/rccm.201902-0334OC.

[21] Ranieri VM, Giuliani R, Fiore T, Dambrosio M, Milic-Emili J. Volume-pressure curve of the respiratory system predicts effects of PEEP in ARDS: "occlusion" versus "constant flow" technique. Am J Respir Crit Care Med. 1994; 149(1): 19 - 27. https://doi.org/10.1164/ajrccm.149.1.8111581.

[22] Grasso S, Stripoli T, De Michele M, Bruno F, Moschetta M, Angelelli G, Munno I, Ruggiero V, Anaclerio R, Cafarelli A, Driessen B, Fiore T. ARDSnet ventilatory protocol and alveolar

hyperinflation: role of positive end-expiratory pressure. Am J Respir Crit Care Med. 2007; 176(8): 761 – 7. https://doi.org/10.1164/rccm.200702-193OC.

[23] Akoumianaki E, Maggiore SM, Valenza F, Bellani G, Jubran A, Loring SH, Pelosi P, Talmor D, Grasso S, Chiumello D, Guérin C, Patroniti N, Ranieri VM, Gattinoni L, Nava S, Terragni PP, Pesenti A, Tobin M, Mancebo J, Brochard L, PLUG Working Group (Acute Respiratory Failure Section of the European Society of Intensive Care Medicine). The application of esophageal pressure measurement in patients with respiratory failure. Am J Respir Crit Care Med. 2014; 189(5): 520 – 31. https://doi.org/10.1164/rccm.201312-2193CI.

[24] Talmor D, Sarge T, Malhotra A, O'Donnell CR, Ritz R, Lisbon A, Novack V, Loring SH. Mechanical ventilation guided by esophageal pressure in acute lung injury. N Engl J Med. 2008; 359(20): 2095 – 104. https://doi.org/10.1056/NEJMoa0708638.

[25] Beitler JR, Sarge T, Banner-Goodspeed VM, Gong MN, Cook D, Novack V, Loring SH, Talmor D, EPVent-2 Study Group. Effect of titrating positive end-expiratory pressure (PEEP) with an esophageal pressure-guided strategy vs an empirical high PEEP-Fio2 strategy on death and days free from mechanical ventilation among patients with acute respiratory distress syndrome: a randomized clinical trial. JAMA. 2019; 321(9): 846 – 57. https://doi.org/10.1001/jama.2019.0555.

[26] Sarge T, Baedorf-Kassis E, Banner-Goodspeed V, Novack V, Loring SH, Gong MN, Cook D, Talmor D, Beitler JR, EPVent-2 Study Group. Effect of esophageal pressure-guided positive end-expiratory pressure on survival from acute respiratory distress syndrome: a risk-based and mechanistic reanalysis of the EPVent-2 trial. Am J Respir Crit Care Med. 2021; 204: 1153. https://doi.org/10.1164/rccm.202009-3539OC.

[27] Cressoni M, Chiumello D, Carlesso E, Chiurazzi C, Amini M, Brioni M, Cadringher P, Quintel M, Gattinoni L. Compressive forces and computed tomography-derived positive end-expiratory pressure in acute respiratory distress syndrome. Anesthesiology. 2014; 121(3): 572 – 81. https://doi.org/10.1097/ALN.0000000000000373.

[28] Puybasset L, Gusman P, Muller JC, Cluzel P, Coriat P, Rouby JJ. Regional distribution of gas and tissue in acute respiratory distress syndrome. III. Consequences for the effects of positive end-expiratory pressure. CT Scan ARDS Study Group. Adult Respiratory Distress Syndrome. Intensive Care Med. 2000; 26(9): 1215 – 27. https://doi.org/10.1007/s001340051340.

[29] Constantin JM, Jabaudon M, Lefrant JY, Jaber S, Quenot JP, Langeron O, Ferrandière M, Grelon F, Seguin P, Ichai C, Veber B, Souweine B, Uberti T, Lasocki S, Legay F, Leone M, Eisenmann N, Dahyot-Fizelier C, Dupont H, Asehnoune K, Sossou A, Chanques G, Muller L, Bazin JE, Monsel A, Borao L, Garcier JM, Rouby JJ, Pereira B, Futier E, AZUREA Network. Personalised mechanical ventilation tailored to lung morphology versus low positive end-expiratory pressure for patients with acute respiratory distress syndrome in France (the LIVE study): a multicentre, single-blind, randomised controlled trial. Lancet Respir Med. 2019; 7(10): 870 – 80. https://doi.org/10.1016/S2213-2600(19)30138-9.

[30] Bouhemad B, Brisson H, Le-Guen M, Arbelot C, Lu Q, Rouby JJ. Bedside ultrasound assessment of positive end-expiratory pressure-induced lung recruitment. Am J Respir Crit Care Med. 2011; 183(3): 341 – 7. https://doi.org/10.1164/rccm.201003-0369OC.

[31] Costa ELV, Borges JB, Melo A, Suarez-Sipmann F, Toufen C Jr, Bohm SH, Amato MBP. Bedside estimation of recruitable alveolar collapse and hyperdistension by electrical impedance tomography. Intensive Care Med. 2009; 35(6): 1132 – 7. https://doi.org/10.1007/s00134-009-

1447-y.

[32] Costa EL, Borges JB, Melo A, Suarez-Sipmann F, Toufen C Jr, Bohm SH, Amato MB. Bedside estimation of recruitable alveolar collapse and hyperdistension by electrical impedance tomography. Intensive Care Med. 2009; 35(6): 1132–7. https://doi.org/10.1007/s00134-009-1447-y.

[33] Bronco A, Grassi A, Meroni V, Giovannoni C, Rabboni F, Rezoagli E, Teggia-Droghi M, Foti G, Bellani G. Clinical value of electrical impedance tomography (EIT) in the management of patients with acute respiratory failure: a single centre experience. Physiol Meas. 2021; 42(7) https://doi.org/10.1088/1361-6579/ac0e85.

[34] Eronia N, Mauri T, Maffezzini E, Gatti S, Bronco A, Alban L, Binda F, Sasso T, Marenghi C, Grasselli G, Foti G, Pesenti A, Bellani G. Bedside selection of positive end-expiratory pressure by electrical impedance tomography in hypoxemic patients: a feasibility study. Ann Intensive Care. 2017; 7(1): 76. https://doi.org/10.1186/s13613-017-0299-9.

[35] Bluth T, Kiss T, Kircher M, Braune A, Bozsak C, Huhle R, Scharffenberg M, Herzog M, Roegner J, Herzog P, Vivona L, Millone M, Dössel O, Andreeff M, Koch T, Kotzerke J, Stender B, Gama de Abreu M. Measurement of relative lung perfusion with electrical impedance and positron emission tomography: an experimental comparative study in pigs. Br J Anaesth. 2019; 123(2): 246–54. https://doi.org/10.1016/j.bja.2019.04.056.

[36] Calfee CS, Delucchi K, Parsons PE, Thompson BT, Ware LB, Matthay MA, NHLBI ARDS Network. Subphenotypes in acute respiratory distress syndrome: latent class analysis of data from two randomised controlled trials. Lancet Respir Med. 2014; 2(8): 611–20. https://doi.org/10.1016/S2213-2600(14)70097-9.

[37] Maddali MV, Churpek M, Pham T, Rezoagli E, Zhuo H, Zhao W, He J, Delucchi KL, Wang C, Wickersham, J. Brennan McNeil, Alejandra Jauregui, Serena Ke, Kathryn Vessel, Antonio Gomez A, Hendrickson CM, Kangelaris KN, Sarma A, Leligdowicz A, Liu KD, Matthay MA, Ware LB, Laffey JG, Bellani G, Calfee CS, Sinha P, for the LUNG SAFE Investigators and the ESICM Trials Group. Machine learning clinical-classifier models identify ARDS subphenotypes in observational cohorts and with differential responses to PEEP. Lancet Respir Med. 2022; S2213-2600(21)00461-6. https://doi.org/10.1016/s2213-2600(21)00461-6.

18 脑损伤患者的机械通气

Mechanical Ventilation in Brain Injured Patients

Lorenzo Peluso, Elisa Bogossian, Chiara Robba

18.1 引言

脑损伤患者经常需要机械通气支持,因为其既保能护气道又可以维持足够的氧合和二氧化碳水平,以尽量减少继发性脑损伤。此外,神经科患者经常出现呼吸系统并发症,如急性呼吸窘迫综合征(acute respiratory distress syndrome,ARDS),其发生率高达20%～38%[1]。脑与肺相互作用背后的病理生理关系是极其复杂的[2]。此外,由于脑损伤的异质性以及缺乏证据,目前尚没有公认能够获益的理想通气策略或确切的气体交换目标。

在本章中,我们将描述和探索可行的神经系统急症患者机械通气管理方法,重点关注其优势和副作用。

18.2 脑损伤患者有创机械通气的适应证

对脑损伤患者制定是否插管的决策应主要取决于保护气道以防止误吸、意识水平和颅内压(intracranial pressure,ICP)水平。尤其是气道保护性反射丧失、格拉斯哥昏迷评分(Glasgow Coma Scale,GCS)≤8、ICP显著增加或有脑疝迹象的患者,应考虑插管。此外,在伴有需要插管的非神经系统指征时,不应延迟插管。

关于脑损伤患者无创通气(non-invasive ventilation,NIV)的使用、适应证和时机的文献很少。NIV有减少有创通气的需求的潜力,但也会增加胸内压力,且不能保护气道、

L. Peluso · E. Bogossian
Department of Intensive Care, Erasme Hospital, Université Libre de Bruxelles, Brussels, Belgium

C. Robba (✉)
Department of Surgical Science and Diagnostic Integrated, Policlinico San Martino Genova, IRCCS for Oncology and Neuroscience, Genoa, Italy

© The Author(s), under exclusive license to Springer Nature Switzerland AG 2022
G. Bellani (ed.), *Mechanical Ventilation from Pathophysiology to Clinical Evidence*, https://doi.org/10.1007/978-3-030-93401-9_18

控制 CO_2 水平。最近,急性脑损伤患者机械通气的共识声明中,专家组指出由于证据质量很低,在该人群中使用无创呼吸支持没有达成共识[3]。然而,对于常规氧疗难以治疗的低氧性呼吸衰竭患者,可考虑使用经鼻高流量氧疗[3]。

18.3 通气策略和目标

18.3.1 呼吸机设置

在呼吸机设置方面目前缺少评估某种通气模式是否优于其他模式的研究,而且大部分研究主要是集中在创伤性脑损伤(traumatic brain injury,TBI)中,研究表明在压力调节容量控制模式下通气的患者 ICP 和 $PaCO_2$ 波动较小[4]。呼气末正压(positive end-expiratory pressure,PEEP)的使用是呼吸衰竭管理和预防肺不张、优化氧合的保护性通气策略的基础。但在脑损伤患者中的 PEEP 应用面临挑战[5],因为它可以增加胸内压并减少颅内静脉回流。不过,只要不引起恶性颅内压升高并能保持血流动力学稳定性,PEEP 的使用似乎是安全的[3]。因此,欧洲重症医学学会(European Society of Intensive Care Medicine,ESICM)建议,无 ARDS 且无 ICP 升高或 ICP 升高对"PEEP 不敏感"的脑损伤患者,应与无脑损伤患者采用相同的 PEEP 水平进行通气[3]。在脑损伤患者中,无论是否患有 ARDS,只要 ICP 没有升高,强烈建议采用低潮气量和低平台压的肺保护性通气策略,以尽量减少呼吸系统并发症。然而在 ICP 不稳定的脑损伤患者中使用该策略仍存在疑问(图 18.1),在这种情况下,通气设置应根据具体情况进行考量,有必要进行进一步的神经系统监测以评估脑代谢状态。

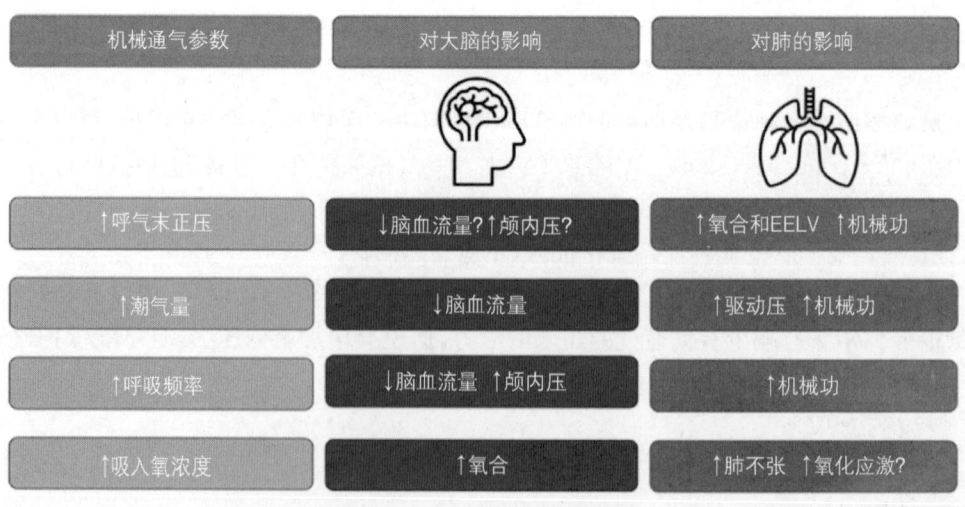

图 18.1 机械通气参数对脑和肺的作用。EELV,呼气末肺容积

18.3.2 氧合和二氧化碳目标

应严密监测血液中的氧(PaO_2)和 CO_2 水平,因为它们在维持大脑内环境稳定中起着

关键作用。外周血氧饱和度应保持＞94%[6]同时避免低氧血症和高氧血症，无论ICP水平如何，PaO_2应维持在80～120 mmHg[3]。

在脑损伤患者中，因为CO_2能够显著改变脑灌注，是脑血流量（cerebral blood flow, CBF）的主要决定因素[7]，所以应对其严格且频繁地监测。如 ESICM 建议中所述，无 ICP 升高的脑损伤患者最佳$PaCO_2$目标是35～45 mmHg。仅当出现难治性 ICP 升高和脑疝征象时，才应使用短期的过度通气[3]。在这种情况下，应保证$PaCO_2$目标为30 mmHg，并应严格监测其对脑灌注的可能影响[8]。

图 18.2 显示了作者提出的急性脑损伤患者通气支持的管理决策树。

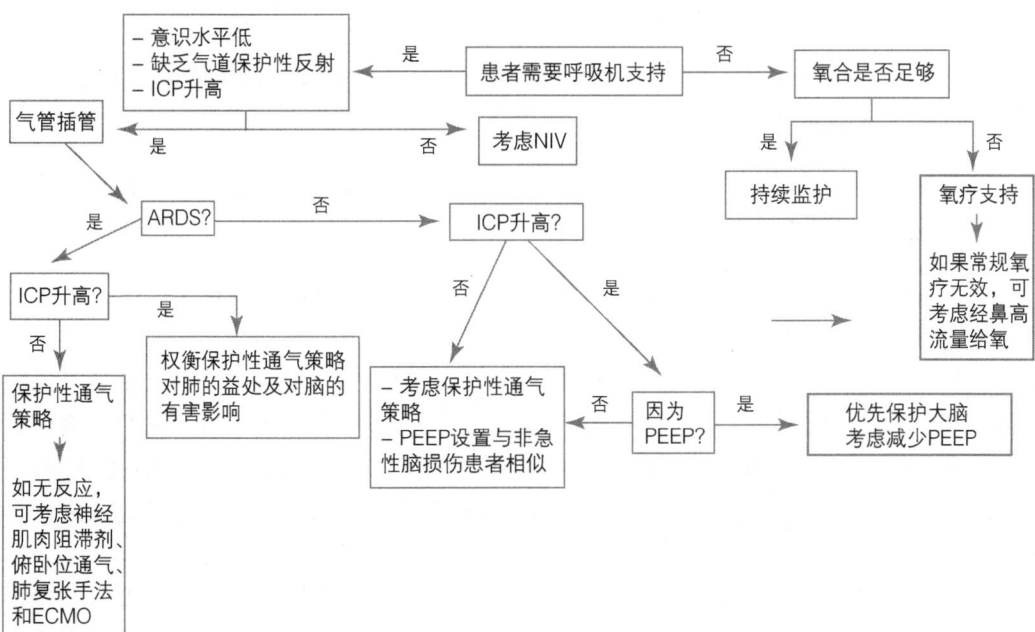

图 18.2 可行的脑损伤患者通气管理流程图。ICP，颅内压；NIV，无创通气；ARDS，急性呼吸窘迫综合征；ECMO，体外膜肺氧合；PEEP，呼气末正压

18.4 难治性呼吸衰竭的抢救干预措施

对于常规治疗无效的呼吸衰竭患者，有几种策略可用于优化通气和氧合，如肺复张手法、俯卧位、使用神经肌肉阻滞剂和体外膜肺氧合（extracorporeal membrane oxygenation, ECMO）。然而，这些策略可能不适用于急性脑损伤患者，因为它们可能对 ICP、脑灌注压和脑血流产生影响。

肺复张手法可改善氧合、复张肺泡并减少通气/灌注不匹配。但是这些操作可能通过影响脑静脉回流而增加自身调节受损患者的颅内压[9]。一项纳入蛛网膜下腔出血（subarachnoid hemorrhage, SAH）或 TBI 合并 ARDS 患者的研究发现，压力控制肺复张手法可改善PaO_2/FiO_2值，且对 ICP 和脑灌注压（cerebral perfusion pressure, CPP）无显著不利影响[9]。然而,由于数据匮乏,最近的 ESICM 指南未就急性脑损伤的肺复张手法提供推荐意见[3],肺复张手法应仅用于继发于肺不张的难治性重度低氧血症的特定病例。

在 ARDS 患者中,俯卧位已被证明可以改善氧合,降低病死率。在急性脑损伤患者中,俯卧位的使用可能具有挑战性,这是因为存在神经监测装置、引流管移位,以及胸内压和 ICP 升高的风险[10]。在 SAH 和 TBI 患者的小型研究中,俯卧位改善了氧合,但 ICP 有不同程度的增加[10,11]。因此在特定情况下,可考虑在严密监测 ICP 的情况下采用俯卧位[3]。

ECMO 是对常规方法无效的 ARDS 患者的一种令人感兴趣的救治策略。然而,ECMO 运行中需要抗凝以避免回路血栓形成,出血仍然是该操作的重要并发症。因此,ECMO 通常在颅内出血患者中禁用。然而,一些病例报告表明,ECMO 可以作为头部损伤 ARDS 患者的挽救性治疗[12,13],使用时减少初始肝素负荷量或避免使用肝素;或用于颅内出血风险较低的病例。

18.5 撤机和气管切开

急性脑损伤患者延迟拔管和拔管失败的疾病负担很高,导致机械通气时间延长,ICU 住院时间延长,病死率高[14]。

急性脑损伤后拔管和(或)使患者脱离通气支持的决策应考虑到几个神经和非神经因素,如患者临床发展的预期、急性脑损伤潜在并发症的预期、意识水平及患者的气道保护能力(充分的咳嗽、呕吐和吞咽反射)[3]。患者还应具备稳定的血流动力学和代谢状态,以及充足的氧合和肺功能[15]。对于机械通气时间＞24 小时的 ICU 人群,通常建议进行自主呼吸测试[15]。

意识水平持续降低的患者和一次或多次尝试拔管失败的患者应进行气管切开造口术,以便于撤机和呼吸治疗。进行气管切开的合适时机尚不清楚,但在急性脑损伤患者中,早期气管切开可能会减少 ICU 和住院时间[16]。

18.6 神经肌肉疾病的通气

大多数神经肌肉疾病会导致进行性呼吸肌无力和呼吸衰竭。急性呼吸衰竭是急性发作性神经肌肉疾病常见的危及生命的并发症,并可能进一步恶化神经肌肉疾病患者的慢性通气不足。标准管理措施包括氧疗、物理治疗、咳嗽辅助,以及在需要时使用抗生素和间歇性正压通气。

长期无创机械通气是通气管理的基本措施,因为它可以改善气体交换、提高生活质量和生存率。有不同的连接接口可供选择,如鼻罩、面罩或全脸设备,具有各种类型和尺寸。便携式呼吸机具有良好的泄漏补偿和多种模式,医院外也可使用。

然而,肌肉无力会导致肺活量减少,再加上用力吸气导致胸廓变形,可能导致无创设备失效,需要有创通气。目前没有相应的临床证据,需要进行应用无创与有创机械通气的随机试验来制定基于循证实践的方案。这些试验应根据病情状况预测治疗反应的变化,特别是根据是否存在延髓功能障碍,预测慢性神经肌肉疾病的急性发作与急性加重。

由于肌无力,撤机失败很常见。在神经肌肉疾病中应用常规撤机策略通常是困难的,可以采用包括"T"管或压力支持通气模式的方案进行撤机。

对于需要有创机械通气或无法保护气道且无法脱离呼吸机的患者,应进行气管切开术。

18.7 总结

在脑损伤患者的机械通气管理方面,仍然缺乏科学证据。尽管如此,一些基于病理生理假设、合并症和临床环境的推荐意见指导临床医生个体化治疗,是管理此类患者的最佳方法。

未来需要进一步的高质量研究来确定可能影响预后的通气策略和气体交换目标。

(高甜甜,周媛 译)

参考文献

[1] Veeravagu A, Chen YR, Ludwig C, Rincon F, Maltenfort M, Jallo J, et al. Acute lung injury in patients with subarachnoid hemorrhage: a nationwide inpatient sample study. World Neurosurg. 2014; 82(1-2): e235-41.

[2] Pelosi P, Rocco PR. The lung and the brain: a dangerous cross-talk. Crit Care. 2011; 15(3): 168.

[3] Robba C, Poole D, McNett M, Asehnoune K, Bosel J, Bruder N, et al. Mechanical ventilation in patients with acute brain injury: recommendations of the European Society of Intensive Care Medicine consensus. Intensive Care Med. 2020; 46(12): 2397-410.

[4] Schirmer-Mikalsen K, Vik A, Skogvoll E, Moen KG, Solheim O, Klepstad P. Intracranial pressure during pressure control and pressure-regulated volume control ventilation in patients with traumatic brain injury: a randomized crossover trial. Neurocrit Care. 2016; 24(3): 332-41.

[5] Huynh T, Messer M, Sing RF, Miles W, Jacobs DG, Thomason MH. Positive end-expiratory pressure alters intracranial and cerebral perfusion pressure in severe traumatic brain injury. J Trauma. 2002; 53(3): 488-92; discussion 92-3.

[6] Chesnut R, Aguilera S, Buki A, Bulger E, Citerio G, Cooper DJ, et al. A management algorithm for adult patients with both brain oxygen and intracranial pressure monitoring: the Seattle International Severe Traumatic Brain Injury Consensus Conference (SIBICC). Intensive Care Med. 2020; 46(5): 919-29.

[7] Bouma GJ, Muizelaar JP. Cerebral blood flow in severe clinical head injury. New Horiz. 1995; 3(3): 384-94.

[8] Gouvea Bogossian E, Peluso L, Creteur J, Taccone FS. Hyperventilation in adult TBI patients: how to approach it? Front Neurol. 2020; 11: 580859.

[9] Nemer SN, Caldeira JB, Azeredo LM, Garcia JM, Silva RT, Prado D, et al. Alveolar recruitment maneuver in patients with subarachnoid hemorrhage and acute respiratory distress

syndrome: a comparison of 2 approaches. J Crit Care. 2011; 26(1): 22-7.

[10] Della Torre V, Badenes R, Corradi F, Racca F, Lavinio A, Matta B, et al. Acute respiratory distress syndrome in traumatic brain injury: how do we manage it? J Thorac Dis. 2017; 9(12): 5368-81.

[11] Towner JE, Rahmani R, Zammit CG, Khan IR, Paul DA, Bhalla T, et al. Mechanical ventilation in aneurysmal subarachnoid hemorrhage: systematic review and recommendations. Crit Care. 2020; 24(1): 575.

[12] Friesenecker BE, Peer R, Rieder J, Lirk P, Knotzer H, Hasibeder WR, et al. Craniotomy during ECMO in a severely traumatized patient. Acta Neurochir. 2005; 147(9): 993-6; discussion 996.

[13] Yen TS, Liau CC, Chen YS, Chao A. Extracorporeal membrane oxygenation resuscitation for traumatic brain injury after decompressive craniotomy. Clin Neurol Neurosurg. 2008; 110(3): 295-7.

[14] Godet T, Chabanne R, Marin J, Kauffmann S, Futier E, Pereira B, et al. Extubation failure in brain-injured patients: risk factors and development of a prediction score in a preliminary prospective cohort study. Anesthesiology. 2017; 126(1): 104-14.

[15] Boles JM, Bion J, Connors A, Herridge M, Marsh B, Melot C, et al. Weaning from mechanical ventilation. Eur Respir J. 2007; 29(5): 1033-56.

[16] Robba C, Galimberti S, Graziano F, Wiegers EJA, Lingsma HF, Iaquaniello C, et al., CENTER-TBI ICU Participants and Investigators. Tracheostomy practice and timing in traumatic brain-injured patients: a CENTER-TBI study. Intensive Care Med 2020; 46(5): 983-994.

19 心力衰竭患者的有创与无创通气
Invasive and Non-invasive Ventilation in Patient with Cardiac Failure
Aurora Magliocca, Giuseppe Ristagno

19.1 引言

急性心力衰竭表现为心功能迅速恶化,常伴有肺淤血和急性呼吸衰竭(acute respiratory failure,ARF),可能危及生命。严重低氧血症常见于急性心源性肺水肿和心源性休克患者,这两种情况需要及时进行呼吸功能支持。基于病理生理学和临床证据的支持,气道正压通气的应用是心力衰竭致 ARF 患者呼吸辅助的基石。

19.2 急性心力衰竭时呼吸衰竭的病理生理

19.2.1 急性心源性肺水肿

心源性肺水肿的特征是肺毛细血管静水压的迅速升高,从而扰乱了 Starling 的平衡机制。实际上,心源性肺水肿的血流动力学特征通常表现为高充盈压(即肺毛细血管楔压)、高血压和正常/低心输出量。因此,可以观察到① 血管周围和支气管周围间质组织中积液,即肺间质水肿;② 直到液体穿过上皮细胞进入肺泡,产生肺泡水肿。

肺泡内的水肿液会改变表面活性剂的功能,增加表面张力。肺容积低时肺泡陷闭的可能性增加,阻碍充满液体的肺泡单位进行通气。在这些肺泡单位的血流灌注保留时,肺内分流增加和通气/灌注不匹配会导致低氧血症。

这种情况下,预示着多种心源性肺水肿引起 ARF 的病理生理学机制。

(1) 肺水肿时肺的压力-容积曲线向右下位移,导致功能残气量(functional residual

capacity,FRC)显著降低,肺僵硬度增加(即顺应性降低)[1]。

(2) 支气管周围区域水肿形成会引起气道阻力的增加。心源性肺水肿的实验模型与非心源性肺水肿的实验模型相比,气道阻力的变化更大[2]。

(3) 这些病理生理改变导致呼吸做功(work of breathing,WOB)的增加和呼吸肌的耗氧量增加,可能会造成氧供和氧耗之间的失衡[3]。事实上,据报道,在心肺疾病患者中,呼吸耗氧量显著增加,可高达总耗氧量的25%(正常为1%～3%)[4]。

19.2.2 心源性休克

如果急性心力衰竭进一步恶化,心输出量下降,会在肺水肿的同时导致组织灌注不足。心源性休克的血流动力学特征为低心输出量、低血压和高充盈压(即中心静脉压和肺毛细血管楔压),外周组织氧输送不足导致混合静脉氧饱和度(mixed venous oxygen saturation,SvO_2)降低和乳酸水平升高。

心源性休克往往同时伴有 ARF。除了前面章节所述呼吸衰竭的病理生理机制外,还存在其他机制。肺灌注减少导致通气/灌注不匹配增加(无效腔增加)。此外,在相同肺内分流率的情况下,混合静脉饱和度的下降会导致更严重的低氧血症。

19.3 心力衰竭患者气道正压的基本原理

应用 PEEP 会增加胸腔内压(intrathoracic pressure,ITP),从而影响呼吸和血流动力学功能,如图 19.1 所示。较高的 ITP 能增加 FRC,促进萎陷的肺泡单元开放,改善肺

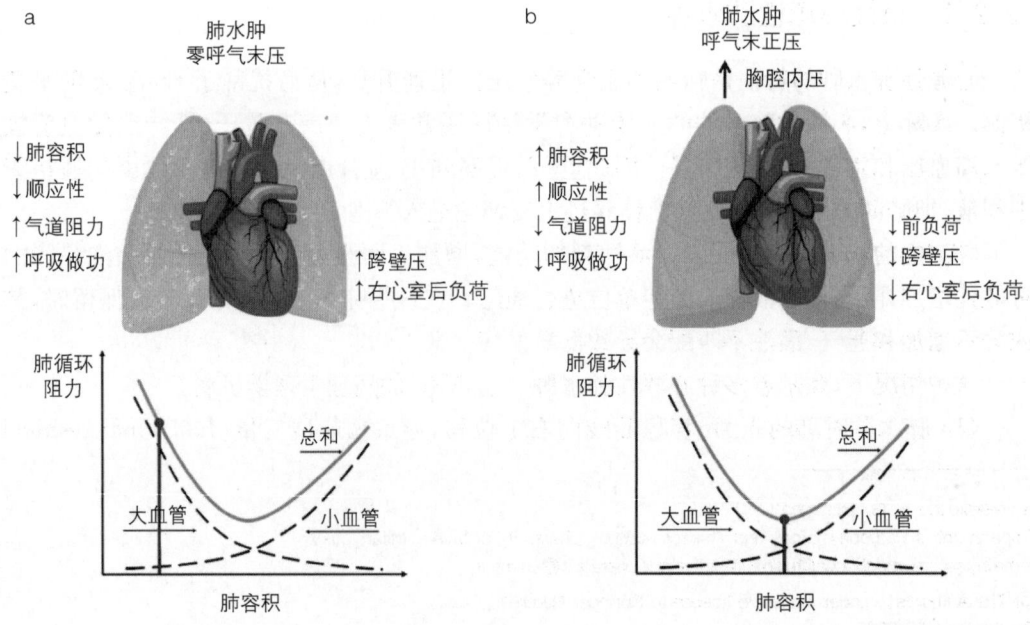

图 19.1　a. 心源性肺水肿时呼吸衰竭的病理生理机制。b. 气道正压通气对呼吸力学和血流动力学的生理效应。ZEEP,零呼气末压;PEEP,呼气末正压;ITP,胸腔内压;RV,右心室;PVR,肺循环阻力(见彩色插图)

顺应性。减少肺内分流和通气/灌注不匹配可以改善氧合。ITP的增加也可以导致气道阻力和WOB显著降低[5]。由于这些机制和呼吸驱动的减少,不同水平PEEP(5和10 cmH$_2$O)的CPAP可减少呼吸肌产生的吸气ITP负向波动(尽管不提供任何"主动"的吸气支持),并且对左心室后负荷也有积极影响[5]。

ITP增加的主要血流动力学效应是减少全身静脉向右心室(right ventricle, RV)回流和降低左心室(left ventricle, LV)系统输出的压力梯度,如下所述。

19.3.1 右心室

气道内正压可能影响RV前负荷和后负荷。右心室静脉回流的压力梯度由体循环平均充盈压(上游压力)与右心房(right atrial pressure, RAP)之间的差值表示(即下游压力)[6]。气道正压通气可同时增加ITP和RAP,减少静脉血流量、右心室充盈和心输出量(图19.2a)[9]。虽然通常情况下,ITP对前负荷的影响主要为增加RAP引起静脉回流压力梯度的降低,但实际机制可能要复杂得多,因为ITP的增加同时伴随着RAP和体循环平均充盈压(mean systemic filling pressure, MSFP)的增加。在心功能正常的情况下,对PEEP的适应性反应已被证明可降低血容量,导致MSFP的增加而对压力梯度(MSFP-RAP)无影响[9],而在心源性肺水肿时,积极控制全身血压也会影响MSFP。

实验数据还表明,血管形变可能是静脉阻力增加的原因,这是ITP对静脉回流的不利影响[10]。最后,RV容积的减小可以使心室壁张力下降,从而降低心脏耗氧量[11]。

ITP对RV后负荷的影响反映了它对肺容积的作用。事实上,肺容积与肺循环阻力(pulmonary vascular resistance, PVR)的U型关系提示PEEP可扩张塌陷的肺泡单位,导致肺容积增加,PVR降低(图19.1b)。在较高的肺容积(即肺泡过度扩张)时,小血管受压增加了PVR,从而增加RV后负荷。

19.3.2 左心室

较高的ITP可以通过降低跨壁压(transmural pressure, P_{TM})来降低LV后负荷[12]:这是LV壁上的压力梯度,是腔内和腔外压力的差值。LV的P_{TM}定义为收缩压(systolic arterial pressure, SAP)减去ITP(LV P_{TM} = SAP−ITP)。

心力衰竭患者应用CPAP可通过降低呼吸肌产生的胸腔负压过度波动来降低左心室跨壁压和后负荷,从而改善左心室功能(图19.2b)[5,13]。ITP增大可增加充血性心力衰竭患者的心输出量[5,13-15]和左心室射血分数[16]。有趣的是,心输出量的增加主要依赖于每搏量的增加,而在使用CPAP期间心率明显下降[5,13-16]。

然而,即使在同一项研究中,患者对PEEP的反应也存在相当大的差异:在不同的患者中观察到心输出量增加、减少或无变化[13-15]。当左心室收缩功能下降且充盈压力较高(即肺毛细血管楔压≥12 mmHg)时,PEEP对心输出量的正向作用最有可能发生[15]。这表明提高ITP的正向血流动力学效应不仅是由于降低了LV P_{TM},LV前负荷的降低也可能使其在顺应性曲线上处于更有利的位置。最后,PEEP在胸内结构的不均匀传输可能进一步导致了所观察到效果的可变性[17]。

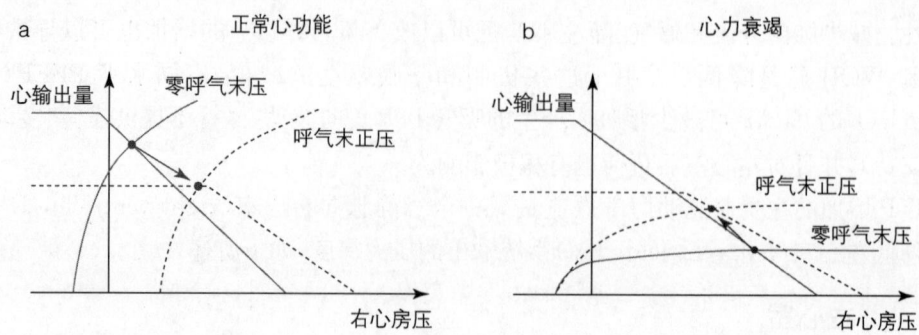

图 19.2 在心功能正常和心力衰竭时,应用气道正压通气对心输出量的影响。基于 Guyton 的模型[6,7],绘制心输出量(曲线)或静脉回流(直线)对右心房压的函数图像。由于心输出量和静脉回流必然相等,唯一可能的"工作"状态为两条线的交点。在心功能正常的情况下(a),PEEP(虚线)使静脉回流曲线向右下移动,因此对于给定的右心房压[临床上通过中心静脉压(CVP)评估],静脉回流较低。此外,心输出量曲线也向右移动,因为这里的右心房压是相对于大气压测量的(壁内压力),而跨壁压更低。当右心房压相对于外壁压力(跨壁压)测量时,即使 PEEP 高达 15 cmH_2O,心功能曲线也不受影响[8]。a 图中的新工作点(黑点)位于新的静脉回流曲线的平台支上,不仅表明心输出量下降,还表明心功能的改善不会进一步增加心输出量。心力衰竭时(b) PEEP 对静脉回流的影响类似。然而,由于 PEEP 降低后负荷,心室功能改善,心输出量曲线更为陡峭,两条曲线在较高的心输出量(或静脉回流)水平交汇

19.4 无创正压通气治疗心源性肺水肿:临床证据

多项随机对照试验(randomized controlled trial,RCT)的结果支持在心力衰竭患者中应用气道正压通气以改善预后[18-20]。无论正压以 CPAP 方式输送还是采用压力支持方式(如 NIV),效果似乎都是相同的,因为没有 RCT 研究显示一种技术比另一种技术明显更有优势[19]。与标准氧疗相比,CPAP 或 NIV 始终能产生更大的生理改善,一项系统性综述纳入的所有研究中都能观察到治疗 1 小时后呼吸频率降低可以证实这一点[19]。

有趣的是,可能是因为呼吸力学的改善,仅靠 CPAP(本质上不增加肺泡通气)就能够降低 $PaCO_2$ 和改善 pH[20]。虽然在这些 RCT 中没有评估心输出量,但气道正压通气的应用改善了整体血液动力学,因为在治疗的第一个小时内动脉血压没有变化,而心率显著降低[18-20]。

关于在心源性肺水肿合并酸中毒(pH<7.35)患者中应用 NIV 疗效最大的多中心 RCT(3CPO 试验)显示,与标准吸氧治疗治疗 1 小时后相比,通过 CPAP(5~15 cmH_2O)或 NIV(吸气压:8~20 cmH_2O;呼气压:4~10 cmH_2O)提供持续 2 小时的呼吸支持可以快速改善呼吸困难,同时减少高碳酸血症、酸中毒的发生和降低心率[18]。但是 NIV 的积极生理效应与插管率和第 7、30 天病死率的降低无关。多项因素,包括高交叉率(约 15% 随机分配到标准氧疗组的患者交叉到 NIV)和患者严重程度低(三组的基线平均 $PaO_2 \approx$ 100 mmHg),是对本试验观察到 NIV 对病死率没有疗效的可能解释。

然而,随后发表的系统综述,包括 3CPO 试验和其他 23 项 RCT(2 664 例患者),显示

NIV 的应用降低了胃内插管率和住院病死率,对住院时长没有确定的效果[19]。与标准药物治疗相比,随机采用无创通气(CPAP 或双水平正压通气)的患者急性心肌梗死的发生率无差异。此外,治疗 1 小时后,两组患者的收缩压、舒张压和平均血压无差异,而通过降低呼吸频率和增加氧合,治疗 1 小时后呼吸窘迫得到改善[19]。在高碳酸血症心源性肺水肿患者亚组中,最佳通气技术及其对预后的影响有待进一步探讨。

关于 NIV 的使用,ERS/ATS 临床实践指南推荐对心源性肺水肿引起 ARF 的患者使用双水平正压通气或 CPAP。2019 年 Cochrane 系统评价显示,与单纯标准药物治疗心源性肺水肿比较,气道正压通气可降低医院病死率($RR=0.65$,95% CI 为 0.51～0.82)和气管插管率($RR=0.49$,95% CI 为 0.38～0.62)。

最后,气道正压通气应用于心源性肺水肿引起 ARF 患者的有益效果也已在院前环境中得到证实[20-22]。院外应用 CPAP 是可行的,可以改善低氧血症,降低气管插管率[20-22]。

19.5 无创和有创正压通气治疗心源性休克

支持心源性休克患者使用 NIV 的证据有限。事实上,2017 年 ERS/ATS 指南并没有提供在这些患者中使用 NIV 的推荐意见[21]。

最近的一项前瞻性登记报告显示,在因心源性休克入住心脏 ICU 的患者中,有创机械通气的使用比例为 49.5%,其中在急性心肌梗死导致心源性休克的患者中这一比例增加至 60.3%;而在混合型休克 ICU 患者中,该比例为 65.9%[23]。

由于缺乏心源性休克的具体证据,根据临床症状调整呼吸支持似乎是合理的。的确,心源性休克的临床特征,如精神状态改变、血流动力学不稳定和低灌注常常损害维持自主呼吸的能力,因此与有创通气相比,NIV 并不是个合适的选择。

19.6 心脏停搏后的通气

自主循环恢复(return of spontaneous circulation,ROSC)后,心脏骤停(cardiac arrest,CA)患者容易出现以全身炎症和多器官功能障碍为特征的再灌注后状态,称为心脏骤停后综合征。在该综合征的临床特征中,缺氧缺血性脑损伤是死亡和长期残疾的主要原因。此外,心脏骤停后肺损伤/肺水肿的发生率很高[24,25],近 50% 心脏停搏幸存者在入院后 48 小时内发生 ARDS[24],反映了肺-脑交互的相关性。

适当的机械通气对减少继发性脑损伤至关重要,其主要目的是将氧气和二氧化碳的分压维持在生理范围内。

复苏后治疗在 ROSC 后立即开始。然而,在院前设置中,最佳的通气策略和具体的氧合目标仍不确定。

在院内,目前的 ERC-ESICM 指南[26]推荐使用基于理想体重(predicted body weight,PBW)以 6～8 mL/kg 标准确定的潮气量(tidal volume,V_T)的肺保护性通气策略。这是基于对 256 名院外 CA 患者数据的倾向调整分析得出的,显示 ROSC 后前 48 小

时内的低 V_T 与良好的神经预后($OR=1.61$,95%CI 为 1.13~2.28)以及更多的无呼吸机和无休克天数独立相关。有趣的是,38%的患者在前 48 小时内的平均 $V_T>8$ mL/kg (PBW),而只有 4%的患者在此期间平均 $V_T\leqslant 6$ mL/kg (PBW)[27]。

ROSC 后推荐的氧合目标为,滴定氧浓度使 SpO_2 维持在 94%~98%或使 PaO_2 维持在 75~100 mmHg[26]。尽管实验研究表明高氧血症与心脏骤停后较差的神经结局相关,但临床研究却显示出相互矛盾的结果[28,29]。在 COMACARE 试验[29]中,在 ROSC 后 48 小时通过血液中神经元特异性烯醇化酶水平来评估神经元损伤,正常血氧组(PaO_2 为 75~113 mmHg)和中度高氧血症组(PaO_2 为 150~188 mmHg)之间没有差异。

最后,$PaCO_2$ 的调节至关重要,因为它是脑血流量和氧气输送的主要决定因素。事实上,低碳酸血症和高碳酸血症分别引起脑血管收缩或舒张,从而影响脑血流量和颅内压(见"18 脑损伤患者的机械通气")。ERC - ESICM 指南建议将 $PaCO_2$ 维持在 35~45 mmHg[26]。有关二氧化碳水平与脑损伤之间相关联的证据存在分歧[29,30],但目前 TAME 试验中正在研究轻度高碳酸血症的神经保护作用,这是一项Ⅲ期多中心 RCT (NCT03114033)。

(邓会标,计恩东 译)

参考文献

[1] Sharp JT, Griffith GT, Bunnell IL, et al. Ventilatory mechanics in pulmonary edema in man. J Clin Invest. 1958; 37: 111 - 7.

[2] Bernard GR, Pou NA, Coggeshall JW, Carroll FE, Snapper JR. Comparison of the pulmonary dysfunction caused by cardiogenic and noncardiogenic pulmonary edema. Chest. 1995; 108(3): 798 - 803.

[3] Aubier M, Trippenbach T, Roussos C. Respiratory muscle fatigue during cardiogenic shock. J Appl Physiol. 1981; 51: 499 - 508.

[4] Field S, Kelly SM, Macklem PT. The oxygen cost of breathing in patients with cardiorespiratory disease. Am Rev Respir Dis. 1982; 126: 9 - 13.

[5] Lenique F, Habis M, Lofaso F, Dubois-Randé JL, Harf A, Brochard L. Ventilatory and hemodynamic effects of continuous positive airway pressure in left heart failure. Am J Respir Crit Care Med. 1997; 155(2): 500 - 5.

[6] Guyton AC, Lindsey AW, Abernathy B, Richardson T. Venous return at various right atrial pressures and the normal venous return curve. Am J Phys. 1957; 189(3): 609 - 15.

[7] Magder S. Bench-to-bedside review: an approach to hemodynamic monitoring—Guyton at the bedside. Crit Care. 2012; 16(5): 236.

[8] Marini JJ, Culver BH, Butler J. Effect of positive end-expiratory pressure on canine ventricular function curves. J Appl Physiol. 1981; 51: 1367 - 74.

[9] Nanas S, Magder S. Adaptations of the peripheral circulation to PEEP. Am Rev Respir Dis. 1992; 146(3): 688 - 93.

[10] Fessler HE, Brower RG, Wise RA, Permutt S. Effects of positive end-expiratory pressure on the canine venous return curve. Am Rev Respir Dis. 1992; 146(1): 4 - 10.

[11] Schuster S, Erbel R, Weilemann LS, et al. Hemodynamics during PEEP ventilation in patients with severe left ventricular failure studied by transesophageal echocardiography. Chest. 1990; 97: 1181-9.

[12] Buda AJ, Pinsky MR, Ingels NB Jr, Daughters GT II, Stinson EB, Alderman EL. Effect of intrathoracic pressure on left ventricular performance. N Engl J Med. 1979; 301: 453-9.

[13] Naughton MT, Rahman MA, Hara K, Floras JS, Bradley TD. Effect of continuous positive airway pressure on intrathoracic and left ventricular transmural pressures in patients with congestive heart failure. Circulation. 1995; 91: 1725-31.

[14] Baratz DM, Westbrooke PR, Shah PK, Mohsenifar Z. Effect of nasal continuous positive airway pressure on cardiac output and oxygen delivery in patients with congestive heart failure. Chest. 1992; 102: 1397-401.

[15] Bradley TD, Holloway RM, McLaughlin PR, Ross BL, Walters J, Liu PP. Cardiac output responses to continuous positive airway pressure in congestive heart failure. Am Rev Respir Dis. 1992; 145: 377-82.

[16] Bendjelid K, Schütz N, Suter PM, et al. Does continuous positive airway pressure by face mask improve patients with acute cardiogenic pulmonary edema due to left ventricular diastolic dysfunction? Chest. 2005; 127: 1053-8.

[17] O'Quin R, Marini JJ. Pulmonary artery occlusion pressure: clinical physiology, measurement, and interpretation. Am Rev Respir Dis. 1983; 128: 319-26.

[18] Gray A, Goodacre S, Newby DE, Masson M, Sampson F, Nicholl J, 3CPO Trialists. Noninvasive ventilation in acute cardiogenic pulmonary edema. N Engl J Med. 2008; 359(2): 142-51.

[19] Berbenetz N, Wang Y, Brown J, Godfrey C, Ahmad M, Vital FM, Lambiase P, Banerjee A, Bakhai A, Chong M. Non-invasive positive pressure ventilation (CPAP or bilevel NPPV) for cardiogenic pulmonary oedema. Cochrane Database Syst Rev. 2019; 4(4): CD005351.

[20] Ducros L, Logeart D, Vicaut E, Henry P, Plaisance P, Collet JP, Broche C, Gueye P, Vergne M, Goetgheber D, Pennec PY, Belpomme V, Tartière JM, Lagarde S, Placente M, Fievet ML, Montalescot G, Payen D, CPAP Collaborative Study Group. CPAP for acute cardiogenic pulmonary oedema from out-of-hospital to cardiac intensive care unit: a randomised multicentre study. Intensive Care Med. 2011; 37(9): 1501-9.

[21] Rochwerg B, Brochard L, Elliott MW, Hess D, Hill NS, Nava S, Paolo Navalesi Members of the Steering Committee, Antonelli M, Brozek J, Conti G, Ferrer M, Guntupalli K, Jaber S, Keenan S, Mancebo J, Mehta S, Suhail Raoof Members of the Task Force. Official ERS/ATS clinical practice guidelines: noninvasive ventilation for acute respiratory failure. Eur Respir J. 2017; 50(2): 1602426.

[22] Foti G, Sangalli F, Berra L, Sironi S, Cazzaniga M, Rossi GP, Bellani G, Pesenti A. Is helmet CPAP first line pre-hospital treatment of presumed severe acute pulmonary edema? Intensive Care Med. 2009; 35: 656-62.

[23] Berg DD, Bohula EA, van Diepen S, Katz JN, Alviar CL, Baird-Zars VM, Barnett CF, Barsness GW, Burke JA, Cremer PC, Cruz J, Daniels LB, DeFilippis AP, Haleem A, Hollenberg SM, Horowitz JM, Keller N, Kontos MC, Lawler PR, Menon V, Metkus TS, Ng J, Orgel R, Overgaard CB, Park JG, Phreaner N, Roswell RO, Schulman SP, Jeffrey Snell R, Solomon MA, Ternus B, Tymchak W, Vikram F, Morrow DA. Epidemiology of shock in contemporary cardiac intensive care units. Circ Cardiovasc Qual Outcomes. 2019; 12(3): e005618.

[24] Johnson NJ, Caldwell E, Carlbom DJ, Gaieski DF, Prekker ME, Rea TD, et al. The acute respiratory distress syndrome after out-of-hospital cardiac arrest: incidence, risk factors, and outcomes. Resuscitation. 2019; 135: 37-44.

[25] Magliocca A, Rezoagli E, Zani D, Manfredi M, De Giorgio D, Olivari D, Fumagalli F, Langer T, Avalli L, Grasselli G, Latini R, Pesenti A, Bellani G, Ristagno G. Cardiopulmonary resuscitation-associated lung edema (CRALE). A translational study. Am J Respir Crit Care Med. 2021; 203(4): 447-57.

[26] Nolan JP, Sandroni C, Bottiger BW, Cariou A, Cronberg T, Friberg H, Genbrugge C, Haywood K, Lilja G, VRM M, Nikolaou N, Olasveengen TM, Skrifvars MB, Taccone F, Soar J. European Resuscitation Council and European Society of Intensive Care Medicine guidelines 2021: post-resuscitation care. Intensive Care Med. 2021; 47: 369-421.

[27] Beitler JR, Ghafouri TB, Jinadasa SP, Mueller A, Hsu L, Anderson RJ, et al. Favorable neuro-cognitive outcome with low tidal volume ventilation after cardiac arrest. Am J Respir Crit Care Med. 2017; 195: 1198-206.

[28] Roberts BW, Kilgannon JH, Hunter BR, et al. Association between early hyperoxia exposure after resuscitation from cardiac arrest and neurological disability: prospective multicenter protocol-directed cohort study. Circulation. 2018; 137: 2114-24.

[29] Jakkula P, Pettila V, Skrifvars MB, Hastbacka J, Loisa P, Tiainen M, Wilkman E, Toppila J, Koskue T, Bendel S, Birkelund T, Laru-Sompa R, Valkonen M, Reinikainen M. Targeting low-normal or high-normal mean arterial pressure after cardiac arrest and resuscitation: a randomised pilot trial. Intensive Care Med. 2018; 44: 2091-101.

[30] Eastwood GM, Schneider AG, Suzuki S, Peck L, Young H, Tanaka A, Martensson J, Warrillow S, McGuinness S, Parke R, Gilder E, McCarthy L, Galt P, Taori G, Eliott S, Lamac T, Bailey M, Harley N, Barge D, Hodgson CL, Morganti-Kossmann MC, Pebay A, Conquest A, Archer JS, Bernard S, Stub D, Hart GK, Bellomo R. Targeted therapeutic mild hypercapnia after cardiac arrest: a phase II multi-Centre randomised controlled trial (the CCC trial). Resuscitation. 2016; 104: 83-90.

20 慢性阻塞性肺疾病和严重哮喘
COPD and Severe Asthma

Lise Piquilloud, Damian Ratano

20.1 病理生理学

阻塞性呼吸系统疾病包括慢性阻塞性肺疾病（chronic obstructive pulmonary disease，COPD）和哮喘。在肺气肿的 COPD 患者中，由于肺实质破坏，肺弹性回缩力下降，可导致呼气时小气道塌陷和呼气气流阻力增加[1]。以呼吸系统症状急性恶化为特征的间歇性急性加重是阻塞性呼吸系统疾病临床过程的一部分，在最严重的情况下可能需要有创机械通气。COPD 急性加重（AE－COPD）的特征是分泌物增加、炎症和一定程度的支气管痉挛。急性哮喘[或哮喘发作（asthma attack，AA）]的主要特征是严重的支气管痉挛导致非常高的气道阻力、一定程度的炎症和气道中存在黏液[2]。尽管 AE－COPD 和 AA 的病理生理不同，但均有两个主要特征：气道阻力增加和气流受限。因此，AE－COPD 和急性哮喘期间的呼吸支持管理非常相似。

气流受限导致在呼气结束时气体被残留在肺泡中。呼气末肺容积高于功能残气量，肺泡压高于大气压（或高于设定的 PEEP）。这种现象被称为动态肺过度充气或动态气体陷闭，呼气结束时高于大气压力（或设定 PEEP）的压力值被称为内源性 PEEP（PEEPi）或自发性 PEEP(autoPEEP)[3]。在临床实践中，增加呼吸驱动、潮气量和呼吸频率（导致呼气时间缩短）会加剧动态肺过度充气。AE－COPD 和 AA 的病理生理如图 20.1 所示。

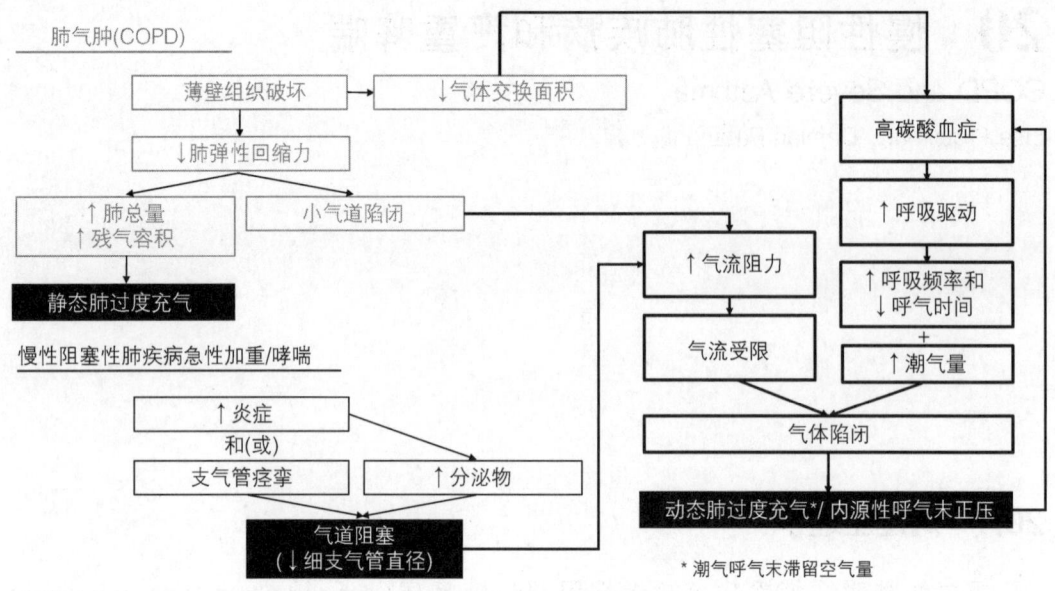

图 20.1 慢性阻塞性肺疾病加重和哮喘发作时呼吸衰竭的病理生理

AE-COPD 和 AA 患者在自主呼吸和控制通气时都有动态肺过度充气的风险。动态肺过度充气具有严重的不良影响,会增加气压伤的风险(由于肺泡内压增加),血流动力学可能改变(由于胸腔内压增加和静脉回流持续减少)[4]。当肺发生过度膨胀时,由于通气/灌注改变导致高碳酸血症和低氧血症,呼吸系统顺应性降低。膈肌收缩功能也因膈肌低平而降低。此外,在辅助呼吸期间,动态肺过度充气会增加 WOB 并导致人-机同步性差(延迟触发、无效努力和呼气周期延迟)。图 20.2 总结了动态肺过度充气在一般情况下和辅助呼吸期间(灰色)的主要不良反应。

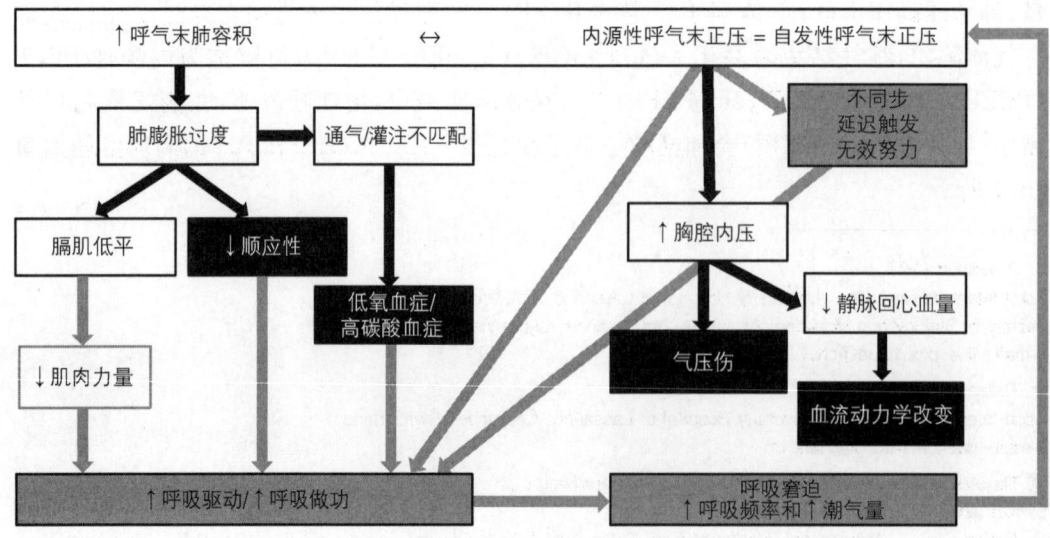

图 20.2 动态肺过度充气的不良后果。灰色表示辅助呼吸

20.2 通用呼吸支持策略

有创机械通气与 AE-COPD 和急性哮喘的高病死率相关[5]。与标准氧疗相比，NIV 可以降低 AE-COPD 患者的插管率和病死率，是一线呼吸支持策略[6,7]。因此，在没有绝对禁忌证或需要即刻插管指征的情况下，推荐将 NIV 作为 AE-COPD 第一步的通气支持手段[8]。值得注意的是，因 NIV 失败而插管的 AE-COPD 患者与先前未尝试 NIV 的患者相比，病死率没有增加[9,10]。AA 的一线治疗是给予大剂量吸入式支气管扩张剂（β_2 受体激动剂）。即使有经验的团队有时会使用 NIV[11]，但 NIV 在 AA 中的作用仍然存在争议，在最新的指南中都不推荐使用[8]。对严重的 AA 患者，插管后会发生严重低血压（由于肺过度充气和低血容量），并且即使进行了插管，哮喘患者的病死率仍然很高。因此，在 AA 中，插管应仅限于有立即危及生命情况的患者［呼吸停止、呼吸减慢、呼吸疲劳和（或）伴有在恰当治疗后仍然存在严重和恶化的高碳酸血症、严重呼吸窘迫或意识水平改变］。

在过去的几十年里，NIV 在 AE-COPD 患者中的广泛应用和吸入式支气管扩张剂对 AA 的积极治疗显著降低了插管率[12]。然而，在最严重的病例中，为了维持充分的气体交换和（或）因为呼吸衰竭仍然需要插管，这种情况更多见于 AE-COPD。由于动态肺过度充气有严重的不良影响，在对插管的阻塞性患者进行通气时，目标是在呼气末尽可能减少肺中的残留气体量，而并不是使气体交换正常化，尤其不能以高碳酸血症恢复正常为目标。因为这会加剧动态肺过度充气。因此，允许性高碳酸血症与阻塞性肺疾病患者严重哮喘状态预后改善有关[13]。

20.3 阻塞性肺疾病患者的有创控制通气：目标、动态气体陷闭的监测和通气策略

在急性加重期，阻塞性肺疾病患者插管后需要采用控制性通气。为了限制动态肺过度充气，可以接受允许性高碳酸血症（和呼吸性酸中毒）。pH 为 7.25～7.30 显然可以被认为是安全的[13]，而更低的 pH 已被证明在长时程机械通气中具有很好的耐受性[13,14]。

动态肺过度充气可以通过呼气末阻断来测量，在此期间，呼吸机的吸气阀和呼气阀关闭。因此，在没有完全关闭气道的情况下，压力达到平衡状态时，在呼吸机回路中测量的压力等于气道和肺泡压力。在阻断后测量的呼气末压称为总 PEEP（$PEEP_{tot}$）。当存在动态气体陷闭时，$PEEP_{tot}$ 高于设定的 PEEP，即存在 PEEPi 或 autoPEEP。$PEEP_{tot}$ 和 PEEPi 与呼气末肺容积高于功能残气量的气体量相关。因此，限制动态肺过度充气意味着尽可能降低 $PEEP_{tot}$ 和 PEEPi 水平。在不进行呼气末阻断的情况下，可以通过观察呼吸机上的流量-时间曲线，初步判断是否存在动态气体陷闭（尽管没有量化）。当流量-时间曲线在呼气结束时不归零时，很可能存在动态气体陷闭。在对阻塞性肺疾病患者进行通气时，另一个重要的监测参数是平台压（plateau pressure，P_{plat}），通过吸气末阻断测量（见"4 控制性机械通气：模式和监测"）。P_{plat} 等于吸气结束时的肺泡压力，取决于呼

吸系统的顺应性、呼吸机提供的辅助量和 PEEP$_{tot}$。控制性通气的目标是使 P_{plat} 保持在 28～30 cmH$_2$O 甚至更低。

和通常的气管插管有创通气患者一样,尚无证据证明选择使用压力还是容量控制的通气模式对阻塞性肺疾病患者的结局有影响[15]。然而,容量控制模式在这种情况下有优势。首先,潮气量和每分钟通气量不因气道阻塞程度改变而受到影响,因此不受支气管痉挛严重程度变化的影响。其次,如果使用恒定的吸气流量,容量控制模式可以相对容易地监测呼吸系统力学,包括气道阻力。不管使用哪种通气模式(压力或容量控制),必须尽量减少每分钟通气量,必须保证足够的呼气时间,以限制动态肺过度通气[16]。这可以通过提供相对较低的潮气量(按理想体重 6～8 mL/kg)和较低的呼吸频率来实现,如 12 次/分的呼吸频率[17,18]。目的是在气道阻塞特别严重时提供最小(10 L/min 或更少)的通气。这种策略被称为控制性低通气,可导致允许性高碳酸血症[14]。需要注意的是,将呼吸频率降低到低于 12 次/分时,虽然有助于限制动态肺过度充气,但在每分钟通气量较低时,仅具有轻微的额外效果[19,20]。只有在最严重的情况下:每分钟通气量已经很低时 P_{plat} 仍然高于 30 cmH$_2$O 和(或)动态肺过度充气相关并发症(如气压伤)已经发生时,才应考虑使用低于 12 次/分的呼吸频率。呼气时间也是对阻塞性肺疾病患者进行通气时的一个关键值。为了提供足够长的呼气时间,除了设定低呼吸频率,降低吸呼比(I∶E)也非常重要,如使 I∶E 为 1∶4,而不是 1∶2 的生理值。这里必须强调的是,对于给定且稳定的每分钟通气量,增加呼气时间对动态肺过度充气的限制作用相对有限[16],降低呼吸频率更为有效。减少吸气暂停时间是另一种增加可用呼气时间的方式,然而,这不利于 P_{plat} 的自动测量,即使在阻力增加的情况下也是一种非常有价值的连续监测工具,尽管它经常高估静态 P_{plat}。只有在最严重的气道梗阻中,才应考虑在容量控制通气期间减少吸气暂停。表 20.1(上半部分)总结了阻塞性肺疾病急性期患者采用控制模式通气时设置呼吸机参数的基本原则。在将潮气量设置为 6～8 mL/kg(理想体重)、呼吸频率设置为 12 次/分,P_{plat} 低于 28 cmH$_2$O 且 PEEP$_{tot}$ 足够低时,就可以考虑缓慢而逐步地增加呼吸频率以改善血气。每次增加呼吸频率时,必须监测 P_{plat} 和 PEEP$_{tot}$。如果这些压力升高,呼吸频率应再次降低。

表 20.1 在对阻塞性肺疾病患者进行控制和压力支持通气时,设置呼吸机参数的基本原则

目的:减少肺过度充气,而不是正常的气体交换=控制低通气/允许高碳酸血症				
	目的: ↓每分钟通气量 到↓呼气量	目的: ↑呼气时间 ↓吸气时间	目的: ↓呼吸做功	监测预警和目标
控制性通气	• 限制潮气量 [6～8 mL/kg(理想体重)] • 低呼吸频率	• ↑吸气流速(VAC) • ↓吸呼比(1∶4 及以下) • 无吸气暂停?(VAC)		• 每分钟通气量<10 L/min • 低 PEEPi • 平台压 28～30 cmH$_2$O

		续 表		
支持性通气	• 限制压力支持水平/无过度辅助 • 低潮气量目标[最大 8 mL/kg(理想体重)]	• 呼气触发阈值 25%～30%（提前打开呼气阀）	• 适当的 PEEPe 水平以避免/减少无效做功	• 低潮气量和每分钟通气量 • 人-机同步

V_T,潮气量；PBW,预测体重；VAC,容量辅助控制模式；PEEPe,外源性呼气末正压；PEEPi,内源性呼气末正压。

关于阻塞性肺疾病患者在控制通气期间的外源性 PEEP(PEEPe)的设置，目前还没有多少研究数据，这仍然是一个有争议的话题。从根本上说，对阻塞性肺疾病患者，在控制呼吸时使用 PEEPe 可降低呼气驱动压，从而降低呼气流量。因此，它可以成为呼气的障碍并增加动态气体陷闭。然而，这主要发生在 PEEPe 高于或接近 PEEPi 时。只要 PEEPe 保持低于 PEEPi 的 80%，至少在患者存在呼气流量受限时，不会由于使用 PEEPe 导致动态肺过度充气加重[21]。此外，在有创通气时，适量的 PEEPe 有助于预防肺不张和改善氧合。当考虑在阻塞性肺疾病有创通气的患者中使用中等水平的 PEEPe 时，患者可以表现出以下 3 种不同反应[22]。第一，对使用中等水平 PEEP 的患者，可良好耐受；且 PEEPe 与 $PEEP_{tot}$ 和 P_{plat} 的增加无关，直到达到一个 PEEPe 阈值。第二，PEEPe 的增加会导致 $PEEP_{tot}$ 和 P_{plat} 增加。第三，适量的 PEEPe 反而使 $PEEP_{tot}$ 和 P_{plat} 下降。虽然最后一种表型仅见于少数阻塞性疾病患者，但在控制通气期间，无法预测患者对中度 PEEPe 水平的反应，因此对每个患者都应进行谨慎的 PEEPe 试验。对阻塞性肺疾病患者而言，一种实用的在控制通气期间设置 PEEPe 的方法是先将 PEEPe 设置为 0 cmH_2O，在监测 $PEEP_{tot}$ 和 P_{plat} 的同时，使用循序渐进的策略逐步增加 PEEPe。一旦 $PEEP_{tot}$ 和 P_{plat} 增加，应停止 PEEPe 滴定，PEEPe 应降低到前一步的值。尽管存在上述风险，但滴定 PEEPe 是为了在患者可耐受的范围内使用 PEEPe 以预防肺不张。然而，这一策略主要适用于 COPD 患者。在哮喘患者中，即使使用少量的 PEEPe，动态肺过度充气加重的风险也比较高，因此，在这种情况下，应尽可能谨慎使用。尽管如此，在非常严格的 $PEEP_{tot}$ 和 P_{plat} 监测下，推荐在哮喘患者中使用低水平的 PEEPe (<5 cmH_2O)[19]。

20.4 阻塞性肺疾病患者的有创辅助通气及撤机策略

机械通气时间过长与预后不良相关[23]。因此，尽早切换到辅助性通气并启动机械通气撤机流程是很重要的。压力支持模式常用于降阶梯治疗的第一步。在这一阶段，通常仍然存在一定程度的气道阻塞，应特别注意保证潮气量不超过 8 mL/kg(预测体重)。应滴定压力支持水平，避免过度支持[24]。存在残余气流阻塞的情况下，在压力支持期间特别关注呼气触发设置是很重要的。因为气流阻塞时，会出现默认设置下(即吸气峰流速的 25%～30%)呼气延迟切换，这会减少呼气可用时间，导致呼吸相延迟，加重动态肺过度充气。将默认呼气触发的流量提高到 45%～50%可以帮助克服这个问题[25]。

当 PEEPi 存在时，患者必须产生相当大的吸气努力来克服 PEEPi，才能触发呼吸机[26]。当存在高 PEEPi 和(或)膈肌无力时,吸气努力不足以克服 PEEPi 以触发呼吸机时,就会发生无效触发[27]。减少吸气努力强度来触发呼吸机的解决办法是设置一个 PEEPe,其可以平衡 PEEPi,促进触发,并改善人-机同步性。但是,PEEPe 同样应保持低于 PEEPi 的 80%。难点在于辅助通气时,PEEPi 不容易在床边测量。实际上,PEEPe 应该逐步滴定,以避免无效呼吸或使无效呼吸最小化。另一个有助于在阻塞性肺疾病患者压力支持期间设置 PEEPe 的临床方法是观察辅助呼吸肌是否参与呼吸,不平衡的 PEEPi 与更强的吸气努力导致的辅助呼吸肌明显收缩有关。值得注意的是,在压力支持通气期间,吸气触发器也必须设置为最足够敏感以有效触发,同时不产生自动触发。表 20.1(下半部分)总结了使用压力支持模式对阻塞性肺疾病患者进行通气时设置呼吸机的基本原则。

对于所有机械通气的患者,应每天评估撤机的条件[28],当达到撤机标准时,应进行自主呼吸试验(spontaneous breathing trial, SBT)。在 SBT 成功且无拔管禁忌证的情况下,应尽快拔管[28]。在 COPD 患者中,拔管后序贯使用 NIV 已被证明可有效降低再插管率[29]。

(邓会标,计恩东 译)

参考文献

[1] Junhasavasdikul D, Telias I, Grieco DL, Chen L, Gutierrez CM, Piraino T, et al. Expiratory flow limitation during mechanical ventilation. Chest. 2018;154(4):948-62.

[2] Oddo M, Feihl F, Schaller MD, Perret C. Management of mechanical ventilation in acute severe asthma: practical aspects. Intensive Care Med. 2006;32(4):501-10.

[3] Vassilakopoulos T, Toumpanakis D, Mancebo J. What's new about pulmonary hyperinflation in mechanically ventilated critical patients. Intensive Care Med. 2020;46(12):2381-4.

[4] Marini JJ. Dynamic hyperinflation and auto-positive end-expiratory pressure: lessons learned over 30 years. Am J Respir Crit Care Med. 2011;184(7):756-62.

[5] Brenner B, Corbridge T, Kazzi A. Intubation and mechanical ventilation of the asthmatic patient in respiratory failure. Proc Am Thorac Soc. 2009;6(4):371-9.

[6] Brochard L, Mancebo J, Wysocki M, Lofaso F, Conti G, Rauss A, et al. Noninvasive ventilation for acute exacerbations of chronic obstructive pulmonary disease. N Engl J Med. 1995;333(13):817-22.

[7] Girou E, Brun-Buisson C, Taille S, Lemaire F, Brochard L. Secular trends in nosocomial infections and mortality associated with noninvasive ventilation in patients with exacerbation of COPD and pulmonary edema. JAMA. 2003;290(22):2985-91.

[8] Rochwerg B, Brochard L, Elliott MW, Hess D, Hill NS, Nava S, et al. Official ERS/ATS clinical practice guidelines: noninvasive ventilation for acute respiratory failure. Eur Respir J. 2017;50(2):1602426.

[9] Demoule A, Girou E, Richard JC, Taille S, Brochard L. Benefits and risks of success or failure of noninvasive ventilation. Intensive Care Med. 2006;32(11):1756-65.

[10] Chandra D, Stamm JA, Taylor B, Ramos RM, Satterwhite L, Krishnan JA, et al. Outcomes of noninvasive ventilation for acute exacerbations of chronic obstructive pulmonary disease in the United States, 1998-2008. Am J Respir Crit Care Med. 2012;185(2):152-9.

[11] Pendergraft TB, Stanford RH, Beasley R, Stempel DA, Roberts C, McLaughlin T. Rates and

characteristics of intensive care unit admissions and intubations among asthma-related hospitalizations. Ann Allergy Asthma Immunol. 2004; 93(1): 29-35.

[12] Penuelas O, Muriel A, Abraira V, Frutos-Vivar F, Mancebo J, Raymondos K, et al. Intercountry variability over time in the mortality of mechanically ventilated patients. Intensive Care Med. 2020; 46(3): 444-53.

[13] Darioli R, Perret C. Mechanical controlled hypoventilation in status asthmaticus. Am Rev Respir Dis. 1984; 129(3): 385-7.

[14] Feihl F, Perret C. Permissive hypercapnia. How permissive should we be? Am J Respir Crit Care Med. 1994; 150(6 Pt 1): 1722-37.

[15] Rittayamai N, Katsios CM, Beloncle F, Friedrich JO, Mancebo J, Brochard L. Pressure-controlled vs volume-controlled ventilation in acute respiratory failure: a physiology-based narrative and systematic review. Chest. 2015; 148(2): 340-55.

[16] Tuxen DV, Lane S. The effects of ventilatory pattern on hyperinflation, airway pressures, and circulation in mechanical ventilation of patients with severe air-flow obstruction. Am Rev Respir Dis. 1987; 136(4): 872-9.

[17] Mancebo J. Assist-control ventilation. In: Tobin M-J, editor. Principles and practice of mechanical ventilation. New York: McGraw Hill; 2013. p. 159-74.

[18] Demoule A, Brochard L, Dres M, Heunks L, Jubran A, Laghi F, et al. How to ventilate obstructive and asthmatic patients. Intensive Care Med. 2020; 46(12): 2436-49.

[19] Leatherman J. Mechanical ventilation for severe asthma. Chest. 2015; 147(6): 1671-80.

[20] Leatherman JW, McArthur C, Shapiro RS. Effect of prolongation of expiratory time on dynamic hyperinflation in mechanically ventilated patients with severe asthma. Crit Care Med. 2004; 32(7): 1542-5.

[21] Tobin MJ, Lodato RF. PEEP, auto-PEEP, and waterfalls. Chest. 1989; 96(3): 449-51.

[22] Caramez MP, Borges JB, Tucci MR, Okamoto VN, Carvalho CR, Kacmarek RM, et al. Paradoxical responses to positive end-expiratory pressure in patients with airway obstruction during controlled ventilation. Crit Care Med. 2005; 33(7): 1519-28.

[23] Beduneau G, Pham T, Schortgen F, Piquilloud L, Zogheib E, Jonas M, et al. Epidemiology of weaning outcome according to a new definition. The WIND study. Am J Respir Crit Care Med. 2017; 195(6): 772-83.

[24] Thille AW, Cabello B, Galia F, Lyazidi A, Brochard L. Reduction of patient-ventilator asynchrony by reducing tidal volume during pressure-support ventilation. Intensive Care Med. 2008; 34(8): 1477-86.

[25] Tassaux D, Gainnier M, Battisti A, Jolliet P. Impact of expiratory trigger setting on delayed cycling and inspiratory muscle workload. Am J Respir Crit Care Med. 2005; 172(10): 1283-9.

[26] Smith TC, Marini JJ. Impact of PEEP on lung mechanics and work of breathing in severe airflow obstruction. J Appl Physiol. 1988; 65(4): 1488-99.

[27] Vassilakopoulos T. Understanding wasted/ineffective efforts in mechanically ventilated COPD patients using the Campbell diagram. Intensive Care Med. 2008; 34(7): 1336-9.

[28] Boles JM, Bion J, Connors A, Herridge M, Marsh B, Melot C, et al. Weaning from mechanical ventilation. Eur Respir J. 2007; 29(5): 1033-56.

[29] Ferrer M, Sellares J, Valencia M, Carrillo A, Gonzalez G, Badia JR, et al. Non-invasive ventilation after extubation in hypercapnic patients with chronic respiratory disorders: randomised controlled trial. Lancet. 2009; 374(9695): 1082-8.

21 肥胖患者的通气

Ventilation in the Obese Patient

Pedro Leme Silva, Paolo Pelosi, Patricia Rieken Macedo Rocco

21.1 引言

正压机械通气（mechanical ventilation，MV）是维持血气交换的生命支持系统。肥胖患者的正压 MV 值得关注。因为与较瘦患者相比，肥胖患者的功能残气量较低、呼吸系统发生改变（由于胸壁和肺力学的变化）、气体交换受损，以及慢性局部和全身性炎症。应仔细调整 MV 参数，并时时监测。输入通气参数可以由医务人员调整，而输出通气参数不仅取决于对呼吸机的调整，还取决于肥胖对肺部状况的影响。本章旨在对肥胖患者的输入、输出通气参数进行详细的叙述（图 21.1）。

21.2 肥胖患者的机械通气需要调整的呼吸机输入参数

21.2.1 潮气量

潮气量（tidal volume，V_T）应根据呼气末肺容积（end-expiratory lung volume，EELV）或深吸气量设定，两者在肥胖情况下都减少[1]。V_T 相较于 EELV 的调整在低呼气末正压（end-expiratory pressure，PEEP）时可能比高 PEEP 时更为准确，因为较高的

输入

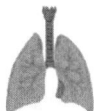
潮气量 = 6~8 mL/kg(预测体重)。理想情况下,潮气量可以根据呼气末肺容积和深吸气量进行设定,但需要是闭环系统。

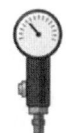
PEEP = 根据安全的驱动压和潮气量进行个体化设置

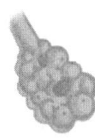
PEEP滴定下逐步肺复张策略。注意低血压。不推荐球囊鼓肺。

输出

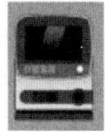
驱动压 < 15 cmH₂O
平台压 < 15 cmH₂O

机械能 < 17J/min
在肥胖患者中没有特定的数据

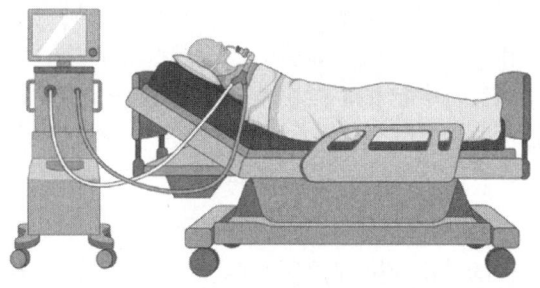

图 21.1　肥胖患者机械通气的示意图。由床旁的医护人员调整呼吸机输入参数如下:① 潮气量(V_T)在保护范围内,根据预测体重以 6~8 mL/kg 设定;② 根据安全的驱动压(ΔP)和 V_T 设定个体化呼气末正压(PEEP);③ PEEP 滴定,逐步实现肺复张;④ 不推荐球囊鼓肺。对于呼吸机输出参数,这些呼吸参数不仅取决于对呼吸机的调整还取决于肥胖导致的肺部状况,如① ΔP_{RS} 应保持≤15 cmH₂O;② 平台压保持≤20 cmH₂O,或特殊情况下＜27 cmH₂O;③ 机械能(MP)应保持＜17 J/min。(由 BioRender.com 制图)

PEEP 会增加 EELV,包括可能的肺复张和(或)过度充气。在对纳入 4 968 名患者的前瞻性多中心研究[2]的二次分析中,发现严重肥胖患者采用基于实际体重的 V_T,以预测体重(predicted body weight,PBW)标化后的 V_T 远高于预期(分别为 5 mL/kg 和 11 mL/kg),增加了呼吸机相关肺损伤的风险。因此,就像非肥胖患者一样,有健康肺的肥胖患者的最合适 V_T 应在 6~8 mL/kg(PBW)内。

21.2.2　呼气末正压

比较肥胖患者术中高和低 PEEP 的保护性通气(PROBESE)试验[3]显示,与 PEEP 为 4 cmH₂O 的患者相比,对 PEEP 为 12 cmH₂O 的患者采用联合肺复张手法(recruitment maneuver,RM)并不能减少术后肺部并发症。在对 PROBESE 试验的二次分析中,发现与固定 PEEP(4 cmH₂O)相比,通过电阻抗断层扫描(electric impedance tomography,EIT)进行个体化 PEEP 设置[中位数(四分位距)为 18cmH₂O(16~22 cmH₂O)]的患者氧合改善,驱动压降低,使肺部重力依赖区的通气重新分布,但未评估临床结局。在之前对 LAS VEGAS 研究的二次分析中,Ball 等发现,总体上为肥胖患者设置的 PEEP 水平相对较低（4 cmH$_2$O）[4]，而对Ⅲ度肥胖患者采用了更高的 PEEP（5 cmH$_2$O）和球囊鼓肺的 RM。在多变量混合 logistic 回归分析中，球囊鼓肺与术后肺部并发症显著相关。

现在有人建议术中 MV 时通过 EIT 进行个体化的 PEEP 设定。Simon 等比较了 EIT 设定的个体化 PEEP 与 PROBESE 试验中的 PEEP 4 和 PEEP 12 对呼吸功能和不良事件的影响[5]，由 EIT 设定的个体化 PEEP 与较高的术中氧合和较低的驱动压（即更好的呼吸系统顺应性）相关，但对液体和血管活性药物的需求较高。这些对呼吸功能的有益影响在 PEEP 停止后消失，提示个体化 PEEP 与固定 PEEP 相比并没有明显优势，但需要进一步的研究来更好地阐明这一重要的临床问题[6]。

21.2.3 肺复张手法

文献报道，不同形式的肺复张手法已应用于无急性肺部疾病的肥胖患者。Pirrone 等研究发现，在内科和外科重症监护病房的病态肥胖患者中，RM 加 PEEP 滴定可改善肺容积、呼吸系统弹性和氧合[7]。RM 以逐步的方式进行，其中基线 PEEP 为 15 cmH$_2$O，每 30 秒 PEEP 增加 5 cmH$_2$O，直至 PEEP 为 30 cmH$_2$O，同时压力控制为 15 cmH$_2$O。Nestler 等[8]比较了 RM 后个体化 PEEP 设置（使用 EIT 滴定）与无 RM 且采用 5 cmH$_2$O 的固定 PEEP 的差异。RM 具体包括调节至 50 cmH$_2$O 的气道峰压，30 cmH$_2$O 的 PEEP，持续约 90 秒的 6 次/分的呼吸频率。研究人员发现，与 5 cmH$_2$O 的固定 PEEP 相比，个体化 PEEP 可改善麻醉期间的氧合、呼吸系统力学、通气分布和 EELV。然而，这些有益的影响在术后早期消失。因此，RM 后个体化 PEEP 设置并不能防止拔管后肺不张的再次发生，这是术后肺部并发症复合结局的要素之一。

21.3 肥胖患者的机械通气需要监测的呼吸机输出参数

21.3.1 驱动压

驱动压是在 MV 期间的气道平台压与 PEEP 之间的差值，也可以被定义为基于呼吸系统顺应性标准化的 V_T（因此，间接地反映了 V_T 与肺容积的比值）。到目前为止，关于肥胖患者 MV 时的安全驱动压，还没有大型研究的数据来得出结论。在这种情况下，一些理论上的比较可能是有价值的，考虑将肥胖患者与正常范围胸廓和肺顺应性的非肥胖患者进行对比。对于一个非肥胖患者，胸廓和肺顺应性平均水平在 200 mL/cmH$_2$O 和 100 mL/cmH$_2$O，其吸气 500 mL 时，分别需要 2.5 cmH$_2$O 和 5 cmH$_2$O 的压力来驱动胸廓和肺部。此时，呼吸系统的驱动压是 7.5 cmH$_2$O。在非肥胖的麻醉患者中，当呼吸系统驱动压超过 13 cmH$_2$O，即相当于跨肺驱动压为 10 cmH$_2$O 时，肺损伤会开始出现[9]。在肥胖患者中，胸廓和肺顺应性平均分别为 100 mL/cmH$_2$O 和 50 mL/cmH$_2$O。同样吸气 500 mL 时，肥胖患者分别需要 5 cmH$_2$O 和 10 cmH$_2$O 的压力来驱动胸廓和肺部。因此，这种差异主要取决于肺的组分，可能与肥胖患者肺的大小有关[10]。为了避免肺损伤，

15 cmH$_2$O 是有创 MV 时肥胖患者可接受的最高呼吸系统驱动压[11]（图 21.2）。尽管 PROBESE 试验显示，与 4 cmH$_2$O 相比，PEEP 为 12 cmH$_2$O 的患者驱动压有所降低，但这并没有改善接受择期手术的肥胖患者的临床结局。也许驱动压对患有急性肺部疾病的肥胖患者（如需要 MV 的 ARDS）具有相应的预后价值。

非肥胖患者：
胸廓顺应性 = 200 mL/cmH$_2$O
肺顺应性 = 100 mL/cmH$_2$O

输入
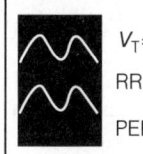
V_T=0.500 L
RR = 18 bpm
PEEP = 5 cmH$_2$O

输出
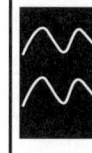
$P_{peak(RS)}$ = 15 cmH$_2$O
$P_{plat(RS)}$ = 12.5 cmH$_2$O
ΔP_{RS} = 7.5 cmH$_2$O
ΔP_L = 5 cmH$_2$O
ΔP_{CW} = 2.5 cmH$_2$O
MP$_{RS}$ = 9.9 J/min

当呼吸系统驱动压 >13 cmH$_2$O
或呼吸系统机械能 > 17 J/min 时发生肺损伤

肥胖患者：
胸廓顺应性 = 100 mL/cmH$_2$O
肺顺应性 = 50 mL/cmH$_2$O

输入
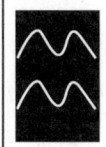
V_T=0.500 L
RR = 18 bpm
PEEP = 5 cmH$_2$O

输出
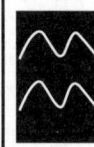
$P_{peak(RS)}$ = 22.5 cmH$_2$O
$P_{plat(RS)}$ = 20 cmH$_2$O
ΔP_{RS} = 15 cmH$_2$O
ΔP_L = 10 cmH$_2$O
ΔP_{CW} = 5 cmH$_2$O
MP$_{RS}$ = 13.2 J/min

当呼吸系统驱动压 >15 cmH$_2$O
或呼吸系统机械能 > 17 J/min 时发生肺损伤

图 21.2 非肥胖和肥胖患者呼吸机输入、输出参数的模拟分析。非肥胖患者的胸廓（CW）和肺（L）顺应性为 200 mL/cmH$_2$O 和 100 mL/cmH$_2$O，在 V_T=0.5 L 时，需要 2.5 cmH$_2$O 和 5 cmH$_2$O 的压力来驱动胸廓（ΔP_{CW}）和肺（ΔP_L）。因此，呼吸系统驱动压力（ΔP_{RS}）为 7.5 cmH$_2$O，气道峰压（$P_{peak(RS)}$）为 15 cmH$_2$O，呼吸系统机械能（MP$_{RS}$）为 9.9 J/min。在机械通气的非肥胖患者中，当 ΔP_{RS} 和 MP$_{RS}$ 分别高于 13 cmH$_2$O 和 17 J/min 时，更容易发生肺损伤。肥胖患者胸廓和肺顺应性平均分别为 100 mL/cmH$_2$O 和 50 mL/cmH$_2$O，因此，要达到相同的 V_T=500 mL，肥胖患者需要压力 ΔP_{CW}=5 cmH$_2$O 和 ΔP_L=10 cmH$_2$O。因此，输出呼吸变量为 $P_{peak(RS)}$ = 22.5 cmH$_2$O，$P_{plat(RS)}$ = 20 cmH$_2$O，ΔP_{RS} = 15 cmH$_2$O，MP$_{RS}$=13.2 J/min。因此，为了避免肺部损伤，肥胖患者有创机械通气时可接受的最高 ΔP_{RS} 和 MP$_{RS}$ 值为 15 cmH$_2$O 和 17 J/min。这是一个以教学为目的模拟计算，迄今为止，尚无肥胖患者机械通气时 MP$_{RS}$ 的安全阈值数据

21.3.2 平台压

呼吸系统平台压($P_{plat(RS)}$)反映了呼吸系统的弹性回缩力。它也可以解释为用来扩张胸壁和肺的压力。因此,在肥胖患者中,$P_{plat(RS)}$升高可能是胸壁和(或)肺变化的结果。计算跨肺或跨胸壁压对于分别判断肺或胸壁的力学改变很重要,能够更好地理解$P_{plat(RS)}$增加的原因。基于$P_{plat(RS)}$对胸壁力学进行判断可能会产生误导,如在肥胖人群中,仅基于$P_{plat(RS)}$得出的肺泡过度膨胀,以及由于肺不张导致通气面积减少的结论是不准确的。

然而,有专家提出了管理肥胖患者$P_{plat(RS)}$的一些建议。无急性肺疾病的肥胖患者的$P_{plat(RS)}$应<20 cmH$_2$O[12]。作者强调,这些患者胸壁顺应性的降低可能与腹腔内压(intra-abdominal pressure,IAP)有关,其可以通过膀胱压力估算。因此,目标$P_{plat(RS)}$可以基于IAP,使用以下公式进行计算:调整后的$P_{plat(RS)}$=目标$P_{plat(RS)}$+IAP—13 cmH$_2$O/2[13]。

21.3.3 能量和机械能

V_T和$P_{plat(RS)}$分别为应变和应力的简单替代测量值。应变定义为V_T与EELV的比值。应力则是肺的扩张力,等于跨肺压。对呼吸系统施加的能量可以根据气道压力-容积曲线进行计算,考虑到在总肺活量区域内该曲线是线性的。因此,可以根据每个呼吸周期的压力-容积曲线下面积计算出施加到呼吸系统的能量。每个频率周期作用于肺部的能量称为机械能,实际上就是每分钟传递的能量[14],与危重症患者的病死率相关[15]:绝对机械能=0.098×V_T×呼吸频率×($P_{peak(aw)}-\Delta P/2$)。

使用机械能来指导肥胖患者的治疗可能特别有意义,因为这个参数依赖于胸壁弹性,在肥胖患者中发生了本质上的改变。在MV患者中,呼吸机诱导肺损伤的应力和能量的指标在病态肥胖患者中受到胸壁和肺共同对整体呼吸力学的影响[16]。着眼于呼吸机诱导肺损伤风险的相关指南必须考虑到病态肥胖时这些弹性特征的变化。专注于控制机械能的研究还应监测ARDS的肥胖患者MV期间胸壁的力学特性和腹腔内压。

21.4 总结

对于MV的肥胖患者,尤其是发生呼吸并发症的高危人群,应仔细控制和监测输入和输出的呼吸机参数。有新的证据提出了气道压力的安全阈值,建议避免一些操作(如球囊鼓肺手法);并确认了新的呼吸机衍生参数,如能量和机械能。

(邓会标,计恩东 译)

参考文献

[1] Babb TG, Wyrick BL, DeLorey DS, Chase PJ, Feng MY. Fat distribution and end-expiratory lung volume in lean and obese men and women. Chest. 2008;134(4):704-11.
[2] Anzueto A, Frutos-Vivar F, Esteban A, Bensalami N, Marks D, Raymondos K, et al. Influence

of body mass index on outcome of the mechanically ventilated patients. Thorax. 2011; 66(1): 66-73.

[3] Bluth T, Serpa Neto A, Schultz MJ, Pelosi P, Gama de Abreu M, Bobek I, et al. Effect of intraoperative high positive end-expiratory pressure (PEEP) with recruitment maneuvers vs low PEEP on postoperative pulmonary complications in obese patients: a randomized clinical trial. JAMA. 2019; 321(23): 2292-305.

[4] Ball L, Hemmes SNT, Serpa Neto A, Bluth T, Canet J, Hiesmayr M, et al. Intraoperative ventilation settings and their associations with postoperative pulmonary complications in obese patients. Br J Anaesth. 2018; 121(4): 899-908.

[5] Simon P, Girrbach F, Petroff D, Schliewe N, Hempel G, Lange M, et al. Individualized versus fixed positive end-expiratory pressure for intraoperative mechanical ventilation in obese patients: a secondary analysis. Anesthesiology. 2021; 134(6): 887-900.

[6] Pereira SM, Tucci MR, Morais CCA, Simoes CM, Tonelotto BFF, Pompeo MS, et al. Individual positive end-expiratory pressure settings optimize intraoperative mechanical ventilation and reduce postoperative atelectasis. Anesthesiology. 2018; 129(6): 1070-81.

[7] Pirrone M, Fisher D, Chipman D, Imber DA, Corona J, Mietto C, et al. Recruitment maneuvers and positive end-expiratory pressure titration in morbidly obese ICU patients. Crit Care Med. 2016; 44(2): 300-7.

[8] Nestler C, Simon P, Petroff D, Hammermuller S, Kamrath D, Wolf S, et al. Individualized positive end-expiratory pressure in obese patients during general anaesthesia: a randomized controlled clinical trial using electrical impedance tomography. Br J Anaesth. 2017; 119(6): 1194-205.

[9] Neto AS, Hemmes SN, Barbas CS, Beiderlinden M, Fernandez-Bustamante A, Futier E, et al. Association between driving pressure and development of postoperative pulmonary complications in patients undergoing mechanical ventilation for general anaesthesia: a meta-analysis of individual patient data. Lancet Respir Med. 2016; 4(4): 272-80.

[10] Pelosi P, Croci M, Ravagnan I, Tredici S, Pedoto A, Lissoni A, et al. The effects of body mass on lung volumes, respiratory mechanics, and gas exchange during general anesthesia. Anesth Analg. 1998; 87(3): 654-60.

[11] Maia LA, Silva PL, Pelosi P, Rocco PRM. Controlled invasive mechanical ventilation strategies in obese patients undergoing surgery. Expert Rev Respir Med. 2017; 11(6): 443-52.

[12] Ball L, Pelosi P. How I ventilate an obese patient. Crit Care. 2019; 23(1): 176.

[13] Regli A, Pelosi P, Malbrain M. Ventilation in patients with intra-abdominal hypertension: what every critical care physician needs to know. Ann Intensive Care. 2019; 9(1): 52.

[14] Gattinoni L, Tonetti T, Cressoni M, Cadringher P, Herrmann P, Moerer O, et al. Ventilator-related causes of lung injury: the mechanical power. Intensive Care Med. 2016; 42(10): 1567-75.

[15] Serpa Neto A, Deliberato RO, Johnson AEW, Bos LD, Amorim P, Pereira SM, et al. Mechanical power of ventilation is associated with mortality in critically ill patients: an analysis of patients in two observational cohorts. Intensive Care Med. 2018; 44(11): 1914-22.

[16] Syed MKH, Selickman J, Evans MD, Dries D, Marini JJ. Elastic power of mechanical ventilation in morbid obesity and severe hypoxemia. Respir Care. 2021; 66(4): 626-34.

22 简单和复杂患者的撤机
Weaning the Simple and Complex Patients

Tài Pham, Martin Dres, Rémi Coudroy

22.1 引言

入住重症监护室的大部分患者都接受一种形式的人工通气治疗,从简单的低流量鼻导管吸氧到需要深镇静、肌肉松弛和俯卧位的有创机械通气(invasive mechanical ventilation, IMV)。自 20 世纪 50 年代脊髓灰质炎流行以来,通气管理是重症医学的里程碑,也是重症医师和呼吸治疗师的特定专业领域。最近 SARS-CoV-2 的暴发,伴随着重症 COVID-19 导致的急性呼吸窘迫综合征(acute respiratory distress syndrome, ARDS)患者的激增,更加突出了适当使用 IMV 的重要性。据估计,在 COVID-19 流行以前,ICU 的 IMV 治疗每年都在增加,而且在 COVID-19 流行高峰时期,全球对呼吸机

T. Pham (✉)
Service de Médecine Intensive-Réanimation, AP-HP, Hôpital de Bicêtre, DMU 4 CORREVE Maladies du Coeur et des Vaisseaux, FHU Sepsis, Groupe de Recherche Clinique CARMAS, Le Kremlin-Bicêtre, France

Université Paris-Saclay, UVSQ, Univ. Paris-Sud, Inserm U1018, Equipe d'Epidémiologie Respiratoire Intégrative, CESP, Villejuif, France
e-mail: tai.pham@aphp.fr

M. Dres
Sorbonne Université, INSERM, UMRS1158 Neurophysiologie Respiratoire Expérimentale et Clinique, Paris, France

Service de Médecine Intensive — Réanimation (Département "R3S"), AP-HP. Sorbonne Université, Hôpital Pitié-Salpêtrière, Paris, France
e-mail: martin.dres@aphp.fr

R. Coudroy
Médecine Intensive Réanimation, Centre Hospitalier Universitaire de Poitiers, Poitiers, France
INSERM CiC 1402, ALIVE Research Group, INSERM, Université de Poitiers, Poitiers, France
e-mail: remi.coudroy@chu-poitiers.fr

© The Author(s), under exclusive license to Springer Nature Switzerland AG 2022
G. Bellani (ed.), *Mechanical Ventilation from Pathophysiology to Clinical Evidence*, https://doi.org/10.1007/978-3-030-93401-9_22

的需求进一步增加[1]。虽然有创通气通常是必要的且用以挽救生命,但它也会引起特定的并发症。启动通气的决策会对患者的预后产生重大影响,同时避免或延迟插管也会使患者面临不利的后果。患者使用 IMV 的持续时间与并发症的风险直接相关,因此成功撤离呼吸机的过程(简称为"撤机")至关重要。据报道,撤机过程可达 IMV 总持续时间的 50%。在这一章中,我们将回顾撤机和患者表型的定义(从简单到困难)。我们将详细介绍不同类型自主呼吸试验(spontaneous breathing test,SBT)的优点和缺点,并提出具体的避免 SBT 失败的处理方法,以及避免重新插管。

22.2 撤机的定义和步骤

22.2.1 什么是撤机,何时开始(以及何时结束)

随着对机械通气及其后果的了解更深入,标准化撤机过程变得越来越重要,但仍有一些基本问题有待解决。撤机过程的步骤和成功的终点没有公认的定义,缺乏统一的定义是不确定和混淆的根源。

2007 年,一个由五个主要科学学会的专家组成的工作组发表了一份关于撤机的会议共识声明[2]。这一宝贵的贡献有助于澄清许多问题,如提出了撤机成功和失败的定义并根据撤机过程提出了分类方案(表 22.1),提出了避免撤机失败的策略。然而,几个重要的缺陷限制了它的广泛应用,只有少数后续研究使用了共识定义,并经常对其修改以提高适用性[3]。为了解决这些局限性,Béduneau 及其同事对 2 729 名接受 IMV 的患者进行了观察性研究(WIND 研究),并提出了不同的定义和分类方案。在这个队列中,作者引入了撤机尝试的概念,可以对所有接受 IMV 的患者进行分类(表 22.1)[4]。相比之下,会议共识的定义未能对该队列中近一半的患者进行分类。但是 WIND 的定义并不完美:当撤机过程结束时对患者进行回顾性分组,撤机终止的主要终点是 IMV 持续时间而不是以患者为中心的结局——撤机终止可能是撤机成功或死亡(从患者的角度来看非常不同)。尽管如此,许多研究仍使用了 WIND 定义[5,6],而且相较于会议共识定义,其在适用性和组间病死率比较方面显示出优势[6]。

表 22.1 会议共识和 WIND 定义

	会议共识定义
自主呼吸试验(SBT)	T 管试验或低水平压力支持($\leqslant 8\ cmH_2O$)
SBT 失败	客观指标:呼吸急促、心动过速、高血压、低血压、低氧血症、酸中毒、心律失常 主观指标:焦虑、痛苦、情绪状态低落、出汗、呼吸做功增加
撤机成功	拔管后 48 小时无通气支持
撤机失败	SBT 失败或再插管和(或)恢复呼吸支持或拔管后 48 小时内死亡

正在撤机	拔管后需要无创通气(NIV)
简单撤机	从开始撤机到第一次拔管成功没有困难的患者
困难撤机	初次撤机失败需要多达 3 次 SBT 或从第一次 SBT 起 7 天内成功撤机的患者
延迟撤机	至少 3 次尝试撤机失败或第一次 SBT 后需要间隔大于 7 天再撤机的患者
WIND 定义	
撤机尝试	对于插管患者:执行 SBT,无论是否拔管;没有执行 SBT 直接拔管(无论是哪种类型、计划或非计划拔管) 对于气管切开的患者:24 小时或更长时间内通过气管切开导管进行自主通气,不进行任何机械通气
成功撤机或撤离	对于插管患者:无论患者是否使用无创呼吸机支持,拔管后 7 天内无死亡或未再插管;ICU 出院后 7 天内没有使用 IMV(两者不分先后,无论满足哪个均视为成功撤机) 对于气管切开的患者:通过气管切开自主呼吸,连续 7 天不需要机械通气治疗;或以自主呼吸方式出院(两者不分先后)
"未撤机"组	从未进行撤机尝试的患者
撤机组 1(简单撤机)	第一次尝试撤机在 1 天内就撤机终止(成功撤机或早期死亡)
撤机组 2(困难撤机)	在第一次尝试撤机后超过 1 天,但 1 周内完成撤机(成功撤机或死亡)
撤机组 3(延迟撤机)	在第一次尝试撤机后 7 天仍未完成撤机(成功撤机或死亡)

考虑到这些定义问题,针对"撤机何时开始"这个问题给出一个明确的答案是相当具有挑战性的。因为对于一个给定的患者,不同的临床医生会考虑在机械通气过程的不同时刻开始撤机过程。不同的标志事件可以被认为是撤机过程的开始:① 镇静剂量降低;② 停用镇静药物;③ 呼吸机支持水平下降(FiO_2 和 PEEP 的降低);④ 低氧血症改善;⑤ 无论在何种通气模式下存在自主呼吸的证据;⑥ 呼吸机切换到支持通气模式;⑦ SBT(图 22.1)。

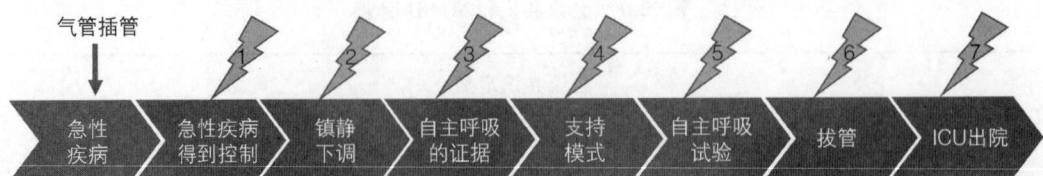

图 22.1 接受机械通气患者病情演变过程中的重要事件和 ICU 住院期间可能发生的不良事件。在机械通气过程中的任何时候,并发事件或并发症都可能发生:① 需要回到上一步(增加镇静,切换到控制模式等);② 意外或自行拔管(1,2,3,4,5);③ 呼吸机相关性肺炎或新发急性病(1,2,3,4,5);④ SBT 失败(6);⑤ 再插管(6,7);⑥ 拔管后呼吸窘迫(6);⑦ 再入重症监护病房(7);⑧ 气管切开术(1,2,3,4,5);⑨ 死亡(1,2,3,4,5,6,7)

这里没有正确或错误的答案，所有这些关键事件在患者撤离机械通气的过程中都是重要的。国际性观察性 WEAN SAFE 研究（世界范围内对患者脱离辅助通气的评估）将提供 IMV 期间患者日常管理的详细数据，特别是撤机过程中的标记事件（NCT03255109，www.esicm.org/trials-group-2/wean-safe/）。

撤机终止仍然是一个有争议的问题，关于其定义的讨论将在下面的"尝试撤机步骤"中进行探讨。

22.2.2 有简单和复杂的患者吗

不同的撤机方法和挑战取决于患者的类型。虽然每个患者都是一个特定的个体，将其分类为"简单"和"复杂"两个不同的群体，可以帮助确定主要的管理内容和明确的目标。一方面，重症医生不应该延迟"简单患者"的撤机，因为早期成功撤机的机会很高；另一方面，理想情况下，应该要尽早确定"复杂患者"何时可以完成撤机。通常情况下，一个"简单患者"是指年轻的（<65 岁）、既往无明显心脏病或呼吸系统疾病史、由于可快速解决的原因接受机械通气（如中毒性昏迷、手术）的患者。延长这些患者机械通气的时间可能会导致不必要的并发症，如镇静副作用、呼吸机相关性肺炎或自行拔管。在这些患者中，甚至可以在不进行 SBT 的情况下进行拔管，特别是当他们的机械通气持续时间没有超过 24～48 h。相反，复杂患者可能会带来特殊的挑战，ICU 管理的每一步都将影响到撤机的时机和结果。合并严重充血性心力衰竭或慢性阻塞性肺疾病的 ARDS 患者通常属于这类"困难患者"。与其他 ARDS 患者相比，COVID-19 相关 ARDS 患者的 IMV 持续时间更长[8-10]，毫无疑问属于"困难患者"组。然而，没有强有力的证据表明在这群患者中需使用不同方法进行撤机（另见"24 COVID-19 中的有创通气"）。最后，神经功能障碍或创伤性脑损伤患者是一个特殊的群体，由于咳嗽或分泌物清除问题，他们的撤机可能具有挑战性，有时需要气管切开术而不是机械通气本身来保护气道。

22.2.3 疾病急性期

一旦患者插管，负责的团队应该考虑可用的策略以尽可能缩短机械通气的总持续时间、限制呼吸机通气相关并发症。因此，实践指南建议使用旨在尽可能减少镇静的方案，并考虑采用早期活动导向的程序化康复方案[11,12]。采用低潮气量、限制驱动压的控制模式进行肺保护性通气联合适用于大多数低氧血症患者的肌松药和俯卧位，已在世界范围内被广泛采用。然而，这种让患者处于被动状态的方法可能会导致延迟撤机，并导致肌肉的废用。最近，专家们提出了"肺和膈肌"保护性通气的概念：通过监测呼吸肌来保持呼吸做功不过度和最小化人-机不同步，从而平衡 VILI 和呼吸机引起的膈肌功能障碍[13]。肺和膈肌保护性通气的概念是诱人的并合乎逻辑，但尚未证明其益处。目前几个研究正在进行中（NCT 03527797、NCT 03612583、NCT 03646266）。

22.2.4 疾病急性期之后

当最初的急性疾病得到控制时，临床医生应尽可能早（和安全）地使患者脱离呼吸机支持。在此期间,呼吸机通常从辅助控制切换到部分支持模式,允许患者的呼吸努力。几种模式可供选择(PSV、成比例辅助通气、神经调节通气辅助等),已在本书的相关章节中进行了讨论,但 PSV 是全球使用最广泛的模式[5]。没有证据表明哪种模式优于其他模式,但是一旦选择了某种支持模式,医生应该优化通气设置,以提供最低限度的支持,保持患者舒适。这需要每天进行多次评估,有证据表明,由护士、呼吸治疗师甚至是计算机组成的呼吸机管理方案可以加快撤机的准备和 SBT 的成功[14,15]。关于促使 SBT 的撤机准备没有达成共识,但我们建议将以下标准作为合理的先决条件:表现出自主呼吸努力,$FiO_2 \leqslant 0.5$,$PEEP \leqslant 10\ cmH_2O$,$PaO_2/FiO_2 > 200\ mmHg$,未接受升压药或接受低剂量升压药[去甲肾上腺素或等效物低于 $0.2\ \mu g/(kg \cdot min)$]。使用浅快呼吸指数(患者断开呼吸机超过 1 分钟)可有助于识别能够成功完成 SBT 的患者[16]。

在未来,人工智能和机器学习能够整合大量现成的数据,也可能有助于促进撤机进程。

22.3 尝试撤机步骤

22.3.1 挑战与陷阱

当最初的急性症状得到控制,患者的呼吸和血流动力学状态似乎稳定时(参考上述撤机准备标准),通常在拔管前进行 SBT[2,4,5,17]。SBT 是一项挑战在没有任何呼吸机辅助条件下的呼吸能力测试。如果患者通过了 SBT,应该考虑拔管,但成功的 SBT 实际上并不总是伴随着拔管成功[4]。这并不奇怪,因为准备好无需辅助呼吸并不一定意味着准备好拔管,拔管还需要适当的意识水平、咳嗽力量,以及没有声门无法关闭的风险。

观察性研究表明,SBT 在常规治疗中的运用并不一致[4,5]。在上述 WIND 队列中,12% 的患者(没有决定限制/放弃治疗)在没有进行 SBT 的情况下拔管[4]。在最近的一项国际流行病学研究中,28% 的患者没有进行 SBT 而直接拔管[5]。然而,这两种策略(拔管是否执行 SBT)的结果相似[4,5]。因此,SBT 与拔管的相关性是值得怀疑的,特别是对于拔管失败风险较低的患者。首先,SBT 可能产生焦虑、缺氧和呼吸困难,而看护人员很难发现这些问题[18]。第二,观察者之间对 SBT 结果的分歧可能导致错误解读和延迟拔管。第三,通过 SBT 后拔管的患者只有 58%[4]。因此,当预先评估失败的概率较低时(如大多数进入撤机过程的患者),进行 SBT 可能会延迟拔管[19]。SBT 预测拔管成功的敏感性和特异性难以估计。拔管失败率约为 15%,即 SBT 预测拔管成功的特异性为 85%[17]。相比之下,尽管 SBT 失败(即用于确定敏感性的假阴性测试结果),但仍能耐受拔管的患者比例不容易评估,因为 SBT 失败的患者通常不会拔管。然而,在自行拔管的患者中(独立于准备撤机标准),只有 40%~60% 的患者需要再次插管[20]。此外,在一项研究 SBT 失败患者拔管结局的试验中,42% 的患者不需要挽救性无创通气来治疗拔管后呼吸衰竭,只有 37% 的患者再次接受插管[21]。SBT 耐受性的判断依赖于客观标准[2],但也取决于临床医生的技能,错误的决定会对患者产生不利的后果。

22.3.2 哪种自主呼吸试验

SBT 有多种形式,但 T 管或无 PEEP 和 0 cmH$_2$O 压力支持水平的 PSV 似乎最能反映没有辅助的自主呼吸(表 22.2)[22]。这两种测试可能比其他测试更具挑战性和符合"生理要求",然而其并不比拔管本身更符合"要求"[22]。在上面提到的 WIND 研究中,半数 SBT 采用最小压力支持加/不加 PEEP(42%)或 T 管(40%)[4],但在最近的一项国际研究中,初始 SBT 最常使用 PSV+PEEP(49%)或 T 管(25%),较少使用 CPAP(11%)或无 PEEP 的 PSV(9%)[5]。SBT 的方式对患者的预后有影响吗?最新的荟萃分析纳入了 10 项随机临床试验(3 165 例患者),显示 T 管和最小压力支持(有/没有 PEEP)在预测危重症患者成功拔管方面具有相似的作用[22]。最大的随机对照试验(包括在本荟萃分析中)纳入了 1 153 例患者,比较了 30 分钟的 PSV 支持的 SBT 和更具挑战性的 2 小时 T 管 SBT,结果前者显示出更高的拔管成功率(82% vs. 74%),结果有利于最短的测试[19]。这些发现证实 PSV 试验比 T 管试验更容易通过,并可能加速拔管的进程,并且没有增加再次插管的风险。然而,在这项研究中,简单撤机(预先评估成功概率高)的患者比例特别高,从而限制了通用性。没有一个测试是完美的,假阴性或假阳性的风险总是存在的。如前所述,试验的预测值很大程度上取决于预先评估的概率,因此也取决于被测试人群的特征。在第一次或进一步撤机尝试失败的人群中,有必要使用更具挑战性的试验,如使用 T 管(连接或不连接到呼吸机),以避免低估后续失败的风险。同样,在拔管失败风险高的患者中,使用 T 管进行初始 SBT 可以避免不恰当的拔管。然而,这一假设并未在一项多中心研究的事后分析中得到证实[23]。

表 22.2 主要自主呼吸试验类型的特点

	T 管	压力支持	无压力支持,无 PEEP
方法	• 断开呼吸机 • 氧气可以直接输入气管内插管(或气管切开处)	• 患者连接呼吸机 • 低水平压力支持,伴或不伴 PEEP • 有时候单独使用 PEEP	• 患者连接呼吸机 • 没有呼吸机辅助通气
合理性	• 模拟"拔管后"呼吸状况	• 通过呼吸机回路补偿呼吸	• 模拟"拔管后"呼吸状况
优点	• 标准化	• 无需断开呼吸机连接 • 监测呼吸模式	• 标准化 • 监测呼吸模式
缺点	• 没有呼吸模式的监测 • FiO$_2$ 的不确定	• 临床异质性(压力支持和 PEEP 组合,取决于呼吸机品牌)	• 没有临床结果的数据

FiO$_2$,吸入氧气浓度,PEEP,呼气末正压。

22.3.3 自主呼吸试验失败的病理生理学

SBT 失败发生在呼吸能力/负荷不平衡的情况下。慢性阻塞性肺疾病患者因气道阻力导致呼吸做功增加,这就解释了该人群 SBT 高失败率的原因[16]。气道阻力增加导致内源性呼气末正压（PEEPi），特别是在患者出现呼吸急促、呼气时间减少时[16]。图 22.2 显示了可能导致撤机诱发肺水肿的主要生理机制，这是 SBT 失败的常见原因。超声心动图可能是诊断撤机引起的心源性肺水肿的最佳工具[24]。正常的左心室射血分数并不能预防撤机引起的心功能障碍，因为左心室舒张功能在其中起着主要作用[25]。撤机引起的心脏水肿也可以通过测量从血管腔向肺泡和间质滤过的液体来诊断[26]。SBT 期间液体转移导致的血浆容量减少可通过血浆蛋白浓度（或红细胞压积）增加超过 5%～6% 来证实[27]。撤机引起的心功能障碍（和肺水肿）的治疗主要依赖于液体清除和降压药物（而不是正性肌力药物）。胸腔积液引起的肺和（或）胸壁顺应性的改变也可能涉及撤机失败的机制，但这仍然存在争议[28]。

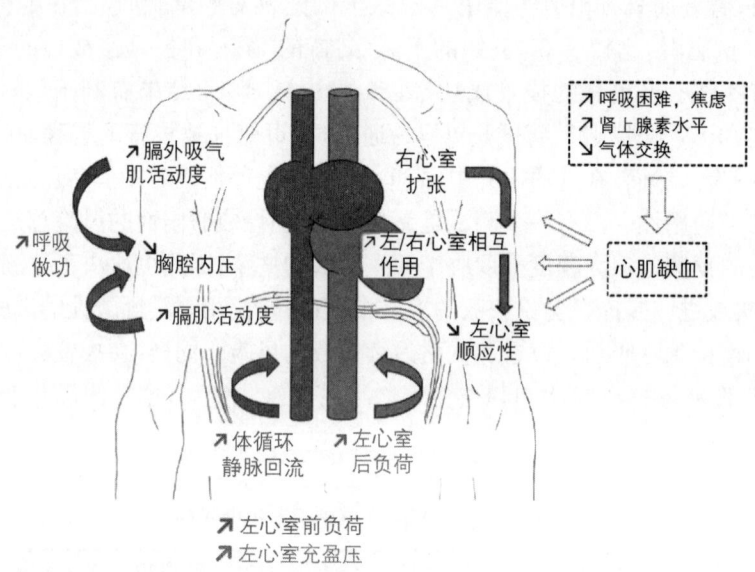

图 22.2　撤机致肺水肿（weaning induced pulmonary oedema，WIPO）的机制。因为心血管和呼吸系统之间的密切相互作用，所有这些机制都可能在慢性阻塞性肺疾病患者中加剧。胸内压降低主要的诱发因素是由机械通气（胸内正压）转为自主呼吸（胸内负压）。静脉回流增加，可能会导致右心室扩张和右/左心室相互作用。胸内压力的降低也会导致左心室后负荷的增加（左心室必须克服胸内压力的下降，才能将血液从胸腔泵出）。此外，还可能发生心肌缺血，使左心室功能恶化。这些机制均可引起 WIPO，导致肺水肿和自主呼吸试验失败。图片来源：Ann. Intensive Care 11, 99 (2021)（见彩色插图）

在呼吸肌力量减弱和（或）呼吸驱动减弱时，呼吸系统的能力会降低。呼吸驱动受损是撤机失败的常见原因，常见于脑卒中、中枢性通气不足和代谢性碱中毒患者。呼吸驱动下降的另一个常见原因是撤机时使用的镇静剂没有（或没完全）中断或者没有被清除，特别是在肾衰竭的情况下。在 SBT 失败的患者中经常能观察到重症相关神经和肌肉病变，同时伴有呼吸肌无力[29]。在撤机时膈肌功能障碍的发生率很高（三分之二的患者），其可能导致撤机失败。尽管如此，部分膈肌功能障碍的患者也通过了 SBT 并成功拔管[29,30]。

因此，在将膈肌功能障碍作为导致撤机失败的主要原因之前，应先排除其他失败原因（特别是撤机诱导的心脏水肿）是至关重要的。

22.4 预防拔管失败

22.4.1 拔管后并发症：流行病学和定义

拔管后呼吸衰竭是计划拔管后最常见的并发症，有25％的患者受到影响[31-33]。尽管其定义尚不明确，但常表现为呼吸频率增加和其他临床症状，如呼吸窘迫、低氧血症或呼吸性酸中毒[31-33]。

45％～80％拔管后呼吸衰竭的患者会再次插管[34]。再次插管的标准存在很大的差异，但与拔管后呼吸衰竭的标准类似：呼吸频率加快、呼吸窘迫的临床表现、低氧血症或呼吸性酸中毒[34]。定义再次插管的时机，尤其是在拔管失败后，也存有争议，从拔管后48小时到7天不等。再次插管不仅导致机械通气时间延长，还增加了25％～50％的病死率[3,20]。考虑到死亡风险的增加，以及拔管1周后重新插管的患者数量较少，大多数研究将拔管失败定义为在拔管后的前7天内需要重新插管[4,33]。

22.4.2 拔管失败的危险因素

气管拔管失败的危险因素在各个患者间存在差异，大多数研究比较预防策略时会根据拔管前的风险水平将患者分层。

与再插管风险增加相关的许多因素已被确定。有些与患者的年龄、肥胖、合并症等特征有关，尤其是潜在的心脏或肺部疾病[20,31]；还有一些与急性疾病有关，如插管原因、累积液体正平衡、呼吸肌功能障碍（使用电磁刺激膈神经、膈肌超声或其替代方案评估）、咳嗽能力弱和分泌物多、ICU获得性虚弱、机械通气时间延长或拔管当天疾病严重程度评分升高有关[20,31]。而其他与SBT本身有关，如一次或多次SBT失败，浅快呼吸指数高，甚至是拔管后才能评估的，如拔管或呼吸困难时出现上呼吸道喘鸣。

然而，考虑全部风险因素可能会导致所有ICU患者被错误地分类为高风险组并采用不恰当的预防拔管失败策略。实用的方法是将具有以下三个特征之一的患者考虑为高风险组：①年龄超过65岁；②有潜在心脏疾病；③慢性呼吸系统疾病。根据最初的观察性队列研究，基于这些易评估的标准，拔管失败高风险患者的再次插管率为28％，而低风险患者的再次插管率为10％[35]。

22.4.3 预防拔管失败的策略

拔管后呼吸衰竭是再次插管的主要原因[36]。因此，预防拔管失败的策略是减少呼吸做功和使气体交换正常化。拔管后有几种氧疗策略，包括标准氧疗、无创通气和经鼻高流量氧疗。

无创机械通气通过一个避免漏气的密封面罩在气道内提供正压通气。呼气时，气道保持正压,增加呼气末肺容积和氧合。在吸气时,额外的压力支持可以减少呼吸频率和呼吸做功。

经鼻高流量氧疗使患者通过鼻导管吸入加热和加湿的空气和氧气混合气体。它可以提供接近100%的高吸入氧浓度,流量可达到60 L/min。在急性低氧性呼吸衰竭患者中,经鼻高流量氧疗增加了呼气末肺容积和氧合,同时降低了呼吸频率和呼吸做功[37]。

22.4.4 预防ICU拔管失败策略有效性的证据总结

比较不同预防再插管策略的临床试验结果汇总在表22.3中。虽然拔管失败高风险的定义不一致,但不同研究的结果是一致的。

在拔管后的所有人群(非特定人群)中,与标准氧疗相比,无创通气和经鼻高流量氧疗均与较低的再插管率无关(分别为14% vs. 9%,10% vs. 13%)。因此,国际临床实践指南不支持在这些患者中使用无创通气来预防拔管失败。

在低拔管失败风险的患者中,与标准氧疗相比,高流量氧疗再次插管率较低(5% vs. 14%)(表22.3)。令人惊讶的是,常规氧疗的对照组再次插管率远高于预期的10%。

在高拔管失败风险的患者中,与常规氧疗和高流量吸氧治疗相比,无创机械通气与较低的再次插管率有关(分别为10% vs. 22%,14% vs. 19%)。唯一一项比较经鼻高流量氧疗与常规氧疗的试验未发现再插管率有任何差异(表22.3)。这些研究使国际临床实践指南对高拔管失败风险的患者推荐使用无创通气来预防拔管失败[58]。

表22.3 比较不同氧合策略预防拔管失败的研究

无创通气 vs. 常规氧疗

第一作者	发表时间	再插管		P
		无创通气组,n(%)	常规氧疗组,n(%)	
未分组				
Su[38]	2012	21/202(10%)	16/204(8%)	NS
Jiang[39]	1999	13/47(28%)	7/46(15%)	NS
总计		34/249(14%)	23/250(9%)	NS
高拔管失败风险				
Nava[40]	2005	4/48(8%)	12/49(24%)	0.03
Ferrer[41]	2006	9/79(11%)	18/83(22%)	NS
Ferrer[42]	2009	6/54(11%)	10/52(19%)	NS
Khilnani[43]	2011	3/20(15%)	5/20(25%)	NS
Mohamed[44]	2013	9/60(15%)	15/60(25%)	0.04

续　表

无创通气 vs. 常规氧疗

		再插管		
Ornico[45]	2013	1/20(5%)	7/18(39%)	0.02
Vargas[46]	2017	6/71(8%)	13/72(18%)	NS
Thanthitaweewat[47]	2018	0/29(0%)	5/29(17%)	NS
	总计	38/381(10%)	85/382(22%)	<0.001

高流量氧疗 vs. 常规氧疗

		再插管		
第一作者	发表时间	高流量氧疗组, n(%)	常规氧疗组, n(%)	P
未分组				
Song[48]	2017	1/30(3%)	3/30(10%)	NS
Matsuda[49]	2020	5/30(17%)	6/39(15%)	NS
	总计	6/60(10%)	9/69(13%)	NS
低拔管失败风险				
Maggiore[50]	2014	2/53(4%)	11/52(21%)	0.005
Hernandez[51]	2016	13/264(5%)	32/263(12%)	0.004
	总计	15/317(5%)	43/315(14%)	<0.001
高拔管失败风险				
Fernandez[52]	2017	9/78(11%)	12/77(16%)	NS

无创通气 vs. 高流量氧疗

		再插管		
第一作者	发表时间	无创通气组, n(%)	高流量氧疗组, n(%)	P
高拔管失败风险				
Hernandez[53]	2016	60/314(19%)	66/290(23%)	NS
Jing[54]	2019	1/20(5%)	2/22(9%)	NS
Thille[55]	2019	41/339(12%)	59/302(20%)	0.02
Theeravit[56]	2020	5/69(7%)	6/71(9%)	NS
Tan[57]	2020	6/42(14%)	6/44(14%)	NS
	总计	113/784(14%)	139/729(19%)	0.02

22.4.5 拔管后呼吸衰竭的治疗

在一项纳入 221 例拔管后呼吸衰竭患者的随机试验中,发现与常规氧疗相比,无创机械通气与较低的再插管率无关(两组均为 48%)[59]。然而,无创机械通气组的病死率高于常规氧疗组(25% *vs.* 14%,$P=0.048$)[59]。这个结果的可能解释为无创机械通气组的患者再次插管前坚持的时间更长(12 小时 *vs.* 2.5 小时,$P=0.02$)[59]。在另一项随机试验中,对 81 例拔管后呼吸衰竭患者进行无创通气与常规氧疗的比较,没有发现这种损害[60]。此外,一项纳入 146 例拔管后呼吸衰竭患者的随机试验事后分析表明,与经鼻高流量氧疗相比,无创机械通气无害,甚至对高碳酸血症亚组的患者有利[34]。

因此,虽然国际临床实践指南不推荐在未经选择的患者中使用无创通气治疗拔管后的呼吸衰竭[58],但特定的亚组人群可能受益于这种技术。拔管后呼吸衰竭的治疗问题尚未解决。

22.5 总结

撤机阶段,作为机械通气总持续时间的重要部分,也是有关预后的关键时期。应尽早识别出"简单患者"并对其拔管(有时不需要 SBT),以避免延迟撤机导致的不良事件。对于"复杂患者",应在插管后立即实施有利于撤机的策略,并在整个机械通气过程中进行优化。

在不同的阶段使用的机械通气模式都可能会影响撤机,但没有证据表明某种模式比其他模式更优越。当满足撤机准备标准时,SBT 可以帮助预测拔管结果,但最合适的 SBT 类型仍有争议。最后,无创机械通气或湿化高流量氧疗可预防特定亚组患者的拔管失败。

尽管对所有接受机械通气的患者至关重要,但撤机过程尚未被完全了解。未来的共识和对撤机过程中每个步骤的研究可能会更好地阐明撤机进程,并为所有这些未解决的问题提供答案。

(邓会标,计恩东 译)

参考文献

[1] Piscitello GM, Kapania EM, Miller WD, Rojas JC, Siegler M, Parker WF. Variation in ventilator allocation guidelines by US State during the coronavirus disease 2019 pandemic: a systematic review. JAMA Netw Open. 2020;3(6):e2012606.

[2] Boles J-M, Bion J, Connors A, Herridge M, Marsh B, Melot C, et al. Weaning from mechanical ventilation. Eur Respir J. 2007;29(5):1033-56.

[3] Peñuelas O, Frutos-Vivar F, Fernández C, Anzueto A, Epstein SK, Apezteguía C, et al. Characteristics and outcomes of ventilated patients according to time to liberation from mechanical ventilation. Am J Respir Crit Care Med. 2011;184(4):430-7.

[4] Béduneau G, Pham T, Schortgen F, Piquilloud L, Zogheib E, Jonas M, et al. Epidemiology of weaning outcome according to a new definition. The WIND Study. Am J Respir Crit Care Med. 2017; 195(6): 772-83.

[5] Burns KEA, Rizvi L, Cook DJ, Lebovic G, Dodek P, Villar J, et al. Ventilator weaning and discontinuation practices for critically ill patients. JAMA. 2021; 325(12): 1173-84.

[6] Jeong B-H, Lee KY, Nam J, Ko MG, Na SJ, Suh GY, et al. Validation of a new WIND classification compared to ICC classification for weaning outcome. Ann Intensive Care. 2018; 8(1): 115.

[7] ARDS Definition Task Force, Ranieri VM, Rubenfeld GD, Thompson BT, Ferguson ND, Caldwell E, et al. Acute respiratory distress syndrome: the Berlin Definition. J Am Med Assoc. 2012; 307(23): 2526-33.

[8] COVID-ICU Group on behalf of the REVA Network and the COVID-ICU Investigators. Clinical characteristics and day-90 outcomes of 4244 critically ill adults with COVID-19: a prospective cohort study. Intensive Care Med. 2021; 47(1): 60-73.

[9] Grasselli G, Zangrillo A, Zanella A, Antonelli M, Cabrini L, Castelli A, et al. Baseline characteristics and outcomes of 1591 patients infected with SARS-CoV-2 admitted to ICUs of the Lombardy Region, Italy. JAMA. 2020; 323(16): 1574-81.

[10] Bellani G, Laffey JG, Pham T, Fan E, Brochard L, Esteban A, et al. Epidemiology, patterns of care, and mortality for patients with acute respiratory distress syndrome in intensive care units in 50 countries. JAMA. 2016; 315(8): 788-800.

[11] Fan E, Zakhary B, Amaral A, McCannon J, Girard TD, Morris PE, et al. Liberation from mechanical ventilation in critically ill adults. An official ATS/ACCP Clinical Practice guideline. Ann Am Thorac Soc. 2017; 14(3): 441-3.

[12] Aitken LM, Bucknall T, Kent B, Mitchell M, Burmeister E, Keogh SJ. Protocol-directed sedation versus non-protocol-directed sedation in mechanically ventilated intensive care adults and children. Cochrane Database Syst Rev. 2018; (11): CD009771.

[13] Goligher EC, Jonkman AH, Dianti J, Vaporidi K, Beitler JR, Patel BK, et al. Clinical strategies for implementing lung and diaphragm-protective ventilation: avoiding insufficient and excessive effort. Intensive Care Med. 2020; 46(12): 2314-26.

[14] Blackwood B, Burns KEA, Cardwell CR, O'Halloran P. Protocolized versus non-protocolized weaning for reducing the duration of mechanical ventilation in critically ill adult patients. Cochrane Database Syst Rev. 2014; (11): CD006904.

[15] Rose L, Schultz MJ, Cardwell CR, Jouvet P, McAuley DF, Blackwood B. Automated versus non-automated weaning for reducing the duration of mechanical ventilation for critically ill adults and children: a cochrane systematic review and meta-analysis. Crit Care Lond Engl. 2015; 19: 48.

[16] Jubran A, Tobin MJ. Pathophysiologic basis of acute respiratory distress in patients who fail a trial of weaning from mechanical ventilation. Am J Respir Crit Care Med. 1997; 155(3): 906-15.

[17] Thille AW, Richard J-CM, Brochard L. The decision to extubate in the intensive care unit. Am J Respir Crit Care Med. 2013; 187(12): 1294-302.

[18] Decavèle M, Similowski T, Demoule A. Detection and management of dyspnea in mechanically ventilated patients. Curr Opin Crit Care. 2019; 25(1): 86-94.

[19] Subirà C, Hernández G, Vázquez A, Rodríguez-García R, González-Castro A, García C, et al.

Effect of pressure support vs T-piece ventilation strategies during spontaneous breathing trials on successful extubation among patients receiving mechanical ventilation: a randomized clinical trial. JAMA. 2019; 321(22): 2175-82.

[20] Thille AW, Harrois A, Schortgen F, Brun-Buisson C, Brochard L. Outcomes of extubation failure in medical intensive care unit patients. Crit Care Med. 2011; 39(12): 2612-8.

[21] Girault C, Bubenheim M, Abroug F, Diehl JL, Elatrous S, Beuret P, et al. Noninvasive ventilation and weaning in patients with chronic hypercapnic respiratory failure: a randomized multicenter trial. Am J Respir Crit Care Med. 2011; 184(6): 672-9.

[22] Sklar MC, Burns K, Rittayamai N, Lanys A, Rauseo M, Chen L, et al. Effort to breathe with various spontaneous breathing trial techniques. A physiologic meta-analysis. Am J Respir Crit Care Med. 2017; 195(11): 1477-85.

[23] Thille AW, Coudroy R, Nay M-A, Gacouin A, Demoule A, Sonneville R, et al. Pressure-support ventilation vs T-piece during spontaneous breathing trials before extubation among patients at high risk of extubation failure: a post-hoc analysis of a clinical trial. Chest. 2020; 158(4): 1446-55.

[24] Caille V, Amiel J-B, Charron C, Belliard G, Vieillard-Baron A, Vignon P. Echocardiography: a help in the weaning process. Crit Care Lond Engl. 2010; 14(3): R120.

[25] Papanikolaou J, Makris D, Saranteas T, Karakitsos D, Zintzaras E, Karabinis A, et al. New insights into weaning from mechanical ventilation: left ventricular diastolic dysfunction is a key player. Intensive Care Med. 2011; 37: 1976.

[26] Teboul J-L, Monnet X, Richard C. Weaning failure of cardiac origin: recent advances. Crit Care Lond Engl. 2010; 14(2): 211.

[27] Dres M, Teboul J-L, Anguel N, Guerin L, Richard C, Monnet X. Extravascular lung water, B-type natriuretic peptide, and blood volume contraction enable diagnosis of weaning-induced pulmonary edema. Crit Care Med. 2014; 42(8): 1882-9.

[28] Dres M, Roux D, Pham T, Beurton A, Ricard J-D, Fartoukh M, et al. Prevalence and impact on weaning of pleural effusion at the time of liberation from mechanical ventilation: a multicenter prospective observational study. Anesthesiology. 2017; 126(6): 1107-15.

[29] Dres M, Dubé B-P, Mayaux J, Delemazure J, Reuter D, Brochard L, et al. Coexistence and impact of limb muscle and diaphragm weakness at time of liberation from mechanical ventilation in medical intensive care unit patients. Am J Respir Crit Care Med. 2017; 195(1): 57-66.

[30] Vivier E, Muller M, Putegnat J-B, Steyer J, Barrau S, Boissier F, et al. Inability of diaphragm ultrasound to predict extubation failure: a multicenter study. Chest. 2019; 155(6): 1131-9.

[31] Hernandez G, Vaquero C, Colinas L, Cuena R, Gonzalez P, Canabal A, et al. Effect of postextubation high-flow nasal cannula vs noninvasive ventilation on reintubation and postextubation respiratory failure in high-risk patients: a randomized clinical trial. JAMA. 2016; 316(15): 1565-74.

[32] Hernández G, Vaquero C, González P, Subira C, Frutos-Vivar F, Rialp G, et al. Effect of postextubation high-flow nasal cannula vs conventional oxygen therapy on reintubation in low-risk patients: a randomized clinical trial. JAMA. 2016; 315(13): 1354.

[33] Thille A, Muller G, Gacouin A, Coudroy R, Decavèle M, Sonneville R, et al. Effect of postextubation high-flow nasal oxygen with noninvasive ventilation vs high-flow nasal oxygen alone on reintubation among patients at high risk of extubation failure: a randomized clinical trial. JAMA. 2019; 322: 1465-75.

[34] Thille AW, Monseau G, Coudroy R, Nay M-A, Gacouin A, Decavèle M, et al. Non-invasive ventilation versus high-flow nasal oxygen for postextubation respiratory failure in ICU: a posthoc analysis of a randomized clinical trial. Crit Care. 2021; 25(1): 221.

[35] Thille AW, Harrois A, Schortgen F, Brun-Buisson C, Brochard L. Outcomes of extubation failure in medical intensive care unit patients. Crit Care Med. 2011; 39(12): 2612-8.

[36] Epstein SK, Ciubotaru RL. Independent effects of etiology of failure and time to reintubation on outcome for patients failing extubation. Am J Respir Crit Care Med. 1998; 158(2): 489-93.

[37] Mauri T, Turrini C, Eronia N, Grasselli G, Volta CA, Bellani G, et al. Physiologic effects of high-flow nasal cannula in acute hypoxemic respiratory failure. Am J Respir Crit Care Med. 2017; 195(9): 1207-15.

[38] Su C-L, Chiang L-L, Yang S-H, Lin H-I, Cheng K-C, Huang Y-CT, et al. Preventive use of noninvasive ventilation after extubation: a prospective, multicenter randomized controlled trial. Respir Care. 2012 Feb; 57(2): 204-10.

[39] Jiang J-S, Kao S-J, Wang S-N. Effect of early application of biphasic positive airway pressure on the outcome of extubation in ventilator weaning. Respirology. 1999 Jun; 4(2): 161-5.

[40] Nava S, Gregoretti C, Fanfulla F, Squadrone E, Grassi M, Carlucci A, et al. Noninvasive ventilation to prevent respiratory failure after extubation in high-risk patients*: Crit Care Med. 2005 Nov; 33(11): 2465-70.

[41] Ferrer M, Valencia M, Nicolas JM, Bernadich O, Badia JR, Torres A. Early Noninvasive Ventilation Averts Extubation Failure in Patients at Risk: A Randomized Trial. Am J Respir Crit Care Med. 2006 Jan 15; 173(2): 164-70.

[42] Ferrer M, Sellarés J, Valencia M, Carrillo A, Gonzalez G, Badia JR, et al. Non-invasive ventilation after extubation in hypercapnic patients with chronic respiratory disorders: randomised controlled trial. The Lancet. 2009 Sep; 374(9695): 1082-8.

[43] Khilnani GC, Galle AD, Hadda V, Sharma SK. Non-invasive ventilation after extubation in patients with chronic obstructive airways disease: a randomised controlled trial. Anaesth Intensive Care. 2011 Mar; 39(2): 217-23.

[44] Mohamed KAE, Abdalla MH. Role of non invasive ventilation in limiting re-intubation after planned extubation. Egypt J Chest Dis Tuberc. 2013 Oct; 62(4): 669-74.

[45] Ornico SR, Lobo SM, Sanches HS, Deberaldini M, Tofoli LT, Vidal AM, et al. Noninvasive ventilation immediately after extubation improves weaning outcome after acute respiratory failure: a randomized controlled trial. Crit Care Lond Engl. 2013 Mar 4; 17(2): R39.

[46] Vargas F., Clavel M., Sanchez-Verlan P., Garnier S., Boyer A., Bui H.-N., et al. Intermittent noninvasive ventilation after extubation in patients with chronic respiratory disorders: a multicenter randomized controlled trial (VHYPER). Intensive Care Med. 2017; 43(11): 1626-36.

[47] Thanthitaweewat V. Targeted-Volume Noninvasive Ventilation Reduces Extubation Failure in Postextubated Medical Intensive Care Unit Patients: A Randomized Controlled Trial. Indian J Crit Care Med. 2018 Sep; 22(9): 639-45.

[48] Song H, Gu J, Xiu H, Cui W, Zhang G. The value of high-flow nasal cannula oxygen therapy after extubation in patients with acute respiratory failure. Clinics. 2017 Sep 10; 72(09): 562-7.

[49] Matsuda W, Hagiwara A, Uemura T, Sato T, Kobayashi K, Sasaki R, et al. High-Flow Nasal Cannula May Not Reduce the Re-Intubation Rate Compared With a Large-Volume Nebulization-Based Humidifier. Respir Care. 2020 May; 65(5): 610-7.

[50] Maggiore SM, Idone FA, Vaschetto R, Festa R, Cataldo A, Antonicelli F, et al. Nasal High-Flow versus Venturi Mask Oxygen Therapy after Extubation. Effects on Oxygenation, Comfort, and Clinical Outcome. Am J Respir Crit Care Med. 2014 Aug; 190(3): 282-8.

[51] Hernández G, Vaquero C, González P, Subira C, Frutos-Vivar F, Rialp G, et al. Effect of Postextubation High-Flow Nasal Cannula vs Conventional Oxygen Therapy on Reintubation in Low-Risk Patients: A Randomized Clinical Trial. JAMA. 2016 Apr 5; 315(13): 1354.

[52] Fernandez R, Subira C, Frutos-Vivar F, Rialp G, Laborda C, Masclans JR, et al. High-flow nasal cannula to prevent postextubation respiratory failure in high-risk non-hypercapnic patients: a randomized multicenter trial. Ann Intensive Care. 2017 Dec; 7(1): 47.

[53] Hernandez G, Vaquero C, Colinas L, Cuena R, Gonzalez P, Canabal A, et al. Effect of Postextubation High-Flow Nasal Cannula vs Noninvasive Ventilation on Reintubation and Postextubation Respiratory Failure in High-Risk Patients: A Randomized Clinical Trial. JAMA. 2016 Oct 18; 316(15): 1565-74.

[54] Jing G, Li J, Hao D, Wang T, Sun Y, Tian H, et al. Comparison of high flow nasal cannula with noninvasive ventilation in chronic obstructive pulmonary disease patients with hypercapnia in preventing postextubation respiratory failure: A pilot randomized controlled trial. Res Nurs Health. 2019 Jun; 42(3): 217-25.

[55] Thille A, Muller G, Gacouin A, Coudroy R, Decavèle M, Sonneville R, et al. Effect of Postextubation High-Flow Nasal Oxygen With Noninvasive Ventilation vs High-Flow Nasal Oxygen Alone on Reintubation Among Patients at High Risk of Extubation Failure: A Randomized Clinical Trial. JAMA. 2019; 322: 1465-75.

[56] Theerawit P, Natpobsuk N, Petnak T, Sutherasan Y. The efficacy of the WhisperFlow CPAP system versus high flow nasal cannula in patients at risk for postextubation failure: A Randomized controlled trial. J Crit Care. 2021 Jun; 63: 117-23.

[57] Tan D, Walline JH, Ling B, Xu Y, Sun J, Wang B, et al. High-flow nasal cannula oxygen therapy versus non-invasive ventilation for chronic obstructive pulmonary disease patients after extubation: a multicenter, randomized controlled trial. Crit Care. 2020 Dec; 24(1): 489.

[58] Rochwerg B, Brochard L, Elliott MW, Hess D, Hill NS, Nava S, et al. Official ERS/ATS clinical practice guidelines: noninvasive ventilation for acute respiratory failure. Eur Respir J. 2017; 50(2): 1602426.

[59] Esteban A, Frutos-Vivar F, Ferguson ND, Arabi Y, Apezteguía C, González M, et al. Noninvasive positive-pressure ventilation for respiratory failure after extubation. N Engl J Med. 2004; 350(24): 2452-60.

[60] Keenan SP, Powers C, McCormack DG, Block G. Noninvasive positive-pressure ventilation for postextubation respiratory distress: a randomized controlled trial. JAMA. 2002; 287(24): 3238-44.

23 COVID-19相关呼吸衰竭的无创氧疗策略

Non-invasive Oxygenation Strategies for COVID-19 Related Respiratory Failure

Michael C. Sklar, Bhakti K. Patel, Laveena Munshi

23.1 引言

2020年3月11日,世界卫生组织(World Health Organization,WHO)宣布COVID-19暴发为全球大流行[1]。从那时起,成千上万的COVID-19患者因严重的急性呼吸衰竭需要收治于ICU。患者的激增使许多地区不堪重负,特别是在危重症患者数量开始超过有限的重症监护资源的时候。在这一危机时期,分诊方案、无创支持策略和医院病房患者的干预措施被紧急制定出来。其中一项策略是使用无创的给氧设备,如经鼻高流量给氧导管、无创通气面罩和头罩。最初,一些医疗中心对使用无创设备感到担忧,因为其对患者和医护人员的安全性(气溶胶)或疗效不确定。然而,在呼吸机数量有限的情况下,必须采

M. C. Sklar
Interdepartmental Division of Critical Care Medicine, University of Toronto, Toronto, ON, Canada

Department of Anesthesia and Pain Medicine, St. Michael's Hospital, Unity Health Toronto and University of Toronto, Toronto, ON, Canada

B. K. Patel
Section of Pulmonary and Critical Care, Department of Medicine, University of Chicago, Chicago, IL, USA

L. Munshi (✉)
Interdepartmental Division of Critical Care Medicine, University of Toronto, Toronto, ON, Canada

Department of Medicine, Sinai Health System and University Health Network, Toronto, ON, Canada

Institute of Health Policy, Management, and Evaluation, Dalla Lana School of Public Health, University of Toronto, Toronto, ON, Canada
e-mail: Laveena.munshi@sinaihealth.ca

© The Author(s), under exclusive license to Springer Nature Switzerland AG 2022
G. Bellani (ed.), *Mechanical Ventilation from Pathophysiology to Clinical Evidence*, https://doi.org/10.1007/978-3-030-93401-9_23

用这些无创设备以应对有限的条件。这些无创氧疗策略减少COVID-19患者所需呼吸机的潜力启发了许多研究。在第10章和第9章分别阐述了高流量氧疗和无创正压通气的应用。在本章中,我们将概述在全球呼吸疾病大流行期间使用这些设备的特殊注意事项,并评估了它们应对COVID-19导致的呼吸衰竭的有效性。

23.2 无创氧疗策略:设备、生理学和非COVID-19证据

23.2.1 设备和生理学

无创氧合策略可以通过传统无创通气(non-invasive ventilation,NIV)连接面罩、NIV连接头罩或高流量鼻导管实施。每种技术都有独特的生理考量和重要的优、缺点,必须理解才能提供安全、有效和个性化的治疗(表23.1)。将合适的患者和临床状况与无创氧疗策略相匹配是获取最佳疗效的必要条件。

表 23.1 常见无创氧疗设备的优缺点

设备	优点	缺点
面罩无创通气	• 提供压力支持改善肺泡通气 • 提供 PEEP 改善氧合 • 可通过降低前、后负荷来改善心功能 • 可监测最大潮气量	• 可能产生气溶胶 • 皮肤溃烂的风险 • 漏气限制了更高的 PEEP 水平 • 不能耐受长时间的治疗 • 高潮气量或自戕性肺损伤的风险 • 转运存在挑战
头罩无创通气	• 提供压力支持改善肺泡通气 • 比面罩 NIV 提供更高的 PEEP 改善氧合 • 可以耐受更长的治疗时间	• 无法监测潮气量 • 发生气道紧急情况时,需要较长时间移除设备 • 在许多机构不如面罩 NIV 熟练 • 转运困难
高流量氧疗仪	• 舒适和耐受性好 • 提供加热和加湿的氧气 • 增强黏膜纤毛清除能力 • 产生低水平的 PEEP • 减少室内空气混入 • 生理无效腔冲刷效应 • 呼吸做功减少	• 可能产生气溶胶 • 转运存在挑战 • 可产生的 PEEP 最小 • 高流量可能会让人不舒服 • 可能无法耐受加热湿化

NIV,无创机械通气;PEEP,呼气末正压。

23.2.1.1 高流量鼻导管

HFNO通过专门的鼻导管接口提供高流量湿化氧气。该装置与一个空气-氧气混合器连接,允许独立设定吸入氧浓度(FiO_2)和流量[2]。该系统允许输送的气流量高达60 L/min(有些设备允许更高的流量),提供的 FiO_2 可达到100%。这些流量具有能匹配

严重呼吸困难患者流量需求的优点,从而防止吸气时空气混入稀释输送的氧气[3]。HFNO 的其他生理学益处包括生理无效腔冲刷效应、降低呼吸做功和改善呼气末肺容积,因此可能会降低肺和膈肌损伤的风险[3,4]。此外,气体湿化能提高黏膜纤毛清除分泌物的能力,防止冷空气引起的支气管痉挛。关于 HFNO 的更多内容,请参阅第 10 章。

23.2.1.2 无创通气

在急性呼吸衰竭的患者中,NIV 常通过全口鼻面罩来实施。近年来,其他的 NIV 接口(包括头罩装置)的应用也受到关注[5]。NIV 是通过双水平气道正压通气,包括吸气相气道正压(inspiratory positive airway pressure,IPAP)和呼气相气道正压(expiratory positive airway pressure,PAP),类似于 PEEP[6]。在生理上,NIV 增加气道压力,改善动脉氧合,增加呼气末肺容量,减少肺内分流和呼气时膈肌的负荷。NIV 也可能通过减少左心室后负荷和左、右心室前负荷来改善心脏功能[6,7]。通过头罩接口给予的 NIV 具有与面罩 NIV 相似的生理学效益,但具有通过颈部密封项圈可以最大限度地减少漏气的优势。这可能产生更有效的肺通气和增强 PEEP 的设置。此外,头罩 NIV 患者耐受性更好,可允许更长的 NIV 治疗时间。有关 NIV 的更多内容,请参阅第 9 章。

23.2.1.3 新发急性呼吸衰竭无创氧疗策略的证据

新发急性呼吸衰竭的最佳无创氧疗策略尚不清楚。其中,部分原因可能是呼吸衰竭的异质性和对其亚表型的认识日益增加[8]。在临床实践中,根据呼吸衰竭的原因、疾病的严重程度和病程,不同的无创治疗方式可能会有不同的治疗反应。

FLORALI 研究发表后,HFNO 的使用迅速增加[9]。这项随机对照试验比较了 313 例呼吸衰竭患者使用标准面罩氧疗、面罩 NIV 与 HFNO 氧疗的治疗效果。结果表明与其他治疗方式相比,使用 HFNO 可显著降低 90 天病死率。标准氧疗与 HFNO 组患者 90 天死亡的风险比为 2.01[95% 置信区间(confidence interval,CI)为 1.01~3.99,$P=0.046$],NIV 与 HFNO 组 90 天死亡的风险比为 2.50(95% CI 为 1.31~4.78,$P=0.006$)。与 HFNO 相比,接受 NIV 的患者病死率更高理论上可能与 NIV 的大潮气量有关。

最近的一项网络荟萃分析比较了所有无创氧疗模式,发现与常规氧疗模式相比,面罩 NIV 显著降低了气管插管率和病死率($RR=0.76$,95%CI 为 0.62~0.90;$RR=0.83$,95%CI 为 0.68~0.99)[10]。然而,在更严重的呼吸衰竭患者中(平均 $PaO_2/FiO_2<200$),面罩 NIV 不再有在病死率上的优势。在同一网络荟萃分析中,发现与常规氧疗相比,头罩 NIV 也与较低的插管风险($RR=0.26$,95%CI 为 0.14~0.45)和病死率($RR=0.40$,95%CI 为 0.24~0.63)相关[10]。有趣的是,与其他模式(HFNO 和面罩 NIV)相比,头罩 NIV 组的病死率和插管率有所下降,但是该分析结果受限于研究过少。

23.3 COVID-19 大流行期间无创氧疗策略的注意事项

COVID-19 大流行的加剧和带来的患者数量激增突显了对于无创氧疗策略在疫情中角色的重要考量。那些因大量患者而不堪重负的医疗中心希望这些设备具有节省呼吸机的潜力。相反,没有该问题的医疗中心对此持谨慎态度,因为关于"早期插管"受益的一些报告,以及对气溶胶风险的不确定性。一旦明确COVID-19相关呼吸衰竭应该采用与大流行前相同的原则进行管理(即没有"早期插管"的标准),各医疗中心立即开始评估无创氧疗设备的安全性、可行性和有效性。在本节和表23.2中强调了在大流行期间使用无创氧疗设备的特殊考量。

表23.2 在呼吸疾病大流行期间使用无创氧疗策略的特殊考虑

了解医院氧气供应情况:确定可同时使用HFNO设备的最大数量
制定关于如何在非传统ICU环境中管理危重症患者的流程
需要培训更多的工作人员在这些非传统场所参与管理危重症患者(即术后康复医护人员)
为管理使用无创氧疗设备患者的医护人员强化个人防护设备
根据正在使用的装置,注意病毒颗粒气溶胶的风险。根据病毒的特性和设备的影响采取适当的保护措施(如N95,必要时使用负压病房)
制定关于如何转运需要无创氧疗支持的危重症患者的方案(如过渡到Tavish面罩,使用医用口罩遮挡设备)

23.3.1 重症监护室外重症患者的管理

通常情况下,无创氧疗设备主要用于ICU中。然而,由于大流行期间重症监护资源有限,导致许多医院制定了在ICU外使用无创氧疗设备的策略。

在普通病房,越来越多地使用HFNO治疗COVID-19重症肺炎[11]。需要考虑两个重要的因素包括:① 医院有足够的氧气供应;② 准确地识别HFNO治疗失败的高风险患者。鉴于HFNO所需的高流量,有报道称,大量使用该设备时,医院的氧气会很快耗尽。当务之急是医院领导与医院工程师一起提前确定在呼吸疾病大流行期间可以同时运行设备的最大数量。

在理想的环境下,HFNO患者应在密切监测的环境中接受治疗。尽管有HFNO,但意外断开或进行性缺氧可能导致严重而快速的血氧饱和度下降。然而,由于资源有限,在ICU环境下管理HFNO并不总是可行的。在疫情大流行期间采取的策略有:① 设置HFNO专用病房,用于不插管的患者;② 设置专用HFNO加护病房,在这里护理/呼吸治疗的占比高于普通病房,但低于ICU;③ 将低风险患者送入普通病房,持续进行脉搏血氧测量和视频监控;④ 根据连续测量的流速、氧气、PaO_2/FiO_2 或独立评分系统制定收住ICU的阈值。准确评估HFNO失败风险以识别可能迫切需要接受有创机械通气的患者至关重要。在COVID-19之前,ROX指数[定义为脉搏氧饱和度/吸入氧浓度(SpO_2/FiO_2)与呼吸频率(RR)的比值]被设计用来识别有HFNO失败风险的患者[12]。在COVID-19之前,12小时ROX指数<4.88被认为与HFNO高失败风险有关。最近,在120例接受HFNO治疗的COVID-19肺炎患者的试验中,对ROX指数进行了评价[13],12 h ROX指数<5.99的阈值与HFNO失败高风险相关(特异性96%,敏感性62%)。对164例HFNO支持的COVID-19肺炎患者进行回顾性分析,应用ROX指数(使用传

统的截断值)预测 HFNO 成功,其敏感性为 85%[14]。NIV 的应用应限于可密切监测单位(ICU 或高依赖单位),以满足滴定 NIV 治疗、治疗失败的识别和插管的专业需求。

23.3.2 气溶胶的风险

自大流行以来,人们对 HFNO 和 NIV 产生气溶胶的风险非常关注。已经有几个模拟研究来确定这些设备的气溶胶风险。在一项模拟研究中,有 8 名健康志愿者被安置在急诊科的房间里,这些房间采用正压通气,每 10 分钟换气一次[15]。受试者戴上无重复呼吸面罩、高流量鼻导管(15 L/min、30 L/min 和 60 L/min)和 CPAP 面罩(10 cmH$_2$O)。在无重复呼吸面罩和高流量鼻导管在受试者中可以使用或不使用外科口罩。研究人员发现,与使用 CPAP 和无重复呼吸面罩相比,高流量鼻导管流速的增加与气溶胶产生的显著增加有关。然而,正如其他研究小组所描述的那样,当受试者戴上外科口罩时,能减少 HFNO 产生的气溶胶[16]。在一项 ICU 模拟研究中,研究人员测量了使用有创通气(通过带气囊的气管内插管与呼吸机连接)、头罩 NIV、面罩 NIV、无重复呼吸面罩、HFNO 和鼻导管的病房中不同位置的颗粒计数[17]。密闭系统通气,即有创机械通气和头罩 NIV,与最低的气溶胶计数相关;而 HFNO 和鼻导管通气与最高气溶胶计数相关。然而,在一项对负压病房中 COVID-19 患者的研究发现(常规氧疗组 $n=7$,HFNO 组 $n=10$),与常规氧疗相比,HFNO 并未增加气溶胶风险[18]。

虽然有关于气溶胶风险的数据存在矛盾,但是在管理 COVID-19 患者时,医护人员应谨慎并遵循当地医院指南。在许多机构,建议医护人员在管理这些患者时穿上防护服,戴上手套、N95 口罩和面屏。有些人还建议使用负压病房,但是这在各机构之间并不一致。对 HFNO 患者使用外科口罩可能会进一步减少病毒传播。在未来的大流行中,气溶胶的风险可能会根据病原体的生物特征而改变,因此建议的安全预防措施必须与当时的证据相匹配。

23.3.3 院内转运

因入住 ICU 或诊断/治疗的目的,患者可能经常需要在医院内转运。转运依赖 HFNO 或 NIV 的 COVID-19 患者是一项特殊挑战,需要考虑到 COVID-19 的独特因素。许多传统的 HFNO 设备依赖于电源,没有电池供电的选项。然而,新的转运呼吸机有能力提供高流量和氧气用于转运。一般转运经 HFNO 通气的患者时需要考虑重要的因素包括:① 确保充足的氧气供应;② 确保呼吸机在转运期间有足够的电量供应。大流行期间的其他考虑因素包括 COVID-19 气溶胶扩散的潜在风险。许多治疗组会首先评估是否可以在不需要 HFNO 的情况下成功转运(即在转运之前试用 Tavish 口罩一段时间)[19]。或者,一些机构在转运使用高流量鼻导管的患者时应用外科口罩,以尽量减少任何潜在的气溶胶风险,而转运团队则穿戴全套个人防护装备,包括 N95 口罩。

23.3.4 无创氧疗支持在 COVID-19 中的证据

与非 COVID-19 呼吸衰竭相似,对于 COVID-19 患者来说,最佳的无创氧疗支持仍然是一个问题。最近的一项随机对照试验比较了 ICU 中头罩 NIV 和 HFNO 在 COVID-19 患者中的应用。研究者评估了早期使用头罩 NIV 是否增加了 28 天内无呼吸支持（HFNO、NIV 或有创通气）的天数[20]。在 110 名患者（每组 55 名）中，无呼吸支持天数没有差异[头罩 NIV 组的 20 天（四分位距为 0～25 天）vs. HFNO 组的 18 天（四分位距 0～22 天）；平均差 2 天，95% CI 为 −2～6 天，$P=0.26$]。有趣的是，在统计学上，头罩 NIV 组的 28 天气管插管率和无有创机械通气天数更占优势。头罩 NIV 组气管插管率为 30%，而 HFNO 组为 51%[−21%（95%CI 为 −38%～−3%）；$P=0.03$]。头罩 NIV 组与 HFNO 组 28 天内无有创机械通气天数的中位数分别为 28 天（IQR 13～28 天）和 25 天（IQR 4～28 天），平均差 3 天，95%CI 为 0～7 天，$P=0.04$。这是第一次直接比较头罩 NIV 和 HFNO 的研究。它表明头罩 NIV 可以减少气管插管的需求，但需要进一步的研究来证实这一次要结果。

RECOVERY-RS 研究进一步支持了提供正压的无创策略，该试验目前还处于预发表阶段[21]。在这项适应性随机对照试验中，1 272 例患者被随机分为 HFNO、面罩 CPAP 或常规氧疗 3 组。主要结局是气管内插管或入组后 30 天内病死率的复合结局。与常规氧疗相比，CPAP（平均值为 10 cmH_2O）显著降低病死率或插管率（未校正的 $OR=0.72$，95%CI 为 0.53～0.96，$P=0.03$），而 HFNO 组与氧疗组相比无显著差异（未校正的 $OR=0.97$，95%CI 为 0.73～1.29，$P=0.85$）。

23.3.5 患者体位

根据强有力的生理和临床证据，俯卧位是中重度急性呼吸窘迫综合征有创通气患者的标准治疗体位[22,23]。有研究报道，在大流行的早期，采用清醒非插管俯卧位治疗方案是成功的。这启发了一系列评估普通病房中轻度低氧患者及 ICU 内中度低氧患者俯卧位治疗的随机研究。一项 1 126 例需要 HFNO 的临床试验评估俯卧位治疗能否改善治疗失败（定义为 28 天内插管或病死）[24]，本试验关注的主要终点为死亡或 28 天内插管。564 例采用清醒俯卧位和 HFNO 的患者中有 223 例（40%）出现治疗失败（主要是因为插管），557 例采用 HFNO 标准治疗的患者中有 257 例（46%）出现治疗失败（$RR=0.86$，95% CI 为 0.75～0.98）。当患者从仰卧位转变到俯卧位时，生理指标（如呼吸频率、ROX 指数和氧合指数）都有所改善。重要的是，两组的不良事件发生率没有差异。更多研究正在评估可行的俯卧位和插管的阈值。没有研究直接将头罩 NIV 和 HFNO 进行比较。然而，应该注意的是，在之前的头罩研究中，60% 的 HFNO 组患者采用了俯卧位治疗，而头罩 NIV 组采用了仰卧位[20]。

23.4 总结

COVID-19 大流行给全球医疗卫生系统带来了前所未有的挑战。通过面罩或头罩的 NIV 和 HFNO 均有生理学和临床证据的支持。治疗必须以一种既对患者有效又优先考虑医疗人员安全的方式提供。在未来的大流行期间采用这些设备时，需要重点考虑设备使用地点、气溶胶和转运问题。

(邓会标,计恩东 译)

参考文献

[1] Ghebreyesus TA. WHO Director-General's opening remarks at the media briefing on COVID-19-2020. 2020.

[2] Papazian L, Corley A, Hess D, Fraser JF, Frat J-P, Guitton C, et al. Use of high-flow nasal cannula oxygenation in ICU adults: a narrative review. Intensive Care Med. 2016; 42(9): 1336 - 49.

[3] Goligher EC, Slutsky AS. Not just oxygen? Mechanisms of benefit from high-flow nasal cannula in hypoxemic respiratory failure. Am J Respir Crit Care Med. 2017; 195(9): 1128 - 31.

[4] Mauri T, Turrini C, Eronia N, Grasselli G, Volta CA, Bellani G, et al. Physiologic effects of high-flow nasal cannula in acute hypoxemic respiratory failure. Am J Respir Crit Care Med. 2017; 195(9): 1207 - 15.

[5] Patel BK, Wolfe KS, Pohlman AS, Hall JB, Kress JP. Effect of noninvasive ventilation delivered by helmet vs face mask on the rate of endotracheal intubation in patients with acute respiratory distress syndrome: a randomized clinical trial. JAMA. 2016; 315(22): 2435 - 41.

[6] Mehta S, Hill NS. Noninvasive ventilation. Am J Respir Crit Care Med. 2001; 163(2): 540 - 77.

[7] Hill NS, Brennan J, Garpestad E, Nava S. Noninvasive ventilation in acute respiratory failure. Crit Care Med. 2007; 35(10): 2402 - 7.

[8] Calfee CS, Delucchi K, Parsons PE, Thompson BT, Ware LB, Matthay MA, et al. Subphenotypes in acute respiratory distress syndrome: latent class analysis of data from two randomised controlled trials. Lancet Respir Med. 2014; 2(8): 611 - 20.

[9] Frat J-P, Thille AW, Mercat A, Girault C, Ragot S, Perbet S, et al. High-flow oxygen through nasal cannula in acute hypoxemic respiratory failure. N Engl J Med. 2015; 372(23): 2185 - 96.

[10] Ferreyro BL, Angriman F, Munshi L, Del Sorbo L, Ferguson ND, Rochwerg B, et al. Association of noninvasive oxygenation strategies with all-cause mortality in adults with acute hypoxemic respiratory failure: a systematic review and meta-analysis. JAMA. 2020; 324(1): 57 - 67.

[11] Tonetti T, Grasselli G, Zanella A, Pizzilli G, Fumagalli R, Piva S, et al. Use of critical care resources during the first 2 weeks (February 24-March 8, 2020) of the Covid-19 outbreak in Italy. Ann Intensive Care. 2020; 10(1): 133.

[12] Roca O, Caralt B, Messika J, Samper M, Sztrymf B, Hernández G, et al. An index combining respiratory rate and oxygenation to predict outcome of nasal high-flow therapy. Am J Respir Crit Care Med. 2019; 199(11): 1368 - 76.

[13] Vega ML, Dongilli R, Olaizola G, Colaianni N, Sayat MC, Pisani L, et al. COVID-19 pneumonia and ROX index: time to set a new threshold for patients admitted outside the ICU. Pulmonology. 2021; 27(5): 475 - 47.

[14] Chandel A, Patolia S, Brown AW, Collins AC, Sahjwani D, Khangoora V, et al. High-flow nasal cannula therapy in COVID-19: using the ROX index to predict success. Respir Care. 2021; 66(6): 909 - 19.

[15] Pearce E, Campen MJ, Baca JT, Blewett JP, Femling J, Hanson DT, et al. Aerosol generation

[16] Li J, Fink JB, Elshafei AA, Stewart LM, Barbian HJ, Mirza SH, et al. Placing a mask on COVID-19 patients during high-flow nasal cannula therapy reduces aerosol particle dispersion. ERJ Open Res. 2021; 7(1): 00519 - 2020.

[17] Avari H, Hiebert RJ, Ryzynski AA, Levy A, Nardi J, Kanji-Jaffer H, et al. Quantitative assessment of viral dispersion associated with respiratory support devices in a simulated critical care environment. Am J Respir Crit Care Med. 2021; 203(9): 1112 - 8.

[18] Bem RA, van Mourik N, Klein-Blommert R, Spijkerman IJ, Kooij S, Bonn D, et al. Risk of aerosol formation during high-flow nasal cannula treatment in critically ill subjects. Respir Care. 2021; 66(6): 891 - 6.

[19] Morin F, Dubie E, Serruys A, Usseglio P, Richard J-C, Douillet D, et al. Interhospital transport of patients with COVID-19 under high-flow nasal cannula (HFNC). Am J Emerg Med. 2021; 50: 791 - 2.

[20] Grieco DL, Menga LS, Cesarano M, Rosà T, Spadaro S, Bitondo MM, et al. Effect of helmet noninvasive ventilation vs high-flow nasal oxygen on days free of respiratory support in patients with COVID-19 and moderate to severe hypoxemic respiratory failure: the HENIVOT randomized clinical trial. JAMA. 2021; 325(17): 1731 - 43.

[21] Perkins GD, Ji C, Connolly BA, Couper K, Lall R, Baillie JK, et al. An adaptive randomized controlled trial of non-invasive respiratory strategies in acute respiratory failure patients with COVID-19. 2021. Available from: https://www.medrxiv.org/content/10.1101/2021.08.02.21261379v1.

[22] Guérin C, Albert RK, Beitler J, Gattinoni L, Jaber S, Marini JJ, et al. Prone position in ARDS patients: why, when, how and for whom. Intensive Care Med. 2020; 46(12): 2385 - 96.

[23] Guérin C, Reignier J, Richard J-C, Beuret P, Gacouin A, Boulain T, et al. Prone positioning in severe acute respiratory distress syndrome. N Engl J Med. 2013; 368(23): 2159 - 68.

[24] Ehrmann S, Li J, Ibarra-Estrada M, Perez Y, Pavlov I, McNicholas B, et al. Awake prone positioning for COVID-19 acute hypoxaemic respiratory failure: a randomised, controlled, multinational, open-label meta-trial Lancet Respir Med. 2021. https://www.ncbi.nlm.nih.gov/pmc/articles/PMC8378833/

24 COVID-19 中的有创通气
Invasive Ventilation in COVID-19

Giacomo Grasselli, Gaetano Florio, Emanuele Cattaneo

24.1 引言

自 2019 年 12 月以来,数百万人感染了严重急性呼吸系统综合征冠状病毒 2 型 (severe acute respiratory syndrome coronavirus 2,SARS-CoV-2),全球范围内已经有超过 450 万例死亡病例。此次的冠状病毒感染(COVID-19)传播范围极其广泛,但最常见的住院原因是 COVID-19 相关性肺炎,随后可进展为由肺泡和内皮细胞损伤导致的急性呼吸衰竭,通常与细胞因子释放引起的促凝现象和过度炎症反应相关。

高达 32% 的 COVID-19 住院患者需要入住 ICU,进行气管插管和机械通气 (mechanical ventilation,MV)[1]。在疫情初期,全球的 ICU 都被需要呼吸支持的 COVID-19 相关严重急性呼吸窘迫综合征(COVID-19 related severe acute respiratory distress syndrome,C-ARDS)患者住满,多种医疗系统都被调整来应对这些数量庞大的患者,因其具有新的呼吸病理机制而没人知道该如何处理。

COVID-19 患者的机械通气设置迅速成为一个"热门"话题,尤其是因为缺乏任何针对 SARS-CoV-2 的特异性治疗。在大流行的第一个月,早期的初步报告描述了 C-ARDS 的一些独特和特定表现[2],提示该疾病存在两种表型,具有不同的呼吸力学特征,可能需要不同的通气方法。然而,随后的研究未能证实这种观点,许多专家倾向于将 C-ARDS 视为与"经典"ARDS 类似[3]。

目前 C-ARDS 的低氧血症的病理生理学仍未完全阐明,尽管通气/灌注不匹配、肺灌注调节失调和分流是最可能的机制[3]。即使自疫情开始以来已经过去近 2 年时间,已经引入了新的疗法和疫苗,但很少有研究专门关注 C-ARDS 患者的呼吸力学、病理生理

G. Grasselli (✉) · G. Florio · E. Cattaneo
Department of Pathophysiology and Transplantation, University of Milan, Milan, Italy
e-mail: giacomo.grasselli@unimi.it

© The Author(s), under exclusive license to Springer Nature Switzerland AG 2022
G. Bellani (ed.), *Mechanical Ventilation from Pathophysiology to Clinical Evidence*, https://doi.org/10.1007/978-3-030-93401-9_24

学和机械通气设置[4,5]。此外,大部分可用的数据来自小型的回顾性病例研究。本章的目的是总结有关 COVID-19 危重症患者有创机械通气(invasive mechanical ventilation, IMV)设置相关的已有证据。

24.2 气管插管和时机选择

大多数需要呼吸支持的 COVID-19 患者最初都采用无创辅助通气,包括高流量鼻导管、持续性气道正压和通过不同接口的无创通气。气管插管的最佳时机仍是一个激烈争论的问题。一项基于非随机队列研究的荟萃分析表明不能确定插管时机对病死率的影响[6]。与对"经典"ARDS 危重症患者的建议类似,对 COVID-19 患者,应该尽一切努力基于以下内容及时判断无创支持的失败,如疾病进展迅速、高风险患者的识别、患者病情的恶化(如低氧血症和高碳酸血症的严重程度、总体呼吸做功、精神状态),以及出现血流动力学不稳定和(或)多器官功能障碍的情况。

为 COVID-19 患者进行气管插管被认为是最危险的操作之一,因为病毒可经飞沫传播,使健康医疗人员暴露于最高的传染风险中。El-Boghdadly 等在疫情初期报道,在插管后 21 天,插管相关 SARS-CoV-2 感染的发生率为 8.5%[7],尽管随后几个月风险有所降低。专家建议使用个人防护设备(如 N95 口罩、防护服、帽子和手套),优化预充氧,避免手动面罩通气,以及通过视频喉镜进行快速插管。

24.3 机械通气设置

机械通气的作用是为肺部"争取时间"从疾病中恢复,同时保持足够的氧合和二氧化碳清除而不造成进一步的伤害,从而最小化通气相关肺损伤(ventilator induced lung injury, VILI)。由于 C-ARDS 与"经典"ARDS 一样,被证明是一种异质性很高的疾病,因此不可能采用"一刀切"的通气设置,建议采用基于生理参数的个体化设定并进行持续监测。

表 24.1 总结了针对 COVID-19 机械通气患者队列分析的文献中报导的通气设置和呼吸力学。数据清楚地显示 COVID-19 导致了中重度 ARDS 表现,PaO_2/FiO_2 中位数常常低于 150 mmHg,通气策略与"经典"ARDS 推荐的策略没有区别。实际上,广泛采用了肺保护性通气设置,包括潮气量(tidal volume, V_T)中位数在 6~8 mL/kg(PBW)之间,并且平台压和气道驱动压处于安全范围内。由于疾病的严重程度,采用的 PEEP 中位数高于 10 cmH_2O;值得注意的是,这个值显著高于在针对"经典"ARDS 患者的 LUNG SAFE 研究中观察到的 8.4 cmH_2O 这一中位数水平[15]。

以下是 C-ARDS 患者 IMV 设置的概述:

(1) 低容积、低压通气:普遍认为让肺休息是有益处的,尤其对于损伤肺,因为这些肺组织更容易受到进一步的损害。开创性的 ARMA 试验表明,在 ARDS 中,与 12 mL/kg(PBW)的 V_T 相比,使用 6 mL/kg(PBW)的 V_T 通气有更好的预后[16]。在 C-ARDS 患

表 24.1　多数相关研究报导的通气设置和呼吸力学参数

研究	样本量	潮气量 [mL/kg(PBW)]	RR (次/分)	PEEP (cmH_2O)	平台压 (cmH_2O)	驱动压 (cmH_2O)	C_{RS} (mL/cmH_2O)	PaO_2/FiO_2 (mmHg)
Schmidt[8]	4 643	6.1 (5.8~6.7)		12 (10~14)	24 (21~27)	13 (10~17)	33 (26~42)	154 (106~223)
Estenssoro[9]	1 990	6.1 (6~7)	24 (20~26)	10 (8~12)	23 (20~26)	12 (10~14)	36 (29~44)	160 (111~218)
Ferrando[10]	742	6.9 (6.3~7.8)	24 (20~30)	12 (11~14)	25 (22~29)	12 (10~16)	35 (27~45)	120 (83~177)
Zanella[11]	707	7.1 (6.4~7.9)	20 (16~22)	12 (10~15)	24 (22~27)	12 (9~14)	41 (33~51)	129 (93~180)
Patel[12]	633	6.8 (6~7.8)	19 (16~22)	10 (8~12)	26 (23~29)			137 (98~189)
Botta[13]	553	6.3 (5.7~7.1)	20 (18~24)	14 (11~15)		14 (11~16)	32 (26~40)	159 (129~201)
Grasselli[1]	301	7 (6.3~7.6)	20 (18~24)	13 (10~15)	24 (22~26)	11 (9~14)	41 (33~52)	124 (89~164)
Cummings[14]	257	6.2 (5.9~7.2)	15 (12~18)	27 (23~31)	15 (11~18)	27 (22~36)		129 (80~203)

PBW，预测体重；RR，呼吸频率；PEEP，呼气末正压；C_{RS}，呼吸系统顺应性；PaO_2/FiO_2，动脉氧分压与吸入氧浓度之比

者中，同样推荐使用低潮气量[6~8 mL/kg(PBW)]，并且必须将气道平台压和驱动压力置于保护性阈值以下，分别为 30 cmH_2O 和 14 cmH_2O。

(2) 呼气末正压：可以使肺部保持膨胀，从而增加呼气末肺容积并减少肺内分流。此外，呼气末正压(positive end-expiratory pressure，PEEP)可以通过减少肺萎陷伤(肺泡在每个呼吸周期中的开放和关闭)来减少 VILI，但是过高的 PEEP 水平可能导致肺过度膨胀，对呼吸和心血管系统都可能产生有害影响。在"经典"ARDS 中，应用高 PEEP 可以改善重度 ARDS 患者的预后，而对轻度低氧血症患者则没有任何益处[17]。如前所述，分流可能是 C-ARDS 低氧血症的主要机制，但肺灌注失调、血管缺氧性收缩的丧失，以及通气/灌注不匹配也可能起到重要作用。此外，一些 C-ARDS 患者，特别是在疾病的早期阶段，尽管呼吸系统顺应性能相对维持，却出现严重低氧。在这种情况下，使用高 PEEP 是有争议的。PEEP 滴定最常用方法之一是使用 ARDSnet 表格，将患者的吸入氧浓度(fraction of inspired oxygen，FiO_2)与特定水平的 PEEP 相匹配。这种方法易于实施，并且在大流行期间可能非常实用，因为大量危重症患者被送入重症监护室，在 ARDS 管理方面缺乏或没有经验的医生可能会参与治疗这些患者。然而，在这种紧急情况之外，应监测肺可复张性(如评估 CT、电阻抗断层成像或计算复张-充气比)，并评估不同 PEEP 水平对气体交换、呼吸力学和血液动力学的影响，采用个性化的 PEEP 滴定方法。

(3) 自主呼吸：在机械通气的 C-ARDS 患者中，一个非常有趣和具有挑战性的问题是明确从控制性通气转换为自主辅助通气的最佳时机。众所周知，保持自主呼吸活动有很多好处，如改善通气/灌注、预防肌肉萎缩或无力、减少镇静药物的需求，以及降低对血流动力学的影响。另一方面，肺"不稳定"的患者过早地转换为自主呼吸可能导致呼吸困难、焦虑、耗氧量增加和更高的通气需求、呼吸机不同步和患者自戕性肺损伤（patient self-inflicted lung injury, P-SILI），最终导致患者呼吸功能恶化。C-ARDS 患者的现有研究表明，其需要长期 IMV，其 MV 持续时间的中位数高于 LUNG SAFE 研究中报导的时间（10 天 vs. 8 天）[1,11,15]。因此，转换为自主呼吸应该非常小心，并且只在有肺愈合的明显迹象，如 PaO_2/FiO_2 的稳定改善、炎症生物标志物的降低和通气的需求减少时才进行。

图 24.1 总结了适合此类患者的呼吸机设置和监护。

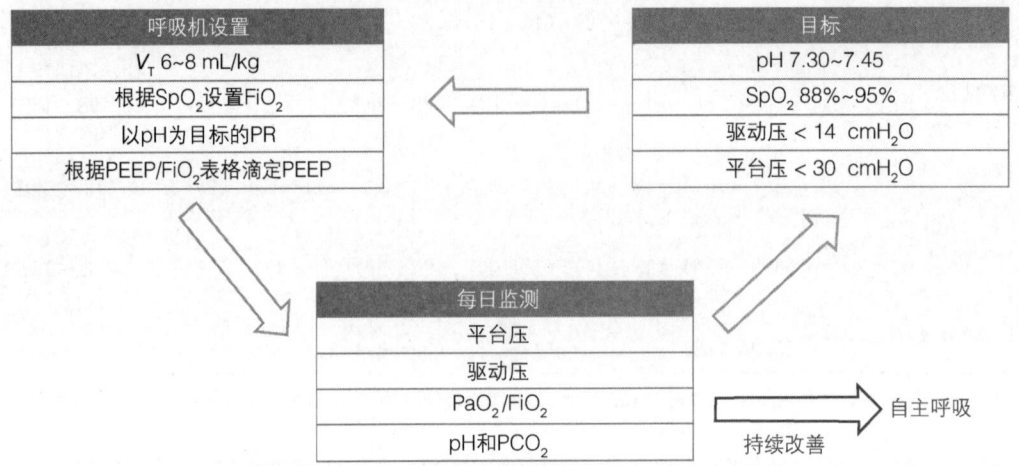

图 24.1 COVID-19 机械通气患者呼吸机设置和监护。FiO_2，吸入氧浓度；RR，呼吸频率；PEEP，呼气末正压；SpO_2，脉搏氧饱和度；PaO_2/FiO_2，动脉氧分压与吸入氧浓度之比

24.4 挽救性治疗

由于 COVID-19 重症患者常出现严重低氧，因此针对难以纠正的低氧血症的挽救性治疗被广泛使用，总结在表 24.2 中。具体而言，在大多数已发表的研究报道中，使用神经肌肉阻滞剂的患者比例高达 88%[1,8,10]，而俯卧位的使用比例则高达 77%[8,10]。当 PaO_2/FiO_2 低于 150 mmHg 时，通常会应用俯卧位通气，这可以减少肺不张并增加通气/灌注，从而提高氧合并降低 VILI 的风险。在早期 ARDS 患者中进行的一项大型随机对照试验表明，应用俯卧位可以显著提高生存率[18]。在 ARDS 的早期阶段使用俯卧位且每天至少持续 12~16 h，应用的效果更好。尽管其在中重度 ARDS 中的疗效明显，但在大流行前期，俯卧位仍未被充分利用：在 LUNG SAFE 研究中，仅有 7.9% 的 ARDS 患者应用了俯卧位[15]。相比之下，最近的研究表明，C-ARDS 患者的俯卧位使用频率要高得多，在一些报道中超过 70%。在意大利进行的一项最新研究中，涉及 24 个 ICU 中 1 000 多名 C-

ARDS 患者,其中有 61% 的患者使用了俯卧位。接受俯卧位的患者中,有 78% 的患者对该治疗方法有积极反应,PaO_2/FiO_2 增加 $\geqslant$ 20 mmHg;此外,与对该挽救性措施无反应的患者相比,有反应亚组的患者 ICU 病死率更低[19]。Mathews 等在最近一项涉及 2 338 名 COVID-19 机械通气患者的多中心观察性研究中发现,早期(入 ICU 的前 2 天内)接受俯卧位治疗的患者与未接受治疗的患者相比,ICU 死亡风险降低[20]。

表 24.2　多数相关研究报道的 COVID-19 机械通气患者低氧的挽救性治疗

研　究	NMBA	俯卧位	肺血管扩张剂	ECMO	死　亡
Schmidt[8]	1 966/2 224 (88%)	1 556/2 223 (70%)	425/2 224 (19%)	235/2 153 (11%)	1 298/4 244 (31%)
Estenssoro[9]		1 176/1 909 (61%)		1/1 909 (<1%)	1 088/1 909 (57%)
Ferrando[10]	536/742 (72%)	564/735 (77%)		21/738 (2.4%)	241/742 (32%)
Zanella[11]	634/752 (84%)	471/1137 (41%)	90/1 137 (8%)	30/1 137 (3%)	428/1 260 (34%)
Patel[12]	434/617 (70%)	273/551 (50%)	128/521 (25%)		274/633 (43%)
Botta[13]	183/487 (38%)	283/530 (53%)		2/553 (<1%)	203/530 (38%)
Cummings[14]	51/203 (25%)	35/203 (17%)	22/203 (11%)	6/203 (3%)	101/257 (39%)

NMBA,神经肌肉阻滞剂;ECMO,体外膜肺氧合。

尽管现有关于神经肌肉阻滞剂在"经典"ARDS 中疗效的证据存在争议,但这些药物通常在最严重的 C-ARDS 患者中使用,这些患者通常需要进行长时间的控制通气。专门关注 C-ARDS 机械通气患者使用神经肌肉阻滞剂的文献数据很少。一项对 COVID-19 患者大型队列的初期回顾性研究(仅以摘要形式发布)表明,使用神经肌肉阻滞剂可能与 28 天病死率增加、机械通气时间延长和 ICU 住院时间延长有关[21]。由于现有证据不能得出任何结论,因此我们建议神经肌肉阻滞剂应该用于难治性低氧血症和(或)人-机不同步患者。

吸入肺血管扩张剂(尤其是一氧化氮)使用较少,为 8%[11]~25%[12]。这些药物可能在重度低氧血症的患者中发挥作用,特别是伴有急性肺动脉高压和右心功能不全时。支持 C-ARDS 机械通气患者使用吸入一氧化氮的数据有限,通常与特定患者群体相关(如自主呼吸者、孕妇)。但是,目前有一项随机对照试验正在进行,以评估其对机械通气患者的临床疗效[22]。

体外膜肺氧合(extracorporeal membrane oxygenation,ECMO)在流行初期很少使

用,其是一项耗时和消耗资源的技术,无法与第一波疫情期间所面对大量的ICU住院需求相匹配。在已发表的系列研究中,C-ARDS患者ECMO的使用频率从1%到11%不等。纳入疫情首月进行的四项中国的研究的荟萃分析显示,在将ECMO与标准治疗进行比较时,病死率没有差异,提示ECMO在C-ARDS患者中可能无获益[23]。然而,近期更多的数据[24]对此发现提出了质疑,表明在有经验的中心,C-ARDS使用ECMO与"经典"ARDS的EOLIA试验有相似的病死率。最新的国际指南建议,应选择特定的患者使用ECMO,如那些在已经使用所有ARDS传统疗法(包括俯卧位)但仍表现为严重的难治性低氧血症的患者[25]。

24.5 气管切开术

气管切开术通常用于需要长期有创通气的患者。目前在气管切开的术式和操作时机方面还存在巨大的异质性,一些证据表明早期气管切开术可能会缩短机械通气时间和ICU住院时间[26]。然而,在COVID-19的早期阶段,大多数指南建议延迟气管切开术(因为医护人员感染风险高),以及在疾病的早期阶段大量使用俯卧位通气[27]。一项涉及18项研究、纳入3 234名患者的荟萃分析显示,晚期(插管14天后或更长时间)气管切开术的累积发生率为71.5%,远高于COVID-19之前观察到的发生率[28]。然而,来自不同中心的最新数据表明,如果严格遵守使用个人防护设备的建议,气管切开术可以在患者的床旁安全地进行[29]。此外,最近一项多中心前瞻性试验对696名重症COVID-19机械通气患者进行了气管切开术的时机评估,结果显示早期气管切开术可能会缩短机械通气时间和ICU住院时间,而不会改变并发症发生率或病死率,因此在可行的情况下可能更倾向于进行早期气管切开[30]。

24.6 总结

目前的证据表明,C-ARDS患者的机械通气管理与"经典"ARDS的管理类似。特别是应在所有C-ARDS患者中实施低潮气量、低平台压和低驱动压的保护性通气策略。在COVID-19相关的急性呼吸衰竭患者中,应根据床旁监测的呼吸力学、气体交换和血流动力学情况,个体化和个性化地设置通气参数。

(张媛,于晨希 译)

参考文献

[1] Grasselli G, Greco M, Zanella A, et al. Risk factors associated with mortality among patients with COVID-19 in intensive care units in Lombardy, Italy. JAMA Intern Med. 2020; 180(10): 1345-55.

[2] Gattinoni L, Coppola S, Cressoni M, Busana M, Chiumello D. Covid-19 does not lead to a

"typical" acute respiratory distress syndrome. Am J Respir Crit Care Med. 2020; 201(10): 1299.

[3] Grasselli G, Tonetti T, Protti A, et al. Pathophysiology of COVID-19-associated acute respiratory distress syndrome: a multicentre prospective observational study. Lancet Respir Med. 2020; 8(12): 1201-8.

[4] Grasselli G, Cattaneo E, Scaravilli V. Ventilation of coronavirus disease 2019 patients. Curr Opin Crit Care. 2021; 27(1): 6-12.

[5] Grasselli G, Cattaneo E, Florio G, et al. Mechanical ventilation parameters in critically ill COVID-19 patients: a scoping review. Crit Care. 2021; 25(1): 115.

[6] Papoutsi E, Giannakoulis VG, Xourgia E, Routsi C, Kotanidou A, Siempos II. Effect of timing of intubation on clinical outcomes of critically ill patients with COVID-19: a systematic review and meta-analysis of non-randomized cohort studies. Crit Care. 2021; 25(1): 121.

[7] El-Boghdadly K, Wong DJN, Owen R, et al. Risks to healthcare workers following tracheal intubation of patients with COVID-19: a prospective international multicentre cohort study. Anaesthesia. 2020; 75(11): 1437-47.

[8] Schmidt M, Hajage D, Demoule A, et al. Clinical characteristics and day-90 outcomes of 4244 critically ill adults with COVID-19: a prospective cohort study. Intensive Care Med. 2021; 47(1): 60-73.

[9] Estenssoro E, Loudet CI, Ríos FG, et al. Clinical characteristics and outcomes of invasively ventilated patients with COVID-19 in Argentina (SATICOVID): a prospective, multicentre cohort study. Lancet Respir Med. 2021; 9(9): 989-98.

[10] Ferrando C, Suarez-Sipmann F, Mellado-Artigas R, et al. Clinical features, ventilatory management, and outcome of ARDS caused by COVID-19 are similar to other causes of ARDS. Intensive Care Med. 2020; 46(12): 2200-11.

[11] Zanella A, Florio G, Antonelli M, et al. Time course of risk factors associated with mortality of 1260 critically ill patients with COVID-19 admitted to 24 Italian intensive care units. Intensive Care Med. 2021; 47(9): 995.

[12] Brijesh V, Haar S, Handslip R, Auepanwiriyakul C, Mei-Ling T, Patel S, Harston JA, Hosking-Jervis F, Kelly D, Sanderson B, Borgatta B, Tatham K, Welters I, Camporota L, Anthony C. Natural history, trajectory, and management of mechanically ventilated COVID-19 patients in the United Kingdom. Intensive Care Med. 2021; 47(5): 549-65. https://doi.org/10.1007/s00134-021-06389-z.

[13] Botta M, Tsonas AM, Pillay J, et al. Ventilation management and clinical outcomes in invasively ventilated patients with COVID-19 (PRoVENT-COVID): a national, multicentre, observational cohort study. Lancet Respir Med. 2020; 9(2): 139-48.

[14] Cummings MJ, Baldwin MR, Abrams D, et al. Epidemiology, clinical course, and outcomes of critically ill adults with COVID-19 in New York City: a prospective cohort study. Lancet. 2020; 395(10239): 1763-70.

[15] Bellani G, Laffey JG, Pham T, et al. Epidemiology, patterns of care, and mortality for patients with acute respiratory distress syndrome in intensive care units in 50 countries. JAMA. 2016; 315(8): 788-800.

[16] Brower RG, Matthay MA, et al. Ventilation with lower tidal volumes as compared with traditional tidal volumes for acute lung injury and the acute respiratory distress syndrome. N Engl J Med. 2000; 342(18): 1301-8.

[17] Briel M, Meade M, Mercat A, et al. Higher vs lower positive end-expiratory pressure in patients

with acute lung injury and acute respiratory distress syndrome. JAMA. 2010; 303(9): 865.

[18] Guérin C, Reignier J, Richard J-C, et al. Prone positioning in severe acute respiratory distress syndrome. N Engl J Med. 2013; 368(23): 2159-68.

[19] Langer T, Brioni M, Guzzardella A, et al. Prone position in intubated, mechanically ventilated patients with COVID-19: a multi-centric study of more than 1000 patients. Crit Care. 2021; 25(1): 128.

[20] Mathews KS, Soh H, Shaefi S, et al. Prone positioning and survival in mechanically ventilated patients with coronavirus disease 2019-related respiratory failure. Crit Care Med. 2021; 49(7): 1026-37.

[21] Li Bassi G, Gibbons K, Suen J, et al. Neuromuscular blocking agents in critically-ill COVID-19 patients requiring mechanical ventilation. 2021. Available from: https://www.atsjournals.org/doi/10.1164/ajrccm-conference.2021.203.1_MeetingAbstracts.A2489

[22] Lei C, Su B, Dong H, et al. Protocol of a randomized controlled trial testing inhaled Nitric Oxide in mechanically ventilated patients with severe acute respiratory syndrome in COVID-19 (SARS-CoV-2). medRxiv Prepr Serv Heal Sci. 2020.

[23] Henry BM, Lippi G. Poor survival with extracorporeal membrane oxygenation in acute respiratory distress syndrome (ARDS) due to coronavirus disease 2019 (COVID-19): pooled analysis of early reports. J Crit Care. 2020; 58: 27-8.

[24] Barbaro RP, MacLaren G, Boonstra PS, et al. Extracorporeal membrane oxygenation support in COVID-19: an international cohort study of the extracorporeal life support organization registry. Lancet. 2020; 396(10257): 1071-8.

[25] Shekar K, Badulak J, Peek G, et al. Extracorporeal life support organization coronavirus disease 2019 interim guidelines: a consensus document from an International Group of Interdisciplinary Extracorporeal Membrane Oxygenation Providers. ASAIO J. 2020; 66(7): 707-21.

[26] Andriolo BN, Andriolo RB, Saconato H, Atallah ÁN, Valente O. Early versus late tracheostomy for critically ill patients. Cochrane Database Syst Rev. 2015; 2017: 6.

[27] McGrath BA, Brenner MJ, Warrillow SJ, et al. Tracheostomy in the COVID-19 era: global and multidisciplinary guidance. Lancet Respir Med. 2020; 8(7): 717-25.

[28] Benito DA, Bestourous DE, Tong JY, Pasick LJ, Sataloff RT. Tracheotomy in COVID-19 patients: a systematic review and meta-analysis of weaning, decannulation, and survival. Otolaryngol Head Neck Surg. 2021; 165: 3.

[29] Avilés-Jurado FX, Prieto-Alhambra D, González-Sánchez N, et al. Timing, complications, and safety of tracheotomy in critically ill patients with COVID-19. JAMA Otolaryngol Neck Surg. 2021; 147(1): 41.

[30] Prats-Uribe A, Tobed M, Villacampa JM, et al. Timing of elective tracheotomy and duration of mechanical ventilation amongst patients admitted to intensive care with severe COVID-19: a multicentre prospective cohort study. SSRN Electron J. 2020; 43: 3743-56.

25 不同手术情境下的机械通气

Mechanical Ventilation in Different Surgical Settings

Luigi Zattera, Adriana Jacas, Carlos Ferrando

25.1 引言

25.1.1 术后肺部并发症

术后肺部并发症（postoperative pulmonary complication，PPC）是全球常见的医疗问题，由于每天进行的手术数量众多，它们的发生率可达到所有手术的5%，并且与ICU入住率、住院时间和病死率增加有关[1]。由于临床定义、疾病严重程度及手术的类型不同，现有研究中其发生率和相关结局的差异性很大。最近发表了一项共识声明，有助于克服这些问题并更好地定义PPC[2]。

PPC的临床表现广泛，包括轻度的术后低氧血症到需要在ICU气管插管和持续机械通气（mechanical ventilation，MV）的重度呼吸衰竭。严重程度差异很大的同时，其病因也是广泛的，主要是由于肺不张、肺炎、吸入性肺炎和急性呼吸窘迫综合征（acute respiratory distress syndrome，ARDS）。也可有其他呼吸系统表现，如胸腔积液、气胸、支气管痉挛，尽管它们的生物学机制不尽相同[2]。

如上所述，PPC的发生率在患者中不一致，多种风险因素与PPC有关，同时包括患者和手术相关的因素，表25.1中总结了这些因素。为了预测PPC开发了多个评分系统：ARISCAT评分[1]基于患者的术前状况和手术特点来预测PPC；而SLIP评分更专注于术后肺损伤和ARDS的风险[3]；最后，LAS VEGAS风险评分同时包括ARISCAT队列风险因素和术中变量[4]。

表 25.1　术后肺部并发症最常见的危险因素

患 者 相 关	手 术 相 关
年龄	上腹部手术
男性	胸部手术
ASA≥Ⅱ级	头颈部手术
虚弱/功能依赖	大血管手术
感觉受损	急诊手术
吸烟	手术时长超过 2 小时
COPD/哮喘	围手术期鼻胃管留置
CHF	残余神经肌肉阻滞
OSA	机械通气策略
肥胖	术中低 SpO_2
酒精滥用	术中使用血管活性药物
慢性肝病	
活动性肿瘤	
术前贫血	
术前低 SpO_2	

ASA,美国麻醉协会体格状态分级系统;COPD,慢性阻塞性肺疾病;CHF,慢性心力衰竭;OSA,阻塞性睡眠呼吸暂停;SpO_2,脉搏氧饱和度。

此外,术后阶段的 Air-Test 评分是一种经过验证的评分系统,它评估了进入术后复苏室前和进入复苏室后 3 小时的基础外周氧合水平,是术中和术后早期筛选 PPC 高风险患者的实用工具[5]。

为了减少 PPC,一旦识别到高风险患者,可以采取多种干预措施,如术前患者预康复优化,调整先前的治疗方案,给予足够的术后镇痛和物理治疗。最后,必须考虑采用保护性机械通气策略,以最小化其对肺功能的负面影响。

25.1.2　保护性机械通气：基本概念

已知绝大多数接受全身麻醉的患者都会发生一定程度的肺不张:膈肌的头侧位移会导致肺基底部塌陷,通常会因气腹或患者肥胖而加重。在这种情况下,机械通气必须将正压通气所造成的损伤最小化,如潮气量过大(即容积伤)和呼气末肺泡周期性萎陷/复张(即肺萎陷伤),尤其表现在肺塌陷区域。通过设置按理想体重(ideal body weight, IBW)计算的低潮气量(tidal volume, V_T),即 6~8 mL/kg,可以减少容积伤;通过应用呼气末正压(positive end-expiratory pressure, PEEP)来防止呼气性肺塌陷,可以减少肺萎陷伤。

25 不同手术情境下的机械通气

此外,全身麻醉引起的肺不张会导致驱动压(driving pressure, DP)增加,意味着肺应变的增加。

换句话说,现今低 V_T 和一定程度 PEEP 的应用已经成为了实践标准。然而,尽管与非保护性策略相比,6 mL/kg(IBW)的 V_T 外加不同程度的 PEEP 应用通常能够减少 PPC[6],但大型随机对照试验(randomized control trial, RCT)研究未能证明对于高危患者和某些手术操作异质性较高的群体,应用 PEEP 可以在 PPC 上获益[7]。因此,需要强调一个观念,即呼吸机设置不能"一刀切":在高危患者和特定手术过程中,如单肺通气(one-lung ventilation, OLV)或腹腔镜手术,患者不能从单一的"低 V_T"策略中获益,必须考虑其他因素,使得保护性机械通气更具针对性。

25.1.3 个性化呼气末正压:肺开放策略

肺开放策略(open lung approach, OLA)是一种新兴的通气策略,旨在根据个体特征滴定 PEEP。它包括进行肺复张手法(recruitment maneuver, RM)来打开塌陷的肺泡,并设置一个 PEEP,以最小化周期性肺萎陷并在安全范围内维持肺开放。几项 RCT 研究了 OLA 在不同手术情境中能否获益(表 25.2)。虽然已经明确,基于应用 PEEP 和低潮气量的保护性机械通气优于零 PEEP 和高潮气量的策略,但比较 OLA 和传统保护性机械通气的研究通常未能显示 OLA 在改善 PPC 临床结局方面的优势,至少在未经选择的人群中。然而,OLA 似乎对气体交换和呼吸力学有益,随后将予讨论。

表 25.2 近期比较不同保护性通气策略的随机对照试验研究

作者 (参考文献)	手术类型	对照组	干预组	结局
Severgnini et al.[34]	腹部开放性手术	• $N=27$ • $V_T=9$ mL/kg(IBW) • 无 RM • PEEP=0 cmH$_2$O	• $N=27$ • $V_T=7$ mL/kg(IBW) • 压力递增法 RM • PEEP=10 cmH$_2$O	低 V_T 及 PEEP 降低 PPC 的发生率
Futier et al.[6]	腹部手术	• $N=200$ • $V_T=11$ mL/kg(IBW) • 无 RM • PEEP=0 cmH$_2$O	• $N=200$ • $V_T=6\sim8$ mL/kg(IBW) • RM=30-30-30 次 • PEEP=6 cmH$_2$O	低 V_T 及 PEEP 降低 PPC 的发生率
Costa Leme et al.[8]	心脏手术(术后)	• $N=163$ • $V_T=6$ mL/kg(IBW) • RM=20-30-3 次 • PEEP=8 cmH$_2$O	• $N=159$ • $V_T=6$ mL/kg(IBW) • RM=45-60-3 次 • PEEP=13 cmH$_2$O	OLA 降低 PPC
Ferrando et al.[9]	腹部手术	• $N=499$ • $V_T=8$ mL/kg(IBW) • 无 RM • PEEP=5 cmH$_2$O	• $N=513$ • $V_T=8$ mL/kg(IBW) • 压力递增法 RM • PEEP 根据最佳 C_{rs}	OLA 降低 PPC(为次要结局)

续表

作者（参考文献）	手术类型	对照组	干预组	结局
Park et al.[10]	胸部手术	• $N=147$ • $V_T=6$ mL/kg(IBW) • 无 RM • PEEP$=5$ cmH_2O	• $N=145$ • $V_T=6$ mL/kg(IBW) • 无 RM • PEEP 根据最低 DP	OLA 降低 PPC
Bluth et al.[11]	肥胖患者	• $N=987$ • $V_T=7$ mL/kg(IBW) • RM • PEEP$=12$ cmH_2O	• $N=989$ • $V_T=7$ mL/kg(IBW) • 无 RM • PEEP$=5$ cmH_2O	无差异
Lagier et al.[12]	心脏手术	• $N=247$ • $V_T=6\sim8$ mL/kg(IBW) • 无 RM • PEEP$=2$ cmH_2O	• $N=246$ • $V_T=6\sim8$ mL/kg(IBW) • RM：重复 30-30 次 • PEEP$=8$ cmH_2O	无差异
Karalapillai et al.[7]	所有手术	• $N=592$ • $V_T=10$ mL/kg(IBW) • 无 RM • PEEP$=5$ cmH_2O	• $N=614$ • $V_T=6$ mL/kg(IBW) • 无 RM • PEEP$=5$ cmH_2O	无差异

V_T，潮气量；IBW，理想体重；RM，肺复张手法；PEEP，呼气末正压；OLA，肺开放策略；PPC，术后肺部并发症。

在应用 OLA 策略之前，必须考虑以下几个方面。

(1) 确定高危患者：除了前面提到的可以用于术前筛查患者的风险评分外，术中 Air-Test 是一种新颖且经过验证的方法。它包括在麻醉诱导后将 FiO_2 降至环境空气水平，并随后检查外周血氧饱和度：如果低于 97%，则存在肺不张引起的分流，患者可能会受益于 OLA[13]。

(2) 手术类型：OLA 可能有益于特别的术式，如减重手术、OLV、腹腔镜手术和头低足高位手术。

(3) 何时实施 RM：通常在手术开始前和拔管前进行，可以在整个手术过程中按时间段或根据更多临床表现（如低氧血症、外周血氧饱和度降低或呼吸力学恶化）实施 RM。

(4) 实施 RM 的方法：RM 旨在复张塌陷的肺部区域，施加的压力要能够使肺泡开放，通常是 40 cmH_2O。经典的 RM 是通过一定时间的 $30\sim40$ cmH_2O 的持续气道正压通气(continuous positive airway pressure，CPAP)实施的。这种方法有几个局限性，现在不推荐使用。首先是因为对患者的血流动力学影响更大，其次是因为此方法无法实现个性化 PEEP 设置。为了实现后者，可以采用压力递增的方法，包括初始复张和随后基于力学变量确定个体化的 PEEP，更为可靠，如图 25.1 所示。PEEP 可以基于平台压(plateau pressure，P_{plat})、DP、呼吸系统顺应性(respiratory system compliance，C_{rs})、环境空气中的氧浓度来滴定[13],或者可以通过新型无创监测技术(如电阻抗成像)、食管探头间接测量跨肺压(transpulmonary pressure,P_{TP})或通过 LUS 评估肺充气来设定。

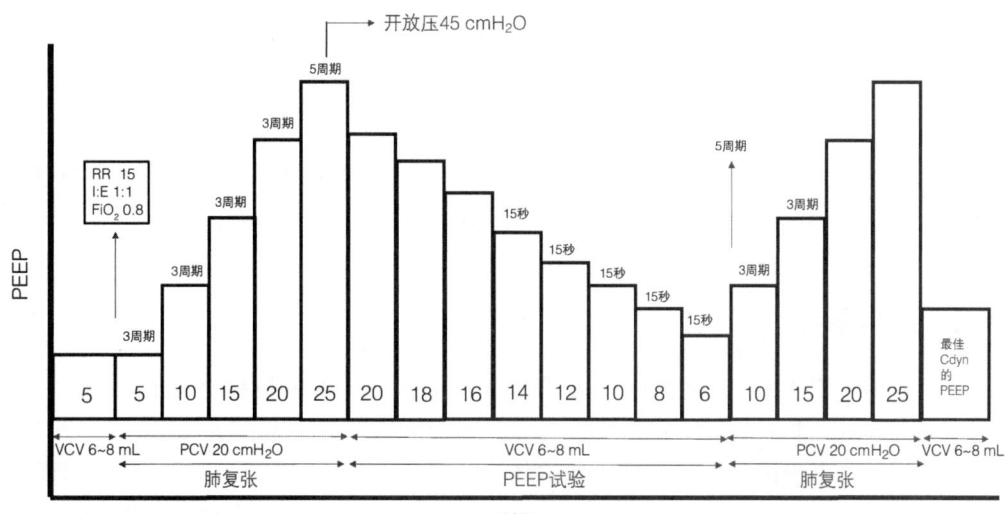

图 25.1 压力递增法实施肺复张：先转换为压力控制模式,将 5 cmH$_2$O 的 PEEP 每次以 5 cmH$_2$O 幅度增加,每次间隔 3 个呼吸周期;DP 设置为固定的 20 cmH$_2$O,直到达到 45 cmH$_2$O 的肺复张吸气压,保持 5 个呼吸周期。在随后的 PEEP 递减滴定试验中,通气模式转换为容量控制,使用与基线相同的参数设定,只是 PEEP 初始值为 20 cmH$_2$O,随后每次下降 2 cmH$_2$O 并每次保持 15 秒。在 PEEP 递减滴定试验中,根据最高的 Cdyn 确定最佳 PEEP。最后,实施一次新的 RM 来重新打开萎陷的肺泡,然后设置滴定的最佳 PEEP,并在术中维持。或者,检测出呼吸力学或氧合变差时再行 RM。VCV,容量控制通气;PCV,压力控制通气;RR,呼吸频率;I∶E,吸呼比;FiO$_2$,吸入氧浓度;PEEP,呼气末正压;Cdyn,动态顺应性

(5) RM 的禁忌证(很少是绝对的):

1) 患有 COPD 或哮喘的患者,特别是存在肺大疱或先前发生过气胸的患者。

2) 血流动力学不稳定:尽管逐步进行的 RM 对患者的血流动力学影响较小,但 TP 的增加可能导致短暂性低血压,特别是在低容量性患者和急性肺心病患者中。在这些患者中,应考虑前期的液体复苏和使用血管活性药物。

3) 急性脑损伤且有颅高压风险的患者,这将在本章后面进行讨论。

4) 开放眼科手术。

25.2 腹腔镜手术

腹腔镜手术(laparoscopic surgery,LPS)由于其微创性而在全球范围内越来越受欢迎。然而,将 CO$_2$ 注入腹腔会导致腹内压力(intra-abdominal pressure,IAP)增加,随后膈肌向头侧位移,增加胸膜腔压力并使 P_{TT} 为负值,最终加重了麻醉引起的肺不张和分流[14],在常用的头低足高位时会更加严重。直接结果是,保护性低潮气量可能不足以维

持 P_{TT} 为正值,因此肺部进一步塌陷。

25.2.1 当前的证据

最近一项大型 RCT 发现,与保护性通气[潮气量 8 mL/kg(IBW),PEEP 5cmH$_2$O]相比,OLA 策略加术后 CPAP 模式显示出了与 PPC 相关的益处(虽然是次要结果),由于研究对象是 LPS(占总数的 40%)和开放性腹部手术的混合人群,可能低估了其对 LPS 人群的影响[9]。在另一项观察性研究中,开放性手术中 5 cmH$_2$O 的 PEEP 能够逆转分流效应,而只有 10 cmH$_2$O 的 PEEP 才能改善 LPS 的分流[15]。

25.3 肥胖患者

与正常体重患者相比,肥胖患者全身麻醉后,膈肌向头侧位移会导致功能残气量(functional residual capacity,FRC)进一步降低,使肥胖患者更容易发生肺不张,无论是在开放性手术还是腹腔镜手术时。此外,在肥胖患者中,存在慢性心脏病和胸壁弹性增加的情况下,肺顺应性可能会进一步降低。最后,在仰卧位或头低足高位下,通常存在呼气气流受限。结果是,在全身麻醉期间,肥胖患者容易出现肺不张和分流,以及产生内源性呼气末正压(PEEPi),使肥胖患者在各种类型手术中都容易发生 PPC。

在减重和非减重腹部手术中越来越多地使用腹腔镜技术,使得这类患者的 PEEP 滴定尤其具有挑战性:由于胸壁弹性增加,在肥胖患者中,DP 和 TP 之间的差异增加,使得 C_{rs}、P_{plat} 和 DP 在监测呼吸力学方面的作用变弱。几种新兴技术,如直接测量 P_{TT}、肺超声和电阻抗成像,似乎在肥胖患者中具有前景。

25.3.1 当前的证据

对于肥胖患者,使用 RM 和武断的高 PEEP 似乎还不足以起效,在最近的 PROBESE 试验中证明了这一点,这是一项大型 RCT 研究,与标准的 5 cmH$_2$O 的 PEEP 相比,RM 外加相对高的 PEEP(12 cmH$_2$O)在非心脏手术和非神经手术术后 PPC 方面未能显示出更好的结果[11]。

再次强调,RM 后设置一个固定的高 PEEP 似乎不是正确的方法:在最近两项初步研究中,发现使用 OLA 和个体化 PEEP 比单独使用 PEEP 显示出更好的氧合和呼吸力学。在一项单中心的研究中,干预组采用 RM 外加根据电阻抗断层扫描测量出的最佳区域通气分布滴定的 PEEP,显示出更好的氧合且潮气量分布更均匀[16]。有趣的是,同一研究小组在比较个体化设置 PEEP 和低 PEEP 以及 RM 后设置 12 cmH$_2$O 的固定 PEEP 时显示了类似的结果,表明个体化设置 PEEP[中位数为 18 cmH$_2$O(因此远高于 12 cmH$_2$O)]与更好的呼吸力学和气体交换有关[17]。

另一项生理学研究采用多模式无创监测,如脉搏血氧仪、呼气末二氧化碳波形、食管压和 C_{rs} 监测,发现 RM 后个体化设置 PEEP 与 8 cmH$_2$O 的相对高 PEEP 相比,显示出更好的呼吸力学效应[18]。最后,基于 LUS 滴定 PEEP 的方法是项有前景的技术,可以进一步帮助监测肥胖患者的 MV[19]。

25.4 胸外科手术

在胸外科手术中,通常采用侧卧位进行 OLV,以便于手术操作。在这种情况下,上肺(即非重力依赖性肺)是塌陷的,而重力依赖肺则被通气。

接受 OLV 的患者由于多种因素而特别容易出现低氧血症和 PPC:首先,由于非重力依赖区肺的残余灌注,加上肺缺氧性血管收缩反射,会产生一定程度的分流;第二,这种现象可能会因合并症和麻醉药物的选择而有所不同;第三,由于全身麻醉和肋骨直接接触手术台导致胸壁顺应性降低,重力依赖区肺会出现肺不张;第四,低 V_T 的保护性通气必须根据依赖区的肺进行调整,V_T 进一步降低会增加肺不张的风险;最后,患者的合并症(如COPD、肺癌等)通常是手术指征的首要因素,通常包括一定范围的肺切除,使他们易于发生 PPC,如 LAS VEGAS 研究的事后分析所述,中高风险患者的 PPC 发生率高达48.1%,会增加住院时间[20]。

25.4.1 当前的证据

在最近的一项大型回顾性研究中,V_T 为 5 mL/kg(IBW) 和 PEEP 为 5 cmH$_2$O 的通气策略未能使 PPC 发生率降低[21],尽管有一项临床试验显示,与高 V_T 和零 PEEP 相比,低 V_T 和 5~8cmH$_2$O 的 PEEP 应用在 OLV 中显示出更好的临床结局,体现在主要的PPC 和住院时间方面[22]。这些结果强调了在 OLV 中,保护性通气的主要决定因素是设置 PEEP。如何设置 PEEP 这一关键问题目前仍不明确,尽管"最低 DP"方法似乎是合理的。Park 等将 292 名患者随机分为两组,接受常规保护性通气[6 mL/kg/(IBW),PEEP为 5 cmH$_2$O,RM]或常规保护性通气加上 OLV 期间基于最低 DP 滴定 PEEP,结果显示后者术后 PPC 更少[10]。

25.5 心脏手术

正压通气增加了平均胸内压,引起多种心脏血液动力学效应,如图 25.2 所示。右心室心输出量由于两种机制减少:其一,右心房压力增加导致前负荷降低;其二,塌陷的重力依赖区域内肺泡内血管塌陷及肺泡周围血管过度扩张导致后负荷增加。左心室前负荷最初因肺泡血管挤压增加,但最终由于右心输出量降低而降低。最后,左心室功能通常由于其跨壁压和后负荷减少而增加。这种相互作用的综合效应主要是由于右心输出量降低而导致心输出量降低。

25.5.1 当前的证据

OLA 策略在心脏手术中并不常见:首先,对于右心室功能储备不佳的患者,RM 可能会进一步恶化右心输出量;此外,心脏手术包括麻醉诱导、体外循环运转和运转结束,麻醉恢复

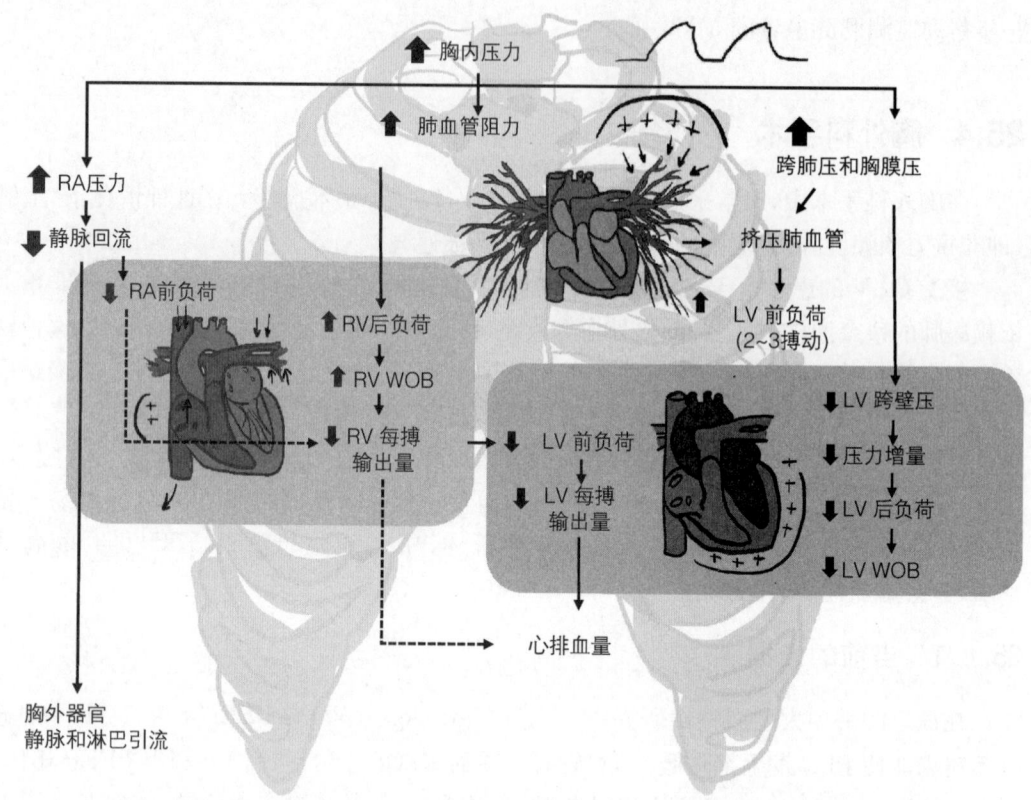

图 25.2　正压机械通气时的心肺交互作用。RA,右心房；RV,右心室；LV,左心室（见彩色插图）

三个不同阶段。这使得研究的解读变得复杂，因为不同阶段可能需要不同的通气策略。

一项小型试验显示，在暂时的血流动力学恶化后，OLA 可以通过打开肺不张中塌陷的血管来改善右心血流动力学和气体交换，提高氧合水平，从而减少缺氧性血管收缩[23]。

在体外循环期间，低潮气量、低 PEEP 的通气策略似乎能够成功减少 PPC，高 DP 是与不良结局最相关的变量[24]，而采用 OLA 的 MV 似乎无法减少 PPC，这在一项纳入近 500 名低水平 PEEP 患者的大型 RCT 中得到证实[12]。

然而，一旦体外循环期结束，OLA 策略可能会带来更好的结果。如一项小型 RCT 所示，在手术结束后进行 RM 及 $10\,cmH_2O$ PEEP 的通气策略，比 $6\,cmH_2O$ PEEP 表现出更好的右心室功能且减少了肺不张[25]，尽管患者人群的心脏基线特征相对较好。

最后，在术后期间，一种强化的 OLA 策略似乎能够减少术后低氧血症患者的 PPC[8]。

25.6　神经外科

MV 对脑内稳态的影响是脑循环、患者特征和手术类型间复杂的交互结果。脑灌注压（cerebral perfusion pressure，CPP）是平均动脉压和颅内压（intracranial pressure，

ICP)差值。根据 Monro－Kellie 理论，ICP 是由脑血流（cerebral blood flow，CBF）、脑实质和脑脊液（cerebrospinal fluid，CSF）之和所决定的。在通气期间，ICP 的改变主要是由 CBF 的变化而引起的，具体表现如下。

（1）$PaCO_2$ 水平的变化会逆向改变 CBF：如果患者出现高碳酸血症，将刺激脑血管扩张，而低碳酸血症则会引起脑血管收缩，因此直接 CO_2 监测（如呼气末 CO_2）成为这类患者通气管理的基石。

（2）低氧血症和呼吸衰竭也能强烈刺激引起脑血管扩张，尤其是当 PaO_2 低于 60 mmHg 时。

（3）PEEP 增加可能会导致颈静脉的回流减少，尤其是处于仰卧位且未倾斜头部的患者，从而导致颅内静脉淤血。

25.6.1 当前的证据

通常认为低潮气量和高 PEEP 可能会与更高的 $PaCO_2$ 和更高的 ICP 相关，并且 RM 可能通过降低 CBF 进一步恶化 CPP，使得在这类患者中，OLA 策略很少使用[26]。但是在神经重症患者中，如果 PEEP 设置在固定的较高水平（15 cmH_2O），似乎不会影响 CPP[27]。另一方面，在神经外科患者中，氧合和 PaO_2/FiO_2 是不良预后和死亡的强有力的预测指标[28]。

此外，尽管采用持续 35cmH_2O CPAP 的 RM 显著增加了硬脑膜下压力并降低了 CPP[29]，但 Nemer 等的研究[30]表明，压力递增的 RM 较经典的 CPAP 的 RM 更安全，并以可逆的方式降低 CPP，能改善蛛网膜下腔出血患者的氧合，这与创伤性脑损伤和 ARDS 患者中 OLA 的结果一致[31]。

最后，与传统的保护性 MV 相比，似乎 6 mL/kg（IBW）的低潮气量加上每 30 分钟一次的 RM 可以减少术后谵妄（并降低胶质纤维酸性蛋白水平，该蛋白是一种新型老年脊柱手术患者脑损伤的生物标志物）[32]。

25.7 总结

由于手术后 PPC 的高发生率，在麻醉期间通常需要考虑采用标准的保护性机械通气策略。

尽管缺乏更具临床意义结果的证据，如 PPC 和死亡，在某些患者人群或手术操作技术中，OLA 似乎是一种安全可行的策略，可以改善手术中的氧合水平和呼吸力学。

最后，基于一项研究事后分析的结果[33]，似乎肺开放状态而不是 OLA 本身是降低发生 PPC 风险的主要因素。因此，在手术室中提出了一个合理的通气策略，如图 25.3 所示：在麻醉诱导后，可以通过 Air－Test、LUS 检查或恶化的呼吸力学（如 C_{rs}、DP）来检测肺泡塌陷。一旦没有 RM 的禁忌证且血流动力学稳定，即可进行 RM 以达到肺泡开放压，然后通过 PEEP 递减法以找到最佳 PEEP。最后，呼吸监测将使临床医生能够检测新的肺泡塌陷并重新进行 RM。

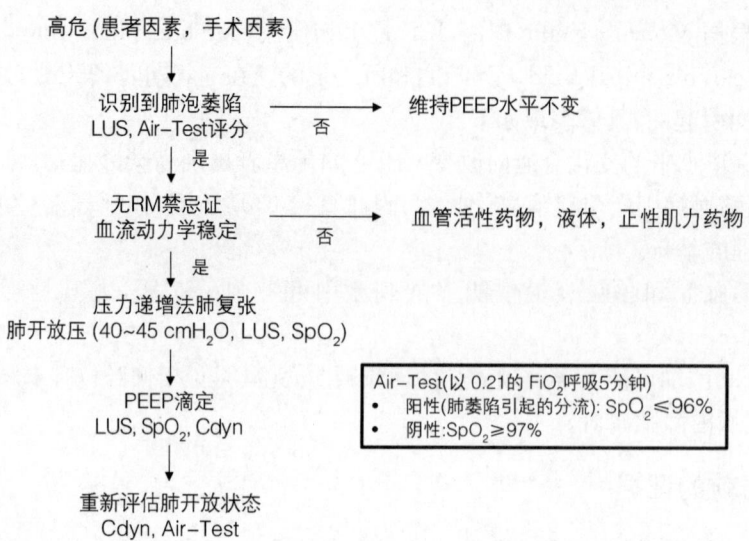

图 25.3 基于 OLA 的通气策略。LUS, 肺部超声; PEEP, 呼气末正压; Cdyn, 动态顺应性

(张媛,于晨希 译)

参考文献

[1] Canet J, Gallart L, Gomar C, Paluzie G, Vallès J, Castillo J, et al. Prediction of postoperative pulmonary complications in a population-based surgical cohort. Anesthesiology. 2010; 113(6): 1338 – 50.

[2] Abbott TEF, Fowler AJ, Pelosi P, Gama de Abreu M, Møller AM, Canet J, et al. A systematic review and consensus definitions for standardised end-points in perioperative medicine: pulmonary complications. Br J Anaesth. 2018; 120(5): 1066 – 79.

[3] Kor DJ, Warner DO, Alsara A, Fernández-Pérez ER, Malinchoc M, Kashyap R, et al. Derivation and diagnostic accuracy of the surgical lung injury prediction model. Anesthesiology. 2011; 115(1): 117 – 28.

[4] Neto AS, da Costa LGV, Hemmes SNT, Canet J, Hedenstierna G, Jaber S, et al. The LAS VEGAS risk score for prediction of postoperative pulmonary complications: an observational study. Eur J Anaesthesiol. 2018; 35(9): 691 – 701.

[5] Ferrando C, Suárez-Sipmann F, Librero J, Pozo N, Soro M, Unzueta C, et al. A noninvasive postoperative clinical score to identify patients at risk for postoperative pulmonary complications: the air-test score. Minerva Anestesiol. 2020; 86(4): 404 – 15.

[6] Futier E, Constantin JM, Paugam-Burtz C, Pascal J, Eurin M, Neuschwander A, et al. A trial of intraoperative low-tidal-volume ventilation in abdominal surgery. N Engl J Med. 2013; 369(5): 428 – 37.

[7] Karalapillai D, Weinberg L, Peyton P, Ellard L, Hu R, Pearce B, et al. Effect of intraoperative low tidal volume vs conventional tidal volume on postoperative pulmonary complications in patients undergoing major surgery: a randomized clinical trial. JAMA. 2020; 324(9): 848 – 58.

[8] Costa Leme A, Hajjar LA, Volpe MS, Fukushima JT, De Santis Santiago RR, Osawa EA, et al.

Effect of intensive vs moderate alveolar recruitment strategies added to lung-protective ventilation on postoperative pulmonary complications: a randomized clinical trial. JAMA. 2017; 317(14): 1422 - 32.

[9] Ferrando C, Soro M, Unzueta C, Suarez-Sipmann F, Canet J, Librero J, et al. Individualised perioperative open-lung approach versus standard protective ventilation in abdominal surgery (iPROVE): a randomised controlled trial. Lancet Respir Med. 2018; 6(3): 193 - 203.

[10] Park M, Ahn HJ, Kim JA, Yang M, Heo BY, Choi JW, et al. Driving pressure during thoracic surgery: a randomized clinical trial. Anesthesiology. 2019; 130(3): 385 - 93.

[11] Bluth T, Serpa Neto A, Schultz MJ, Pelosi P, Gama de Abreu M, Bobek I, et al. Effect of intraoperative high positive end-expiratory pressure (PEEP) with recruitment maneuvers vs low peep on postoperative pulmonary complications in obese patients: a randomized clinical trial. JAMA. 2019; 321(23): 2292 - 305.

[12] Lagier D, Fischer F, Fornier W, Huynh TM, Cholley B, Guinard B, et al. Effect of open-lung vs conventional perioperative ventilation strategies on postoperative pulmonary complications after on-pump cardiac surgery: the PROVECS randomized clinical trial. Intensive Care Med. 2019; 45(10): 1401 - 12.

[13] Ferrando C, Tusman G, Suarez-Sipmann F, León I, Pozo N, Carbonell J, et al. Individualized lung recruitment maneuver guided by pulse-oximetry in anesthetized patients undergoing laparoscopy: a feasibility study. Acta Anaesthesiol Scand. 2018; 62(5): 608 - 19.

[14] Andersson LE, Bååth M, Thörne A, Aspelin P, Odeberg-Wernerman S. Effect of carbon dioxide pneumoperitoneum on development of atelectasis during anesthesia, examined by spiral computed tomography. Anesthesiology. 2005; 102(2): 293 - 9.

[15] Spadaro S, Karbing DS, Mauri T, Marangoni E, Mojoli F, Valpiani G, et al. Effect of positive end-expiratory pressure on pulmonary shunt and dynamic compliance during abdominal surgery. Br J Anaesth. 2016; 116(6): 855 - 61.

[16] Nestler C, Simon P, Petroff D, Hammermüller S, Kamrath D, Wolf S, et al. Individualized positive end-expiratory pressure in obese patients during general anaesthesia: a randomized controlled clinical trial using electrical impedance tomography. Br J Anaesth. 2017; 119(6): 1194 - 205.

[17] Simon P, Girrbach F, Petroff D, Schliewe N, Hempel G, Lange M, et al. Individualized versus fixed positive end-expiratory pressure for intraoperative mechanical ventilation in obese patients: a secondary analysis. Anesthesiology. 2021; 134(6): 887 - 900.

[18] Tusman G, Acosta CM, Ochoa M, Böhm SH, Gogniat E, Martinez Arca J, et al. Multimodal non-invasive monitoring to apply an open lung approach strategy in morbidly obese patients during bariatric surgery. J Clin Monit Comput. 2020; 34(5): 1015 - 24.

[19] Elshazly M, Khair T, Bassem M, Mansour M. The use of intraoperative bedside lung ultra-sound in optimizing positive end expiratory pressure in obese patients undergoing laparo-scopic bariatric surgeries. Surg Obes Relat Dis. 2021; 17(2): 372 - 8.

[20] Uhlig C, Neto AS, van der Woude M, Kiss T, Wittenstein J, Shelley B, et al. Intraoperative mechanical ventilation practice in thoracic surgery patients and its association with postoperative pulmonary complications: results of a multicenter prospective observational study. BMC Anesthesiol. 2020; 20(1): 179.

[21] Colquhoun DA, Leis AM, Shanks AM, Mathis MR, Naik BI, Durieux ME, et al. A lower tidal volume regimen during one-lung ventilation for lung resection surgery is not associated with

reduced postoperative pulmonary complications. Anesthesiology. 2021; 134(4): 562-76.

[22] Marret E, Cinotti R, Berard L, Piriou V, Jobard J, Barrucand B, et al. Protective ventilation during anaesthesia reduces major postoperative complications after lung cancer surgery: A double-blind randomised controlled trial. Eur J Anaesthesiol. 2018; 35(10): 727-35.

[23] Reis Miranda D, Gommers D, Struijs A, Meeder H, Schepp R, Hop W, et al. The open lung concept: effects on right ventricular afterload after cardiac surgery. Br J Anaesth. 2004; 93(3): 327-32.

[24] Mathis MR, Duggal NM, Likosky DS, Haft JW, Douville NJ, Vaughn MT, et al. Intraoperative mechanical ventilation and postoperative pulmonary complications after cardiac surgery. Anesthesiology. 2019; 131(5): 1046-62.

[25] Longo S, Siri J, Acosta C, Palencia A, Echegaray A, Chiotti I, et al. Lung recruitment improves right ventricular performance after cardiopulmonary bypass: a randomised controlled trial. Eur J Anaesthesiol. 2017; 34(2): 66-74.

[26] Robba C, Hemmes SNT, Serpa Neto A, Bluth T, Canet J, Hiesmayr M, et al. Intraoperative ventilator settings and their association with postoperative pulmonary complications in neurosurgical patients: post-hoc analysis of LAS VEGAS study. BMC Anesthesiol. 2020; 20(1): 73.

[27] Nemer SN, Caldeira JB, Santos RG, Guimarães BL, Garcia JM, Prado D, et al. Effects of positive end-expiratory pressure on brain tissue oxygen pressure of severe traumatic brain injury patients with acute respiratory distress syndrome: a pilot study. J Crit Care. 2015; 30(6): 1263-6.

[28] Robba C, Asgari S, Gupta A, Badenes R, Sekhon M, Bequiri E, et al. Lung injury is a predictor of cerebral hypoxia and mortality in traumatic brain injury. Front Neurol. 2020; 11: 771.

[29] Flexman AM, Gooderham PA, Griesdale DE, Argue R, Toyota B. Effects of an alveolar recruitment maneuver on subdural pressure, brain swelling, and mean arterial pressure in patients undergoing supratentorial tumour resection: a randomized crossover study. Can J Anaesth. 2017; 64(6): 626-33.

[30] Nemer SN, Caldeira JB, Azeredo LM, Garcia JM, Silva RT, Prado D, et al. Alveolar recruitment maneuver in patients with subarachnoid hemorrhage and acute respiratory distress syndrome: a comparison of 2 approaches. J Crit Care. 2011; 26(1): 22-7.

[31] Wolf S, Plev DV, Trost HA, Lumenta CB. Open lung ventilation in neurosurgery: an update on brain tissue oxygenation. Acta Neurochir Suppl. 2005; 95: 103-5.

[32] Wang J, Zhu L, Li Y, Yin C, Hou Z, Wang Q. The potential role of lung-protective ventilation in preventing postoperative delirium in elderly patients undergoing prone spinal surgery: a preliminary study. Med Sci Monit. 2020; 26: e926526.

[33] Ferrando C, Librero J, Tusman G, Serpa-Neto A, Villar J, Belda FJ, et al. Intraoperative open-lung condition and postoperative pulmonary complications. A secondary analysis of iPROVE and iPROVE-O_2 trials. Acta Anaesthesiol Scand. 2021. https://doi.org/10.1111/aas.13979.

[34] Severgnini P, Selmo G, Lanza C, Chiesa A, Frigerio A, Bacuzzi A, et al. Protective mechanical ventilation during general anesthesia for open abdominal surgery improves postoperative pulmonary function. Anesthesiology. 2013; 118(6): 1307-21.

26 患者的长期随访

Following Up the Patients at Long Term

Nicola Latronico, Simone Piva, Frank Rasulo

26.1 引言

　　治疗重症患者需要整体评估多个器官功能,整合复杂的信息并迅速采取行动。掌握生理学和生物化学知识、热爱临床医学,熟悉有创生命支持措施和复杂监测的高级技能,以及基于献身精神、热情、同理心和同情心建立模范医患关系,是做好重症医学的关键[1]。随着对培训的不断投入和技术的持续改进,在过去 50 年中,重症医学已经实现了多种疾病短期病死率实质性的降低。然而,随着病死率的下降,重症医学界开始了解到重症疾病,以及用于器官功能支持的侵入性治疗的"遗留效应"。许多 ICU 幸存者可能会经历长期持久的健康问题,这些问题被统称为 ICU 后综合征(post-intensive care syndrome, PICS),并定义为在重症疾病后新发的或恶化的生理、心理和认知障碍,经过急性期住院治疗后仍持续存在[2]。疼痛、肌肉无力、呼吸困难、抑郁症状、焦虑和创伤后应激,以及注意力和记忆问题是患者在急性期幸存后数月乃至数年仍被常常诉说的问题[1]。PICS 的症状对幸存者的健康相关生命质量(health-related quality of life, HRQoL)和他们日常生

N. Latronico (✉) · F. Rasulo
Department of Anesthesia, Intensive Care and Emergency, Spedali Civili University Hospital, Brescia, Italy

Department of Medical and Surgical Specialties, Radiological Sciences and Public Health, University of Brescia, Brescia, Italy

"Alessandra Bono" Interdepartmental Research Center for LOng-Term Outcome (LOTO) in Survivors of Critical Illness, University of Brescia, Brescia, Italy
e-mail: nicola.latronico@unibs.it

S. Piva
Department of Anesthesia, Intensive Care and Emergency, Spedali Civili University Hospital, Brescia, Italy

Department of Medical and Surgical Specialties, Radiological Sciences and Public Health, University of Brescia, Brescia, Italy

© The Author(s), under exclusive license to Springer Nature Switzerland AG 2022
G. Bellani (ed.), *Mechanical Ventilation from Pathophysiology to Clinical Evidence*, https://doi.org/10.1007/978-3-030-93401-9_26

活行为(activities of daily living，ADL)和返回工作的能力有显著影响，与医疗资源和成本的增加相关[3,4]。事实上，ICU 社区正在意识到我们需要超越旨在减少短期病死率的急性期治疗，以减少长期持久的残疾，并改善 ICU 幸存者及其家庭的生活质量[5]。

在本章中，我们提出了一个模型，使用全面的临床方法对急性疾病幸存的患者进行随访，并分享我们在随访门诊中的长期经验。我们还回顾了 PICS 相关的临床特征、出现 ICU 后障碍的危险因素和及时检测识别的策略。

26.1.1 协助 ICU 幸存者的逻辑和文化框架

大多数关于重症疾病后长期结局的研究都是在 ARDS 幸存者中进行的。作为一种具有异常炎症反应和多器官功能障碍的急性疾病原型，ARDS 代表了一种高风险疾病，即在原发疾病治愈后发展为具有持久缺陷的疾病。我们提出，"ARDS"的"A"也应该表示"之后"，强调"需要重视早期的幸存者护理以预防 ICU 后的残疾，与治疗急性肺损伤以减少病死率一样，给予相同的优先级"[6]。然而，与其他危重疾病相比，ARDS 幸存者并未表现出特定的损伤模式[7]。此外，脓毒症[8]、ICU 获得性虚弱[9]和其他在 ICU 住院期间发生的并发症，特别是在处于持续重症状态的患者中(即 ICU 停留超过 10 天)，它们本身就会导致长期的损伤，并且在许多危重病情中普遍存在。因此，我们更倾向于将 PICS 描述为全球 ICU 幸存者的主要健康问题，而不是某个特定类别的危重症患者。

26.2 随访门诊和 PICS 框架

PICS 的症状通常被归类于躯体、认知和心理健康方面(表 26.1)。然而，随着研究的进展，已在 ICU 幸存者中发现了新状况，并被建议作为 PICS 的追加组成部分。例如，伴有吸入性肺炎和营养不良风险的吞咽障碍、导致脆性骨折风险增加的骨代谢紊乱、内分泌和代谢障碍(包括新发糖尿病、一过性皮质醇和垂体前叶激素的改变)、性功能障碍和睡眠障碍[11]。此外，常见多个症状同时存在(即存在两个或更多领域的症状)[12]。因此，临床实践中对 ICU 后患者的处理必须是多维度和多专业的(图 26.1)[13]。在英国，建议对在 ICU 住院超过 4 天且有发病风险的所有成年人进行 ICU 后综合征的评估[14]，而 2006 年的一项调查显示，在 266 个 ICU 中有 30% 提供随访门诊，其中的 55% 由护士负责[15]。只有 59% 的随访门诊得到资助，主要来自 ICU 的预算。

表 26.1 重症监护后综合征的症状分类、评估结果及工具

PICS 分类	评估结果	评估工具
躯体方面		
身体机能	• 肌肉无力 • 危重神经肌病 • 乏力	• MRC 量表，握力测试 • EMG • FSS，FACIT - F

续 表

PICS 分类	评估结果	评估工具
活动能力	• 基于表现的活动限制 • 自我报告的活动限制	• 6分钟步行测试,定时起立行走测试 • SF-36 生理功能量表
社会参与	• 参与受限	• ADL,IADL,返回工作岗位 • SF-36 生理功能量表
认知方面		
	• 主观报告认知损害 • 客观报告认知损害:筛查试验 • 客观报告认知损害:一组认知测试	• 患者及其看护者报告的认知结果 • MoCA • RBANS
心理健康领域		
	• 抑郁障碍	• HADS-抑郁障碍
	• 焦虑障碍	• HADS-焦虑障碍
	• PTSD	• DSM-5 的 PTSD 检查表,IES

评估工具列介绍了一些例子,并没有提供完整的可用的评估测试清单,更多信息请见参考文献[10](见文章内容)。MRC,医学研究委员会;EMG,肌电图;FSS,疲劳严重度评分;FACIT-F,慢性病治疗功能评估-疲劳量表;SF-36,36个项目健康状况调查问卷;ADL,日常生活活动;IADL,日常生活的工具性活动;MoCA,蒙特利尔认知评估量表;RBANS,神经心理状态评估可重复性系列测试;HADS,医院焦虑和抑郁量表;PTSD,创伤后应激障碍;IES,事件冲击量表。

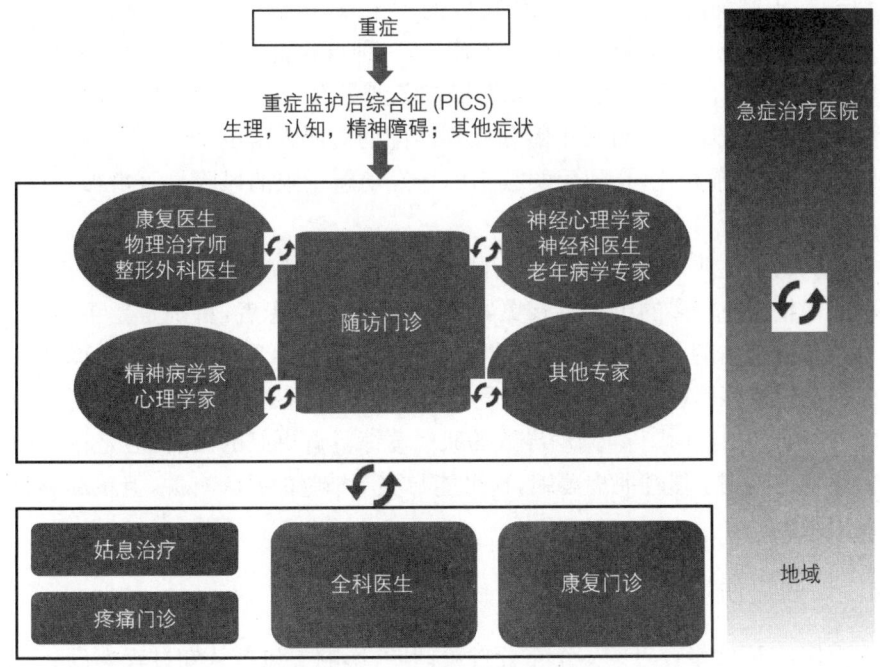

图 26.1　随访门诊与急救医院的院内外医疗专家和机构的互动

我们的随访门诊位于布雷西亚的 Spedali Civili 医院,一家大型的大学附属医院,为意大利北部的 120 万人提供服务。随访门诊建立于 2012 年,已逐渐增加到每个工作日开放,每周共 30 小时的工作时间。最初,在第 6 个月和第 12 个月对 ICU 患者进行面对面评估,后来我们增加了第 3 个月的随访,以便早期照料 COVID-19 患者。最近增加了第 24 个月的随访,延长观察期以评估对长期症状干预治疗的有效性。治疗小组由重症医生和护士组成,他们接受训练,用工具来评估 PICS 症状以及计算 ADL 和 HRQoL 量表(表 26.1)。随访门诊为患者提供直接的临床支持,负责转诊给其他专科,并作为研究 PICS 发展史和治疗干预的平台。

26.2.1 躯体损伤

实现正常的躯体功能需通过身体功能和结构层面、整个个体(活动)层面以及环境(社会环境中的完整个体)层面之间的相互作用(表 26.1)。躯体残疾往往涉及一个或多个层面的功能失调。重症相关的肌病和神经病变是身体层面结构损伤的一个例子,代表了肌肉的外周神经功能障碍,导致肌肉无力和持续的躯体障碍[16]。6 分钟步行测试表现的下降是整个个体层面功能障碍的一个例子,因为该测试评估所有步行相关系统的综合反应,包括神经肌肉单元、肌肉代谢、肺部和心血管系统、血液,也包括关节(运动范围)、大脑(本体感觉、平衡、认知)和心理(动机)。

躯体功能改变在 ICU 幸存者中很常见,患者受影响的比例从 20% 到 80% 不等。这种变异性可能是由于患者人群、评估的具体躯体层面、使用的工具和阈值,以及随访评估时间的差异[4,7,13]。躯体损伤可能会在离开 ICU 后持续数年,并且一些患者可能永远无法恢复到进入 ICU 前的状态[17]。在出 ICU 的 1 年内,几乎 40% 的内科和急诊手术 ICU 患者出现了新发的或加重的躯体问题[4]。疲劳,一种自我报告式临床结局,对生活质量有严重影响,70% 的 ARDS 幸存者在 1 年内报告了疲劳[18]。在 5 年内,ARDS 幸存者 6 分钟行走测试的中位数距离是与其年龄和性别匹配的对照人群的 76%[17]。脓毒症的老年患者住院后,与住院前相比,在随后的数年中新发功能受限的风险显著增加,没有功能受限基础的患者平均新增 1.6 个限制[8]。

在危重疾病急性期,肌肉量的丢失可以是显著的,约为肌肉总量的 15%~20%。年轻患者和肌肉量储备较多的患者将有更好的预后,但一些患者,特别是老年、有合并症的虚弱患者或急性期病情严重的患者,可能永远无法恢复到 ICU 前的状态。ICU 获得性肌肉无力是长期躯体障碍和病死率增加的危险因素[19],特别是当其由危重多发性神经病变或多发性神经肌病引起时[16]。制动导致的肌肉萎缩具有更好的预后,但是在肌肉再生能力下降的患者中出现了慢性肌肉萎缩,这可能与卫星细胞的丢失有关,卫星细胞是肌肉再生的肌肉干细胞[20]。

26.2.2 认知损伤

认知损伤是 ICU 幸存者的一个重要健康问题,影响了包括认知过程速度、记忆、注意力和执行功能在内的各种认知领域。损伤可以持续很长时间,总体认知得分在出院后 1

年仍然有所降低,并且与那些持续中度创伤性颅脑损伤或有轻度阿尔茨海默病的患者相当[21]。损伤并不仅限于老年患者或既往有认知障碍的患者,实际上在各个年龄段的人群中都有报道[21]。

对认知受损发生率的估计不太精确,6%的择期手术、11%的内科和13%的急诊手术患者在1年后表现出全面的认知功能下降。ARDS幸存者报导的认知受损发生率要高得多,为30%~46%。ARDS幸存者1年后的认知受损发生率为46%~80%,2年后为20%~47%,5年为20%[17]。这种异质性可以归因于研究的患者群体和评估的时间不同;然而,评价认知工具的类型,包括主观或客观评估、筛查测试或全面的神经心理测试,在很大程度上影响了认知障碍的检测。例如,在3个月后,患者本人或照护者报告的主观认知障碍的频率为35%(95% CI为29%~41%),用各种神经心理测试评估的客观认知障碍的频率为54%(95%CI为51%~57%)[10]。简易精神状态量表(Mini Mental State Examination, MMSE)是一种筛查测试,其检测到的认知障碍的患病率低于使用神经心理测试检测到的患病率。实际上,MMSE在检测ICU幸存者认知障碍时的敏感性非常低,康复早期的认知障碍被归类为轻度,12个月后为没有认知障碍。因此,MMSE不推荐作为筛查测试使用,而可以使用Montreal认知评估测试进行筛查[22]。关于认知筛查测试、综合的神经心理测试和主观认知障碍的更全面的讨论已经在其他地方发表[23]。谵妄、苯二氮䓬类药物的使用、脓毒症、低氧血症、ARDS和休克是ICU后认知损伤的关键风险因素[22]。首次社区获得性脓毒症患者,与脓毒症前状态相比,认知衰退速度加快了近7倍[24]。因严重脓毒症住院的老人出院数年后,中重度认知损伤的概率增加了3倍[8]。长时间的谵妄与3个月后和12个月后随访时的全面认知恶化独立相关。每日监测、恰当的预防和治疗谵妄、最小化镇静和及时治疗脓毒症不仅对于降低短期病死率,还对减轻长期认知障碍的负担至关重要。

26.2.3 心理健康受损

ICU幸存者承受着相当大的心理病理负担,包括抑郁症状、严重的普遍性焦虑和创伤后应激障碍(post-traumatic stress disorders, PTSD)。这些是ICU幸存者中很常见的问题,并且在大多数患者中,容易同时出现2个或3个不同领域的精神问题[25]。

荟萃分析中有重要临床意义的抑郁症状发生率在2~3个月时为29%(95%CI为22%~36%),6个月时为34%(95%CI为24%~43%),12~14个月时为29%(95%CI为23%~34%),症状在出ICU后的前12个月持续存在[26]。在英国进行的大型多中心关于自我报告抑郁障碍的邮寄调查中,有抑郁症状的患者在出ICU后的前2年病死率比无抑郁症状的患者高47%[25]。ARDS幸存者既往的抑郁障碍和心理困扰与ICU后持续心理疾病的风险密切相关[27]。相反,性别和年龄与ICU后抑郁症状的出现没有一致的关联,不同于总体人群,女性和40~59岁的人更容易出现抑郁症状。疾病的严重程度和ICU入住时间也与抑郁障碍无关。这意味着筛查计划应该包含大范围ICU幸存者群体,包括所有性别、各个年龄段和各种临床严重程度[26]。抑郁症状更常表现为躯体症状(即身体上的抱怨,如疼痛、身体功能限制、头晕、心悸、疲劳),而不是认知-情感症状(即与思维和情绪有关的抱怨)[28]。躯体型抑郁症状可能对精神药物治疗起部分反应[28],因此患者可能无法完全缓解,从而降低了他们对治疗的依从性,增加了早期复发、疾病加重和慢性化的风险。"给患者一颗药片"是对于一个复杂问题的过于简单化的解决方案。相反,应该跨学科进行躯体和职业康复治疗、充分的疼痛和其他躯体症状的治疗、适当地将心理压力和社会经济限制一并考量,结合精神科会诊和抗抑郁药物治疗,以实现最佳的照护。

荟萃分析显示,焦虑障碍的患病率在2~3个月时为32%(95%CI为27%~38%),6个月时为40%(95%CI为33%~46%),12~14个月时为34%(95%CI为25%~42%)[29]。重复评估相同人群的纵向研究表明,在出院后的第一年中,焦虑严重程度或患病率并没有显著变化[29]。与抑郁障碍一样,年龄和性别与焦虑障碍无关。而与总体人群相对比,焦虑障碍更常见于女性和30~44岁的患者。疾病的严重程度、ICU入住时间和ICU入院诊断也与焦虑障碍无关。在ARDS中,急性疾病发作前的既往心理障碍与ICU后持续焦虑和抑郁障碍有强烈的关联[27]。

PTSD属于《精神疾病诊断与统计手册》(*Diagnostic and Statistical Manual of Mental Disorders*)(DSM-5)中的"创伤和应激相关障碍"类别,是暴露于灾难性事件后最常见的精神病理后果[30]。诊断标准包括直接接触或目睹实际或威胁性死亡、严重伤害或性暴力,侵入症状,持续回避刺激,认知和心境的负面改变,以及唤醒与反应性严重改变,伴随着睡眠障碍和与创伤事件相关的过度警觉。持续时间往往超过1个月并导致显著的痛苦或严重的功能受损。在ICU幸存者中,22%~24%的患者在出ICU后的12个月内出现严重的PTSD症状,并且HRQoL量表的分值显著降低。既往的心理疾病、苯二氮䓬镇静和痛苦ICU经历的早期记忆与PTSD有关。值得注意的是,疾病的严重程度、入院诊断、机械通气和ICU入住时间与PTSD并无必然关联。与苯二氮䓬的关联可能是假的,这可能反映了严重焦虑的ICU患者对抗焦虑药物需求的增加;然而,这再次强调了需要谨慎使用苯二氮䓬和其他镇静药物以避免深度镇静。

26.3 总结

PICS是ICU幸存者及其家庭所面临的主要健康问题,对患者的生活质量和整个社会产生了巨大影响。随着过去几十年观察到的ICU病死率降低,预计存活患者的数量将会增加,同时存活患者中伴随长期躯体功能、认知和心理健康障碍的数量也将增加[31]。影响危重疾病幸存患者的症状和体征在不断更新,很可能不久以后需要拓宽PICS的定义以涵盖新的情况。重症医学界应该将此作为一项重要的优先事项,培养新一代的重症监护医生,不仅能拯救生命,还要能够负责处理PICS。

(张媛,于晨希 译)

参考文献

[1] Sprung CL, Cohen R, Marini JJ. The top attributes of excellence of intensive care physicians.

Intensive Care Med. 2015; 41(2): 312-4.

[2] Needham DM, Davidson J, Cohen H, Hopkins RO, Weinert C, Wunsch H, et al. Improving long-term outcomes after discharge from intensive care unit: report from a stakeholders' conference. Crit Care Med. 2012; 40(2): 502-9.

[3] Study AC. Annals of internal medicine article one-year trajectories of care and resource utilization for recipients of prolonged mechanical ventilation. 2010.

[4] Geense WW, Zegers M, Peters MAA, Ewalds E, Simons KS, Vermeulen H, et al. New physical, mental, and cognitive problems 1-year post-ICU: a prospective multicenter study. Am J Respir Crit Care Med. 2021; 203(12): 1512-21.

[5] Stevens RD, Hart N, Herridge MS. Textbook of post-ICU medicine: the legacy of critical care. 1st ed. Oxford: Oxford University Press; 2014.

[6] Latronico N, Minelli C, Eikermann M. Prediction of long-term outcome subtypes in ARDS: first steps towards personalised medicine in critical care. Thorax. 2017; 72(12): 1067-8.

[7] Bein T, Weber-Carstens S, Apfelbacher C. Long-term outcome after the acute respiratory distress syndrome: different from general critical illness? Curr Opin Crit Care. 2018; 24(1): 35-40.

[8] Iwashyna TJ, Ely EW, Smith DM, Langa KM. Long-term cognitive impairment and functional disability among survivors of severe sepsis. JAMA. 2010; 304(16): 1787-94.

[9] Latronico N, Herridge M, Hopkins RO, Angus D, Hart N, Hermans G, et al. The ICM research agenda on intensive care unit-acquired weakness. Intensive Care Med. 2017; 43(9): 1270-81.

[10] Honarmand K, Lalli RS, Priestap F, Chen JL, McIntyre CW, Owen AM, et al. Natural history of cognitive impairment in critical illness survivors. A systematic review. Am J Respir Crit Care Med. 2020; 202(2): 193-201.

[11] Rousseau A-F, Prescott HC, Brett SJ, Weiss B, Azoulay E, Creteur J, et al. Long-term outcomes after critical illness: recent insights. Crit Care. 2021; 25(1): 108.

[12] Marra A, Pandharipande PP, Girard TD, Patel MB, Hughes CG, Jackson JC, et al. Co-occurrence of post-intensive care syndrome problems among 406 survivors of critical illness. Crit Care Med. 2018; 46(9): 1393-401.

[13] Rasulo FA, Piva S, Latronico N. Long-term complications of COVID-19 in ICU survivors: what do we know? Minerva Anestesiol. 2021. https://doi.org/10.23736/S0375-9393.21.16032-8.

[14] National Institute for Health and Clinical Excellence. Rehabilitation after critical illness. London: National Institute for Health and Clinical Excellence; 2017.

[15] Griffiths JA, Barber VS, Cuthbertson BH, Young JD. A national survey of intensive care follow-up clinics. Anaesthesia. 2006; 61(10): 950-5.

[16] Latronico N, Bolton CF. Critical illness polyneuropathy and myopathy: a major cause of muscle weakness and paralysis. Lancet Neurol. 2011; 10(10): 931-41.

[17] Herridge MS, Tansey CM, Matté A, Tomlinson G, Diaz-Granados N, Cooper A, et al. Functional disability 5 years after acute respiratory distress syndrome. N Engl J Med. 2011; 364(14): 1293-304.

[18] Neufeld KJ, Leoutsakos J-MS, Yan H, Lin S, Zabinski JS, Dinglas VD, et al. Fatigue symptoms during the first year following ARDS. Chest. 2020; 158(3): 999-1007.

[19] Vanhorebeek I, Latronico N, Van den Berghe G. ICU-acquired weakness. Intensive Care Med. 2020; 46(4): 637-53.

[20] Dos Santos C, Hussain SNA, Mathur S, Picard M, Herridge M, Correa J, et al. Mechanisms of

chronic muscle wasting and dysfunction after an intensive care unit stay: a pilot study. Am J Respir Crit Care Med. 2016; 194(7): 821-30.

[21] Pandharipande PP, Girard TD, Jackson JC, Morandi A, Thompson JL, Pun BT, et al. Long-term cognitive impairment after critical illness. N Engl J Med. 2013; 369(14): 1306-16.

[22] Mikkelsen ME, Still M, Anderson BJ, Bienvenu OJ, Brodsky MB, Brummel N, et al. Society of Critical Care Medicine's International Consensus Conference on prediction and identification of long-term impairments after critical illness. Crit Care Med. 2020; 48(11): 1670-9.

[23] Roebuck-Spencer TM, Glen T, Puente AE, Denney RL, Ruff RM, Hostetter G, et al. Cognitive screening tests versus comprehensive neuropsychological test batteries: a national academy of neuropsychology education paper. Arch Clin Neuropsychol. 2017; 32(4): 491-8.

[24] Wang HE, Kabeto MM, Gray M, Wadley VG, Muntner P, Judd SE, et al. Trajectory of cognitive decline after sepsis. Crit Care Med. 2021; 49(7): 1083-94.

[25] Hatch R, Young D, Barber V, Griffiths J, Harrison DA, Watkinson P. Anxiety, depression and post traumatic stress disorder after critical illness: a UK-wide prospective cohort study. Crit Care. 2018; 22(1): 310.

[26] Rabiee A, Nikayin S, Hashem MD, Huang M, Dinglas VD, Bienvenu OJ, et al. Depressive symptoms after critical illness: a systematic review and meta-analysis. Crit Care Med. 2016; 44(9): 1744-53.

[27] Bienvenu OJ, Friedman LA, Colantuoni E, Dinglas VD, Sepulveda KA, Mendez-Tellez P, et al. Psychiatric symptoms after acute respiratory distress syndrome: a 5-year longitudinal study. Intensive Care Med. 2018; 44(1): 38-47.

[28] Jackson JC, Pandharipande PP, Girard TD, Brummel NE, Thompson JL, Hughes CG, et al. Depression, post-traumatic stress disorder, and functional disability in survivors of critical illness in the BRAIN-ICU study: a longitudinal cohort study. Lancet Respir Med. 2014; 2(5): 369-79.

[29] Nikayin S, Rabiee A, Hashem MD, Huang M, Bienvenu OJ, Turnbull AE, et al. Anxiety symptoms in survivors of critical illness: a systematic review and meta-analysis. Gen Hosp Psychiatry. 2016; 43: 23-9.

[30] Shalev A, Liberzon I, Marmar C. Post-traumatic stress disorder. N Engl J Med. 2017; 376(25): 2459-69.

[31] Latronico N, Peli E, Calza S, Rodella F, Novelli MP, Cella A, et al. Physical cognitive and mental health outcomes in 1-year survivors of COVID-19-associated ARDS. Thorax. thoraxjnl-2021-218064. https://doi.org/10.1136/thoraxjnl-2021-218064.

27 有限资源环境下的机械通气

Mechanical Ventilation in Limited Resource Settings

Theogene Twagirumugabe

27.1 引言

尽管面临不同的挑战,对在资源匮乏的 ICU 中机械通气危重症患者的管理,与在资源充分的环境中一样至关重要。在资源有限的条件下,机械通气主要用于各种原因引起的呼吸衰竭、意识水平降低的患者的气道保护,以及循环衰竭(旨在维持重要器官的功能)。不幸的是,在资源匮乏的环境下,不是所有设计用于 ICU 的区域和床位都配备了功能完备的呼吸机。因此,在低资源国家,接受机械通气的患者比例变化取决于呼吸机可获得性的差异,以及入院患者的组成或引起入院的疾病的严重程度[1-4]。

在资源匮乏的 ICU 中,获得机械通气可能有助于降低危重症患者的病死率,尽管如果不满足所有先决条件,干预措施可能会因为并发症带来损害。在资源匮乏国家有关机械通气操作和接受机械通气患者结局的证据很少。本章旨在揭示这些环境中有限的现有证据,并描述这些环境下的机械通气实践状态。

27.2 有限资源环境下的机械通气设施

在资源有限的医院中,本已有限的 ICU 床位因为缺乏适当管理危重症患者所需的关键设备,包括呼吸机,而更加受限。值得注意的是,在这些环境中,不到 50% 的可用 ICU 床位配备有呼吸机。2020 年,在非洲进行的一项调查中,受访结果显示每 10 万人平均有 3.1 个 ICU 床位,远低于高收入国家每 10 万人平均 12.79 个 ICU 床位,而像美国和意大

T. Twagirumugabe (✉)
University of Rwanda, College of Medicine and Health Sciences, Kigali, Rwanda
University Teaching Hospital of Butare, Huye, Rwanda
e-mail: twagirumugabe@chub.rw

© The Author(s), under exclusive license to Springer Nature Switzerland AG 2022
G. Bellani (ed.), *Mechanical Ventilation from Pathophysiology to Clinical Evidence*, https://doi.org/10.1007/978-3-030-93401-9_27

利这样的国家甚至每 10 万人拥有超过 25 个 ICU 床位[5]。此外,在非洲,并不是所有的 ICU 床位都配有呼吸机。据估计,每 10 万人配备的呼吸机数量为 0.97 个。这个差距在非洲的低收入国家中更为显著,每 10 万人只有 0.53 个 ICU 床位和 0.14 个呼吸机,而非洲的中高收入国家相应的呼吸机数量为每 10 万人 2.49 个,并且现有的呼吸机主要集中在城市,使得偏远和农村地区几乎没有任何办法来治疗这些有需求的患者[1,2]。在资源有限的环境中,呼吸支持的限制可能会对三级医院或转诊医疗机构产生更加负面的影响,因为将近 80% 入住 ICU 的患者可能需要进行机械通气[4]。这给医疗服务提供者带来了一个伦理挑战,即选择谁应该被收治和进行机械通气。在具备救治重症患者资质人员严重缺乏的环境中,这对工作人员是一种心理负担。由于有效利用呼吸机所需的必要基础设施,如持续不间断的电力和足够的供氧系统常常不稳定,因此这种复杂性进一步加剧[6,7]。

呼吸机数量和 ICU 床位数间的差距是资源有限国家长期存在的现实,这在 COVID-19 大流行期间变得更加显著。一些制造业公司与西方大学合作,启动了以设计和制造出经济实惠且易于使用的呼吸机的项目,也可用于资源有限的环境。然而,这个难题的重要部分似乎被忽视了,或者至少没有得到适当的关注[8-10],即包括足够的氧气生产(或供应)、对工程师的培训使其掌握对这些呼吸机的维护,以及对终端用户的正式培训。事实上,在 2010 年由世界卫生组织在 12 个西非和东非国家进行的一项调查中,只有 43% 的卫生设施能够获得氧气,氧气仅由氧气钢瓶或制氧机供应,并且只有三分之一被调查的设备配备不间断的电力[11]。这种情况在 10 年后也没有太大的变化,正如在 COVID-19 大流行期间所证明的那样[10]。

27.3　资源可变环境下机械通气的适应证

与世界其他地区类似,资源有限的 ICU 中,入院的主要原因和机械通气适应证是脓毒症和脓毒症休克、创伤、中毒、术后恢复和围产期并发症,但在不同的环境中存在一些差异[3,12,13]。由于难以达到诊断标准,急性呼吸衰竭的极端表现,也就是急性呼吸窘迫综合征(acute respiratory distress syndrome, ARDS),长期以来一直被忽视,但通过使用 Kigali 修改的 ARDS 柏林定义(表 27.1),已经表明 ARDS 在有限资源环境中也存在,其占比与充分资源环境中相似[14,15]。然而,鉴于床位数量有限,只有三分之一的 ARDS(或高度怀疑为 ARDS 的)患者可以被收治到 ICU 中[14]。人们也许会认为,由于缺乏对此状况的认识,ARDS 患者可能无法从适当的治疗中受益,特别是在呼吸机参数设置方面,这可能会对患者造成伤害并增加其病死率。

表 27.1　基于 ARDS 柏林定义的 Kigali 修订版[14]

	柏 林 定 义	基于柏林定义的 Kigali 修订版
发病时机	已知诱因的、新出现的或原有呼吸系统症状加重后一周内发病	已知诱因的、新出现的或原有呼吸系统症状加重后一周内发病

	柏 林 定 义	基于柏林定义的 Kigali 修订版
氧合	$PaO_2/FiO_2 \leqslant 300$	$SpO_2/FiO_2 \leqslant 315$
PEEP 需求	有创机械通气条件下最小 5 cmH_2O 的 PEEP（轻度 ARDS 可以用无创通气）	不需要 PEEP
肺部影像学	双肺透亮度减低，且不能完全用胸腔积液、肺叶不张或结节解释，通过胸部 X 线摄影或 CT 观察	双肺透亮度减低，且不能完全用胸腔积液、肺叶不张或结节解释，通过胸部 X 线摄影或 CT 观察
肺水肿的来源	无法用心脏衰竭或液体负荷过多解释的呼吸衰竭（如果没有危险因素，则需要客观评估，如心脏超声，排除静水压升高的肺水肿）	无法用心脏衰竭或液体负荷过多解释的呼吸衰竭（如果没有危险因素，则需要客观评估，如心脏超声，排除静水压升高的肺水肿）

PEEP，呼气末正压；SpO_2，脉搏氧饱和度；PaO_2，由血气测定的动脉氧分压；FiO_2，吸入氧浓度；CT，计算机断层扫描。

27.4 资源有限环境下的机械通气模式

考虑到机械通气的适应证，相对于不需要气管插管的无创通气（non-invasive ventilation, NIV），通过气管插管进行的经典有创机械通气（invasive mechanical ventilation, IMV）在资源有限环境中可能是最常用的通气方式[3,12,13]。然而，有创通气在技术上需要更多的资源，需要镇静，还需要有经验的麻醉提供者进行气管插管，并预见可能发生的心肺并发症，这些并发症可能会在约 40% 的病例中发生[16]。因此，在资源有限的机构中，IMV 可能会与通气患者的病死率增加相关，但缺乏设计良好（考虑患者病情严重程度以允许客观比较并确定可归因病死率）的研究。有时 IMV 的高病死率会被用作支持在低资源环境中使用 NIV（作为安全的呼吸支持替代方案）的论据，但并非所有患者都符合条件[17]。

NIV 确实是令人感兴趣的选择，因为它可以避免由气管插管引起的潜在并发症。此外，当决定开始 IMV 时，NIV 也可以是预防气管插管相关并发症的一种方式，可以用于预充氧。选择适当的患者，如急性心源性肺水肿和（或）COPD 急性加重导致急性呼吸窘迫，在这些情况下 NIV 是单独而有效的呼吸支持选项[18]。NIV 也被评估是否可用于 ARDS 患者在诊断后 48 小时内的管理，但随着低氧血症的严重程度增加，其失败率也增加，并且 NIV 模式治疗的重度 ARDS 患者的 ICU 死亡风险显著增加[19]。

在资源有限环境中，NIV 的适应证和结果都不为人知。然而，不同的研究报告了这些环境中 NIV 设施和设备的可用性，但主要来自大学附属医院[20,21]。除全脸面罩外，其他设备（如鼻罩、头罩和高流量鼻导管）基本上在资源有限环境中没有记录。这些环境中 NIV 使用的相关证据仅限于在新生儿和小儿患者中使用的基本气泡式低流量 CPAP，该技术似乎带来了更好的结果[22,23]。对于资源有限环境中其他 NIV 模式或接口的使用经验及其优于 IMV 的报告很少（如果有的话）。

27.5 资源有限环境下的机械通气并发症

NIV 或范围更大的 IMV 可因各种并发症而增加负担。呼吸机相关的并发症或事件可以被认为是 MV 治疗质量的可靠指标。事实上,根据患者异常的肺部力学,适当设置呼吸机参数,可以避免大多数并发症。呼吸机相关肺损伤(ventilator-induced lung injury,VILI)是一种已经被理解得很好的并发症,可能是患者自主呼吸与呼吸机不匹配和(或)呼吸机的参数设置不适合需要呼吸支持的病理生理模式所致。由于 ICU 中缺乏熟练的工作人员,在资源有限环境中 VILI 可能变得更为重要。VILI 可源自不同的机制,如容积伤、气压伤、肺萎陷伤或生物性损伤,在低资源环境很重要,然而关于它的发生率、发病机制和对患者结果的影响的证据仍然很少被探索和报道[24]。

VILI 可以通过应用肺保护性通气来限制,包括低潮气量、限制平台压和最佳的 PEEP,但在资源有限环境中的依从性是未知的。然而,一项在 10 个亚洲中等收入国家的 ICU 进行的研究揭示,这些环境中最佳实践的依从性达到中等至良好的水平[21]。在低资源国家的 ICU 中,如非洲,对这种策略的低依从性是否是造成通气患者更高的并发症发生率和病死率的原因尚不清楚[13]。

除 VILI 外,MV 的另一个严重且最普遍的并发症是呼吸机相关性肺炎(ventilator-associated pneumonia,VAP)。机械通气患者的 VAP 发病率随通气时间的延长而增加,而在低资源环境中,VAP 更为普遍,几乎达到每 1 000 呼吸机日 116 例,而且在撒哈拉以南的非洲国家,这种发病率更高[25,26]。VAP 会给通气患者带来更高的死亡负担,特别是当涉及多重耐药微生物时,尤其是在这些微生物对碳青霉烯类耐药时[26,27]。

这些高 VAP 发病率背后的原因之一是中等收入国家对"呼吸机集束化策略"(有助于减少 VAP 的发生率)的依从性不高[21],低收入国家可能也是如此,但缺乏数据。

减少 VAP 发生率的另一种策略,从缩短机械通气持续时间的角度出发,依赖于预防性气管切开术,这可以实现恰当的口腔卫生、经口喂养,并避免持续的喉部创伤。

27.6 长期机械通气患者气管切开的实践

在机械通气第一周结束时进行早期气管切开可能会缩短机械通气时间、住院时间,并可能减少 VAP 的发病率。然而,对 ICU 和住院病死率的影响仍不清楚[28]。

有关低资源环境的 ICU 中长期机械通气患者实施气管切开的现有数据显示,绝大多数为晚期的气管切开,术后并发症的发生率高,40% 的病例发生气管狭窄,对 ICU 和住院病死率没有影响[29,30]。

27.7 总结

在资源有限的环境中,机械通气的实践主要依赖于 IMV,但在大学附属医院中,有一些 NIV 设施可用，尽管这种方法主要是在儿童中应用气泡式 CPAP。

即使机械通气的适应证可能与资源充分的国家不同，但在资源有限环境中也存在 ARDS 患者（或有 ARDS 风险）。对这些患者肺保护策略的依从性在中等收入国家是中等到良好的水平，但在低资源国家中没有记录。

资源有限环境中机械通气很复杂，并发 VAP 的发生率很高，长期机械通气的患者常在晚期接受气管切开手术，而在拔管后气管狭窄的发生率很高。

（张媛，于晨希 译）

参考文献

[1] Murthy S, Leligdowicz A, Adhikari NK. Intensive care unit capacity in low-income countries: a systematic review. PLoS One. 2015; 10(1): e0116949.

[2] Craig J, Kalanxhi E, Hauck S. National estimates of critical care capacity in 54 African countries. medRxiv. 2020. https://doi.org/10.1101/2020.05.13.20100727.

[3] Dünser MW, Towey RM, Amito J, Mer M. Intensive care medicine in rural sub-Saharan Africa. Anaesthesia. 2017; 72(2): 181-9. https://doi.org/10.1111/anae.13710.

[4] Riviello ED, Kiviri W, Fowler RA, Mueller A, Novack V, et al. Predicting mortality in low-income country ICUs: the Rwanda mortality probability model (R-MPM). PLoS One. 2016; 11(5): 0155858. https://doi.org/10.1371/journal.pone.0155858.

[5] Sen-Crowe B, Sutherland M, McKenney M, Elkbuli A. A closer look into global hospital beds capacity and resource shortages during the COVID-19 pandemic. J Surg Res. 2021; 260: 56-63.

[6] Kershaw C, Williams M, Kilaru S, Zash R, Kalenga K, Masole F, et al. Audit of early mortality among patients admitted to the general medical ward at a district Hospital in Botswana. Ann Glob Health. 2019; 85(1): 1354. https://doi.org/10.5334/aogh.1354.

[7] Murthy S, Adhikari NK. Global health care of the critically ill in low-resource settings. Ann Am Thorac Soc. 2013; 10(5): 509-13. https://doi.org/10.1513/AnnalsATS.201307-246OT.

[8] Mantena S, Rogo K, Burke TF. Re-examining the race to send ventilators to low-resource settings. Respir Care. 2020; 65(9): 1378-81. https://doi.org/10.4187/respcare.08185.

[9] Madzimbamuto F. Ventilators are not the answer in Africa. Afr J Prm Health Care Fam Med. 2020; 12(1): a2517. https://doi.org/10.4102/phcfm.

[10] Navuluri N, Sour ML, Kussin P, Murdoch DM, MacIntyre NR, Que LG, et al. Oxygen delivery systems for adults in Sub-Saharan Africa: a scoping review. J Glob Health. 2021; 11: 04019. https://doi.org/10.7189/jogh.11.04019.

[11] Belle J, Cohen H, Shindo N, Lim M, Verazquez-Berumen A, N'dihokubwayo JB, et al. Influenza preparedness in lowresource settings: a look at oxygen delivery in 12 African countries. J Infect Dev Ctries. 2010; 4(7): 419-24.

[12] Adhikari NKFR, Bhagwanjee S, Rubenfeld GD. Critical care and the global burden of critical illness in adults. Lancet. 2010; 376(9749): 1339-46.

[13] Parker RK, Mwachiro EB, Mwachiro MM, Pletcher J, Parker AS, Many HR. Mortality prediction in rural Kenya: a cohort study of mechanical ventilation in critically ill patients. Crit Care Explorat. 2019; 1: 12.

[14] Riviello ED, Kiviri W, Twagirumugabe T, Mueller A, Banner-Goodspeed VM, Officer L, et al.

Hospital incidence and outcomes of the acute respiratory distress syndrome using the Kigali modification of the berlin definition. Am J Respir Crit Care Med. 2016; 193(1): 52-9.

[15] Riviello ED, Pisani L, Schultz MJ. What's new in ARDS: ARDS also exists in resource-constrained settings. Intensive Care Med. 2016; 42(5): 794-6.

[16] Simpson GD, Ross MJ, McKeown DW, Ray DC. Tracheal intubation in the critically ill: a multi-centre national study of practice and complications. Br J Anaesth. 2012; 108(5): 792-9. https://doi.org/10.1093/bja/aer504.

[17] Inglis R, Ayebale E, Schultz MJ. Optimizing respiratory management in resource-limited settings. Curr Opin Crit Care. 2019; 25(1): 45-53. https://doi.org/10.1097/mcc.0000000000000568.

[18] Rochwerg B, Brochard L, Elliott MW, Hess D, Hill NS, Nava S, et al. Official ERS/ATS clinical practice guidelines: noninvasive ventilation for acute respiratory failure. Eur Respir J. 2017; 50: 2.

[19] Bellani G, Laffey JG, Pham T, Madotto F, Fan E, Brochard L, et al. Noninvasive ventilation of patients with acute respiratory distress syndrome. Insights from the LUNG SAFE Study. Am J Respir Crit Care Med. 2017; 195(1): 67-77.

[20] Vincent J-L, Sakr Y, Singer M, Martin-Loeches I, Machado FR, Marshall JC, et al. Prevalence and outcomes of infection among patients in intensive care units in 2017. JAMA. 2020; 323: 15.

[21] Pisani L, Algera AG, Serpa Neto A, Ahsan A, Beane A, Chittawatanarat K, et al. Epidemiological characteristics, ventilator management, and clinical outcome in patients receiving invasive ventilation in intensive care units from 10 Asian middle-income countries (PRoVENT-iMiC): an international, multicenter, prospective study. Am J Trop Med Hyg. 2021; 104(3): 1022-33.

[22] Baud O, Kawaza K, Machen HE, Brown J, Mwanza Z, Iniguez S, et al. Efficacy of a low-cost bubble CPAP system in treatment of respiratory distress in a neonatal ward in Malawi. PLoS ONE. 2014; 9: 1.

[23] Hansmann A, Morrow BM, Lang H-J. Review of supplemental oxygen and respiratory support for paediatric emergency care in sub-Saharan Africa. Afr J Emerg Med. 2017; 7: 10.

[24] Saini PC, Atina J. Ventilator induced lung injury (VILI) in acute respiratory distress syndrome (ARDS). "barotrauma" to "biotrauma": case report. East Afr Med J. 2017; 94(5): 391-7.

[25] Magira E, Kharel S, Bist A, Mishra SK. Ventilator-associated pneumonia among ICU patients in WHO Southeast Asian region: a systematic review. PLoS One. 2021; 16: 3.

[26] Waweru-Siika W, Chokwe TM. Ventilator-associated pneumonia in critically ill African patients on stress ulcer prophylaxis. East Afr Med J. 2015; 92(1): 1-5.

[27] Crivellari M, Bento Talizin T, de Maio D, Carrilho CM, Grion MC, Tibery Queiroz Cardoso L, Toshiyuki Tanita M, et al. Polymyxin for treatment of ventilator-associated pneumonia in a setting of high carbapenem resistance. PLoS One. 2020; 15: 8.

[28] Terragni PP, Antonelli M, Fumagalli R, Faggiano C, Berardino M, Pallavicini FB, et al. Early versus late tracheotomy for prevention of pneumonia in mechanically ventilated adult ICU patients a randomized controlled trial. JAMA. 2010; 303(15): 1483-9.

[29] Prin M, Kaizer A, Cardenas J, Mtalimanja O, Kadyaudzu C, Charles A, et al. Tracheostomy practices for mechanically ventilated patients in Malawi. World J Surg. 2021; 45(9): 2638-42.

[30] Khazbak A, Maaty A, Shawadfy M, El-Anwar M, Nofal A. Tracheostomy in the intensive care unit: a university hospital in a developing country study. Int Arch Otorhinolaryngol. 2016; 21(1): 33-7.

28 患者转运期间的机械通气

Mechanical Ventilation During Patient's Transferral

Susan Wilcox, Raymond Che

28.1 概述

机械通气患者的转运是一个需要大量的准备工作、熟练的转运人员且伴有一定不良事件风险的复杂过程[1-6]。其中，对患者临床状态的维持，或是改善，需要转运及接收机构投入大量的资源[7]。因此，转运的获益必须超过其风险[3,4,7,8]。除了对风险因素进行识别以外，与具有高技能的临床医生共同进行转运可以减少不良事件的发生[1-11]。虽然认识到医院内部及医院之间转运的差异很重要，但本章的原则可以适用于以上两种情况。

28.2 转运对患者生理的影响

在转运过程中，主要存在三种机制影响患者的生理状况。第一种机制是包括床位的转运、位置的改变以及加速/减速在内的患者移动。低氧性呼吸衰竭患者可能存在不稳定的通气/灌注（ventilation/perfusion，V/Q）匹配，通常伴有大面积的分流。移动可导致血流重新分配到通气不良的区域，从而改变了基于缺氧性血管收缩的匹配，进而导致血氧饱和度下降。事实上，28％的低氧性呼吸衰竭患者在转运过程中表现出血氧饱和度的下降[12]。

第二种机制涉及患者支持的任何突然变化，如短期停泵或更换为转运呼吸机。即使是微小的环境变化也可能使患者应激和不适[2]。临床医生可以通过良好的实践将这些变化的影响最小化,如确保药物已经准备好可以进行更换,或在更换转运呼吸机前设置好呼吸机等。考虑到典型的转运患者群体已经处于院内死亡的高风险状态,临床医生应尽量减少这些因素,从而减少转运期间的生理损害[9]。

最后,如果患者采用空中运输,大气压力的变化可能会影响其氧合。随着海拔高度的增加,氧分压逐渐降低,进而导致氧气扩散至肺泡所需的分压差减少。在海拔10 000英尺(3 048米)时,氧饱和度将由在海平面的98%降至87%[13]。此外,氧分压的降低会导致每次呼吸吸入的氧分子减少。因此,在海拔8 000英尺(2 438米)处呼吸的环境空气相当于在海平面上呼吸15%浓度的氧气。

在大约8 000英尺的高度时,固定翼运输机通常会对机舱加压。然而,直升机通常不会加压。没有基础呼吸衰竭的患者,在直升机中通常不会出现显著的临床变化。然而,已经出现低氧血症的患者,可能会出现显著的病情恶化。

此外,Boyle's定律指出,气体的体积与其所受压力成反比。大气压力随着海拔高度的增加而降低,导致气体膨胀,这可能导致气胸的扩大和由于肠道气体膨胀所致的功能残气量减少。

28.3 设置转运呼吸机

尽管转运呼吸机各不相同,但大多数的型号允许类似于ICU呼吸机的参数设置和监测。作为重症监护转运的目标,即保持治疗等同于或甚至高于转出机构的水平,呼吸机应提供所有的常见模式,包括辅助控制-容量控制通气或压力控制通气、压力支持和任何其他不同区域所使用的模式。所有转运呼吸机都能提供呼气末正压(positive end-expiratory pressure, PEEP),尽管许多机器都限制于20 cmH$_2$O或22 cmH$_2$O的水平;可以调整吸入氧浓度,并根据模式设置呼吸频率;可以监测吸气峰压(peak inspiratory pressure, PIP),测量平台压的功能因品牌而异。大多数呼吸机也可以监测内源性PEEP。

肺保护性、低潮气量、低压策略适用于大多数患者[8]。虽然缺乏转运中呼吸机管理的试验,但已发现运输中的潮气量影响接收急诊科和重症监护室的潮气量[14]。在大多数情况下,以预测体重的6 mL/kg为目标设置潮气量和小于15 cmH$_2$O的驱动压较为合适。PEEP可以通过氧合及患者的顺应性进行滴定。考虑到运输的不稳定性,可能需要增加患者的FiO$_2$。滴定设置由团队自行决定。然而,5%~32%的患者使用了不恰当的呼吸机设置[2,11]。转运团队有机会通过适当降低潮气量、增加PEEP和增加FiO$_2$来积极影响通气设置。然而,为实现这一点,工作人员必须接受培训并且准备好在途中进行正确的呼吸机调整。

28.4 肺部和气道并发症

低氧血症是转运过程中最常见的并发症,影响高达29%的转运患者[1],主要归因于由于移动产生的分泌物、患者体位的变化或 PEEP 的丧失[2,5]。这些移动产生的效应可能导致转运期间肺不张的风险增加三倍[4]。这突出了吸痰的重要性,可以改善氧合、减少肺不张、降低呼吸机压力,并可能降低呼吸机相关性肺炎的风险。PEEP 大于 6 cmH_2O 或 FiO_2 大于 0.5 的患者被认为是转运的高危人群,因其与氧合并发症的风险增加有关[2,4,7]。在转运过程中经常提高 FiO_2,以提供所谓的安全保障或暂时处理患者呼吸恶化的问题,而不考虑病理生理变化和解决问题的根本原因。这种做法可能会因为吸收性肺不张导致肺泡进一步塌陷。另一种可行的选择是考虑更高水平的 PEEP,针对患者个体化滴定,因为在转运患者中,PEEP 的应用通常是保守的[11]。

过度通气通常发生于使用手动通气设备(如球囊通气)时。因此,临床医生应尽可能使用具有设置参数的机械通气。避免手动球囊通气是许多转运组织的质量指标。在转运过程中,焦虑、疼痛和移动可能会导致患者在呼吸机上触发额外的呼吸。因此,应优先考虑给予充分的镇静,尤其是在人-机不同步时。

除了镇静以外,神经肌肉阻滞剂(neuromuscular blockade,NMBA)经常在转运中使用[2,7,11]。先前的研究发现,在中度至重度 ARDS 患者中,NMBA 的使用与 90 天病死率的改善有关。然而,在最近的一项更大的试验中发现,NMBA 与病死率的益处无关[15]。因此,在治疗低氧血症患者时,NMBA 不再被常规推荐使用。然而,当患者镇静后仍与呼吸机不同步时,NMBA 适合用来降低呼吸机相关肺损伤的风险。许多转运组织在高风险转运时,会在充分镇静后使用 NMBA,以减少一个潜在的风险变量——患者产生的移动。此外,在转运过程中使用 NMBA 与改善氧合有关[7]。

由于气道移位、阻塞或位置不当,可导致低通气,这是转运患者的风险[2]。其次,使用镇静或神经肌肉阻滞的同时呼吸机设置不恰当也可能导致低通气。当转运团队降低潮气量以减少呼吸机相关肺损伤的风险时,他们还必须增加呼吸频率以维持每分钟通气量。先前的研究表明,在转运中可能会忘记增加呼吸频率,从而导致呼吸性酸中毒的加重[7]。值得注意的是,许多肺部并发症通常归因于设备故障和人为错误[4]。

28.5 心血管并发症

在转运过程中,血流动力学的改变仍然是最常见的并发症。最常见的是低血压,其次是有意义的心率变化和心律失常[1,4,6,11]。因为体液转移,转运时低血压很常见,根据经验,患者的血管活性药物需求越高,移动时严重恶化的风险就越大。气胸的扩大虽然罕见,也可导致低血压[4]。相反,应激、疼痛和焦虑可能导致高血压,这强调了在患者转运过程中充分维持镇静的重要性。心脏停搏是转运过程中罕见但灾难性的事件,许多病例是由于无人监督或未经培训的工作人员对患者的监测不足[4,6,7]。

28.6 设备故障、注意事项和人为错误

设备故障或工作人员培训不足也是转运过程中紧急事件的重要因素[1,2]。例如,ECG

导联故障、监测器故障、静脉注射通路丢失和呼吸机脱落[4]。不良事件是否发生取决于团队的组成和专业能力。当不具备充分培训的工作人员时,专业医师的存在可能会显著降低不良事件的风险[1]。另一方面,具有专业培训和远程医师会诊能力的熟练团队可以降低风险。无论转运团队成员自身是何学科或专业,所有人都必须认识到,转运医学是一种专业的医学实践。在无法获取医院的资源时,团队必须在保证患者和工作人员安全的同时,应对移动的影响。因此,无论临床专业技能如何,临床医生不应该在没有对转运环境的适当培训或监督下承担运输任务。重要的是,要提前建立一个转运体系,分配合适的工作人员和资源以满足患者的需求[10]。

在转运过程中,由于呼吸回路的固定,患者与呼吸机的连接可能会意外断开[4]。虽然通常可以迅速被发现,但是即使间隔的时间很短暂,高度敏感的患者也会因与呼吸机连接中断造成肺去复张,V/Q 不匹配,可能需要调高呼吸机参数来逆转。连续呼气末 CO_2 监测是呼吸机和气道状态的一种可靠(且未被充分利用)的监测工具,因为它可以立即检测呼吸机故障和意外脱管[2]。在计划转运时,充分考虑患者对呼吸机中断的耐受性非常重要。

28.7 检查清单的重要性

降低不良事件风险的最佳方法是采用并严格遵守系统化的检查清单[1-4,10]。转运过程中的检查清单可以分为三个不同的阶段:① 转运前;② 转运过程中;③ 转运后。然后,每个阶段可以细分为四个类别:① 组织和规划;② 监护设备;③ 生理指标;④ 药物[1]。表 28.1 为转运前检查清单的示例。

表 28.1 运输前检查清单的示例

转运前呼吸机检查清单	
	确定或数值
组织和规划	
转运前	
确定转运的必要性	
确定患者身份	
通知接收机构	
转运前患者评估	
基线生命体征记录	
监护设备	
气道	
确认 ETT 放置位置/深度记录	

续 表

转运前呼吸机检查清单	
	确定或数值
导管支架或胶带固定气道	
紧急/疑难插管箱	
手术气道包	
备用气管造口套管/造口器（如适用）	
呼吸机设备	
备用电路	
备用 HME	
全套电池/备用电池/充电器	
吸引装置和配件	
$EtCO_2$ 监测	
氧气瓶充满和备用	
带有 PEEP 阀的手动复苏装置	
生理指标	
呼吸机参数	
与送出机构确认初始设置	
最近的血气值	
预测体重（PBW）	
呼出潮气量[mL/kg(PBW)]	
每分钟通气值	
平台压＜30 cmH_2O	
警报设定	
触发器设置适当	
药物	
药物和设备	
足够的静脉注射药物	
额外的镇静剂/镇痛剂	
血管加压/正性肌力药	
备用输液泵	
备用静脉输液	

在转运前阶段,应对患者进行评估,以确定是否存在任何转运禁忌证,包括未能建立和维持气道,或监测资源不足。此时,应评估风险与收益比。一旦决定转运,根据患者的敏感性,必须选择至少两名合格的工作人员(不包括车辆操作员)。转运机构和接收机构之间应进行沟通(护士与护士之间,医生与医生之间)。适当的设备/监护设备应予以说明,并进行功能测试。然后对患者进行转运准备,整理好管路,确保气道安全,并将药物放在容易拿到的地方。在转运过程中,通过维持ICU级别的管理、持续监测生命体征,优先确保患者保持稳定状态。到达接收医院后,如转运后阶段,必须将患者放回ICU设备上。应提供一份详细的关于生命体征、给药、发生事件和干预措施的报告。设备应清洁、充电并准备下一次使用[1-3,10]。

28.8 总结

患者转运的过程涉及评估患者的危险因素,清晰地了解其收益,并仔细实施标准化的检查清单。设备必须与患者的需求相一致。虽然患者的生理状况复杂,是在转运前无法解决的因素,但仍需了解最常见的并发症并进行额外的培训,以便工作人员应对这些在转运过程中发生的情况。

(张媛,于晨希 译)

参考文献

[1] Brunsveld-Reinders AH, Arbous MS, Kuiper SG, de Jonge E. A comprehensive method to develop a checklist to increase safety of intra-hospital transport of critically ill patients. Crit Care. 2015;19(1):214. https://doi.org/10.1186/s13054-015-0938-1. Published 2015 May 7.

[2] Fanara B, Manzon C, Barbot O, Desmettre T, Capellier G. Recommendations for the intra-hospital transport of critically ill patients. Crit Care. 2010;14(3):R87. https://doi.org/10.1186/cc9018.

[3] Warren J, Fromm RE Jr, Orr RA, Rotello LC, Horst HM, American College of Critical Care Medicine. Guidelines for the inter- and intrahospital transport of critically ill patients. Crit Care Med. 2004;32(1):256-62. https://doi.org/10.1097/01.CCM.0000104917.39204.0A.

[4] Knight PH, Maheshwari N, Hussain J, et al. Complications during intrahospital transport of critically ill patients: focus on risk identification and prevention. Int J Crit Illn Inj Sci. 2015;5(4):256-64. https://doi.org/10.4103/2229-5151.170840.

[5] Singh JM, MacDonald RD, Ahghari M. Critical events during land-based interfacility transport. Ann Emerg Med. 2014;64(1):9-15.e2. https://doi.org/10.1016/j.annemergmed.2013.12.009.

[6] Schwebel C, Clec'h C, Magne S, et al. Safety of intrahospital transport in ventilated critically ill patients: a multicenter cohort study*. Crit Care Med. 2013;41(8):1919-28. https://doi.org/10.1097/CCM.0b013e31828a3bbd.

[7] Wilcox SR, Saia MS, Waden H, Frakes M, Wedel SK, Richards JB. Mechanical ventilation in critical care transport. Air Med J. 2016;35(3):161-5. https://doi.org/10.1016/j.amj.2016.

01.004.

[8] Wilcox SR, Richards JB, Genthon A, et al. Mortality and resource utilization after critical care transport of patients with hypoxemic respiratory failure. J Intensive Care Med. 2018; 33(3): 182-8. https://doi.org/10.1177/0885066615623202.

[9] Durairaj L, Will JG, Torner JC, Doebbeling BN. Prognostic factors for mortality following interhospital transfers to the medical intensive care unit of a tertiary referral center. Crit Care Med. 2003; 31(7): 1981-6. https://doi.org/10.1097/01.CCM.0000069730.02769.16.

[10] Kiss T, Bölke A, Spieth PM. Interhospital transfer of critically ill patients. Minerva Anestesiol. 2017; 83(10): 1101-8. https://doi.org/10.23736/S0375-9393.17.11857-2.

[11] Singh JM, Ferguson ND, MacDonald RD, Stewart TE, Schull MJ. Ventilation practices and critical events during transport of ventilated patients outside of hospital: a retrospective cohort study. Prehosp Emerg Care. 2009; 13(3): 316-23. https://doi.org/10.1080/10903120902935264.

[12] Wilcox SR, Saia MS, Waden H, Genthon A, Gates JD, Cocchi MN, McGahn SJ, Frakes M, Wedel SK, Richards JB. Improved oxygenation after transport in patients with hypoxemic respiratory failure. Air Med J. 2015; 34(6): 369-76. https://doi.org/10.1016/j.amj.2015.07.006. PMID: 26611225.

[13] Tourtier JP, Astaud C, Domanski L. Specificity of desaturation during air transport. J Trauma Acute Care Surg. 2012; 73(3): 778-9. https://doi.org/10.1097/TA.0b013e31826601ce. PMID: 22929508.

[14] Stoltze AJ, Wong TS, Harland KK, Ahmed A, Fuller BM, Mohr NM. Prehospital tidal volume influences hospital tidal volume: a cohort study. J Crit Care. 2015; 30(3): 495-501. https://doi.org/10.1016/j.jcrc.2015.02.013. Epub 2015 Mar 3. PMID: 25813548; PMCID: PMC4414869.

[15] National Heart, Lung, and Blood Institute PETAL Clinical Trials Network, Moss M, Huang DT, Brower RG, Ferguson ND, Ginde AA, Gong MN, Grissom CK, Gundel S, Hayden D, Hite RD, Hou PC, Hough CL, Iwashyna TJ, Khan A, Liu KD, Talmor D, Thompson BT, Ulysse CA, Yealy DM, Angus DC. Early neuromuscular blockade in the acute respiratory distress syndrome. N Engl J Med. 2019; 380(21): 1997-2008. https://doi.org/10.1056/NEJMoa1901686. Epub 2019 May 19. PMID: 31112383; PMCID: PMC6741345.

第三部分
机械通气的辅助手段

29 俯卧位通气

Prone Position

Claude Guérin

俯卧位通气到目前已经有近50年的历史(图29.1),其效果在COVID-19大流行中得到了进一步的验证。事实上,俯卧位通气的使用率从经典急性呼吸窘迫综合征(acute respiratory distress syndrome,ARDS)患者中的10%~30%[1,2]跃升至COVID-19相关ARDS中的超过70%[3]。这一发现是在这两个时期的相同证据水平下观察到的结果。本章将介绍俯卧位通气的原理、时机、一些实际问题和临床结果,包括COVID-19大流行期间观察到的临床结果。

29.1 基本原理

对俯卧位通气机制的认识已经从使气管插管伴有严重低氧血症的ARDS患者获得更好的氧合深入到了呼吸机诱发的肺损伤(ventilator-induced lung injury,VILI)的预防。此外,最近强调了俯卧位可以维持甚至可以提高心输出量的事实。

29.1.1 对氧合的作用

应用俯卧位后,氧合改善(有时甚至是显著的)的发生机制是需要考虑的重要事项。俯卧位时氧合改善是由于肺内分流的减少和更好的通气/灌注。基本且典型的机制是靠近脊柱区域的肺(俯卧位时转变为非重力依赖)通气增加,这部分肺持续接受大部分肺血流灌注(至少在非COVID-19的ARDS患者中如此)。事实上,俯卧位促进了肺背侧区域的肺复张(肺组织得到充气),但不会明显地减少肺背侧区域的血流。这种

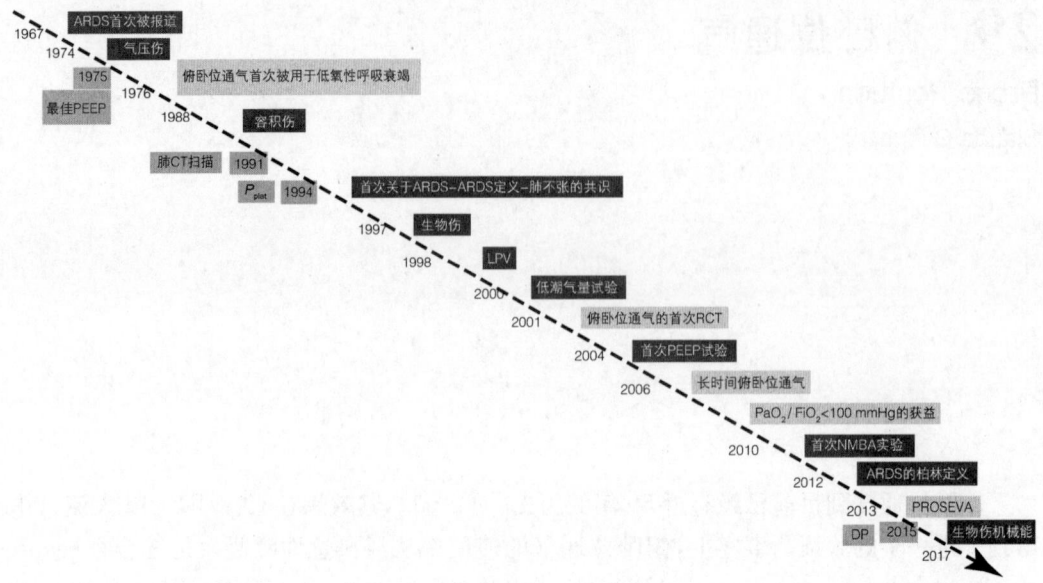

图29.1 急性呼吸窘迫综合征管理的主要进展时间轴(未按比例显示)。红框表示机械通气,蓝框表示生理监测,绿框表示俯卧位。P_{plat},平台压;LPV,肺保护性通气;PEEP,呼气末正压;DP,驱动压;RCT,随机对照试验;NMBA,神经肌肉阻滞剂(见彩色插图)

情况下也可以改善二氧化碳潴留。俯卧位可以增强吸入一氧化氮对氧合的改善作用。

29.1.2 预防呼吸机诱发肺损伤

由于氧合目标应当适度,并且VILI的预防成为了对ARDS实施机械通气的主要目标,因此更好氧合的核心作用变得没那么重要,然而俯卧位仍然具有重要的价值。一项标志性的研究通过CT测量了肺气体-组织比[4],表明在俯卧位时整体肺应力(跨肺压)和应变(由驱动压代替)降低,更为重要的是,气体在整个肺中的分布变得更加均匀[5](图29.2)。这意味着,在其他条件相同的情况下,潮气量导致"婴儿肺"过度膨胀的风险降低。对于给定的潮气量,呼气末正压(positive end-expiratory pressure,PEEP)不再会显著改变应变的分布[5]。与仰卧位相比,俯卧位可以增加胸壁回弹力[6]。因此,呼吸系统回弹力的变化不一定反映肺回弹力的变化。俯卧位时肺回弹力降低进而促进肺复张,其降低幅度应高于胸壁回弹力增加的幅度,可能会使呼吸系统总回弹力保持不变。增加胸壁回弹力可以减少肺过度膨胀,也可以起到肺保护作用[7]。

29.1.3 血流动力学影响

俯卧位通气可以通过更好的气体交换和增加呼气末肺容积来降低肺血管阻力,从而减轻右心室负荷。最近的研究表明,俯卧位可以增加心输出量,特别是在仰卧位时前负荷依赖的患者中[8]。

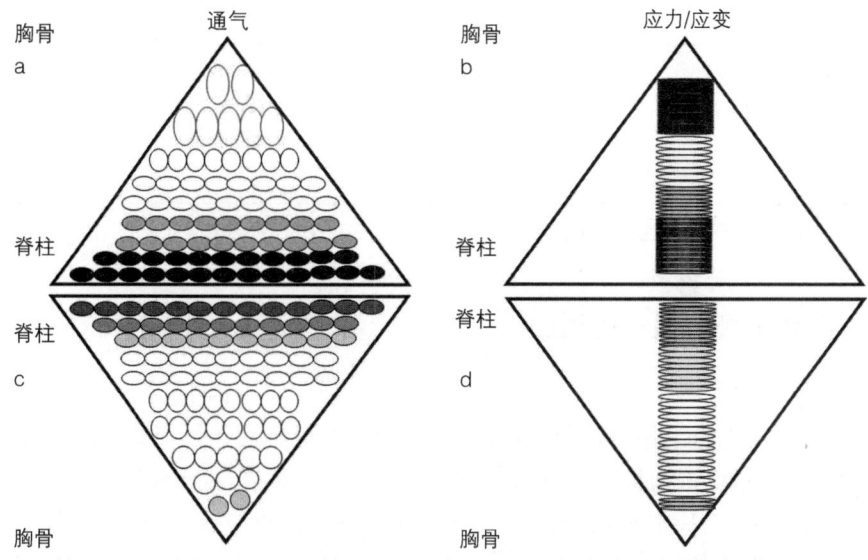

图 29.2　仰卧位(a,b)和俯卧位(c,d)的 ARDS 肺通气和应力/应变分布示意图。黑色椭圆是肺无效腔,由于不通气而无应力。灰色椭圆为部分通气的肺区域。靠近肺无效腔的部分通气肺区域有很高的应力,而距离较远的部分通气肺区域承受较低但高于正常的应力。白色椭圆是正常通气的肺区域,即婴儿肺,承受正常的应力。最后,红色空心椭圆是过度膨胀的肺区域,存在着较高应力。当转向俯卧位时肺复张并且减少了过度膨胀。整个肺的压力/应变降低,在肺内的分布更加均匀(见彩色插图)

29.2　俯卧位的启动时机

29.2.1　急性呼吸窘迫综合征中启动俯卧位的 PaO_2/FiO_2 阈值

一项纳入四个多中心研究的荟萃分析表明,在随机分组时 $PaO_2/FiO_2 < 100$ mmHg 人群中,俯卧位通气是有效的[9](表 29.1),专家也证实了这一阈值[10]。然而,随后一项在 $PaO_2/FiO_2 < 150$ mmHg 的中重度 ARDS 患者中采用俯卧位的试验表明俯卧位组 90 天病死率显著降低[11](表 29.1)。

表 29.1　五个大型的比较急性呼吸窘迫综合征俯卧位和仰卧位通气的随机对照试验

第一作者	意大利	法国	西班牙	意大利	法国和西班牙
病例数(SP/PP)	152/152	378/413	60/76	174/168	229/237
% ARDS 占比(SP/PP)	93.3/94.7	28/33.9	100/100	100/100	100/100
PaO_2/FiO_2 (mmHg)	127	150	147	113	100
潮气量(mL/kg)	10.3 MBW	8 MBW	8.4 PBW	8 PBW	6.1 PBW
PEEP (cmH_2O)	10	8	12	10	10

续 表

第一作者	意大利	法国	西班牙	意大利	法国和西班牙
俯卧位时间	7	8	17	18	17
病死率（SP/PP）(%)	25/21.1	31.5/32.4	58/43	32.8/31	32.8/16

SP，仰卧位；PP，俯卧位；ARDS，急性呼吸窘迫综合征；PEEP，呼气末正压；MBW，测定体重；PBW，预测体重。

29.2.2 启动俯卧位通气的时机

PROSEVA试验[11]要求在纳入患者之前有一个12~24小时的稳定期，纳入实验组的患者将在1小时内进行俯卧位通气，旨在患者确诊ARDS后尽早使其进行俯卧位通气。同时，排除极其严重低氧血症需要即刻进行俯卧位通气的患者，或者临床症状迅速改善的患者。ARDS被识别、稳定和确诊后的早期俯卧位通气是有效的、安全的。在COVID-19疫情期间，大型观察性数据库显示，与较晚使用俯卧位相比，早期使用俯卧位通气（即插管后2天内）有更好的预后[12]。在动物模型研究中，早期（ARDS后第1天）俯卧位促进的复张的背侧区域明显大于晚期（第2天）[13]。

29.2.3 俯卧位通气的终止时机

俯卧位通气的终止时机和启动时机一样重要。在PROSEVA试验中[11]，预定标准是基于先前仰卧位时的氧合、PEEP和FiO_2来决定的。因此，氧合方面对俯卧位的反应性是通过比较俯卧位前后仰卧位时的氧合来定义的，而不是俯卧位过程中的氧合变化。这意味着，即使不满足这些标准，即无论患者有没有表现出氧合改善，抑或无任何变化，俯卧位仍将持续进行。当连续两次俯卧位导致氧合恶化超过20%时，即终止俯卧位通气，以此作为安全防护措施。这一策略的目的是将俯卧位的主要益处定位于预防VILI而不是改善氧合。这个问题可能非常重要，但在文献中导致了一些混淆，并且在实践中也是如此。在典型的ARDS中，没有可靠的数据显示对俯卧位通气有反应者（在氧合改善方面）比无反应者表现更好。对PROSEVA试验的事后分析发现，患者的预后与俯卧位的早期或晚期（对PaO_2或$PaCO_2$的）反应之间没有相关性[14]，这与其他人先前的研究一致[15]。然而，在COVID-19的ARDS患者中，两项观察性研究表明氧合改善与患者预后存在显著相关性[16,17]。

29.2.4 俯卧位持续时间

在西班牙、意大利和法国进行的最后三次研究延长了俯卧位通气时间，远远超过了连续的12小时[18]。长时间治疗的基本原理是尽量减少因实际问题而导致的体位改变，但要记住，体位改变也是俯卧位治疗的组成部分。另一个基本原理是更加符合生理学：假设俯卧位能减少VILI的发生，俯卧的时间越长，机械通气中VILI减少的可能性就越大。在COVID-19中延长俯卧位时间被证实是可行和有效的[19]。

29.3 实际问题

29.3.1 人员配置

在绝大多数情况下，使用患者自己的床和床垫、3~4 名工作人员，其中一人必须位于患者头部来控制保护人工气道。COVID-19 导致大量俯卧位患者、俯卧位的肥胖患者及 ECMO 下实施俯卧位，这些对护理团队和设备带来了巨大挑战。用于患者和护理人员的外骨骼辅助支持装置有利于俯卧位通气的实施、提高其安全性，并减少对护理人员的伤害[20,21]。

29.3.2 腹部支撑

腹部是否应该被支撑并没有明确的答案。在妊娠后期，建议腹部无支撑，同时监测胎儿心率。

29.3.3 俯卧位时的镇静和神经肌肉阻滞

大部分俯卧位通气的 ARDS 患者接受持续静脉镇静及神经肌肉阻滞治疗。ARDS 在俯卧位通气中使用无神经肌肉阻滞的最小镇静是当前的热门话题，但目前尚无关于俯卧位 ARDS 患者有或无神经肌肉阻滞镇静的研究发表。

29.3.4 俯卧位时呼吸机的设置

由于俯卧位通气时有更好的氧合，通常呼吸机设置的改变是 FiO_2 的减少。如何设置俯卧位通气时的 PEEP 仍是一个仍然悬而未决的问题。在 PROSEVA 试验中[11]，PEEP 由 PEEP-FiO_2 表决定，并且在俯卧位时会降低。俯卧时低 PEEP 可能是导致实施俯卧位 2 天内心血管器官功能障碍少于仰卧组的原因。另外两个因素则支持俯卧时更高的 PEEP，一个是俯卧时胸壁回弹力增加，另一个是肺复张。如果俯卧位确实促进肺复张，当患者回到仰卧位时，应根据"肺开放并保持开放"的理念设置较高的 PEEP。通过食管压来指导 PEEP 设置将是一个很有吸引力的策略，因为假设在仰卧位时重力和肺、纵隔和心脏的重量对传感器的压迫较小，俯卧位时食管压的相关性将比仰卧位更好。然而，对于给定的呼气末跨肺压目标，基于相同的基线 PEEP，使用食管压并未导致俯卧位与仰卧位时设置的 PEEP 发生显著变化[23]。然而，此法可以实现基于患者个体水平滴定 PEEP。

29.3.5 禁忌证

对 ARDS 实施俯卧位通气的唯一绝对禁忌是不稳定的脊柱骨折[18]。以下是需要根据个体情况评估风险获益比的相对禁忌证：休克、颅内压升高、外科或内科腹部问题。肥胖，甚至病态肥胖，都不是禁忌证。肥胖患者应该能从实施俯卧位中受益，因为俯卧位并选择恰当 PEEP 可以缓解肥胖患者重要的闭合容积。事实上,怀孕并不是上述俯卧位的禁忌证。

29.4 临床证据

29.4.1 对经典 ARDS 气管插管患者生存的作用

如前所述,一些比较仰卧位和俯卧位的研究没有发现任何显著的预后获益,但一项单独的荟萃分析得出了第一个积极信号,支持在大多数低氧血症患者中使用俯卧位[18]。然后 PROSEVA 试验首次证明了俯卧位能显著改善临床结局,因此 $PaO_2/FiO_2 <$ 150 mmHg 的 ARDS 患者实施俯卧位获得了证据支持。该阈值得到了一些专家的条件性推荐[10],并在经典 ARDS 中得到了其他专家的强烈推荐[24]。在 COVID-19 疫情期间也得到了推荐[25]。

29.4.2 在 COVID-19 中的发现

COVID-19 相关 ARDS 的病理生理研究有两个主要发现:① 与经典 ARDS 相比,低氧血症严重程度与保留的肺通气存在差异,表现出更好的呼吸系统顺应性;② 肺循环受累(肺毛细血管内的微血栓,低氧时肺血管收缩能力受损)导致 PEEP 作用下的肺血流再分布。并且在俯卧位时也与经典的 ARDS 不同,无效腔通气高于经典 ARDS。然而,COVID-19 相关 ARDS 的治疗建议与传统的 ARDS 的治疗方法相同,包括采用俯卧位通气,如前所述,COVID-19 使俯卧位的使用数量激增。另一个特点是在清醒非插管的重症 COVID-19 肺炎患者中大量使用俯卧位,不仅在重症监护室(intensive care unit,ICU),也在急诊室和病房使用。这样做的目的是节省稀缺的 ICU 资源,这对最严重的患者来说是至关重要的。通过这种方式,临床医生希望能改善患者氧合,有助于争取时间并避免插管,这一策略在氧气短缺的发达国家特别常见。这样做的风险在于延迟插管。我们正在等待进行中的几项研究的最终结果,这些研究旨在探讨,相较于仰卧位,让未行气管插管的重症 COVID-19 肺炎患者采用俯卧位,是否可以避免插管并降低病死率。需要注意的是,清醒患者的俯卧位如果能减少患者的吸气努力从而降低跨肺压,可能会起到肺保护作用。

29.5 总结

如无禁忌证,则应对 ARDS 中 $PaO_2/FiO_2 <$ 150 mmHg 的患者实施俯卧位。COVID-19 大流行清楚地显示,即使证据水平与大流行之前相同,临床医生也普遍采纳了这一策略。大流行结束后,这种俯卧位的广泛使用是否会继续目前还有待确定。

需要进一步的研究来证明俯卧位通气是否可以改善 $PaO_2/FiO_2 >$ 150 mmHg ARDS 患者的预后(法国正在准备的一项试验);如果选择有反应性的患者使用俯卧位,需要对俯卧位的反应性进行标准化的定义;并且探讨清醒俯卧位在 COVID-19 之外的应用价值。

(王蕊,戴清霞 译)

参考文献

[1] Guerin C, Beuret P, Constantin JM, Bellani G, Garcia-Olivares P, Roca O, et al. A prospective international observational prevalence study on prone positioning of ARDS patients: the APRONET (ARDS Prone Position Network) study. Intensive Care Med. 2018; 44(1): 22-37.

[2] Bellani G, Laffey JG, Pham T, Fan E, Brochard L, Esteban A, et al. Epidemiology, patterns of care, and mortality for patients with acute respiratory distress syndrome in intensive care units in 50 countries. JAMA. 2016; 315(8): 788-800.

[3] Covid-ICU Group. Clinical characteristics and day-90 outcomes of 4244 critically ill adults with COVID-19: a prospective cohort study. Intensive Care Med. 2021; 47(1): 60-73.

[4] Gattinoni L, Pelosi P, Vitale G, Pesenti A, D'Andrea L, Mascheroni D. Body position changes redistribute lung computed-tomographic density in patients with acute respiratory failure. Anesthesiology. 1991; 74(1): 15-23.

[5] Scaramuzzo G, Ball L, Pino F, Ricci L, Larsson A, Guérin C, et al. Influence of PEEP titration on the effects of pronation in ARDS: a comprehensive experimental study. Front Physiol. 2020; 11: 179.

[6] Mezidi M, Guerin C. Effect of body position and inclination in supine and prone position on respiratory mechanics in acute respiratory distress syndrome. Intensive Care Med. 2019; 45(2): 292-4.

[7] Rezoagli E, Bastia L, Grassi A, Chieregato A, Langer T, Grasselli G, et al. Paradoxical effect of chest wall compression on respiratory system compliance: a multicenter case series of patients with ARDS, with multimodal assessment. Chest. 2021; 160(4): 1335-9.

[8] Jozwiak M, Teboul JL, Anguel N, Persichini R, Silva S, Chemla D, et al. Beneficial hemodynamic effects of prone positioning in patients with acute respiratory distress syndrome. Am J Respir Crit Care Med. 2013; 188(12): 1428-33.

[9] Gattinoni L, Carlesso E, Taccone P, Polli F, Guerin C, Mancebo J. Prone positioning improves survival in severe ARDS: a pathophysiologic review and individual patient meta-analysis. Minerva Anestesiol. 2010; 76(6): 448-54.

[10] Fan E, Del Sorbo L, Goligher EC, Hodgson CL, Munshi L, Walkey AJ, et al. An Official American Thoracic Society/European Society of Intensive Care Medicine/Society of Critical Care Medicine clinical practice guideline: mechanical ventilation in adult patients with acute respiratory distress syndrome. Am J Respir Crit Care Med. 2017; 195(9): 1253-63.

[11] Guérin C, Reignier J, Richard J-C, Beuret P, Gacouin A, Boulain T, et al. Prone positioning in severe acute respiratory distress syndrome. N Engl J Med. 2013; 368(23): 2159-68.

[12] Mathews KS, Soh H, Shaefi S, Wang W, Bose S, Coca S, et al. Prone positioning and survival in mechanically ventilated patients with coronavirus disease 2019-related respiratory failure. Crit Care Med. 2021; 49(7): 1026-37.

[13] Xin Y, Martin K, Morais CCA, Delvecchio P, Gerard SE, Hamedani H, et al. Diminishing efficacy of prone positioning with late application in evolving lung injury. Crit Care Med. 2021; 49(10): e1015-24.

[14] Albert RK, Keniston A, Baboi L, Ayzac L, Guérin C. Prone position-induced improvement in gas exchange does not predict improved survival in the acute respiratory distress syndrome. Am J Respir Crit Care Med. 2014; 189(4): 494-6.

[15] Protti A, Chiumello D, Cressoni M, Carlesso E, Mietto C, Berto V, et al. Relationship between gas exchange response to prone position and lung recruitability during acute respiratory failure. Intensive Care Med. 2009; 35(6): 1011-7.

[16] Langer T, Brioni M, Guzzardella A, Carlesso E, Cabrini L, Castelli G, et al. Prone position in intubated, mechanically ventilated patients with COVID-19: a multi-centric study of more than 1000 patients. Crit Care. 2021; 25(1): 128.

[17] Scaramuzzo G, Gamberini L, Tonetti T, Zani G, Ottaviani I, Mazzoli CA, et al. Sustained oxygenation improvement after first prone positioning is associated with liberation from mechanical ventilation and mortality in critically ill COVID-19 patients: a cohort study. Ann Intensive Care. 2021; 11(1): 63.

[18] Guerin C, Albert RK, Beitler J, Gattinoni L, Jaber S, Marini JJ, et al. Prone position in ARDS patients: why, when, how and for whom. Intensive Care Med. 2020; 46(12): 2385-96.

[19] Carsetti A, Damia Paciarini A, Marini B, Pantanetti S, Adrario E, Donati A. Prolonged prone position ventilation for SARS-CoV-2 patients is feasible and effective. Crit Care. 2020; 24(1): 225.

[20] Kimmoun A, Levy B, Chenuel B, Group DV-T. Usefulness and safety of a dedicated team to prone patients with severe ARDS due to COVID-19. Crit Care. 2020; 24(1): 509.

[21] Settembre N, Maurice P, Paysant J, Theurel J, Claudon L, Kimmoun A, et al. The use of exoskeletons to help with prone positioning in the intensive care unit during COVID-19. Ann Phys Rehabil Med. 2020; 63(4): 379-82.

[22] Chanques G, Constantin JM, Devlin JW, Ely EW, Fraser GL, Gelinas C, et al. Analgesia and sedation in patients with ARDS. Intensive Care Med. 2020; 46(12): 2342-56.

[23] Mezidi M, Parrilla FJ, Yonis H, Riad Z, Bohm SH, Waldmann AD, et al. Effects of positive end-expiratory pressure strategy in supine and prone position on lung and chest wall mechanics in acute respiratory distress syndrome. Ann Intensive Care. 2018; 8(1): 86.

[24] Papazian L, Aubron C, Brochard L, Chiche JD, Combes A, Dreyfuss D, et al. Formal guidelines: management of acute respiratory distress syndrome. Ann Intensive Care. 2019; 9(1): 69.

[25] Alhazzani W, Evans L, Alshamsi F, Moller MH, Ostermann M, Prescott HC, et al. Surviving sepsis campaign guidelines on the management of adults with coronavirus disease 2019 (COVID-19) in the ICU: first update. Crit Care Med. 2021; 49(3): e219-34.

30 静脉-静脉体外膜肺氧合和体外二氧化碳清除
Veno-Venous ECMO and ECCO$_2$R

Marco Giani, Christophe Guervilly, Giuseppe Foti

30.1 严重呼吸衰竭的病理生理：肺内分流和肺泡无效腔

最严重的急性呼吸窘迫综合征（acute respiratory distress syndrome，ARDS）患者会表现出危及生命的低氧血症和（或）呼吸性酸中毒。ARDS 肺组织病理改变复杂，包括肺泡渗出、肺泡塌陷、微血管血栓形成[1]。这些变化导致了分流和无效腔，导致通气-灌注关系的两个极端表现。分流发生在有血流但无通气的肺泡-毛细血管单元，导致增加吸入氧浓度（inspiratory oxygen fraction，FiO$_2$）不能改善的低氧血症。

出现分流时，肺通气区域相对灌注不足，与微血管血栓形成共同引起肺泡无效腔的增加，导致需要更多的每分钟通气量来清除二氧化碳（CO$_2$），这是由于在没有灌注的肺泡通气而造成"浪费"。

30.2 为什么要采用体外气体交换

40 多年以来，静脉-静脉体外膜肺氧合（veno-venous extracorporeal membrane oxygenation，V-V ECMO）可以用来替代功能衰竭的肺的气体交换功能，被认为是一种有效的挽救性治疗方法[2,3]。体外气体交换的基本原理是提供氧合、清除 CO$_2$ 并大幅减少肺自身的通气。在某种程度上,V-V ECMO 是一种"对症"治疗,为肺康复争取时间。

V-V ECMO 既可作为低氧血症的挽救治疗[2],也可通过体外 CO_2 清除(extracorporeal removal of CO_2,$ECCO_2R$)来降低通气负荷[4-6]。为了实现第一个目标,需要高流量的静脉-静脉体外支持(即 3~6 L/min 的血流量)来提供足够的氧合。相反,通过 $ECCO_2R$,只需要较低的体外血流量(即 500~1 500 mL/min),因为与 O_2 相比,CO_2 在膜肺(membrane lung,ML)中的溶解性和弥散性更高[7]。从而纠正或预防呼吸性酸中毒,减轻通气负荷。这种差异是 O_2 和 CO_2 交换的生理机制不同所导致的。氧合主要依赖体外血流量[8],而 CO_2 交换主要取决于 ML 上设定的气流量[9,10]。

如上所述,提高吸入氧浓度不能纠正肺内分流增加导致的低氧血症。V-V ECMO 可以增加混合静脉血氧含量,这样就使"分流"的血液也被氧合了。因此,在实施了低潮气量通气、使用中到高水平的呼气末正压(positive end-expiratory pressure,PEEP)、持续神经肌肉阻滞和至少一次俯卧位尝试情况下仍存在危及生命的低氧血症时,建议使用 V-V ECMO[11]。

另一方面,$ECCO_2R$ 的适应证值得更多的讨论。肺功能的损害越严重,则需要越高的气道压和每分钟通气量来维持足够的氧分压和二氧化碳分压。此外,肺部病变导致肺顺应性下降,因此需要更高的通气压力,但这种高通气负荷可能加重肺部炎症[即呼吸机诱发的肺损伤(ventilator induced lung injury,VILI)]导致恶性循环。此外,同时存在的缺氧性肺血管收缩、高碳酸血症和高通气压引起了肺血管阻力和肺动脉压的增加(即右心室后负荷),最终导致右心室功能障碍或衰竭[12]。

在实验模型中,$ECCO_2R$ 可以将通气负荷降低到接近呼吸暂停的水平,从而减少组织学上的肺损伤和纤维增生[13]。在第 31 章中将详细讨论 ECMO 期间的机械通气。简单地说,体外气体交换开始后呼吸机如何设置在各 ECMO 中心之间存在很大的差异[14]。一般来说,潮气量通常降低到 3~6 mL/kg(基于理想体重计算)以达到低于 25 cmH_2O 的平台压和低于 12~15 cmH_2O 驱动压。此外,为了进一步减少通气负荷,许多中心将呼吸频率降低到 10~15 次/分。图 30.1 展示了我们中心 36 例 ARDS 患者 ECMO 启动后最初 20 分钟内通气量减少的数据(未发表的数据)。

通过将潮气量从 (5.6 ± 1.8) mL/kg 减少到 (4.5 ± 2) mL/kg($P<0.001$)和呼吸频率从 (30 ± 5) 次/分减少到 (10 ± 2) 次/分($P<0.001$)以实现每分钟通气量的减少。潮气量的减小导致驱动压降低 4 cmH_2O,从 (14 ± 3) cmH_2O 降至 (10 ± 3) cmH_2O。

因此,在 ECMO 启动后机械能(即呼吸机传递给受损肺的总能量)也相应地显著下降,如图 30.2 所示(ASST Monza 的 66 例 ARDS V-V ECMO 患者,未发表数据)。

根据临床经验,V-V ECMO 启动后血流动力学明显改善是非常常见的。动脉中氧和二氧化碳水平正常化、胸内压力的降低决定了肺血管阻力的降低和右心室负荷卸载[15],从而降低了急性肺心病(可见于多达 22% 的严重 ARDS 患者,并与病死率密切相关)的发生风险[16]。

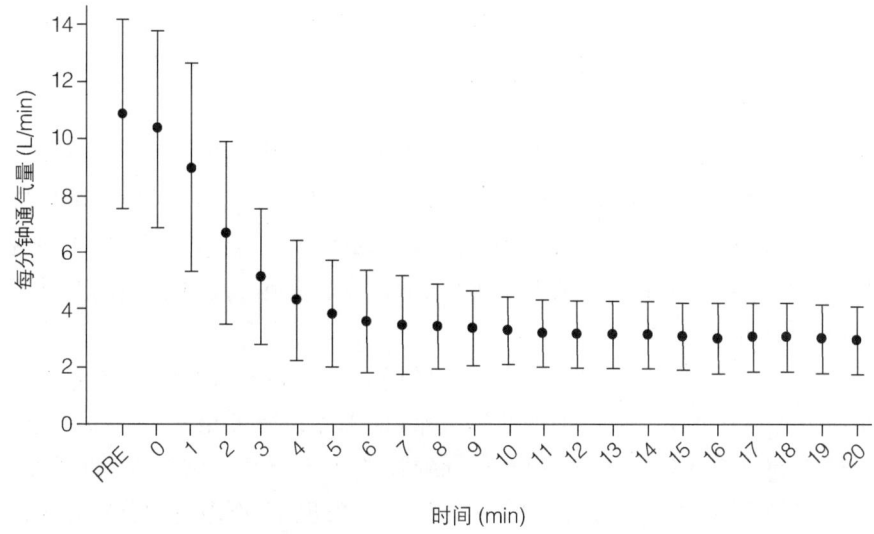

图 30.1 ECMO 启动前后的每分钟通气量。点代表平均值,误差线代表标准差。* $P<0.05$,与上机前(PRE)比较

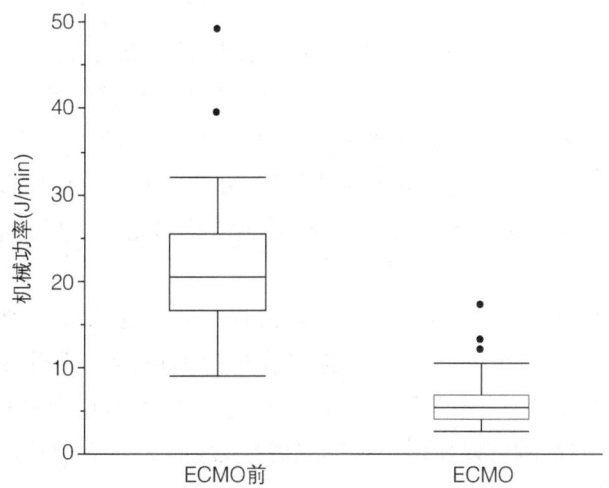

图 30.2 ECMO 启动前后的机械能。ECMO,体外膜肺氧合

30.3 "全"流量静脉-静脉体外膜肺氧合与低流量体外二氧化碳清除

通常情况下,对于非常严重的需要体外气体交换的 ARDS 患者,高流量 V - V ECMO 是首选的技术。严重低氧血症即 PaO_2/FiO_2 低于 50～80 mmHg(FiO_2 100%)和严重呼吸性酸中毒(pH<7.25)是体外支持临床试验的主要纳入标准[2,17-19]。然而,Gattinoni 等质疑了动脉血氧分压过低决定组织缺氧的观点,并提出几乎所有严重的 ARDS 患者都可以用低流量体外系统来治疗。事实上,动脉血氧分压低于 60 mmHg 时似乎没有任何器

官损伤[10]。在 EOLIA 试验中,发现 ECMO 最大的获益是在呼吸性酸中毒达到一定程度无法实施保护性通气的患者人群(ECMO 组的病死率为 24%,对照组为 55%)[17]。这一发现表明 ECMO 的益处可能更多在于预防 VILI,而不是改善动脉血氧。

当体外气体交换的需求是减少机械通气的负荷时,采用创伤性较小的 $ECCO_2R$ 可能是一个合理的选择。然而,定义通气负荷下限来实施 $ECCO_2R$ 可能具有挑战性。事实上,最近的一项关于 $ECCO_2R$ 和超保护性肺通气的研究——SUPERNOVA 研究——使用氧合指数而不是通气负荷作为纳入标准[20],通过比较采用低或中流量的两种不同的装置,仅发现平台压略有降低。

$ECCO_2R$ 系统(管路尺寸、泵和膜表面)限制了可实现的最大血流量,在危及生命的低氧血症情况下无治疗效果。超保护性通气策略(即潮气量降低至 6 mL/kg 以下)旨在降低危重 ARDS 患者的 VILI。然而,这往往导致肺去复张,从而使缺氧进一步恶化[21]。

事实上,在关于 $ECCO_2R$ 安全性的一项研究中,发现 15 例患者中分别有 2 例需要俯卧位和 4 例转换为高流量 V-V ECMO 以挽救危及生命的低氧血症[22]。此外,由于膜肺对呼吸熵的调节,$ECCO_2R$ 可使患者暴露于反常低氧血症[23,24]。

过去我们团队提出并验证了一个 V-V ECMO 过程中氧合的数学模型[8],该模型具有较高的准确性和预测能力。通过该模型我们回顾性分析了我院 76 例高流量 V-V ECMO 患者的数据。在这些患者中,30 例(39%)患者的血流下降到 $ECCO_2R$ 范围(即 1 L/min)存在严重的低氧饱和度(即外周氧饱和度低于 85%),尽管呼吸机的 FiO_2 为 100%(未发表数据)。由于这些数据存在回顾性、初步性和计算机模拟的特点,需要进一步的研究来确定在严重 ARDS 患者中单纯 $ECCO_2R$ 技术相对于高流量 V-V ECMO 的安全性和可行性。

如上所述,需要 500~1 500 mL/min 的体外血流量来清除绝大部分的 CO_2 总产量(VCO_2)。实验性技术已经被开发出来以提高膜肺的体外 CO_2 清除效率,其目的是从非常低的血流量中提取高达一半的 VCO_2,比如在肾脏替代治疗中使用的血流量(150~300 mL/min),这样的话就可以使用小型的双腔导管(如 12~14 Fr)。理论上,甚至可以使用局部柠檬酸抗凝。

血液酸化已经作为提高膜肺的 CO_2 清除能力的一种实验技术[25]。酸化作用将碳酸氢盐转化为 CO_2,增加了 CO_2 的转移[26,27]。最近,呼吸性电透析被认为是一种有效实施 $ECCO_2R$ 的新实验技术[28,29]。与传统 $ECCO_2R$ 相比,呼吸性电透析使膜肺 CO_2 清除量增加了一倍,并且将每分钟通气量减半。由于这些都是非常初步的实验结果,需要进一步的研究。

30.4 急性呼吸窘迫综合征患者体外气体交换的循证证据

如上所述,V-V ECMO 是难治性低氧血症无可争议的挽救性治疗方法,并且在需要高平台压力和(或)潮气量时有坚实的生理学机制支持其使用。然而,目前尚不清楚如何定义必须启动 V-V 体外支持的氧合和通气负荷阈值。

最近，两项重要的研究改变了 V-V ECMO 使用的证据。

大约 10 年前，CESAR 试验[18]清楚地表明，最严重的 ARDS 患者应该转移到具有 ECMO 能力的中心以显著提高生存率而不造成严重残疾。即使只有 75% 的患者接受了 ECMO 治疗，使用 ECMO 极有可能对生存率产生影响。

最近的 EOLIA 试验[17]随机分配 249 名严重 ARDS 患者接受早期 V-V ECMO 或常规限制潮气量（tidal volume, V_T）和压力的通气策略（包括后期将 ECMO 作为挽救性治疗）。尽管没能确定生存获益（ECMO 组和对照组的病死率分别为 35% 和 46%，$P=0.09$），但从常规治疗组转到 ECMO 组进行挽救性治疗的重症患者比例较高（28%），这支持在危及生命的低氧血症中使用 V-V ECMO。此外，按照研究方案的分析和贝叶斯后验分析为研究结果提供了更有利的解读[30,31]。因此，一项针对 EOLIA 和 CESAR 试验的患者个体数据荟萃分析[30]发现，与常规治疗相比，ECMO 支持的患者 90 天病死率显著降低。

与单独机械通气（mechanical ventilation, MV）相比，联合使用 $ECCO_2R$ 和 MV 已被证明是可行的[7,20,22]。尽管如此，使用 $ECCO_2R$ 的获益需要能抵消这项技术的风险。最近发布的 REST 试验[21]旨在确定与标准治疗相比，$ECCO_2R$ 联合超保护性通气可改善全因死亡率。这项研究由于无效和可行性问题被提前中止了。实验组（低潮气量通气＋$ECCO_2R$）90 天病死率为 41.5%，而标准治疗组为 39.5%（$P=0.68$）。然而 $ECCO_2R$ 组有更少的无呼吸机天数和更严重的不良事件。$ECCO_2R$ 组的不良事件包括 9 例患者颅内出血（4.5%，对照组为 0%），以及其他部位出血（3.0%，对照组为 0.5%）。本研究存在一些相关的局限性，包括没有达到实验预设的潮气量目标（3 mL/kg）。基于上述这些结果，$ECCO_2R$ 目前还不能推荐作为改善 ARDS 患者预后的一种策略。

30.5 静脉-静脉体外膜肺氧合治疗急性呼吸窘迫综合征患者的预后

体外生命支持组织（extracorporeal life support organization, ELSO）定期收集并发布 ECMO 运行次数及其结果。总体而言，接受 V-V ECMO 治疗的成年患者的住院存活率为 59%[32]。在过去 10 年里，ECMO 的运行例数增加至原来的 3 倍[32]，最近的 SARS-CoV-2 大流行导致 V-V ECMO 在全球范围内的使用进一步增加。在中国早期报告 ECMO 治疗 COVID-19 患者非常高的病死率之后[33]，后续一些大型观察性研究中发现 ECMO 显示出令人满意的结果。这项来自 ELSO 注册中心的大型观察性研究纳入 1 035 名 COVID-19 患者，90 天病死率为 37%[34]。后来纳入 2020 年秋季的第二波 COVID-19 患者的研究[35-37]显示病死率呈上升的趋势（48%～60%）。这一发现只能部分地由患者的基线特征来解释。作者认为插管前过长的（失败的）无创通气策略和增加的肺损伤可能已经影响了这一糟糕的结果[36]。这凸显了在急性呼吸窘迫的情况下，V-V ECMO 只应被用作一种过渡至恢复的治疗，而不应在肺损伤不可逆的情况下使用。

30.6 是否应该增加体外膜肺氧合中心的数量

在过去的 10 年中,ECMO 中心的数量在稳步增加[32]。人们可能会认为每家医院/ICU 都应该具备 ECMO 能力,以便能够面对任何传统治疗难以治愈的严重呼吸(或心脏)衰竭。然而,开展 ECMO 技术需要一个具有特定技能的多学科团队(即医生、护士、灌注师),这些技能难以在短时间内培养出来且需要大量病例来维持熟练度。多项研究表明,ECMO 患者预后的一个主要决定因素是中心病例数量[38,39]。因此,建立区域中心与辐射点的组织架构似乎能够提供最好的结果[39]。在许多 ECMO 中心都有 24/7 的移动 ECMO 团队值班,可以安全地转运患者,并获得良好的预后。CESAR 试验[18]明确显示,将严重但可能可逆的呼吸衰竭患者集中到具有 ECMO 能力的中心可显著提高生存率。周边的"辐射点"医院必须发展早期识别和管理有 ARDS 恶化风险患者的精细技能,并应及时咨询 ECMO 中心,因为长期机械通气(特别是非保护性的)已被证明是不良预后的独立预测因素[39]。

30.7 总结

简而言之,V-V ECMO 提供氧合并允许更具保护性的通气策略[14,40]。考虑到其强有力的理论基础和最近的随机试验结果[30],当其他疗法(如俯卧位)失败时,应考虑在经验丰富的 ECMO 中心应用于最严重的 ARDS 患者。然而,肺休息的适当水平、机械通气的设置,以及体外支持时辅助呼吸的作用还有待进一步研究。

(王蕊,戴清霞 译)

参考文献

[1] Ware LB, Matthay MA. The acute respiratory distress syndrome. N Engl J Med. 2000; 342(18): 1334-49.

[2] Zapol WM, Snider MT, Hill JD, Fallat RJ, Bartlett RH, Edmunds LH, et al. Extracorporeal membrane oxygenation in severe acute respiratory failure. A randomized prospective study. JAMA. 1979; 242(20): 2193-6.

[3] Gattinoni L, Agostoni A, Pesenti A, Pelizzola A, Rossi GP, Langer M, et al. Treatment of acute respiratory failure with low-frequency positive-pressure ventilation and extracorporeal removal of CO_2. Lancet. 1980; 2(8189): 292-4.

[4] Gattinoni L, Kolobow T, Tomlinson T, Iapichino G, Samaja M, White D, et al. Low-frequency positive pressure ventilation with extracorporeal carbon dioxide removal (LFPPV-ECCO2R): an experimental study. Anesth Analg. 1978; 57(4): 470-7.

[5] Gattinoni L, Pesenti A, Mascheroni D, Marcolin R, Fumagalli R, Rossi F, et al. Low-frequency positive-pressure ventilation with extracorporeal CO_2 removal in severe acute respiratory failure. JAMA. 1986; 256(7): 881-6.

[6] Terragni PP, Del Sorbo L, Mascia L, Urbino R, Martin EL, Birocco A, et al. Tidal volume lower than 6 mL/kg enhances lung protection: role of extracorporeal carbon dioxide removal. Anesthesiology. 2009; 111(4): 826-35.

[7] Combes A, Tonetti T, Fanelli V, Pham T, Pesenti A, Mancebo J, et al. Efficacy and safety of lower versus higher CO_2 extraction devices to allow ultraprotective ventilation: secondary analysis of the SUPERNOVA study. Thorax. 2019; 74(12): 1179-81.

[8] Zanella A, Salerno D, Scaravilli V, Giani M, Castagna L, Magni F, et al. A mathematical model of oxygenation during venovenous extracorporeal membrane oxygenation support. J Crit Care. 2016; 36: 178-86.

[9] Schmidt M, Tachon G, Devilliers C, Muller G, Hekimian G, Bréchot N, et al. Blood oxygenation and decarboxylation determinants during venovenous ECMO for respiratory failure in adults. Intensive Care Med. 2013; 39(5): 838-46.

[10] Gattinoni L, Vassalli F, Romitti F, Vasques F, Pasticci I, Duscio E, et al. Extracorporeal gas exchange: when to start and how to end? Crit Care. 2019; 23(Suppl 1): 203.

[11] Papazian L, Aubron C, Brochard L, Chiche J-D, Combes A, Dreyfuss D, et al. Formal guidelines: management of acute respiratory distress syndrome. Ann Intensive Care. 2019; 9(1): 69.

[12] Zochios V, Parhar K, Tunnicliffe W, Roscoe A, Gao F. The right ventricle in ARDS. Chest. 2017; 152(1): 181-93.

[13] Araos J, Alegria L, Garcia P, Cruces P, Soto D, Erranz B, et al. Near-apneic ventilation decreases lung injury and fibroproliferation in an acute respiratory distress syndrome model with extracorporeal membrane oxygenation. Am J Respir Crit Care Med. 2019; 199(5): 603-12.

[14] Schmidt M, Pham T, Arcadipane A, Agerstrand C, Ohshimo S, Pellegrino V, et al. Mechanical ventilation management during extracorporeal membrane oxygenation for acute respiratory distress syndrome. An international multicenter prospective cohort. Am J Respir Crit Care Med. 2019; 200(8): 1002-12.

[15] Reis Miranda D, van Thiel R, Brodie D, Bakker J. Right ventricular unloading after initiation of venovenous extracorporeal membrane oxygenation. Am J Respir Crit Care Med. 2015; 191(3): 346-8.

[16] Mekontso Dessap A, Boissier F, Charron C, Bégot E, Repessé X, Legras A, et al. Acute cor pulmonale during protective ventilation for acute respiratory distress syndrome: prevalence, predictors, and clinical impact. Intensive Care Med. 2016; 42(5): 862-70.

[17] Combes A, Hajage D, Capellier G, Demoule A, Lavoué S, Guervilly C, et al. Extracorporeal membrane oxygenation for severe acute respiratory distress syndrome. N Engl J Med. 2018; 378(21): 1965-75.

[18] Peek GJ, Mugford M, Tiruvoipati R, Wilson A, Allen E, Thalanany MM, et al. Efficacy and economic assessment of conventional ventilatory support versus extracorporeal membrane oxygenation for severe adult respiratory failure (CESAR): a multicentre randomised controlled trial. Lancet. 2009; 374(9698): 1351-63.

[19] Morris AH, Wallace CJ, Menlove RL, Clemmer TP, Orme JF, Weaver LK, et al. Randomized clinical trial of pressure-controlled inverse ratio ventilation and extracorporeal CO_2 removal for adult respiratory distress syndrome. Am J Respir Crit Care Med. 1994; 149(2 Pt 1): 295-305.

[20] Combes A, Fanelli V, Pham T, Ranieri VM. European Society of Intensive Care Medicine Trials Group and the "strategy of ultra-protective lung ventilation with extracorporeal CO_2 removal for

new-onset moderate to severe ARDS" (SUPERNOVA) investigators. Feasibility and safety of extracorporeal CO_2 removal to enhance protective ventilation in acute respiratory distress syndrome: the SUPERNOVA study. Intensive Care Med. 2019; 45(5): 592-600.

[21] McNamee JJ, Gillies MA, Barrett NA, Perkins GD, Tunnicliffe W, Young D, et al. Effect of lower tidal volume ventilation facilitated by extracorporeal carbon dioxide removal vs standard care ventilation on 90-day mortality in patients with acute hypoxemic respiratory failure: the REST randomized clinical trial. JAMA. 2021; 326(11): 1013-23.

[22] Fanelli V, Ranieri MV, Mancebo J, Moerer O, Quintel M, Morley S, et al. Feasibility and safety of low-flow extracorporeal carbon dioxide removal to facilitate ultra-protective ventilation in patients with moderate acute respiratory distress sindrome. Crit Care. 2016; 10(20): 36.

[23] Diehl J-L, Mercat A, Pesenti A. Understanding hypoxemia on ECCO2R: back to the alveolar gas equation. Intensive Care Med. 2019; 45(2): 255-6.

[24] Cipriani E, Langer T, Bottino N, Brusatori S, Carlesso E, Colombo SM, et al. Key role of respiratory quotient to reduce the occurrence of hypoxemia during extracorporeal gas exchange: a theoretical analysis. Crit Care Med. 2020; 48(12): e1327-31.

[25] Zanella A, Patroniti N, Isgrò S, Albertini M, Costanzi M, Pirrone F, et al. Blood acidification enhances carbon dioxide removal of membrane lung: an experimental study. Intensive Care Med. 2009; 35(8): 1484-7.

[26] Zanella A, Mangili P, Giani M, Redaelli S, Scaravilli V, Castagna L, et al. Extracorporeal carbon dioxide removal through ventilation of acidified dialysate: an experimental study. J Heart Lung Transplant. 2014; 33(5): 536-41.

[27] Zanella A, Mangili P, Redaelli S, Scaravilli V, Giani M, Ferlicca D, et al. Regional blood acidification enhances extracorporeal carbon dioxide removal: a 48-hour animal study. Anesthesiology. 2014; 120(2): 416-24.

[28] Zanella A, Castagna L, El Aziz A, El Sayed DS, Scaravilli V, Ferlicca D, Magni F, et al. Extracorporeal CO_2 removal by respiratory electrodialysis: an in vitro study. ASAIO J. 2016; 62(2): 143-9.

[29] Zanella A, Castagna L, Salerno D, Scaravilli V, El Aziz A, El Sayed DS, Magni F, et al. Respiratory electrodialysis. A novel, highly efficient extracorporeal CO2 removal technique. Am J Respir Crit Care Med. 2015; 192(6): 719-26.

[30] Combes A, Peek GJ, Hajage D, Hardy P, Abrams D, Schmidt M, et al. ECMO for severe ARDS: systematic review and individual patient data meta-analysis. Intensive Care Med. 2020; 46(11): 2048-57.

[31] Goligher EC, Tomlinson G, Hajage D, Wijeysundera DN, Fan E, Jüni P, et al. Extracorporeal membrane oxygenation for severe acute respiratory distress syndrome and posterior probability of mortality benefit in a post hoc Bayesian analysis of a randomized clinical trial. JAMA. 2018; 320(21): 2251-9.

[32] Extracorporeal Life Support Organization. ELSO international summary [Internet]. 2021. https://www.elso.org/Registry/Statistics/InternationalSummary.aspx.

[33] Zeng Y, Cai Z, Xianyu Y, Yang BX, Song T, Yan Q. Prognosis when using extracorporeal membrane oxygenation (ECMO) for critically ill COVID-19 patients in China: a retrospective case series. Crit Care. 2020; 24(1): 1-3.

[34] Barbaro RP, MacLaren G, Boonstra PS, Iwashyna TJ, Slutsky AS, Fan E, et al. Extracorporeal membrane oxygenation support in COVID-19: an international cohort study of the extracorporeal

life support organization registry. Lancet. 2020；396(10257)：1071-8.

[35] Barbaro RP, MacLaren G, Boonstra PS, Combes A, Agerstrand C, Annich G, et al. Extracorporeal membrane oxygenation for COVID-19：evolving outcomes from the international extracorporeal life support organization registry. Lancet. 2021；398(10307)：1230-8.

[36] Schmidt M, Langouet E, Hajage D, James SA, Chommeloux J, Bréchot N, et al. Evolving outcomes of extracorporeal membrane oxygenation support for severe COVID-19 ARDS in Sorbonne hospitals, Paris. Crit Care. 2021；25(1)：355.

[37] Riera J, Roncon-Albuquerque R, Fuset MP, Alcántara S, Blanco-Schweizer P, Riera J, et al. Increased mortality in patients with COVID-19 receiving extracorporeal respiratory support during the second wave of the pandemic. Intensive Care Med. 2021；47(12)：1490-3. https://doi.org/10.1007/s00134-021-06517-9.

[38] Barbaro RP, Odetola FO, Kidwell KM, Paden ML, Bartlett RH, Davis MM, et al. Association of hospital-level volume of extracorporeal membrane oxygenation cases and mortality. Analysis of the extracorporeal life support organization registry. Am J Respir Crit Care Med. 2015；191(8)：894-901.

[39] Lebreton G, Schmidt M, Ponnaiah M, Folliguet T, Para M, Guihaire J, et al. Extracorporeal membrane oxygenation network organisation and clinical outcomes during the COVID-19 pandemic in Greater Paris, France：a multicentre cohort study. Lancet Respir Med. 2021；9(8)：851-62.

[40] Marhong JD, Telesnicki T, Munshi L, Del Sorbo L, Detsky M, Fan E. Mechanical ventilation during extracorporeal membrane oxygenation. An international survey. Ann Am Thorac Soc. 2014；11(6)：956-61.

31 体外膜肺氧合时的机械通气参数设置
Mechanical Ventilation Setting During ECMO
Luigi Camporota, Eddy Fan

31.1 引言

31.1.1 急性呼吸窘迫综合征的机械通气策略

对于急性呼吸窘迫综合征（acute respiratory distress syndrome，ARDS）患者，在接受原发病治疗时常采用机械通气支持气体交换和呼吸做功。然而，现已明确，呼吸机产生的机械力可以损害小而不均一的病变肺，被称为呼吸机诱发的肺损伤（ventilator-induced lung injury，VILI），也是导致肺外器官衰竭发展的因素[1,2]。

基于对 VILI 的认识，在过去的 50 年里，机械通气的目标逐渐从专注于实现接近正常的动脉氧和二氧化碳分压（PaO_2 和 $PaCO_2$）水平（不惜以气道压和潮气量放开为代价）转变为最小化施加于肺的机械能量强度（机械能）。在此背景下，尤其关注将呼吸频率设置得尽可能低（基于 $PaCO_2$）[3]、使用适度的呼气末正压（positive end-expiratory pressure，PEEP）、避免常规使用肺复张手法（recruitment manoeuvre，RM）[2,4]，以及与静息肺容积成比例的潮气量（应变）。最后一项反映在驱动压的测量上，它表示潮气量与呼吸系统顺应性之间的比值[5]。

31.1.2　重度急性呼吸窘迫综合征患者接受体外膜肺氧合时的机械通气策略

机械能的不同组成部分[6]与临床结局之间的关联对于接受体外膜肺氧合（extracorporeal membrane oxygenation，ECMO）治疗重度 ARDS 的患者尤为重要[1]，因为非常低的肺容积和更严重的不均一性使得肺实质更易受到机械应力和应变的影响，从而导致 VILI。

一些研究也证实了肺保护通气和 ECMO 在 ARDS 患者中的价值[7]。迄今为止的证据似乎表明，一旦患者接受 ECMO 治疗，采用较低的驱动压（潮气量）和呼吸频率进行通气是可行的[8-12]，并且能改善预后[13,14]。

在本章中，我们将回顾一些 ECMO 期间机械通气的相关证据和一些实践建议。

31.1.3　体外膜肺氧合对气体交换和与原生肺功能交互的作用

静脉-静脉（"呼吸"）ECMO 使从中心静脉流出的缺氧血，经过充分的氧合、二氧化碳清除，以足够的流量（3~7 L/min）被重新注入腔静脉或右心房，从而实现满足代谢需求的氧输送。

在无 ECMO 的 ARDS 患者中，动脉氧含量（CaO_2）取决于原生肺的分流比例和混合静脉血的氧含量：

$$CaO_2 = CcO_2 \times \left(1 - \frac{Q_s}{Q_t}\right) + \left(CvO_2 \times \frac{Q_s}{Q_t}\right) \tag{31.1}$$

公式中，$1-(Q_s/Q_t)$ 是经过通气肺实质的心输出量占比，Q_s/Q_t 是经过未通气肺区域的心输出量占比。

在完全依赖 ECMO（即无残余原生肺功能）的患者中，CaO_2（最简单的形式，未考虑再循环）为：

$$CaO_2 = C_{post\text{-}oxy}O_2 \times ECBF + CvO_2 \times (CO - ECBF) \tag{31.2}$$

这个公式类似于公式（31.1），其中 ECMO 血流量记为 ECBF，CO 是患者的心输出量，CvO_2 是静脉血氧含量，$C_{post\text{-}oxy}O_2$ 是氧合器出口血含氧量。

通过重新排列，得到公式（31.2）：

$$CaO_2 = \left(\frac{ECBF}{CO}\right) \times C_{post\text{-}oxy}O_2 + \left[1 - \left(\frac{ECBF}{CO}\right)\right] \times CvO_2 \tag{31.3}$$

使用这个公式,可用 ECBF 与心输出量之间的比值表示氧含量,类似于原生肺的分流方程。

显然,氧含量不仅取决于 ECMO 血流量和静脉血中的氧含量,还取决于 ECBF 与患者心输出量之间的比值。为了理解这个概念,我们必须考虑静脉回流(等于患者心输出量)是如何分成两个组成部分的:① 一部分(等于 ECBF)将通过氧合器,因此将成为完全氧合的静脉血回到右心房($S_{post-oxy} = 100\%$;$P_{post-oxy}O_2$ 可达 $60 \sim 70$ kPa 或 $450 \sim 525$ mmHg);② 第二部分是超过 ECBF 的流量(即 CO - ECBF),为原本静脉血的氧饱和度。因此,患者的混合静脉(肺动脉中)的血氧合水平将是两者的混合"加权平均值",其比例将取决于:ECBF 与 CO 的比、静脉氧合水平和膜肺的功能(即充分氧合静脉血的能力)。

31.1.4　原生肺与人工肺之间的相互作用

从上述原理可以清楚地看出,除非 ECBF 恰好等于(或大于——如果考虑到再循环)心输出量,否则患者的动脉饱和度将低于 100%,通常为 85%~92%。在这种情况下,需要采用恰当的通气策略对原生肺进行管理以维持一定程度的原生肺功能。因此,值得反思的是一旦患者接受 ECMO 治疗,原生肺功能可能会因两个主要生理现象而恶化:

(1) 消除低氧性肺血管收缩(由于混合静脉血高氧合)导致原生肺生理性分流增加。

(2) 膜肺清除的 CO_2 导致肺泡氧分压降低、肺泡 CO_2(P_AO_2)减少(表现为呼气末 CO_2 降低)。根据肺泡气体方程,P_AO_2 的降低导致原生肺呼吸熵降低,P_AO_2 逐渐下降:

$$PAO_2 = [FiO_2 - P_{atm-H_2O}] - \left(\frac{PaCO_2 \times VO_2}{VCO_{2NL}}\right) \tag{31.4}$$

其中,VO_2 是耗氧量,VCO_{2NL} 是每分钟通过原生肺排出的 CO_2 量。值得注意的是,超保护性通气策略(严重低通气伴正常碳酸血症)可能导致再吸收性肺不张,而吸气压力的减少可导致呼气末肺容积显著降低,以及由于压力性肺不张引起肺塌陷。所有这些情况都可以通过使用适当水平的 PEEP 来避免。

随着 ECMO 启动后血流动力学的变化,这些生理机制和呼吸机设置的变化导致原生肺分流比例增加和气体交换恶化(图 31.1)。

31.1.5　体外膜肺氧合的机械通气：一般原则

在不同的国际 ECMO 中心,重度 ARDS 患者在 ECMO 上的通气设置差异很大,并且没有普遍接受达成共识的最佳策略。尽管大多数中心报告采用低潮气量的"肺休息"策略[15],但在 PEEP 设置、滴定和肺复张手法的使用方面存在很大的差异[16],不到三分之一的中心为 ECMO 患者制定了明确的机械通气方案[16]。这种实践差异一方面反映了缺乏来自随机对照试验(randomized controlled trial, RCT)的有力证据,另一方面也反映了每个 ECMO 中心在背景、专业知识和病例组合方面的差异。

然而,在 ECMO 期间机械通气的主要目标应该是避免 VILI,同时促进肺休息和愈合[7]。因此,机械通气应在最大程度上保护肺,而气体交换则由 ECMO 支持。

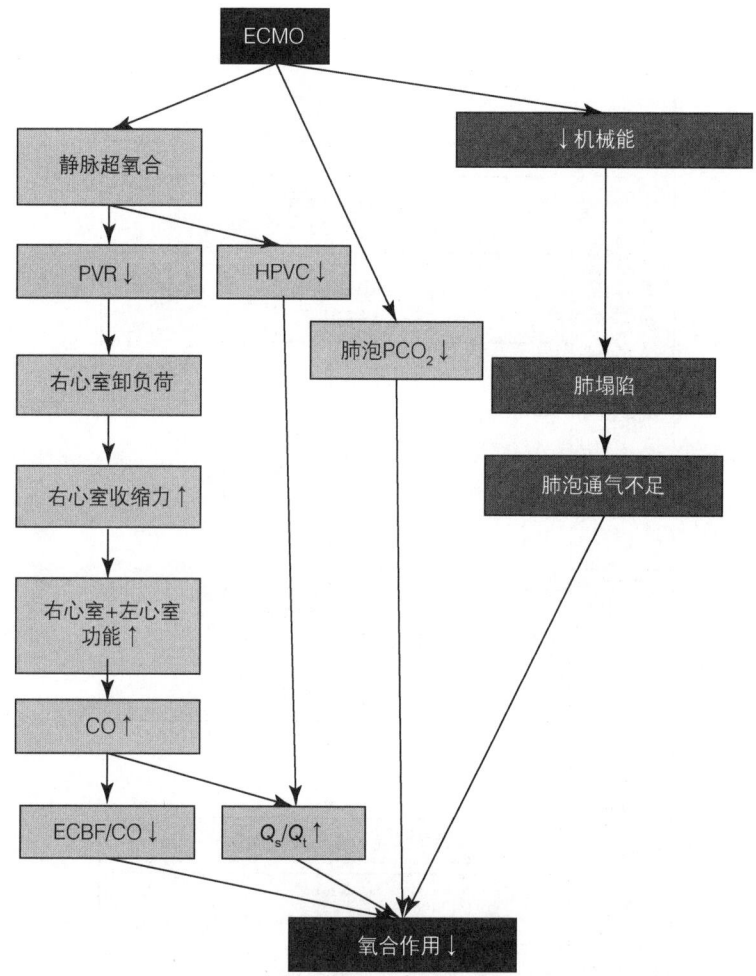

图 31.1 ECMO 启动后可能影响动脉氧合的病理生理变化。V-V ECMO 增加静脉氧合，允许降低机械能。ECMO 产生静脉超氧合，从而降低肺血管阻力（PVR）和缺氧性肺血管收缩（HPVC）。这改善了右心室功能、心输出量并增加了分流（Q_s/Q_t）。心输出量（CO）改善并降低了体外循环血流量（ECBF）和心输出量之间的比值。所有这些变化可以导致动脉氧分压降低。Q_s/Q_t，肺内分流率

CESAR 研究中[17]使用的"标准"通气设置如下：将 FiO_2 降低至 0.3（或尽可能最低）；潮气量为 2~4 mL/kg（基于预测体重计算）；限制平台压在 20~25 cmH_2O；PEEP 最初设置为保持平均气道压的水平，然后逐渐降低至 10 cmH_2O，得到 10 cmH_2O 的驱动压。呼吸频率维持在 10 次/分。最近的 EOLIA 试验[18]采用了类似策略，但呼吸频率为 10~30 次/分。

尽管在接受 ECMO 支持的患者中 RCT 数据较为有限，但过去 20 年来在 ARDS 管理方面积累的证据可以提供一些安全指导原则，同样可以外推应用于 ECMO 患者。

如果我们考虑到单一指导原则，即 VILI 的决定因素（从定义上讲）——由呼吸机向肺输送的总能量（在控制通气的条件下），那么减少 VILI 的最佳方法是尽量降低机械能方程的每个组成部分：呼吸频率、（基于潮气量的）驱动压、吸气流速和 PEEP[6,19]（图 31.2）。

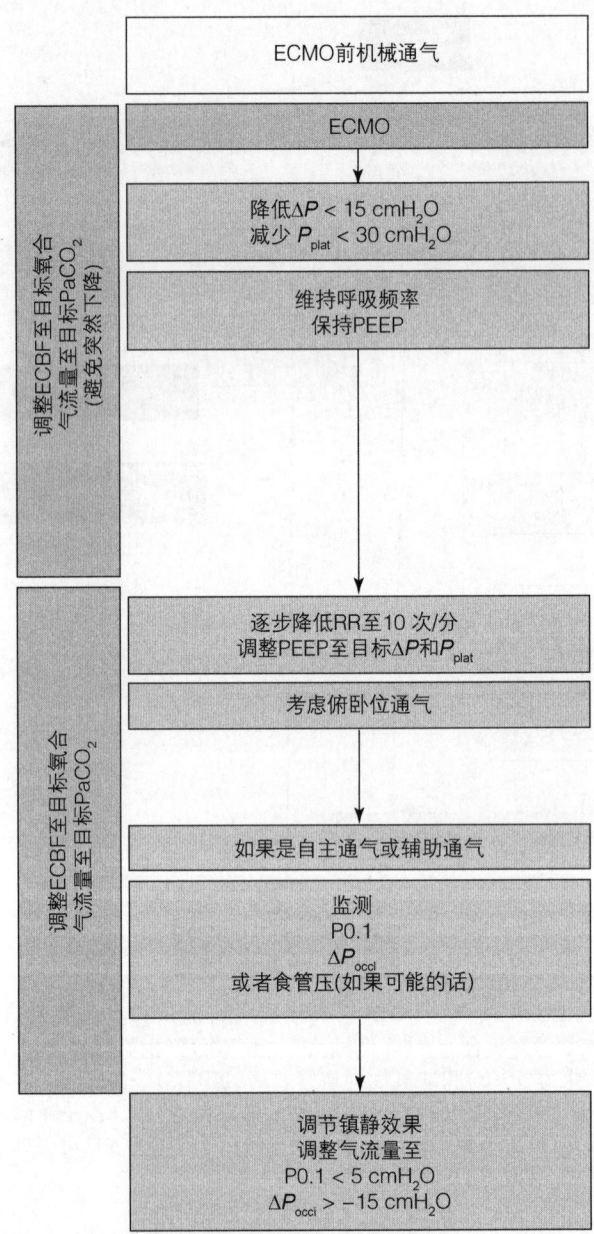

图 31.2　ECMO 时机械通气：步骤和目标

31.1.6　体外膜肺氧合期间的机械通气设置

31.1.6.1　潮气量

尽管关于基于预测体重的最佳潮气量（tidal volume，V_T）是多少的问题（6 mL/kg vs. 4 mL/kg vs. 3 mL/kg）仍存在争议，但越来越多生理学机制支持的有力证据证明容积伤的决定因素是肺应变——测量方法为潮气量与静息肺容积[功能残气量（functional residual capacity，FRC）]的比值。

在无法床旁测量 FRC 的情况下，可以使用 V_T（可通气肺容积，即"婴儿肺"）和呼吸系统顺应性（compliance of the respiratory system，C_{RS}）之间的关系来估计应变水平（公式 31.5），从而以 V_T 是否适合 FRC 的大小对最合适的潮气量做出临床判断。

$$\text{Strain} = \frac{V_T}{\text{FRC}};\ \text{FRC} \propto C_{RS} \to \text{Strain} \approx \frac{V_T}{C_{RS}} \qquad (31.5)$$

$$\text{Strain} = \frac{V_T}{\dfrac{V_T}{P_{\text{plateau}} - \text{PEEP}}} = P_{\text{plateau}} - \text{PEEP} \qquad (31.6)$$

当 C_{RS} 代替 FRC 输入应变方程（公式 31.5 和 31.6）时，可以看到驱动压（平台压减去 PEEP）可以代表肺应变。因此，无论 ARDS 的严重程度如何，均可使用驱动压来设置潮气量[3,20]。ECMO 可以使驱动压降低到 14 cmH$_2$O 以下，超过这个阈值死亡风险会增加[3,5]。

一项多中心前瞻性队列研究对 23 个国际 ICU 中接受 ECMO 治疗的 ARDS 患者进行为期一年的研究，发现 ECMO 启动后，V_T 从 (6.4±2.0) mL/kg(PBW) 减少到 (3.7±2.0) mL/kg(PBW)，驱动压从 (20±7) cmH$_2$O 减少到 (14±4) cmH$_2$O，同时呼吸频率降低，机械能从 (26.1±12.7) J/min 明显降低到 (6.6±4.8) J/min[8]。EOLIA 试验[18]和一项多中心观察性研究[11]也实现了类似的机械能下降。在 ECMO 患者中，潮气量和驱动压的降低与病死率密切相关，驱动压每增加 1 cmH$_2$O，住院死亡风险增加 6%（风险比 1.06，95%CI 为 1.03~1.1）[12]。

31.1.6.2 呼吸频率

呼吸频率可能是 VILI 最容易被忽视的决定因素。在未接受 ECMO 治疗的 ARDS 患者中，呼吸频率通常会增加，以补偿低潮气量和控制高碳酸血症。通过膜肺清除 CO$_2$，可以将呼吸频率降低到非常低的水平。这种策略可以减少炎症和肺损伤[21,22]。根据现有数据，建议 ECMO 期间尽可能降低呼吸频率：可以使用 CESAR 方案[17]：10 次/分，或者按照 ELSO 的建议[23]在 4~15 次/分的范围内设置。

31.1.6.3 呼气末正压

关于 ECMO 期间 PEEP 设置的建议更为多变，可能取决于肺复张的能力和 ECMO 前的平均气道压[24]。虽然过低的 PEEP 水平可能引起肺逐步塌陷、肺不张形成，导致进展为肺实变和纤维化，但过高的 PEEP 水平可能导致静态容积伤、肺应力和应变增加、血流动力学受损和 ECMO 导管引流不足。因此，在将平台压和驱动压保持在安全范围内的前提下，PEEP 设置为 10~15 cmH$_2$O 是一个合理的折中方案。

31.1.7 其他注意事项

31.1.7.1 俯卧位

在 ECMO 中使用俯卧位是可行的，尽管它可能与更长的 ECMO 持续时间相关[26]，但观察研究的数据表明它与预后改善相关[25,26]。虽然尚待确凿证据，但 ECMO 中的俯卧位似乎是一种有用的策略，可以保护肺部并在 ECMO 后最大限度地减少肺去复张。在操作过程中需要采取重要的防范措施,以保护受压的区域,以及避免插管阻塞/扭曲,这将影响甚至中断体外循环的血流。

31.1.7.2 呼吸努力

与 ECMO 患者通气相关的一个潜在问题是从控制通气到自主/辅助通气之间的过渡。尽管气体交换相对正常,但 ECMO 患者主要是在肺回弹力高的刺激下产生强烈的呼吸驱动和吸气努力,导致流量饥饿和呼吸窘迫。这些症状可能无法通过气管切开术改善,特别是在疾病的早期阶段[27],并且如果患者完全依赖 ECMO 或存在凝血功能障碍,可能与并发症相关[28]。增加的呼吸努力可能导致胸腔内压大幅变化,从而导致局部跨肺压不受控制地增加,引起肺损伤和气压伤,这个过程被称为患者自戕性肺损伤(patient self-inflicted lung injury,P-SILI)[29]。

临床医生应注意这种损伤的可能性,并使用诸如 P0.1、阻断压(P_{occ})[30]或侵入性的方法,如食管压或膈肌电活动(electrical activity of the diaphragm,EAdi)来监测吸气努力。可以使用呼气末阻断的方法,可以很容易进行阻断压测定。闭合压是阻断后第一次呼吸过程中 PEEP 与气道压力波动最低值的差值。理想情况下,管理患者使其能够维持 P0.1 在 4~5 cmH$_2$O,阻断压 > −15 cmH$_2$O[31]。

31.2 总结

在 ECMO 期间,通气的一般原则是在体外膜肺维持气体交换的同时最大限度地保护肺。在控制通气期间,密切关注和监测驱动压、呼吸频率,以及 PEEP 选择至关重要,同时监测吸气努力和驱动压可以降低 P-SILI 发生的风险。

利益声明:作者声明无利益冲突。

资金支持:无。

(王蕊,戴清霞 译)

参考文献

[1] Brodie D, Slutsky AS, Combes A. Extracorporeal life support for adults with respiratory failure and related indications: a review. JAMA. 2019; 322(6): 557-68.

[2] Tonetti T, Vasques F, Rapetti F, Maiolo G, Collino F, Romitti F, et al. Driving pressure and mechanical power: new targets for VILI prevention. Ann Transl Med. 2017; 5(14): 286.

[3] Costa ELV, Slutsky AS, Brochard LJ, Brower R, Serpa-Neto A, Cavalcanti AB, et al. Ventilatory variables and mechanical power in patients with acute respiratory distress syndrome. Am J Respir Crit Care Med. 2021; 204(3): 303-11.

[4] Cavalcanti AB, Suzumura EA, Laranjeira LN, Paisani DM, Damiani LP, Guimaraes HP, et al. Effect of lung recruitment and titrated positive end-expiratory pressure (PEEP) vs low PEEP on mortality in patients with acute respiratory distress syndrome: a randomized clinical trial. JAMA. 2017; 318(14): 1335-45.

[5] Amato MB, Meade MO, Slutsky AS, Brochard L, Costa EL, Schoenfeld DA, et al. Driving

[6] Gattinoni L, Tonetti T, Cressoni M, Cadringher P, Herrmann P, Moerer O, et al. Ventilator-related causes of lung injury: the mechanical power. Intensive Care Med. 2016; 42(10): 1567-75.

[7] Aoyama H, Uchida K, Aoyama K, Pechlivanoglou P, Englesakis M, Yamada Y, et al. Assessment of therapeutic interventions and lung protective ventilation in patients with moderate to severe acute respiratory distress syndrome: a systematic review and network meta-analysis. JAMA Netw Open. 2019; 2(7): e198116.

[8] Schmidt M, Pham T, Arcadipane A, Agerstrand C, Ohshimo S, Pellegrino V, et al. Mechanical ventilation management during extracorporeal membrane oxygenation for acute respiratory distress syndrome. An international multicenter prospective cohort. Am J Respir Crit Care Med. 2019; 200(8): 1002-12.

[9] Combes A, Schmidt M, Hodgson CL, Fan E, Ferguson ND, Fraser JF, et al. Extracorporeal life support for adults with acute respiratory distress syndrome. Intensive Care Med. 2020; 46(12): 2464-76.

[10] Quintel M, Busana M, Gattinoni L. Breathing and ventilation during extracorporeal membrane oxygenation: how to find the balance between rest and load. Am J Respir Crit Care Med. 2019; 200(8): 954-6.

[11] Schmidt M, Stewart C, Bailey M, Nieszkowska A, Kelly J, Murphy L, et al. Mechanical ventilation management during extracorporeal membrane oxygenation for acute respiratory distress syndrome: a retrospective international multicenter study. Crit Care Med. 2015; 43(3): 654-64.

[12] Serpa Neto A, Schmidt M, Azevedo LC, Bein T, Brochard L, Beutel G, et al. Associations between ventilator settings during extracorporeal membrane oxygenation for refractory hypoxemia and outcome in patients with acute respiratory distress syndrome: a pooled individual patient data analysis: mechanical ventilation during ECMO. Intensive Care Med. 2016; 42(11): 1672-84.

[13] Munshi L, Walkey A, Goligher E, Pham T, Uleryk EM, Fan E. Venovenous extracorporeal membrane oxygenation for acute respiratory distress syndrome: a systematic review and meta-analysis. Lancet Respir Med. 2019; 7(2): 163-72.

[14] Goligher EC, Tomlinson G, Hajage D, Wijeysundera DN, Fan E, Juni P, et al. Extracorporeal membrane oxygenation for severe acute respiratory distress syndrome and posterior probability of mortality benefit in a post hoc Bayesian analysis of a randomized clinical trial. JAMA. 2018; 320(21): 2251-9.

[15] Marhong JD, Telesnicki T, Munshi L, Del Sorbo L, Detsky M, Fan E. Mechanical ventilation during extracorporeal membrane oxygenation. An international survey. Ann Am Thorac Soc. 2014; 11(6): 956-61.

[16] Camporota L, Nicoletti E, Malafronte M, De Neef M, Mongelli V, Calderazzo MA, et al. International survey on the management of mechanical ventilation during ECMO in adults with severe respiratory failure. Minerva Anestesiol. 2015; 81(11): 1170-83, 77 p following 83.

[17] Peek GJ, Mugford M, Tiruvoipati R, Wilson A, Allen E, Thalanany MM, et al. Efficacy and economic assessment of conventional ventilatory support versus extracorporeal membrane oxygenation for severe adult respiratory failure (CESAR): a multicentre randomised controlled trial. Lancet. 2009; 374(9698): 1351-63.

[18] Combes A, Hajage D, Capellier G, Demoule A, Lavoue S, Guervilly C, et al. Extracorporeal membrane oxygenation for severe acute respiratory distress syndrome. N Engl J Med. 2018;

378(21): 1965-75.

[19] Giosa L, Busana M, Pasticci I, Bonifazi M, Macri MM, Romitti F, et al. Mechanical power at a glance: a simple surrogate for volume-controlled ventilation. Intensive Care Med Exp. 2019; 7(1): 61.

[20] Goligher EC, Costa ELV, Yarnell CJ, Brochard LJ, Stewart TE, Tomlinson G, et al. Effect of lowering V_T on mortality in acute respiratory distress syndrome varies with respiratory system elastance. Am J Respir Crit Care Med. 2021; 203(11): 1378-85.

[21] Grasso S, Stripoli T, Mazzone P, Pezzuto M, Lacitignola L, Centonze P, et al. Low respiratory rate plus minimally invasive extracorporeal CO_2 removal decreases systemic and pulmonary inflammatory mediators in experimental acute respiratory distress syndrome. Crit Care Med. 2014; 42(6): e451-60.

[22] Araos J, Alegria L, Garcia P, Cruces P, Soto D, Erranz B, et al. Near-apneic ventilation decreases lung injury and fibroproliferation in an acute respiratory distress syndrome model with extracorporeal membrane oxygenation. Am J Respir Crit Care Med. 2019; 199(5): 603-12.

[23] Tonna JE, Abrams D, Brodie D, Greenwood JC, Rubio Mateo-Sidron JA, Usman A, et al. Management of adult patients supported with venovenous extracorporeal membrane oxygenation (VV ECMO): guideline from the extracorporeal life support organization (ELSO). ASAIO J. 2021; 67(6): 601-10.

[24] Camporota L, Caricola EV, Bartolomeo N, Di Mussi R, Wyncoll DLA, Meadows CIS, et al. Lung recruitability in severe acute respiratory distress syndrome requiring extracorporeal membrane oxygenation. Crit Care Med. 2019; 47(9): 1177-83.

[25] Zaaqoq AM, Barnett AG, Griffee MJ, MacLaren G, Jacobs JP, Heinsar S, et al. Beneficial effect of prone positioning during venovenous extracorporeal membrane oxygenation for coronavirus disease 2019. Crit Care Med. 2021.

[26] Giani M, Martucci G, Madotto F, Belliato M, Fanelli V, Garofalo E, et al. Prone positioning during venovenous extracorporeal membrane oxygenation in acute respiratory distress syndrome. A multicenter cohort study and propensity-matched analysis. Ann Am Thorac Soc. 2021; 18(3): 495-501.

[27] Schmidt M, Fisser C, Martucci G, Abrams D, Frapard T, Popugaev K, et al. Tracheostomy management in patients with severe acute respiratory distress syndrome receiving extracorporeal membrane oxygenation: an international multicenter retrospective study. Crit Care. 2021; 25(1): 238.

[28] Dimopoulos S, Joyce H, Camporota L, Glover G, Ioannou N, Langrish CJ, et al. Safety of percutaneous dilatational tracheostomy during veno-venous extracorporeal membrane oxygenation support in adults with severe respiratory failure. Crit Care Med. 2019; 47(2): e81-8.

[29] Yoshida T, Amato MBP, Kavanagh BP, Fujino Y. Impact of spontaneous breathing during mechanical ventilation in acute respiratory distress syndrome. Curr Opin Crit Care. 2019; 25(2): 192-8.

[30] Bertoni M, Telias I, Urner M, Long M, Del Sorbo L, Fan E, et al. A novel non-invasive method to detect excessively high respiratory effort and dynamic transpulmonary driving pressure during mechanical ventilation. Crit Care. 2019; 23(1): 346.

[31] Esnault P, Cardinale M, Hraiech S, Goutorbe P, Baumstrack K, Prud'homme E, et al. High respiratory drive and excessive respiratory efforts predict relapse of respiratory failure in critically ill patients with COVID-19. Am J Respir Crit Care Med. 2020; 202(8): 1173-8.

第四部分
机械通气监测

第四部分

机械通气监测

32 呼吸系统的超声评估
Ultrasound Assessment of the Respiratory System

Mark E. Haaksma, Marry R. Smit, Pieter R. Tuinman

32.1 引言

床旁即时超声是一种非常重要的临床诊断和监测工具,它可对整个呼吸系统进行快速评估。通过反复的练习和扎实的解剖学知识,以及对超声模式的理解,操作者可以在床旁获得大量的信息,而且不会增加患者的负担和费用。因此,强烈建议在日常的临床实践中常规使用。在机械通气患者中,肺部疾病往往是机械通气的原因或后果,因此必须快速发现和治疗。在本章中,我们将讨论肺、膈肌和辅助呼吸肌超声检查的关键概念及其在重症监护中的临床应用。

32.2 肺部超声

32.2.1 简介

本节和图 32.1 将简要说明肺部超声最常见的图像并展示其在临床上的应用。

M. E. Haaksma (✉) · P. R. Tuinman
Department of Intensive Care Medicine, Amsterdam University Medical Centers, Location VUmc, Amsterdam, The Netherlands

Amsterdam Leiden Intensive Care Focused Echography (ALIFE), Amsterdam, The Netherlands

Amsterdam Cardiovascular Sciences Research Institute, Amsterdam UMC, Amsterdam, The Netherlands
e-mail: m.haaksma@amsterdamumc.nl; p.tuinman@amsterdamumc.nl; https://www.alifeofpocus.com; https://www.alifeofpocus.com

M. R. Smit
Department of Intensive Care Medicine, Amsterdam University Medical Centers, Location AMC, Amsterdam, The Netherlands
e-mail: m.r.smit@amsterdamumc.nl

© The Author(s), under exclusive license to Springer Nature Switzerland AG 2022
G. Bellani (ed.), *Mechanical Ventilation from Pathophysiology to Clinical Evidence*, https://doi.org/10.1007/978-3-030-93401-9_32

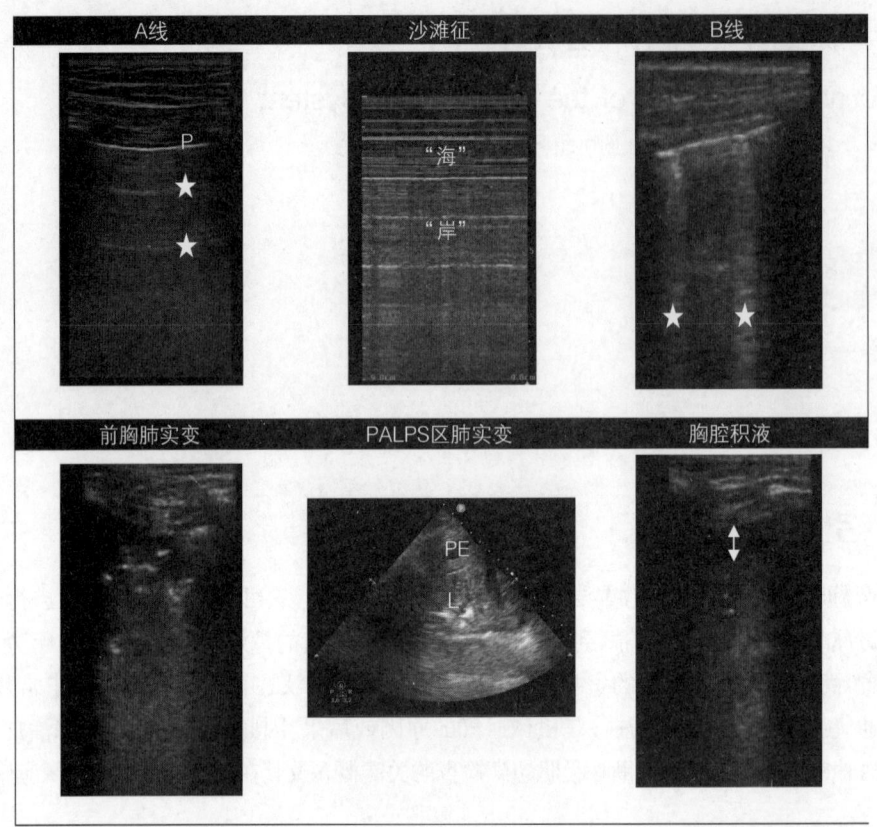

图32.1 肺超声检查中观察到的伪影和征象。P,胸膜;PE,胸膜积液;L,肺;星形,B线;箭头,胸腔积液

32.2.1.1 胸膜

胸膜是胸壁组织(富含液体)和肺部(富含空气)之间的界面。壁层胸膜和脏层胸膜不能相互区分,超声图像上显示为一条水平的、高回声的亮线。在呼吸周期中,表现为亮线滑动,称为肺滑移征。肺滑移征的缺失是病理性的,提示各种病理改变,如肺炎、单侧插管或其他合并症。如果临床医生不能确定是否存在肺滑移征,M超是一个有用的模式工具,它可以显示出沙滩征(存在肺滑移征)或条码征(无肺滑移征)。

32.2.1.2 A 线

A线是超声波在胸膜和探头之间来回反射产生的水平混响伪影。它们的存在表明胸壁与胸膜下组织之间的声阻抗存在很大差异,如软组织与空气。因此,它们的存在表明胸膜下组织含气量较多,比如充气的肺组织或气胸。

32.2.1.3 B 线

B线是由于小叶间隔增厚形成的,表现为垂直的彗星尾状伪影。B线的形成是由于液体外渗导致肺组织气-液比例改变,比如炎症反应或者静水压升高。1~2条B线的存在通常是生理性的,只有在一个肋间内出现两条以上的B线时才会被认为是病理性的,即所谓的间质综合征。在ICU,双侧间质性综合征最常见的原因是心源性肺水肿或ARDS;

至于单侧,肺炎是最可能的解释。

32.2.1.4 实变

如果肺部完全失去通气,超声波会轻易穿过肺实质,产生类似组织样或实变样图像。肺部组织出现的非伪像图像往往是病理性的,通常在肺不张、肺炎或 ARDS 中看到。在肺前部可以表现为"碎片征"(胸膜碎裂的形态学表现),或者表现为完全的实变(最常见于肺后下部)。

32.2.1.5 胸腔积液

胸腔积液可以表现为脏层和壁层胸膜之间的一层低回声区。通常情况下,其厚度随呼吸周期变化,即所谓的正弦征,并随重力分布。

32.2.2 临床应用

超声评估肺部是一门仍在发展的学科。因此,在临床实践中应用时,在一些方面存在异质性。虽然认识到差异是很重要的(我们也在后面罗列了这些内容),但应注意的是,一般来说,没有任何一种机器、探头或技术在各个方面都存在明显优势。因此,这些差异是可以接受的,而医生的个人偏好与习惯在其中也起着重要作用。

从超声机器本身开始,即使是最基础的版本通常也能满足使用,有时甚至因其缺少伪影消除和其他滤波软件的功能而更适合使用于肺部。不管是哪种类型或版本的机器,仔细检查能否停用消除伪影的软件或存在特殊的"肺模式"是很重要的。超声探头的选择取决于医生的偏好和可视化的目标,频率较高的探头可以更准确地检测出胸膜病变,而频率较低的探头可以提供更宽广的视野。探头应根据所执行的操作流程而放置在不同位置(稍后讨论),但通常应该垂直放置在肺表面并正好横跨肋间隙。但是图像深度和增益的进一步设置仍需要更多讨论来明确,通常建议使用至少几厘米的深度,以充分显示 A 线和 B 线等伪影。

32.2.2.1 急性呼吸衰竭的诊断

通常采用"BLUE"流程(图 32.2)来识别急性呼吸衰竭的最常见的原因[2]。为此,将肺部超声检查中观察到的超声图像和伪影与深静脉血栓的超声扫查相结合,用于诊断急性呼吸衰竭的常见原因。简而言之,每侧胸部扫查三个点(两个前点和一个后点)。前点根据肺滑移征和主要的超声图像进行评估,以确定图像特征。

(1) A 或 A′图像:A 线为主(A′,没有肺滑移征)。

(2) B 或 B′图像:B 线为主(B′,没有肺滑移征)。

(3) A/B 图像:单侧 A 线和对侧 B 线。

(4) C 图像:任何前点出现组织样图像。

后点只需表示存在(如胸腔积液、实变肺组织)或不存在(显示未受影响的肺部呼吸运动)。

从这一步开始,根据先前的步骤,可以通过一个分级决策树来建立诊断,或者需要分析深静脉血栓的可能性。决策树的终点有:肺炎、气胸、肺栓塞、肺水肿,以及慢性阻塞性肺疾病或哮喘。

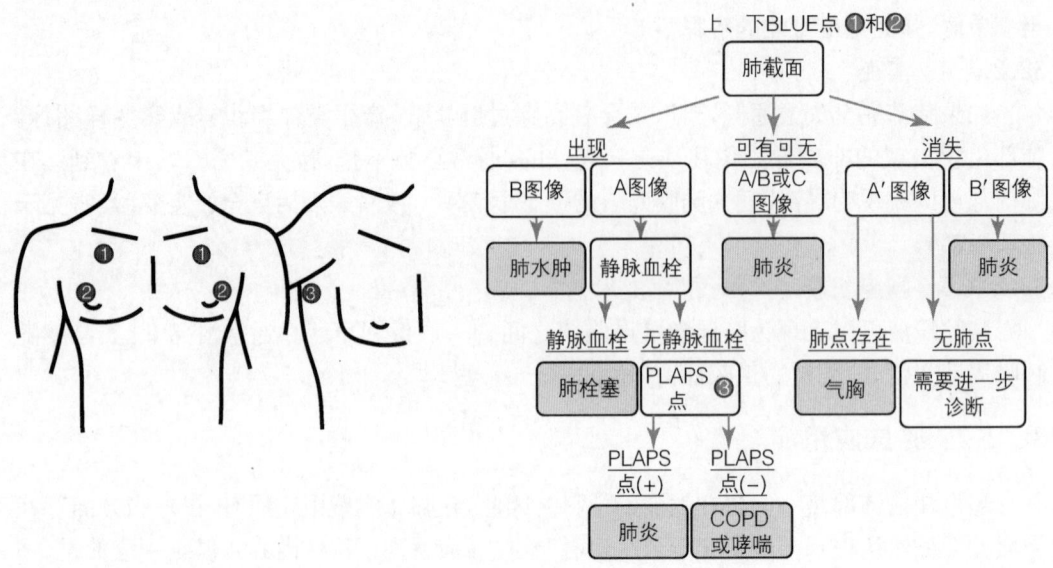

图 32.2 BLUE 流程。左：前点探头扫查位置(1 和 2)和 PLAPS 点位置(3)。右：BLUE 流程图

应该指出的是，这只是对流程的简化解释，更详细的描述请参考原始论文[2]。此外，该方案是在急诊室制定的(因此包括了该环境中最普遍的疾病)，而不是针对 ICU 患者。尽管如此，这不应阻碍其使用，它不仅可以提供重要的提示，而且在机械通气的患者中也适用。有建议采用彩色多普勒成像、支气管充气征和胸膜异常表现对流程进行补充，这是有意义的展望，但超出了本章范围[3]。

32.2.2.2 监测肺通气

在机械通气的患者中，肺通气的不足导致气体交换障碍是一种常见的现象。原因很多，包括机械性、感染性和静水压力等。因此，对于它的识别、治疗和监测是日常临床实践的重要组成部分，而这三个方面都可以通过超声来实现。通过超声扫查 12 个肺区，并根据每个评估点观察到的图像计算出总肺部超声评分(Lung Ultrasound Score，LUS)。图像类型与肺超声总分对应关系如下(图 32.3)。

(1) A 线图像(只有 A 线)=0。
(2) B1 线图像(B 线，≥3 条，界线清晰)=1。
(3) B2 线图像(B 线，≥3 条，融合成片)=2。
(4) C 线图像(实变肺组织)=3。

LUS 为每个区域扫描所得分数的总和，值为 0~36。研究表明，该评分与胸部 CT 有很好的相关性，因此被认为是可行的、侵入性较低的、更具成本效益的选择[4-6]。这种方法也可用于指导 ICU 的液体管理。研究显示，定期使用超声检查可降低总的液体平衡[7]。目前正在进行评估标准化方法及其对临床结果影响的研究。

32.2.2.3 肺部超声指导下的机械通气

如上所述，超声定期评估肺通气也可用于指导呼吸机设置[8]。一般来说，肺前区通气不足呈弥漫性分布的患者，往往对 PEEP 有反应。那些背外侧有通气不足而肺前区未受

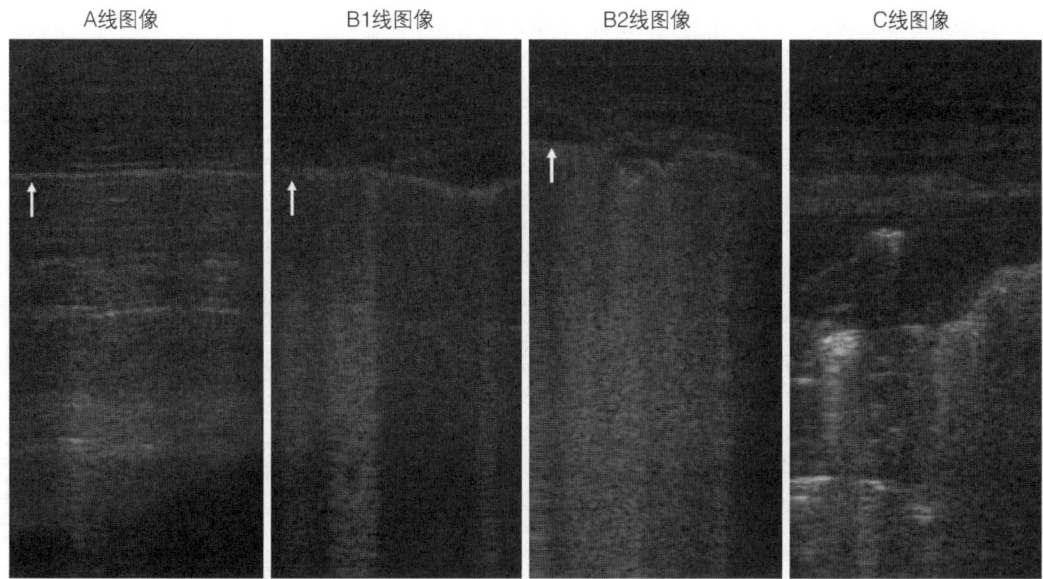

图 32.3 肺超声评分图像。白色箭头表示超声图像中的胸膜

影响的患者,增加 PEEP 可能导致肺部过度膨胀[8]。但是这两类患者都可能从俯卧位中获益。

32.2.2.4 胸腔积液的识别和引流

可以通过超声轻松识别和定量胸腔积液。目前存在几种方法,然而,没有一种方法被证明优于其他方法[9,10]。最简单的方法是患者采取仰卧位,将探头放置在背外侧,在最大吸气时测量脏层和壁层胸膜之间的最大距离。然后将测量值(以毫米为单位)乘以 20,得出以毫升为单位的积液量[胸腔积液体积(毫升)=测得距离(毫米)×20]。

虽然有研究认为通过超声来鉴别胸腔积液的性质可行的,漏出液呈低回声和均匀,而渗出液呈稍高回声和不均匀。然而,最近的证据显示往往并非如此[11]。因此,基于超声来评估积液的性质应谨慎,最好结合其他临床参数一起进行评估。

32.3 膈肌

32.3.1 简介

在生理情况下,膈肌是主要的呼吸肌。其收缩导致膈肌缩短、增厚和向腹部位移。这些变化可以通过超声清楚地显示(图 32.4),并有助于识别病理性的膈肌位移或增厚,特别是在机械通气的患者中[12,13]。然而需要注意的是,正压通气和呼气末正压(positive end-expiratory pressure, PEEP)会导致膈肌被动位移。因此,在评估膈肌活动和厚度时,需要记住这些局限。

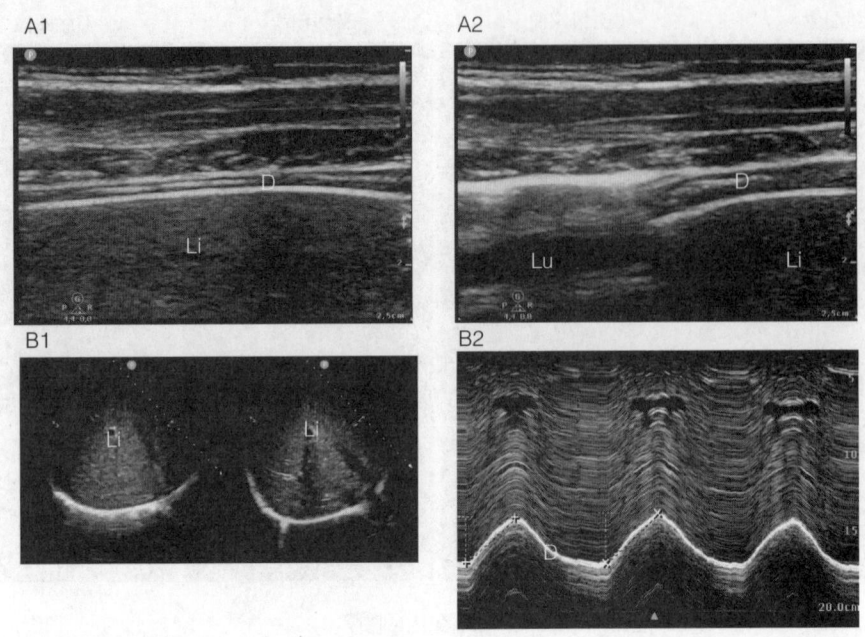

图 32.4 膈肌超声。A1. 呼气末的膈肌(B 型);A2. 呼气末的膈肌(B 型);B1. 膈肌位移(B 型);B2. 膈肌位移(M 型)。D,膈肌;L,肺;Li,肝

32.3.1.1 位移

膈肌位移是从肋下进行测量(双侧腋前线或锁骨中线与肋缘交界处),用低频探头(如心脏或腹部探头)对准膈肌的穹顶。图像上膈肌显示为一条高回声的线性结构。通常情况下,由于肝脏作为声窗,使得右侧膈肌更容易被显现。在左侧,充满气体的肠道会导致无法获得清晰图像,因此需要从更偏背外侧的角度进行观察。吸气时,膈肌将会朝向探头移动,而呼气时,膈肌将松弛并恢复到原来的位置。通常使用 M 超对膈肌位移的幅度进行量化。膈肌位移的正常参考值差异较大(低于 1～2.7 cm 提示功能障碍)[14,15]。对于定性信息,例如,膈肌麻痹或人-机不同步,B 超可能就足够了。

32.3.1.2 厚度和增厚率

膈肌厚度在腋中线处测量,大约位于第 8 肋和第 11 肋之间[12]。这个区域也被称为并行区,因为此处膈肌紧贴着胸壁。使用高频探头,显示膈肌为三层结构,周围被高回声的胸膜和腹膜所包围,肌肉内还有一层额外的高回声层。用于测量其厚度的标记应被放置于胸膜和腹膜之间。如果在呼气末和吸气末重复测量厚度,可以计算出所谓的增厚率[(吸气末厚度−呼气末厚度)/呼气末厚度]。这是一种量化膈肌功能的方法,可用于调整呼吸机设置或指导撤机拔管。存在自主呼吸的机械通气患者中,增厚率低于 30%～36% 提示膈肌功能障碍[16-18]。

32.3.2 临床应用

32.3.2.1 膈肌保护性通气

虽然肺保护性通气已成为重症医学实践中的常识,但膈肌保护性通气的概念却远不

为人所知。其基本理念是调节呼吸机设置,既不对膈肌过度辅助以防止失用性萎缩,也不因为辅助不足引起膈肌疲劳相关的损伤(另见"6　辅助通气过程中患者的监测")。事实上,研究表明,膈肌厚度和功能的丧失与更糟糕的临床结局有关,突显了这个理念的重要性[19]。然而,由于收缩的正常生理水平差异很大,到目前为止尚未明确定义膈肌收缩过度和不足的临界值,使得在临床实践中难以实施[20]。此外,虽然膈肌保护性通气可被视为肺部保护性通气的补充策略,但这两种策略的结果并不总是一致的。常见的一个例子是临床上需对呼吸驱动过度的患者进行深度镇静和肌肉松弛,虽然从肺保护的角度来看这是有益的,但膈肌却丧失了所有的活动,因此容易迅速萎缩[21]。

32.3.2.2　人-机不同步

人-机不同步发生于呼吸机对患者的呼吸需求反应不足的情况下。这是一个临床上的常见问题,但也往往被忽视。及时识别和处理是很重要的,因为不同步与不良预后和患者的不适感有关[22]。膈肌的超声评估可能是一个有价值的方法,但要在临床实践中实施还需要更多的证据。因此,本章不作进一步讨论,但我们推荐感兴趣的读者参阅最近的一篇综述,其总结了重要的不同步现象及其与超声图像的对应关系[13]。

32.3.2.3　撤机

将患者从机械通气中解放出来(参见"22　简单和复杂患者的撤机")是一项艰巨的任务,需要优化肺部、呼吸肌和心脏对撤机后病理生理变化的适应能力[1]。通过超声可以便捷地对这些系统进行评估,从而提供了监测撤机过程和评估失败原因的可能性。这些评估的内容和方法被总结为"ABCDE法",其中每个字母对应撤机过程的一个重要步骤[13]。

A:通气评分和胸腔积液。肺通气的丧失可以采用上述LUS进行评估。通气评分>17与拔管后的呼吸窘迫相关[23]。此外,如果在自主呼吸试验前和结束时计算四个肺前区的B线,B线增加超过6条也与自主呼吸试验失败相关[24]。需要明确胸腔积液的存在及其范围,并根据病情做相应治疗。

B:膈肌下方。腹部疾病可能会破坏理想的呼吸力学,因此会产生重要影响。

C:心脏。评估心功能是一个宽泛的术语,其程度主要取决于医生的专业技能。直接的方法包括目测法评估左心室功能和测量三尖瓣环收缩期位移法评估右心室收缩功能。同时,随着临床经验的积累,舒张功能也可以通过E/A来确定。

D:膈肌。通过超声测量膈肌增厚率和位移。这些指标的数值越低,拔管失败风险越高,下一节将详细介绍。

E:其他呼吸肌。当呼吸负荷高或膈肌疲劳时,这些呼吸肌会被积极利用。可以通过胸骨旁肋间肌和腹外侧肌的增厚进行评估[1,25]。

32.3.2.4　预测拔管结局

膈肌增厚率是研究得最充分的超声参数,用以预测拔管结果。第一批标志性的研究发现,如果将成功拔管的增厚率临界值设定在30%~36%以上,则具有很强的预测性[16-18]。然而,在过去的几年中,一些研究出现了相互矛盾的证据,之前认为它是一个良好预测因子的看法受到了挑战[26,27]。因此,目前还没有可靠的证据来建议支持或反对将其用于预测撤机失败。如果希望在临床实践中应用,最可行的方法可能是把它用作识别撤机失败潜在病因的工具，这在上面的章节中有所介绍。

32.4 辅助呼吸肌

辅助呼吸肌（最重要的是腹外侧肌、腹直肌和肋间肌）是呼吸肌泵的重要组成部分，但常常被忽视。它们对于有效清除气道、预防肺不张和在高呼吸强度情况下协助膈肌至关重要[28,29]。它们与膈肌及肺一样都是相对容易使用超声测量的，因此有可能被纳入完整的呼吸系统超声评估方案中。

目前，尽管研究证据有所增长，但仍然非常匮乏。对于区分生理和病理状态的参考值，以及在临床实践中的具体应用[30]还知之甚少。未来可能应用于早期识别过强的呼吸努力或预测困难撤机方面[25]。

32.5 局限性

肺部超声存在局限性，这是超声的固有物理特性所决定的。如前所述，气体和组织之间阻抗的巨大差异导致所有超声波在气体-组织界面上形成反射。因此，只有当肺部病变接近胸膜时才能被发现。此外，手术敷料或任何其他物理屏障如皮下气肿也会限制其使用。膈肌超声局限性在于膈肌的运动改变和增厚可能是机械通气导致的，以及需要使用皮肤标记以确保不同天数和不同操作人员测量的可重复性。因此，在解释测量结果时，仔细评估呼吸机设置是至关重要的。对于肺部和膈肌超声，还应该注意的是，需要一定的经验才能够正确解释图像。对初学者而言，超声图像会带来一种虚假的安全感，病变很容易被忽视。

32.6 总结

在本章中，我们概述了呼吸系统超声评估的基本概念及其在临床实践中的应用。再结合前面几章的呼吸生理学知识，它可以成为帮助重症医学医生监测机械通气患者的有力工具。同时还可以作为诊断和监测肺部病变、人-机不同步的工具，甚至有可能为调整呼吸机设置提供指导。

（魏东坡，周芳庆　译）

参考文献

[1] Haaksma ME, Tuinman PR, Heunks L. Weaning the patient: between protocols and physiology. Curr Opin Crit Care. 2021; 27(1): 29-36.

[2] Lichtenstein DA, Mezière GA. Relevance of lung ultrasound in the diagnosis of acute respiratory failure: the BLUE protocol. Chest. 2008; 134(1): 117-25.

[3] Haaksma ME, Smit JM, Heldeweg MLA, Nooitgedacht JS, de Grooth H-J, Jonkman AH, et al. Extended lung ultrasound to differentiate between pneumonia and atelectasis in critically ill patients: a diagnostic accuracy study. Critical Care Medicine. 2021. https://doi.org/10.1097/CCM.0000000000005303.

[4] Chiumello D, Mongodi S, Algieri I, Vergani GL, Orlando A, Via G, et al. Assessment of lung aeration and recruitment by CT scan and ultrasound in acute respiratory distress syndrome patients. Crit Care Med. 2018; 46(11): 1761-8.

[5] Smit MR, Pisani L, de Bock EJE, van der Heijden F, Paulus F, Beenen LFM, et al. Ultrasound versus computed tomography assessment of focal lung aeration in invasively ventilated ICU patients. Ultrasound Med Biol. 2021; 47(9): 2589-97.

[6] Heldeweg MLA, Lopez Matta JE, Haaksma ME, Smit JM, Elzo Kraemer CV, de Grooth H-J, et al. Lung ultrasound and computed tomography to monitor COVID-19 pneumonia in critically ill patients: a two-center prospective cohort study. Intensive Care Med Exp. 2021; 9(1): 1.

[7] Heldeweg MLA, Jagesar AR, Haaksma ME, Smit JM, Paulus F, Schultz MJ, et al. Effects of lung ultrasonography-guided management on cumulative fluid balance and other clinical outcomes: a systematic review. Ultrasound Med Biol. 2021; 47(5): 1163-71.

[8] Bouhemad B, Brisson H, Le-Guen M, Arbelot C, Lu Q, Rouby J-J. Bedside ultrasound assessment of positive end-expiratory pressure-induced lung recruitment. Am J Respir Crit Care Med. 2011; 183(3): 341-7.

[9] Balik M, Plasil P, Waldauf P, Pazout J, Fric M, Otahal M, et al. Ultrasound estimation of volume of pleural fluid in mechanically ventilated patients. Intensive Care Med. 2006; 32(2): 318.

[10] Eibenberger KL, Dock WI, Ammann ME, Dorffner R, Hörmann MF, Grabenwöger F. Quantification of pleural effusions: sonography versus radiography. Radiology. 1994; 191(3): 681-4.

[11] Shkolnik B, Judson MA, Austin A, Hu K, D'Souza M, Zumbrunn A, et al. Diagnostic accuracy of thoracic ultrasonography to differentiate transudative from exudative pleural effusion. Chest. 2020; 158(2): 692-7.

[12] Haaksma ME, Atmowihardjo L, Heunks L, Spoelstra-de Man A, Tuinman PR. Ultrasound imaging of the diaphragm: facts and future. A guide for the bedside clinician. Neth. J Crit Care. 2018; 26(2): 6.

[13] Tuinman PR, Jonkman AH, Dres M, Shi Z-H, Goligher EC, Goffi A, et al. Respiratory muscle ultrasonography: methodology, basic and advanced principles and clinical applications in ICU and ED patients—a narrative review. Intensive Care Med. 2020; 46(4): 594-605.

[14] Houston JG, Angus RM, Cowan MD, McMillan NC, Thomson NC. Ultrasound assessment of normal hemidiaphragmatic movement: relation to inspiratory volume. Thorax. 1994; 49(5): 500-3.

[15] Llamas-Álvarez AM, Tenza-Lozano EM, Latour-Pérez J. Diaphragm and lung ultrasound to predict weaning outcome. Chest. 2017; 152(6): 1140-50.

[16] DiNino E, Gartman EJ, Sethi JM, McCool FD. Diaphragm ultrasound as a predictor of successful extubation from mechanical ventilation. Thorax. 2014; 69(5): 423-7.

[17] Ferrari G, De Filippi G, Elia F, Panero F, Volpicelli G, Aprà F. Diaphragm ultrasound as a new index of discontinuation from mechanical ventilation. Thorax. 2014; 69(5): 431-5.

[18] Farghaly S, Hasan AA. Diaphragm ultrasound as a new method to predict extubation outcome in

mechanically ventilated patients. Aust Crit Care. 2016; 30(1): 37 - 43.

[19] Goligher EC, Dres M, Fan E, Rubenfeld GD, Scales DC, Herridge MS, et al. Mechanical ventilation-induced diaphragm atrophy strongly impacts clinical outcomes. Am J Respir Crit Care Med. 2018; 197(2): 204 - 13.

[20] Seok JI, Kim SY, Walker FO, Kwak SG, Kwon DH. Ultrasonographic findings of the normal diaphragm: thickness and contractility. Ann Clin Neurophysiol. 2017; 19(2): 131.

[21] Zambon M, Beccaria P, Matsuno J, Gemma M, Frati E, Colombo S, et al. Mechanical ventilation and diaphragmatic atrophy in critically ill patients: an ultrasound study. Crit Care Med. 2016; 44(7): 1347 - 52.

[22] Vaporidi K, Babalis D, Chytas A, Lilitsis E, Kondili E, Amargianitakis V, et al. Clusters of ineffective efforts during mechanical ventilation: impact on outcome. Intensive Care Med. 2017; 43(2): 184 - 91.

[23] Soummer A, Perbet S, Brisson H, Arbelot C, Constantin J-M, Lu Q, et al. Ultra-sound assessment of lung aeration loss during a successful weaning trial predicts postextubation distress*. Crit Care Med. 2012; 40(7): 2064 - 72.

[24] Ferré A, Guillot M, Lichtenstein D, Mezière G, Richard C, Teboul J-L, et al. Lung ultra-sound allows the diagnosis of weaning-induced pulmonary oedema. Intensive Care Med. 2019; 45(5): 601 - 8.

[25] Dres M, Dubé B-P, Goligher E, Vorona S, Demiri S, Morawiec E, et al. Usefulness of parasternal intercostal muscle ultrasound during weaning from mechanical ventilation. Anesthesiology. 2020; 132(5): 1114 - 25.

[26] Vivier E, Muller M, Putegnat J-B, Steyer J, Barrau S, Boissier F, et al. Inability of diaphragm ultrasound to predict extubation failure. Chest. 2019; 155(6): 1131 - 9.

[27] Haaksma ME, Smit JM, Heldeweg ML, Nooitgedacht JS, Atmowihardjo LN, Jonkman AH, et al. Holistic ultrasound to predict extubation failure in clinical practice. Respir Care. 2021; 66(6): 994 - 1003.

[28] Arora NS, Gal TJ. Cough dynamics during progressive expiratory muscle weakness in healthy curarized subjects. J Appl Physiol. 1981; 51(2): 494 - 8.

[29] Parthasarathy S, Jubran A, Laghi F, Tobin MJ. Sternomastoid, rib cage, and expiratory muscle activity during weaning failure. J Appl Physiol. 2007; 103(1): 140 - 7.

[30] Shi Z-H, de Vries H, de Grooth H-J, Jonkman AH, Zhang Y, Haaksma M, et al. Changes in respiratory muscle thickness during mechanical ventilation: focus on expiratory muscles. Anesthesiology. 2021; 134(5): 748 - 59.

33 电阻抗体断层成像技术
Electrical Impedance Tomography
Inéz Frerichs

33.1 引言

电阻抗断层成像(electrical impedance tomography，EIT)是20世纪80年代初发明的一种成像方法[1]。由生物医学和电气工程师、物理学家、数学家和生理学家完成的相关研究在EIT前20年的发展中占据重要地位。研究的重点是对其技术的改进和对有效性的验证。

有两个决定性因素推动了EIT的后期发展，并大大增加了其临床接受度和使用度，使其主要用于监测接受呼吸机治疗的患者。第一个因素是对于EIT提供的信息存在临床需求；第二个因素是技术的成熟，能够允许在临床环境中使用已批准的EIT设备对患者进行可靠的检查。

当应用于胸部时，EIT可以测量局部肺通气和通气的瞬时变化。这些信息与临床息息相关，因为机械通气不仅是挽救生命的一种治疗方法，还是导致呼吸机相关肺损伤的原因。而促进肺生物伤的因素，如肺泡过度膨胀、肺不张、周期性肺复张和塌陷，也在推动EIT的应用中发挥了关键性作用。

目前已经采取相关措施来最小化机械通气的有害影响，包括采用新的通气模式和强化患者监测的肺保护性通气策略。尽管如此，机械通气对于局部肺充气的即时作用、呼吸周期中气体的动态分布和区域通气/灌注的匹配，这些信息依然不能在床旁获得。这些信息具有重要意义，因为肺通气、复张和血流灌注存在生理学上的空间和时间不均匀性，而且受到年龄、体位、肺部疾病，以及包括机械通气在内的治疗方案等因素的影响。

I. Frerichs (✉)
Department of Anesthesiology and Intensive Care Medicine, University Medical Center Schleswig-Holstein, Campus Kiel, Kiel, Germany
e-mail: inez.frerichs@uksh.de

© The Author(s), under exclusive license to Springer Nature Switzerland AG 2022
G. Bellani (ed.), *Mechanical Ventilation from Pathophysiology to Clinical Evidence*, https://doi.org/10.1007/978-3-030-93401-9_33

通过提供局部肺通气、复张、呼吸力学和血流灌注，以及过度膨胀、肺不张、周期复张和塌陷的实时信息，EIT 会对患者的肺功能状态和所选呼吸机设置是否恰当产生实时反馈。通过监测设定的通气参数对肺组织局部的直接作用，EIT 为个体化和优化呼吸机支持策略提供了指导。

本章专门介绍胸部 EIT 及其在机械通气患者监测中的应用。它首先描述了 EIT 的测量原理并解释了 EIT 监测是如何进行的。然后讨论了 EIT 数据分析的方法，并详细介绍了 EIT 衍生功能成像的生成和数字 EIT 测量方法。最后，解释了在临床环境中运用 EIT 信息的方式，还包括了一些临床实例。

33.2　电阻抗断层成像的基础

EIT 的基本原理是基于生物电阻抗的测量。生物电阻抗是一种组织学特性，定义为组织对交流电传播的阻力。EIT 通过施加极小且不易察觉的电流来探测人体，并测量其表面产生的电压。

需要在胸部多个位置施加激励电流，才能提供足够的信息用于生成胸腔内电生物阻抗分布的图像。因此，应围绕胸壁放置一圈电极，可以绕横截面或略微倾斜（图 33.1 顶部所示）。目前商用的 EIT 设备使用 16 个或 32 个电极的阵列。这些电极被集成到胸带、背心或条带中，而早期的设备则使用单个自粘电极。

EIT 中使用的典型电流幅度为几毫安，频率约为 $50 \sim 200\ kHz$。这些电流依次通过不同的电极对施加。在每次电流施加期间，测量胸部所有其他被动电极对上产生的电压。在完成一次完整的旋转电流施加和电压测量后所获取的原始数据被称为"帧"。生成一张原始 EIT 图像需要一帧数据。EIT 设备的帧速率，即扫描速率，表示每秒可获得的原始 EIT 图像数量。目前的 EIT 设备扫描速率约每秒 50 张图像。

原始 EIT 图像是由一系列帧（图 33.1，左中）计算出的电生物阻抗构成的区域（像素）值的二维图，该过程称为图像重建。需要说明的是，当前的 EIT 设备不会生成绝对电生物阻抗数值的图像，而是相对于参考阻抗的阻抗差异图像。因此，EIT 数据是无量纲的，通常以"任意单位"表示。EIT 图像通常包含约 1 000 个像素，这取决于所使用的图像重建算法。

肺组织的电阻抗取决于其中的气体、血液和液体的含量，以及细胞屏障的完整性。因此，EIT 可以显示所有影响这些因素的生理和病理过程。最大的阻抗变化是由气体含量的变化引起的，这就解释了为什么 EIT 主要用于监测区域肺通气和复张。较高的气体量扩张肺组织，使应用电流需要通过的途径变长，从而导致测得的阻抗增加。区域气体量的下降则产生了相反的效果。因为血液电导率高，所以在心脏收缩期肺血容量增加时会使测得的电阻抗降低。静脉输注的电解质溶液会导致肺整体阻抗下降，而液体局部积聚，如胸腔积液，将导致其区域性电阻抗下降。

了解 EIT 的基本原理和影响测量电阻抗的因素，有助于使用者正确解释 EIT 的结果。

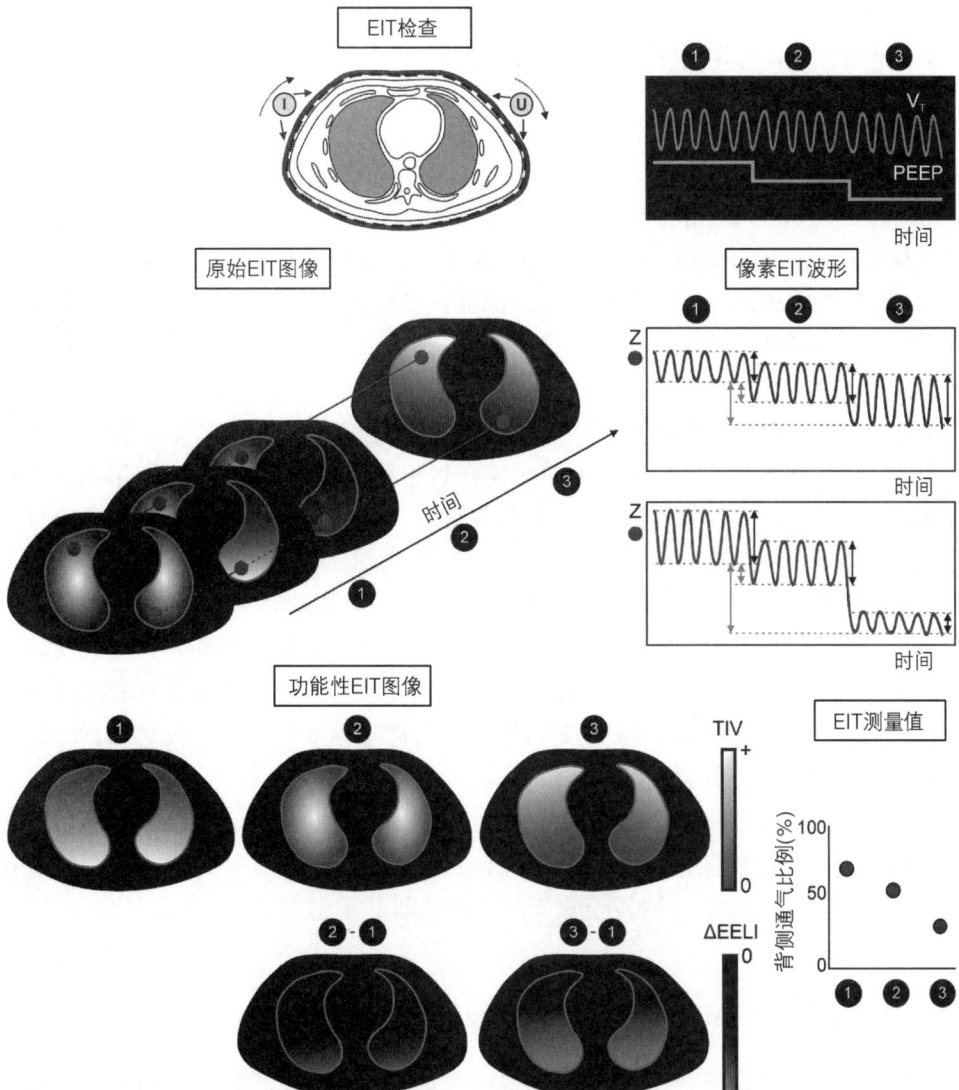

图 33.1 电阻抗断层成像(EIT)的测量原理和 EIT 数据采集和分析的不同步骤。在 EIT 检查期间(左上角),一个集成电极的 EIT 条带作为接口(带有短黑条的紫色线)被放置在胸壁周围。所有电极依次经历快速施加短暂且微小的交流电流(I)和测量施加的电流产生的电压(U)差这两个过程。EIT 数据可以在机械通气过程中获得,如在三个呼气末正压(PEEP)水平下进行恒定潮气量(V_T)的通气过程中(右上)。原始 EIT 数据产生了一系列原始 EIT 图像(左中)。其中,两个图像被标记出来,一个在右肺的非重力依赖区(蓝色),另一个在左肺的重力依赖区(红色)。区域像素阻抗(Z)波形(右中)显示了在三个不同 PEEP 时选定像素的周期阻抗变化(TIV)(黑色箭头)。第一个和其他两个 PEEP 水平间的呼气末肺阻抗(ΔEELI)的变化也被显示出来(橙色箭头)。所有像素中 TIV 和 ΔEELI 的计算值可以绘制在各自的位置上,从而生成两种不同类型的功能性 EIT 图像(左下)。顶部的蓝白色图像显示了 V_T 的空间分布,底部的黑橙图像显示了呼气末肺容积的区域性下降。在功能性图像中得到的值可以用于计算 EIT 相关定量指标。例如,测量背侧肺通气比例,即背侧 TIV 相对于整个图像的占比。图中给出了它在三个 PEEP 时的值(右下)(见彩色插图)

33.3　使用电阻抗断层成像监测患者

EIT 是一种安全、无创的成像方法,目前没有已知的危害。其使用只有少数禁忌证,如大面积胸部伤口或多个胸腔引流导致不能在胸部正确放置电极。此外,不建议在植入带电医疗设备(如起搏器和除颤器)的患者中进行 EIT 检查。在手术室内对机械通气患者应用 EIT 是可能的,但在使用电刀期间应将 EIT 设备断开。

EIT 检查始于胸部放置电极接口。这些接口是特定供应商的产品,通常由聚硅氧烷或纺织物制成,与集成电极结合,可以重复或一次性使用。EIT 电极必须与皮肤良好地贴合,因此,应选择与患者胸围匹配的电极接口。电极接口有不同的尺寸供选择,适合胸围 17~150 厘米的患者。根据电极接口的类型,可以通过使用水、盐水、电极凝胶或特殊接触喷雾来提高信号质量。电极接口不应放置在过于靠近腹部的位置,比如第六肋间隙以下。这一点很重要,尤其当患者处于平躺的姿势时。EIT 监测可以在电极接口放置在胸部后立即开始,但是,建议短暂延迟数分钟以使电极预热。

一旦开始 EIT 监测,数据采集可以持续 24~72 小时,具体取决于所使用的设备类型。使用者需要确定长时间的监测是有意义的,或者较短的 EIT 使用时间是否更方便且适用于打算通过 EIT 解决的临床问题。例如,如果猜测在新生儿通气中主支气管的气管插管位置太深,那么几分钟的 EIT 监测就足以确定重新调整导管位置是否改善了胸部的通气分布。如果通过递减法滴定"最佳 PEEP",则需要略低于半小时的监测。如果评估俯卧位对局部肺复张的影响,那么持续超过 1 小时的监测是有意义的。如果需要密切监测早产儿呼吸窘迫综合征患者使用表面活性剂后通气和复张情况,并及时发现气胸的潜在发生,那么可能会选择持续数小时甚至数天的连续长期 EIT 监测。

33.4　电阻抗断层成像评估局部肺通气和通气变化

在通气过程中获得的一系列原始 EIT 图像记录了区域电阻抗的瞬时变化。这些与通气相关的变化可以以动态图像流或波形的形式呈现而实时可视。像素阻抗波形(图 33.1,右中)可为进一步分析奠定基础。为了可视化的目的,可以对整个图像的值求和,并实时显示"全局"或感兴趣的区域的阻抗波形,通常按象限、腹背分层,或以对半区域的形式呈现。

像素、ROI 和全局阻抗波形允许分析区域周期性阻抗变化(TIV)、对应区域潮气量(V_T),以及区域呼气末肺阻抗的变化(ΔEELI)[主要显示呼气末肺容积(end-expiratory lung volume,EELV)的变化]。如图 33.1(右中)所示,像素 TIV 和 ΔEELI 存在区域差异。在这个记录示例中,容量控制通气期间 PEEP 降低了两次。来自非重力依赖区像素的 EIT 波形在最高的 PEEP 时显示出最低的 TIV。这是区域过度膨胀和顺应性降低造成的。在随后的过程中,因为随着 PEEP 的降低过度膨胀得到了缓解,所以 TIV 随之增加。相比之下,来自重力依赖区域像素的波形显示,由于去复张 TIV 幅度随着 PEEP 的下降而下降。第二次 PEEP 变化后 ΔEELI 的大幅下降也证实了肺泡塌陷。

如果将从 EIT 检查示例中的三个阶段计算得出的 TIV 像素值绘制在其各自的位置上,采用彩色编码绘制图像,即为"功能性"EIT 图像,展示了胸部横断面中的 V_T 分布(图 33.1,左下,前三幅图)。在最高 PEEP 水平下,由于腹侧过度膨胀,吸入气体优先流向肺的重力依赖区。第一次 PEEP 降低后,通气分布变得更加均匀。第二次 PEEP 降低则导致了背侧塌陷和偏向肺非重力依赖区的不均一通气分布。另一种类型的功能性 EIT 图像是将 ΔEELI 的像素值按比例以不同的颜色绘制而成的图像(图 33.1,左下,最后两幅图)。显示随着 PEEP 的降低,肺重力依赖区的局部肺通气减少更为明显。

图 33.2 和图 33.3 显示了对 COVID-19 相关 ARDS 患者进行 EIT 监测的临床病例。一种肺复张手法增加了肺通气(见图 33.2,上图中的整体 EIT 波形),但在随后的 PEEP 降低的过程中逐步下降。尽管如此,这种肺复张手法还是取得了很好的效果。腹侧和背侧区域的 ΔEELI(图 33.2,左下)显示背侧区域的通气量增加较多。图 33.3 顶部的功能性 EIT 图像显示了该患者在各个 PEEP 阶段的通气分布情况,从一开始时的背侧

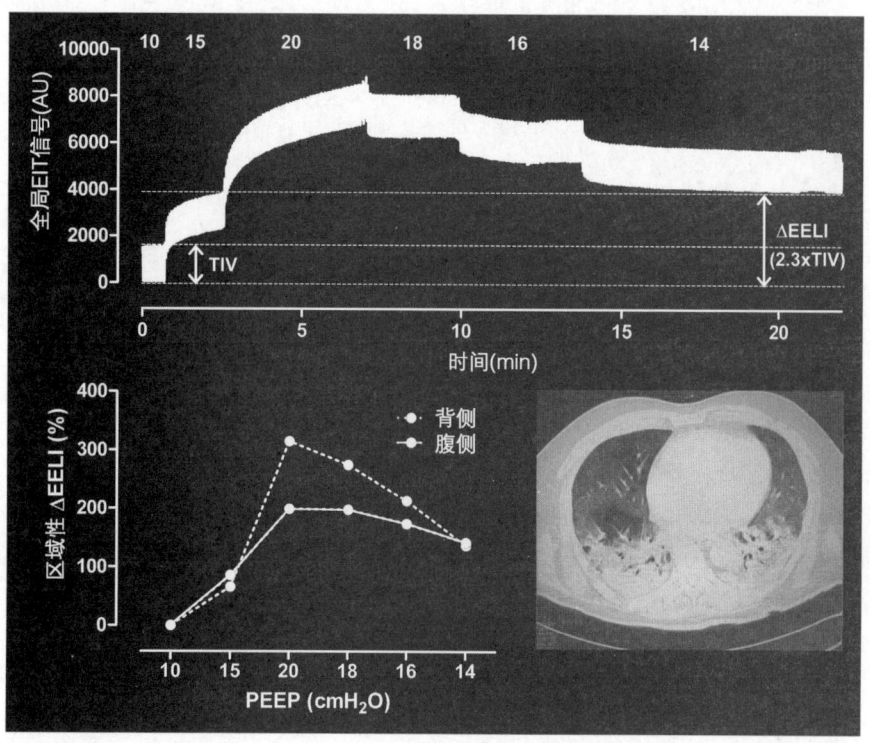

图 33.2 这是获取自 64 岁 COVID-19 相关 ARDS 患者的全局 EIT 信号波形(即完整图像),采用相对单位(AU)表示,用 EIT 监测了两次呼气末正压(PEEP)增加和四次递减步骤的完整过程(上)。在 ICU 入院的第二天进行了 EIT 检查。蓝色箭头表示通气中初始 PEEP 下周期性阻抗变化(TIV)的幅度,以及最后一个 PEEP 值下呼气末肺阻抗的变化(ΔEELI)。波形上的数字表示设定 PEEP 值,以 cmH_2O 为单位。肺腹侧和背侧区域的 ΔEELI 值相对于最低 PEEP(左下)的初始值,在 PEEP 增加后肺依赖区 ΔEELI 增加更明显,这意味着肺复张。胸部 CT 于入 ICU 的第一天进行(右下)(引自参考文献[2])

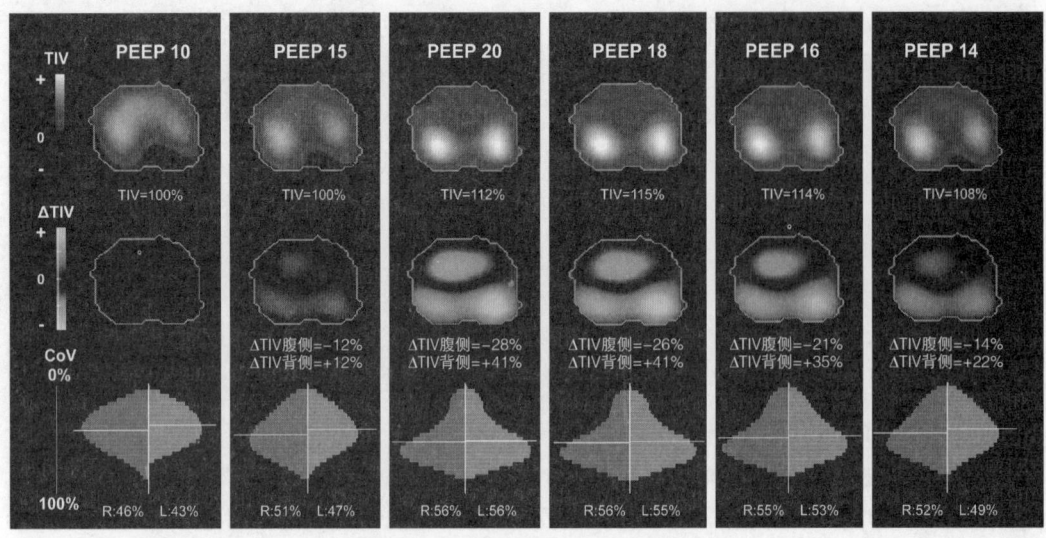

图 33.3 使用 EIT 分析采用俯卧位的 COVID-19 相关 ARDS 患者的区域肺通气。检查也如图 33.2 所示,在呼气末正压(PEEP)的两次增加和四个递减步骤的完整过程中进行。在功能性 EIT 图像上区域周期性阻抗变化(TIV)(上)显示了胸部横断面中的潮气量分布。通气区域以白色和蓝色表示,图像下面的数字给出了 TIV 值,以 10 cmH$_2$O PEEP 时 TIV 初始值为基线按比例显示的全局 TIV 值总和。与初始最低 PEEP 值相比,展示区域 TIV 变化(ΔTIV)(中)的功能性 EIT 图像显示了各个 PEEP 值下通气的局部增加(浅蓝色区域)和减少(橙色区域)。图像下面的数字说明了与操作开始时的初始 TIV 分布相比,肺腹侧和背侧区域的 TIV 的相对变化。通气分布图(下)显示了左、右肺的区域通气分布。每个图中的白色水平线表示通气中心(CoV)的位置,对应的值绘制在每个图像的下面。数值小于 50% 意味着通气分布偏向腹侧区域。CoV,通气中心(引自参考文献[2])(见彩色插图)

通气很少,到最高 PEEP 时背侧通气得到改善(同时腹侧区域通气减少);而在 PEEP 递减的最后阶段,通气分布相对均匀。

对展示区域 TIV 分布的功能性 EIT 图像经常需要进行进一步的定量分析,旨在通过测量的数值来描述通气分布的均匀性。一种简单而直观的方法是计算背侧区域的通气比例,如图 33.1 中的理论模型(右下)所示,可见依赖区的通气逐渐减少。一个临床病例(图 33.4d)的图像显示了由于气胸导致的肺左腹侧象限低通气。另一种方法是确定 TIV 像素值的离散度,如通过变异系数或全局不均一指数[4]。此外,还有通气中心这个参数,可以评估通气在左、右侧和腹、背侧的分布。图 33.3(下)显示了肺复张过程中,该参数是如何从偏向腹侧到偏向背侧,并在结束时达到相对居中的位置的。

由于其高扫描率,EIT 还允许对肺部区域性充气和排空进行动态评估,无论是在潮气式呼吸还是特定操作(如恒定低流量吸气和呼气)期间。区域阻抗波形的呼吸周期内或吸气相/呼气相分析,能够计算通气开始时的区域延迟[5]、区域呼吸时间常数[6]或者呼吸摆动[7]。当结合气道压测量时,可以确定区域呼吸顺应性[8,9]和区域的开放压、闭合压[10]。

总体而言,EIT 在确定通气相关阻抗变化方面是非常稳健的,并且从潮式通气和特殊操作获得的参数是可靠的、可重复的。然而,EIT 使用者在解释 ΔEELI 时应谨慎,因为它不仅反映 EELV 的变化,还会受到其他因素的影响,如液体治疗[11]、患者的移动[12]或脉冲治疗期间的电极皮肤接触产生的波动[13]。

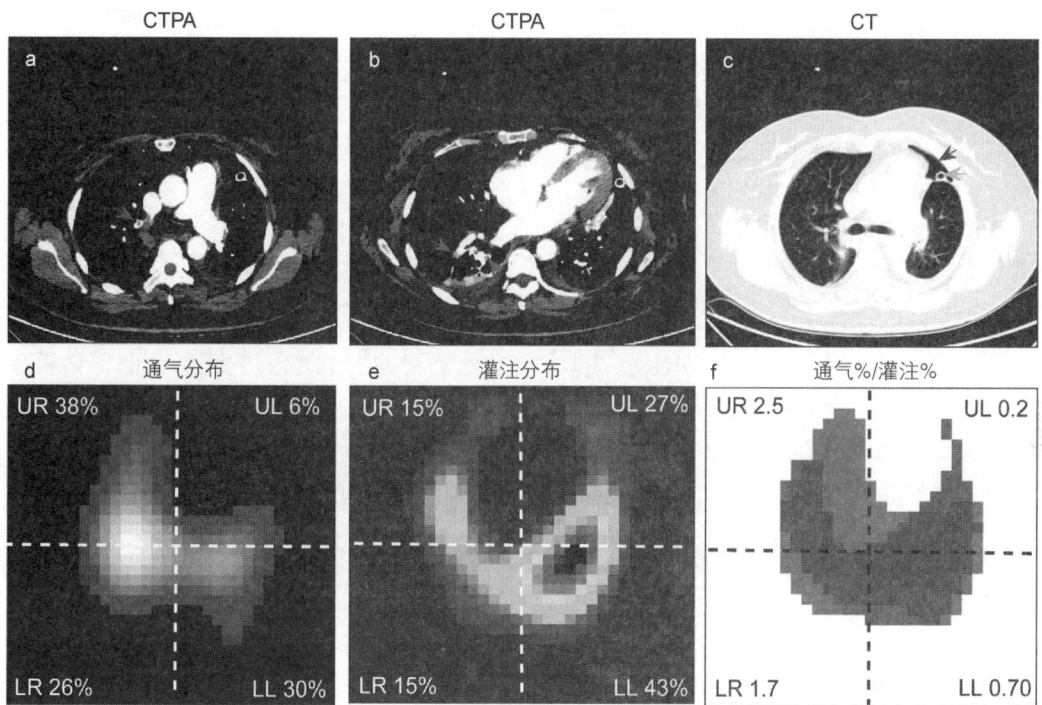

图 33.4 47 岁的仰卧位女性在胸部手术后 1 天进行了计算机断层成像(CT)、CT 肺动脉造影(CTPA)和电阻抗断层成像(EIT),显示了通气和灌注受损。CTPA 显示右肺动脉分支有多个栓塞(a 和 b 中的红色箭头)。CT 发现左腹侧有少量气胸(c 中的蓝色箭头)。胸腔内可见引流管(绿色箭头)。通气分布的功能性 EIT 图像(d)显示深蓝色为低通气区域,白色为高通气区域。图像四个角中的值给出了相应象限中的通气百分比。灌注分布的功能性 EIT 图像中红色为高灌注区域,蓝色为低灌注区域(e)。图像四个角中的值给出了相应象限的灌注百分比。显示区域通气/灌注分布的功能 EIT 图像(f)中:灰色为高通气和低灌注区域(像素点对应的区域有通气而无灌注),红色为低通气和高灌注区域(像素点对应的区域有灌注而无通气),蓝色为良好的通气/灌注匹配(像素点对应的区域在通气和灌注这两个方面都有良好表现)。每个象限显示的区域通气/灌注对应于相应象限的通气分布(以%显示)超过灌注分布(以%显示)的值。LL,左下肺;LR,右下肺;UL,左上肺;UR,右上肺(经美国胸科学会许可,转载自参考文献[3]。版权所有:© 2021 美国胸科学会。保留所有权利)(见彩色插图)

大量的描述性和系统性综述(如参考文献[14-20])以及关于胸部 EIT[17] 的专家共识声明都记录了 EIT 在通气监测方面的进展。最近有 ARDS 的前瞻性临床研究采用了基于 EIT 的个体化 PEEP 滴定方案[21](是其在随机研究设计中的首次应用),以及基于 EIT 同时设置 PEEP 和 V_T[22] 的方案。

33.5 电阻抗断层成像评估局部肺灌注

心脏的收缩和舒张导致肺血容量的周期性变化,以及与心跳同步的区域电生物阻抗的变化可以被 EIT 所记录。虽然这种 EIT 信号成分已被用于评估局部灌注,但其振幅较低,对血流的特异性不如基于高渗盐水注射的方法。生理盐水可以作为对比剂,形成稀释曲线,以测量区域血流[23]。局部灌注的功能性 EIT 图像(图 33.4,下图中部)与通气图像进行比较,可评估局部通气/灌注匹配情况(图33.4,下图右侧)。最近的临床研究证实了该方法在患者通气监测中的安全性和可靠性,并记录了通气/灌注不匹配与不良结局之间的关联[24,25]。这种方法的局限性在于它是间断的,需要让患者在接受向中心静脉注射盐水到测量结束期间屏气。

33.6 总结

  EIT监测能在床旁提供实时、连续的局部肺功能信息。它可以早期识别患者状态的变化,并能对治疗和护理进行个性化调整。与其他监测方法相结合,它可以全面评估机械通气的有效性和危害性。通气和灌注分布的均一性,有害现象的出现,如肺泡过度膨胀、肺不张形成、肺泡循环开放和关闭,通气/灌注不匹配、呼吸摆动或气胸的发生,这些信息是充分指导和优化呼吸机治疗所必需的。EIT的临床接受度和使用程度将受益于标准化检查,包括在特定临床情况下EIT的应用协议、自动目标导向的分析和决策支持工具的提供。

(魏东坡,周芳庆　译)

参考文献

[1] Barber DC, Brown BH, Freeston IL. Imaging spatial distributions of resistivity using applied potential tomography. Electron Lett. 1983; 19(22): 933 - 5. https://doi.org/10.1049/el: 19830637.

[2] Shono A, Kotani T, Frerichs I. Personalization of therapies in COVID-19 associated acute respiratory distress syndrome, using electrical impedance tomography. J Crit Care Med. 2021; 7(1): 62 - 6. https://doi.org/10.2478/jccm-2020-0045.

[3] He H, Long Y, Frerichs I, Zhao Z. Detection of acute pulmonary embolism by electrical impedance tomography and saline bolus injection. Am J Respir Crit Care Med. 2020; 202(6): 881 - 2. https://doi.org/10.1164/rccm.202003-0554IM.

[4] Zhao Z, Moller K, Steinmann D, Frerichs I, Guttmann J. Evaluation of an electrical impedance tomography-based global inhomogeneity index for pulmonary ventilation distribution. Intensive Care Med. 2009; 35(11): 1900 - 6. https://doi.org/10.1007/s00134-009-1589-y.

[5] Muders T, Hentze B, Kreyer S, Wodack KH, Leonhardt S, Hedenstierna G, et al. Measurement of electrical impedance tomography-based regional ventilation delay for individualized titration of end-expiratory pressure. J Clin Med. 2021; 10 (13): 2933. https://doi.org/10.3390/jcm10132933.

[6] Karagiannidis C, Waldmann AD, Roka PL, Schreiber T, Strassmann S, Windisch W, et al. Regional expiratory time constants in severe respiratory failure estimated by electrical impedance tomography: a feasibility study. Crit Care. 2018; 22(1): 221. https://doi.org/10.1186/s13054-018-2137-3.

[7] Yoshida T, Torsani V, Gomes S, De Santis RR, Beraldo MA, Costa EL, et al. Spontaneous effort causes occult pendelluft during mechanical ventilation. Am J Respir Crit Care Med. 2013; 188(12): 1420 - 7. https://doi.org/10.1164/rccm.201303-0539OC.

[8] Costa EL, Borges JB, Melo A, Suarez-Sipmann F, Toufen C Jr, Bohm SH, et al. Bedside estimation of recruitable alveolar collapse and hyperdistension by electrical impedance tomography. Intensive Care Med. 2009; 35(6): 1132 - 7. https://doi.org/10.1007/s00134-009-1447-y.

[9] Dargaville PA, Rimensberger PC, Frerichs I. Regional tidal ventilation and compliance during a stepwise vital capacity manoeuvre. Intensive Care Med. 2010; 36(11): 1953 - 61. https://doi.org/10.1007/s00134-010-1995-1.

[10] Pulletz S, Adler A, Kott M, Elke G, Gawelczyk B, Schadler D, et al. Regional lung opening and closing pressures in patients with acute lung injury. J Crit Care. 2012; 27(3): 323.e11 - 8. https://doi.org/10.1016/j.jcrc.2011.09.002.

[11] Becher T, Wendler A, Eimer C, Weiler N, Frerichs I. Changes in electrical impedance tomography findings of ICU patients during rapid infusion of a fluid bolus: a prospective observational study. Am J Respir Crit Care Med. 2019; 199(12): 1572 - 5. https://doi.org/10.1164/rccm.201812-2252LE.

[12] Vogt B, Mendes L, Chouvarda I, Perantoni E, Kaimakamis E, Becher T, et al. Influence of torso and arm positions on chest examinations by electrical impedance tomography. Physiol Meas. 2016; 37(6): 904 - 21. https://doi.org/10.1088/0967-3334/37/6/904.

[13] Frerichs I, Pulletz S, Elke G, Gawelczyk B, Frerichs A, Weiler N. Patient examinations using electrical impedance tomography-sources of interference in the intensive care unit. Physiol Meas. 2011; 32(12): L1 - 10. https://doi.org/10.1088/0967-3334/32/12/F01.

[14] Frerichs I, Becher T, Weiler N. Electrical impedance tomography. In: Heunks L, Schultz MJ, editors. ERS practical handbook of invasive mechanical ventilation. Lausanne: European Respiratory Society; 2019. p. 129 - 35. https://doi.org/10.1183/9781849841221.029518.

[15] Kobylianskii J, Murray A, Brace D, Goligher E, Fan E. Electrical impedance tomography in adult patients undergoing mechanical ventilation: a systematic review. J Crit Care. 2016; 35: 33 - 50. https://doi.org/10.1016/j.jcrc.2016.04.028.

[16] Shono A, Kotani T. Clinical implication of monitoring regional ventilation using electrical impedance tomography. J Intensive Care. 2019; 7: 4. https://doi.org/10.1186/s40560-019-0358-4.

[17] Frerichs I, Amato MB, van Kaam AH, Tingay DG, Zhao Z, Grychtol B, et al. Chest electrical impedance tomography examination, data analysis, terminology, clinical use and recommendations: consensus statement of the TRanslational EIT developmeNt stuDy group. Thorax. 2017; 72(1): 83 - 93. https://doi.org/10.1136/thoraxjnl-2016-208357.

[18] Bachmann MC, Morais C, Bugedo G, Bruhn A, Morales A, Borges JB, et al. Electrical impedance tomography in acute respiratory distress syndrome. Crit Care. 2018; 22(1): 263. https://doi.org/10.1186/s13054-018-2195-6.

[19] Frerichs I. Bedside lung imaging methods (electrical impedance tomography). In: Rimensberger PC, editor. Pediatric and neonatal mechanical ventilation. Berlin: Springer-Verlag; 2015. 978-3-642-01218-1 (ISBN). p. 457 - 71.

[20] Vasques F, Sanderson B, Barrett NA, Camporota L. Monitoring of regional lung ventilation using electrical impedance tomography. Minerva Anestesiol. 2019; 85(11): 1231 - 41. https://doi.org/10.23736/S0375-9393.19.13477-3.

[21] He H, Chi Y, Yang Y, Yuan S, Long Y, Zhao P, et al. Early individualized positive end-expiratory pressure guided by electrical impedance tomography in acute respiratory distress

syndrome: a randomized controlled clinical trial. Crit Care. 2021; 25(1): 230. https://doi.org/10.1186/s13054-021-03645-y.

[22] Becher T, Buchholz V, Hassel D, Meinel T, Schadler D, Frerichs I, et al. Individualization of PEEP and tidal volume in ARDS patients with electrical impedance tomography: a pilot feasibility study. Ann Intensive Care. 2021; 11(1): 89. https://doi.org/10.1186/s13613-021-00877-7.

[23] Frerichs I, Hinz J, Herrmann P, Weisser G, Hahn G, Quintel M, et al. Regional lung perfusion as determined by electrical impedance tomography in comparison with electron beam CT imaging. IEEE Trans Med Imaging. 2002; 21(6): 646-52. https://doi.org/10.1109/TMI.2002.800585.

[24] He H, Chi Y, Long Y, Yuan S, Frerichs I, Moller K, et al. Influence of overdistension/recruitment induced by high positive end-expiratory pressure on ventilation-perfusion matching assessed by electrical impedance tomography with saline bolus. Crit Care. 2020; 24(1): 586. https://doi.org/10.1186/s13054-020-03301-x.

[25] Spinelli E, Kircher M, Stender B, Ottaviani I, Basile MC, Marongiu I, et al. Unmatched ventilation and perfusion measured by electrical impedance tomography predicts the outcome of ARDS. Crit Care. 2021; 25(1): 192. https://doi.org/10.1186/s13054-021-03615-4.

34 食管压监测
Esophageal Pressure Monitoring

Evangelia Akoumianaki，Katerina Vaporidi

食管压（esophageal pressure，P_{es}）是在食管下部测量的压力，可作为胸膜腔内压（P_{pl}）的替代值[1]。监测食管压可以评估施加在肺部的力、肺和胸壁的力学特性，以及呼吸肌产生的压力。

34.1 引言

食管压可通过将可充气气囊的导管以类似插鼻胃管的方式插入食管来测量。有几种商用食管气囊导管可供选择，通过将导管的开口连接到专用采集系统、标准患者监护仪或机械通气机上的充气压力传感器来获得 P_{es} 监测的结果。通过食管导管进行可靠的胸膜腔内压监测需要食管导管的气囊位置恰当并适量充气，并且胸腔内的压力分布相对均匀。当气囊被放置于理想位置时，可以用 P_{es} 反映 P_{pl}，在气道阻断期间 P_{es} 和 P_{aw} 两者变化量的比值（$\Delta P_{es}/\Delta P_{aw}$）应接近 1，$P_{es}$ 摆动应该与潮气量波动相似，并且 P_{es} 与潮气量的关系应该是线性的[2]。

图 34.1 描述了插入和检查食管导管充气是否适量、位置是否恰当的技术（Baydur 试验）。过度充气的气囊能准确传递 P_{es} 的变化，但会高估 P_{es} 的绝对值。充气不足的气囊既会低估 P_{es} 绝对值，又会低估呼吸时 P_{es} 波动。在最佳充气量时，气囊不会产生弹性回弹力。市场上可获得的导管充气的容积因导管长度、直径和顺应性，以及气囊周围压力的不同而有所不同[1,2]。较大和较长的气囊具有更高的最大充气量和更广泛的最佳充气量范围，使精确测量更容易[1]。值得注意的是，目前制造商建议的充气量都是在大气压下验证的。然而，当胸腔压为负值时，如在自主呼吸时，气囊可能需要低于推荐的充气量，而当

E. Akoumianaki · K. Vaporidi (✉)
Department of Intensive Care, University Hospital of Heraklion and School of Medicine, University of Crete, Heraklio, Greece

© The Author(s), under exclusive license to Springer Nature Switzerland AG 2022
G. Bellani (ed.), *Mechanical Ventilation from Pathophysiology to Clinical Evidence*, https://doi.org/10.1007/978-3-030-93401-9_34

胸腔压增加时(高 PEEP，ΔP)，最佳充气量可能会高于推荐值[1,2]。所以，定期检查充气量是很重要的，特别是在胸内压发生重大变化后。偶尔，在食管下 1/3 处，由于纵隔和膈肌的压力叠加，P_{es} 假性升高，导致肺中部的 P_{pl} 被高估了约 5 cmH$_2$O[1,2]。

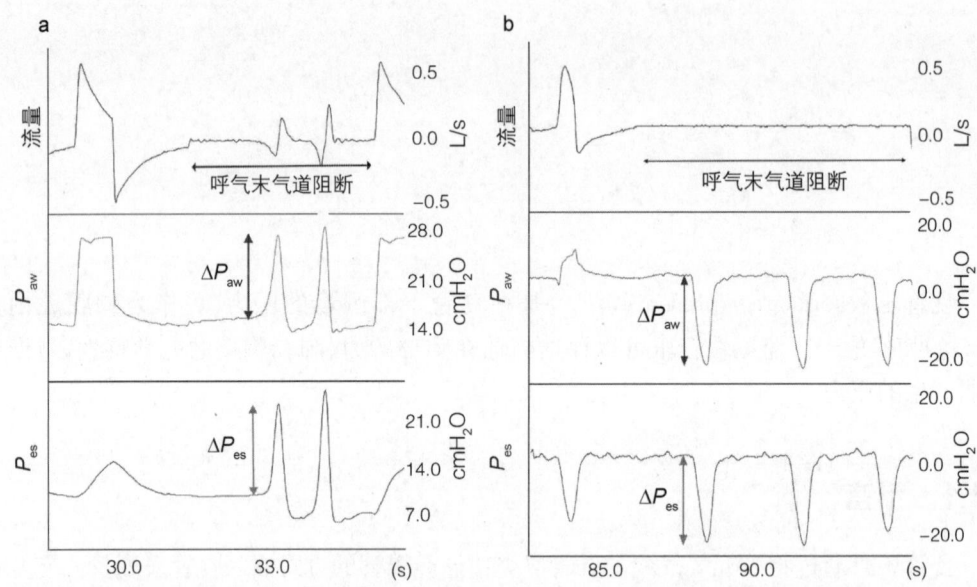

图 34.1 食管导管的放置及气囊填充和位置的评估。食管导管像鼻胃管一样放置，经鼻或经口，通常深度为 40~55 厘米。远端部分连接到压力传感器上，用空气对气囊充气。气囊在食管中的位置可通过 P_{es} 波形中出现呼吸与心脏搏动波形来确定。气囊充气包括以下步骤：① 使气囊完全放气，以精确计算充气体积；② 通过短暂的断开连接使其与大气压平衡；③ 充入允许的最大气体量（根据每种气囊的具体规定），以均匀地展开气囊；④ 放气至推荐的气体量。优化充气量可以进一步通过逐步 (0.5 mL) 注入气囊来实现，选择与 P_{es} 潮气量最大波动相关的最低体积。随后，通过比较呼气末气道阻断时的 P_{aw} 波形和 P_{es} 波形来确定气囊的正确位置：在肺容积不变的情况下，跨肺压不变，因此 P_{es} 的变化应该等于 P_{aw} 的变化，反之亦然。理想情况下，$\Delta P_{es}/\Delta P_{aw}$ 应该接近 1，但 0.8~1.2 也是可接受的。本图从上到下依次为，气流量、气道压 (P_{aw}) 和食管压 (P_{es}) 随时间的波形图。a. 在控制模式下，胸部施加两次轻柔的压力会在 P_{aw} 和 P_{es} 中产生相似的正向压力波动（红色和蓝色箭头）。b. 在辅助模式下（此处为压力支持），在呼气末阻断期间，患者对抗阻断气道的吸气努力在气道压和食管压中产生相似的负向压力波动（红色和蓝色箭头）（见彩色插图）

此外，使用 P_{es} 替代 P_{pl} 是假定 P_{pl} 在胸腔内各处都是相似的，并且 P_{pl} 的变化在胸腔内均匀分布。然而，在健康肺中，由于重力作用，静态 P_{pl} 从非重力依赖区到重力依赖区增加了 0.25 cmH$_2$O/cm，而在急性呼吸窘迫综合征（acute respiratory distress syndrome，ARDS）患者中几乎翻倍，可以达到 10 cmH$_2$O[3]。在任何体位下，P_{es} 的值反映了肺中部到重力依赖区的 P_{pl}[1,2]。实验数据表明，在受损肺中，重力依赖区的 P_{pl} 变化可能大于非重力依赖区[4]；但在不对称的肺损伤中，损伤和非损伤肺的 P_{pl} 变化相似[5]。

34.2 食管压衍生变量的测量

34.2.1 跨肺压

跨肺压(P_L)是指整个肺的压差。假设肺泡压和气道压相等（当没有气道塌陷时），在被动、静态（无气流）的条件下，P_L等于肺的弹性回缩力[6]。肺的弹性回缩力是实际扩张肺所克服的压力。可以通过在吸气末和呼气末进行气道阻断分别测算吸气末($P_{L,\text{end-insp}}$)和呼气末($P_{L,\text{end-exp}}$)的静态P_L，如图34.2所示。另一种方法是通过气道压乘以肺与呼吸系统弹性的比值来估算跨肺压，以避免测量P_{es}绝对值需要留置导管的缺点[1,2]。这种基于弹性推导的方法假设在呼气末P_{pl}、P_L和P_{aw}为零（大气压），并且在呼吸过程中呈线性相关。然而，在危重症患者中，P_{alv}和P_{pl}往往高于零（卧位气道闭合、主动呼气、肺泡积液），压力-容积关系可能不是线性的，特别是在ARDS中。直接法和弹性法提供的P_L值存在显著差异，临床实践中哪种方法更优仍存在争议[7]。一项对人体尸体的研究表明，直接测量的$P_{L,\text{end-exp}}$是准确的，可用于调整PEEP，而弹性推导的$P_{L,\text{end-insp}}$则更好地代表了非重力依赖区吸气结束时的真实P_L[8]。

在危重症患者中偶尔会出现呼气末高食管压($P_{es,\text{end-exp}}$)且$P_{L,\text{end-exp}}$为负值的情况。这时的P_L并不代表肺部的弹性回缩力，可能有以下几个原因。首先，由于纵隔的重量，$P_{es,\text{end-exp}}$可能被高估，因此建议从测量的P_{es}中减去5 cmH$_2$O。其次，P_{pl}在整个胸腔空间的分布可能是不均匀的。P_{es}仅反映肺中部的P_{pl}，而在非重力依赖区P_{pl}较低且P_L为正值。最后，塌陷或积液可引起肺不张，影响P_{alv}和P_{aw}平衡，此时P_{alv}等于局部的P_{pl}[9]。

在辅助通气过程中，动态P_L等于P_{aw}（正值）和P_{es}（负值）之间的差值（图34.2），代表了两个压力组成部分：弹性回缩力和气道阻力。静态的吸气末和呼气末P_L无法可靠地评估，因为气道闭塞操作时无法保证呼吸肌松弛。呼气肌活动可以通过测量胃内压来监测。

34.2.2 吸气努力和动态过度充气指数

吸气努力测量的金标准包括食管压(P_{es})（反映所有呼吸肌）或跨膈压（反映膈肌）的压力-时间乘积（pressure-time product，PTP）和呼吸做功，两者均基于P_{es}计算，如图34.3所示。所有呼吸肌在任何时候产生的压力(P_{mus})都等于胸壁静态回弹力(E_{cw})与P_{es}之间的差值。假设E_{cw}在被动呼吸和主动呼吸之间保持不变，它就可以在静态条件下通过潮气量引起的P_{es}变化值获得，或者以每增加4%预测肺活量的潮气量E_{cw}增加1 cmH$_2$O来估算。膈肌产生的压力，即跨膈压(P_{di})，可通过胃内压(P_{gas})减去P_{es}来估算，P_{gas}可同P_{es}一样通过在胃部放置气囊导管来测量。

P_{mus}与潮气量乘积积分用于计算每次呼吸的呼吸做功（work of breathing，WOB），单位为J/L或J/min[1]。自主呼吸时P_{es}波动的幅度也大致反映了吸气肌努力的大小（另

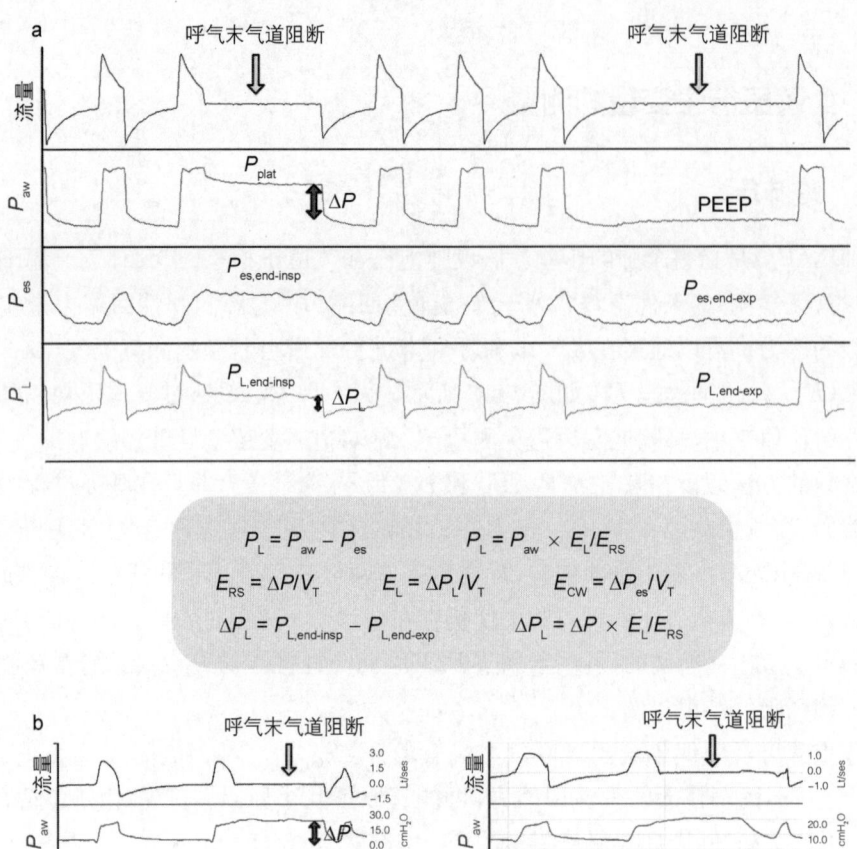

图 34.2 控制性通气（a）和辅助性通气（b）期间的跨肺压和肺部力学计算。a. 从上到下依次为：被动通气患者的流量、气道压（P_{aw}）、食管压（P_{es}）和跨肺压（P_L）随时间变化的波形图。P_L 通过计算 P_{aw} 和 P_{es} 间的差值得出。图中可见吸气末和呼气末气道阻断的操作。在气道阻断期间假设所有的气道都是开放的，此时 P_{alv} 与 P_{aw} 达到平衡。因此，在没有呼吸肌活动的情况下，吸气末的 P_{aw}（P_{plat}）和呼气末阻断时的 P_{aw}（PEEP）被认为分别近似于吸气末和呼气末的静态 P_{alv}。肺的弹性回缩力（流量为零时的 P_L）是肺在高于功能残气量时的不同肺容积时所克服的实际压力。如图所示，使用 P_{es} 的绝对值可以计算静态吸气末 P_L（$P_{L,end-insp}$）和呼气末 P_L（$P_{L,end-exp}$）。呼吸系统的驱动压（ΔP）可通过 P_{plat} 和 PEEP 的差值计算得出，呼吸系统的弹性（E_{rs}）为 ΔP 与 V_T 的比值。如图所示，P_{es} 的计算允许将 E_{rs} 拆分为肺弹性（E_L）和胸壁弹性（E_{CW}）。ΔP_L 称为跨肺驱动压，反映了 V_T 引起的肺应力变化。跨肺压也可以用 P_{aw} 乘以 E_L 与 E_{rs} 之比（弹性推导法）进行计算。因此，该方法只需要 P_{es} 的变化值，而不需要绝对值。b. 从上到下依次为：辅助通气患者在压力支持期间的流量、气道压（P_{aw}）、食管压（P_{es}）、胃内压（P_{gas}）、跨膈压（P_{di}）和动态跨肺压（P_L）随时间变化的波形图。通过 P_{gas} 减去 P_{es} 来计算跨膈压。通过吸气末阻断以测量静态吸气末气道压（P_{plat}）和跨肺压（$P_{L,end-insp}$）。b 左侧图中，无呼吸肌收缩保证了测量 P_{plat} 和 ΔP 的可靠性；而在右侧图中，呼气肌收缩，表现为呼气末 P_{gas} 升高（绿色箭头），P_{plat} 和 ΔP 的测量是无效的（见彩色插图）

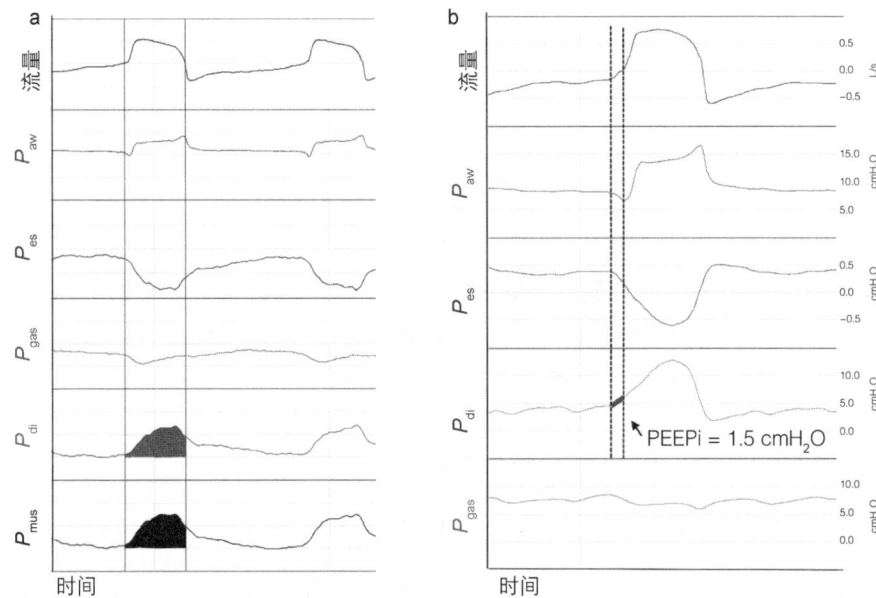

图34.3 压力-时间乘积和内源性PEEP计算。a. 压力支持通气时压力-时间乘积（PTP）的计算。从上到下依次为：压力支持通气期间流量、气道压（P_{aw}）、食管压（P_{es}）、胃内压（P_{gas}）、跨膈压（P_{di}）和肌肉压力（P_{mus}）随时间变化的波形图。膈肌产生的压力，即P_{di}，可以用P_{gas}和食管压之差来计算（$P_{di} = P_{gas} - P_{es}$）。所有呼吸肌产生的压力（$P_{mus}$）可以用公式计算：$P_{mus} = V \times E_{CW} - P_{es}$，其中$V$为即时容积；$E_{CW}$为胸壁弹性，在被动条件下测量或通过公式估算。吸气时P_{mus}或P_{di}波形下的面积（阴影区域）是相应压力下每次呼吸的PTP。每分钟的压力-时间乘积（PTP/min）可以通过每次呼吸的PTP乘以呼吸频率来估算。在没有呼气肌收缩的情况下，用该方法估算的P_{mus}和$PTP_{P_{mus}}$是有效的。
b. 计算内源性PEEP（PEEPi）。从上到下依次为：压力支持通气期间的流量、气道压（P_{aw}）、食管压（P_{es}）、P_{gas}随时间变化的波形图。内源性PEEP（PEEPi）的计算方法是P_{di}或P_{es}从吸气努力开始到零流量点（虚线）的变化。需要注意的是，在有呼气肌活动的情况下，从吸气努力开始至零流量点的P_{es}下降包含了呼气肌的松弛，导致对PEEPi的高估，因此应改为使用P_{di}的变化进行估算

见"6 辅助通气过程中患者的监测"）。如图34.2c和34.3b所示，测量P_{gas}和P_{di}能够评估呼气肌的收缩，并且可以通过测量内源性PEEP（PEEPi）来量化动态过度充气。

34.3 监测食管压力指导机械通气

机械通气时可间歇或连续进行食管压监测。对跨肺压和患者努力的评估可以提供有价值的信息，促进呼吸机设置的个性化调整。下文介绍了使用P_{es}衍生变量滴定通气设置以实现肺和膈肌保护性通气的目标[10,11]，其中包括：① 避免呼气末肺萎陷；② 最小化肺泡过度膨胀；③ 优化患者-呼吸机的相互作用。

34.3.1 监测呼气末跨肺压滴定呼气末正压防止肺泡塌陷

滴定PEEP的目的是防止呼气末肺泡塌陷，同时避免过度膨胀和损害血流动力学，这

对 ARDS 患者尤其具有挑战性。在实验和临床实践中，PEEP 滴定至 $2\sim4$ cmH_2O 的 $P_{L,\,end\text{-}exp}$ 已被证明可最大限度地减少肺泡塌陷[8,12]。第一项在 ARDS 患者中采用基于呼气末跨肺压的 PEEP 滴定研究（根据预先制定的 $P_{L,\,end\text{-}exp}$ - FiO_2 表）发现[13]，该方法与较高的 PEEP、改善的氧合和顺应性相关。在一项针对 ARDS 患者[14]更大规模的多中心研究中，对照组同样使用了 $P_{L,\,end\text{-}exp}$ 导向的 PEEP 滴定方案，但采用了不同的对照表——高 PEEP - FiO_2 表。研究发现两组的 PEEP 设置没有差异，在改善生存率或撤机方面也没有差异，尽管干预组因难治性低氧血症需要挽救性治疗的患者较少。本研究的结果表明可能只有一小部分 PEEP 滴定困难的患者需要基于 $P_{L,\,end\text{-}exp}$ 来设定 PEEP，比如胸壁顺应性异常的患者。事实上，最近一项针对急性呼吸衰竭肥胖患者的研究[12]显示，与基线 PEEP 设置相比，以 $P_{L,\,end\text{-}exp}$ 正压为目标滴定 PEEP，与更高的呼气末肺容积、更好的肺顺应性和氧合有关。

34.3.2 监测呼气末跨肺压和跨肺驱动压滴定潮气量/吸气压防止肺过度膨胀

肺保护性通气的前提是低潮气量，许多研究表明，低潮气量可以通过最小化肺过度膨胀来降低病死率[10,11]。潜在过度膨胀的指标包括高 P_{pl}（>30 cmH_2O）和 ΔP（>15 cmH_2O）[10,11,15]。尽管如此，肺损伤是由 $P_{L,\,end\text{-}exp}$ 和 ΔP_L 直接介导的，并且在胸壁弹性高的患者中，高 ΔP 并不一定与损伤性高 $P_{L,\,end\text{-}exp}$ 和 ΔP_L 相对应。一项针对 ARDS 患者的研究[16]显示 ΔP 和 ΔP_L 之间呈线性相关，但相关系数仅为 0.7，$\Delta P>15$ cmH_2O 的患者中约有三分之一 $\Delta P_L<11$ cmH_2O。此外，在 ARDS 患者中，E_L 与 E_{RS} 的比值为 $0.2\sim0.8$，对应 ΔP 为 15 cmH_2O 时，ΔP_L 为 $3\sim12$ cmH_2（$\Delta P_L=\Delta P\times E_L/E_{RS}$，图 34.2）[17]。

以 $P_{L,\,end\text{-}exp}$ 和 ΔP_L 的特定阈值为目标的通气策略，其效果尚未在临床研究中得到验证。在食管压导向的 PEEP 滴定[13]研究中，采用 25 cmH_2O 作为 ΔP_L 的"安全"阈值，但并未实际观察到过。对健康肺患者建议 $\Delta P_L<20$ cmH_2O，对 ARDS 患者建议 ΔP_L 为 $10\sim12$ cmH_2O[10,11]。这些阈值是基于几项生理和实验观察得出的。首先，根据肺的静态压力-容积曲线，在肺总量下，$P_{L,\,end\text{-}exp}$ 通常约为 30 cmH_2O，并且在 20 cmH_2O 时曲线的斜率会减小。其次，实验数据表明，当机械通气引起的应变（$\Delta V/FRC$）大于 $1.5\sim2$ 时，健康肺可受到损伤[18]。应力（ΔP_L）与应变之间的比例常数（k）为 $12\sim13$ cmH_2O，因此当应力（ΔP_L）为 $18\sim26$ cmH_2O 时，健康肺可发生损伤性应变。对于 ARDS 患者，建议降低应变阈值，因为由于肺的不均匀性，局部应力可能是全局应力的两倍[19]。此外，经验证的 ΔP 阈值（15 cmH_2O）相当于 ΔP_L 为 10 cmH_2O，这是基于 E_L/E_{RS} 通常为 0.7 的观测结果[17]。

在辅助通气过程中也可能出现损伤性高 P_L。由于早期辅助呼吸对避免膈肌萎缩是可取的，因此监测有害 $\Delta P/\Delta P_L$ 的需求正在增加。在自主呼吸的患者中，无法可靠地获得用于测量驱动压的被动条件[20]，因此当用吸气阻断测量的 ΔP 很高时，直接测量 ΔP_L 可以更准确地估算肺部应力。

34.3.3　监测自主呼吸努力防止辅助过度或不足,以及优化人-机协调

膈肌保护性通气策略需要促进膈肌主动收缩,避免过高和过低的吸气努力,并使机械与中枢吸气时间相匹配,以防止膈肌偏心收缩,尽管具体的方案和阈值尚未在临床研究中得到验证。

正常安静呼吸时,PTP 和 WOB 的范围分别为 (80 ± 20) cmH$_2$O·s/min 和 (0.35 ± 0.1) J/L[21]。一些研究[21-23]表明,成功的撤机与呼吸努力达到接近正常范围的两倍(PTP<200 cmH$_2$O·s/min 和 WOB<1 J/L)有关。在床边监测吸气努力的简单工具是潮式呼吸时 P_{es} 或 P_{di} 的波动。平静呼吸时 P_{es} 和 P_{di} 的摆动范围是 (7 ± 3) cmH$_2$O[21]。最近的两项研究[24,25]描述了 P_{es}/P_{di} 波动和吸气努力(以 PTP 或 WOB 表示)之间的相关性,发现 P_{es} 摆动 14~18 cmH$_2$O 与吸气努力增加有关(PTP 150~200 cmH$_2$O·s/min)[24]。

避免吸气努力过低是非常重要的,因为辅助通气的患者有过度辅助和膈肌萎缩的风险[10,11]。建议调整辅助水平使 PTP 维持在 40~50 cmH$_2$O·s/min 的水平[10,11]。根据目前可用的数据,通过 P_{es} 摆动监测患者的努力,可以将其调整到略大于正常范围的水平,一般为 5~15 cmH$_2$O[10,11,24]。

监测 P_{es} 比检查压力和流量波形更能清楚和准确地识别人-机不同步的情况(图 34.4)。触发延迟,被定义为从患者开始努力吸气到呼吸机开始加压之间的时间[26],可以通过 P_{es} 来量化。触发延迟是由呼吸机的特性决定的,但也受到患者努力程度的影响,在努力较弱的患者中可以观察到较长的延迟[27]。自动触发是另一种形式的不同步,在没有监测 P_{es} 的情况下通常很难与吸气努力较弱相区分[26]。

无效努力是最常见的不同步,并与患者更糟糕的预后相关[28]。当患者的努力不足以触发呼吸机时,就会发生无效努力,原因可能是努力低,也可能是存在内源性 PEEP。虽然检查压力和流量波形有助于识别无效努力,但监测 P_{es} 和 P_{di} 可以准确地量化吸气努力和 PEEPi(图 34.3 和图 34.4)。

呼吸夹带或反向触发是指由于机械呼吸而发生的膈肌收缩[29]。在肺部受损的患者中,夹带现象可以通过呼吸叠加(输送双倍潮气量)造成肺过度膨胀或通过呼吸摆动现象(呼吸时一定量的气体从肺非依赖区转移到依赖区)造成局部过度牵拉[4]。夹带的特征是机械呼吸和中枢呼吸开始之间存在稳定的时间差,这可以从 P_{es} 波形中计算出来(图 34.4)。在呼气阻断或 CPAP 试验中,若缺乏吸气努力,则区分反向触发与自发努力。

监测 P_{es} 可以准确评估中枢吸气时间,并且有助于识别和纠正与加压阶段持续时间、延迟和过早的吸-呼切换有关的不同步现象[26]。当直接通过 P_{es} 波形观察中枢吸气时间时,可在床旁调节吸-呼切换规则,从而轻松实现机械吸气时间与中枢吸气时间的匹配。避免这种不同步对保护性通气很重要[11],因为过早的吸-呼切换,无论是否存在双触发,都可能通过增加肺部应力使膈肌发生偏心收缩,从而促使肺和膈肌损伤。而延迟的吸-呼

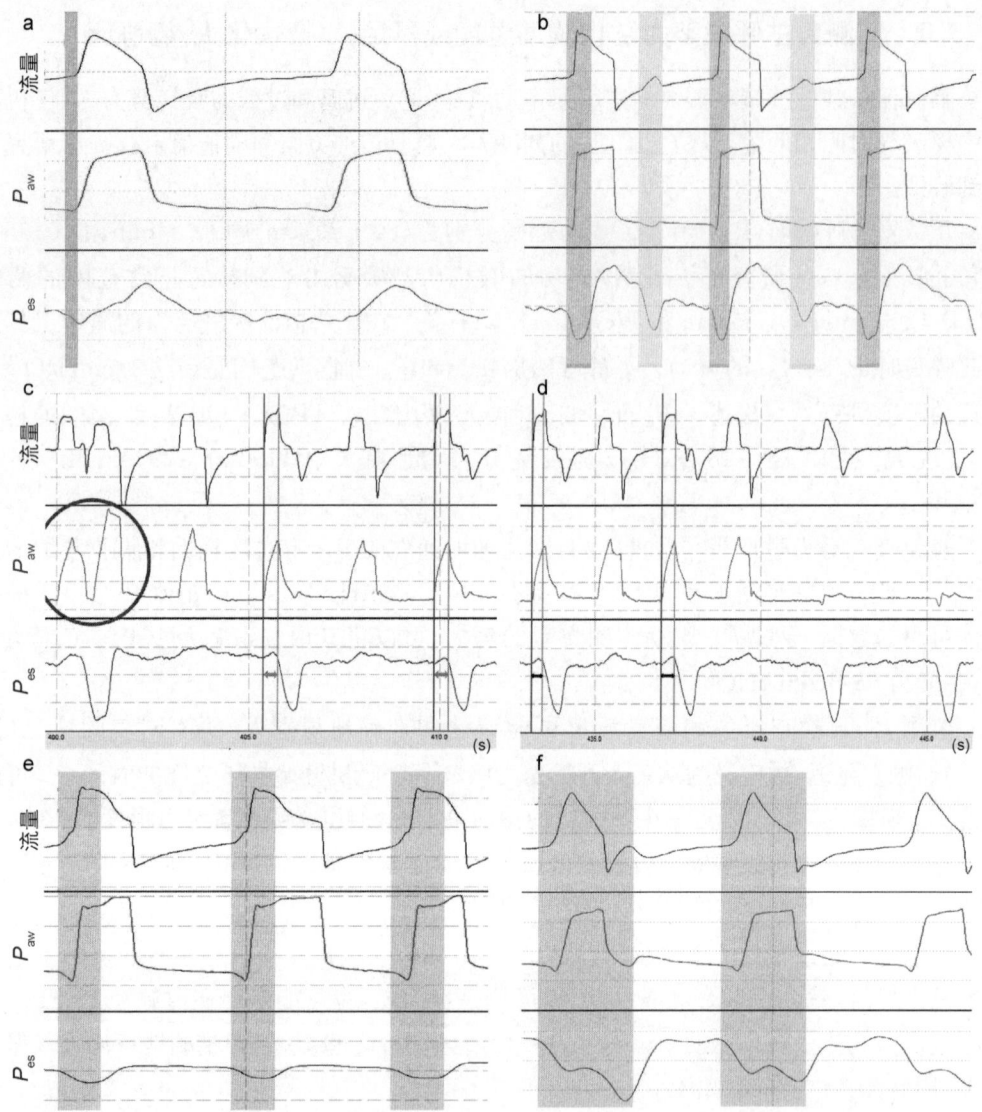

图 34.4 识别不同步现象。从上到下依次为：流量、气道压（P_{aw}）和食管压（P_{es}）随时间变化的波形图。a. 触发延迟和自动触发：在压力支持模式下，患者小幅努力会触发第一次呼吸，随后吸气肌放松，表现为 P_{es} 上移（与被动通气一样）。触发延迟（显示为蓝色）为 120 毫秒，在这种情况下，几乎与患者努力时间一样长。第二次呼吸是自动触发的呼吸，因为在 P_{es} 波形中没检测到任何努力。这种自动触发在 P_{aw} 波形中无法识别。b. 高水平压力支持下的无效努力：患者的努力可以在 P_{es} 波形上识别出来，第一、第三和第六次努力触发了呼吸机送气（显示为蓝色），而第二和第四次努力是无效的（显示为黄色）。呼气流速波形的轻度变形表明存在无效努力，但 P_{es} 波形可以更清楚地识别患者的努力。c. 辅助容量控制通气中的呼吸叠加和夹带（反向触发）：延伸到机器呼气时间的吸气努力触发了呼吸机输送第二次的叠加呼吸，增加了潮气量带来的应力（红圈）。这种患者努力可能是夹带的结果，其特征是与机器呼吸（紫色箭头）保持稳定的时间关系，可以使用 P_{es} 波形进行测量。d. 在控制模式下的自发努力可与夹带表现相似，可以通过与机器呼吸缺乏稳定的时间关系（黑色箭头）和 CPAP 试验中存在吸气努力进行区分。e, f. 机器和中枢吸气时间不匹配：在压力支持模式下，中枢吸气时间（显示为橙色）可能比机器吸气时间短，表现为吸-呼切换延迟（e）；也可能比机械时间长，表现为吸-呼切换过早（f）（见彩色插图）

切换则与过度辅助有关，可能促进PEEPi的产生和导致无效努力。

34.4　总结

综上所述，P_{es}监测是一种有价值的工具，易于床旁应用，有助于提供个体化的保护性通气。具备智能报警功能的先进监测设备和更大规模的临床研究有望在未来将个体化通气的生理机制转化为患者受益的结果。

（魏东坡，周芳庆　译）

参考文献

[1] Akoumianaki E, Maggiore SM, Valenza F, Bellani G, Jubran A, Loring SH, et al. The application of esophageal pressure measurement in patients with respiratory failure. Am J Respir Crit Care Med. 2014; 189(5): 520-31.

[2] Mojoli F, Torriglia F, Orlando A, Bianchi I, Arisi E, Pozzi M. Technical aspects of bedside respiratory monitoring of transpulmonary pressure. Ann Transl Med. 2018; 6(19): 377.

[3] Pelosi P, D'Andrea L, Vitale G, Pesenti A, Gattinoni L. Vertical gradient of regional lung inflation in adult respiratory distress syndrome. Am J Respir Crit Care Med. 1994; 149(1): 8-13.

[4] Yoshida T, Torsani V, Gomes S, De Santis RR, Beraldo MA, Costa ELV, et al. Spontaneous effort causes occult pendelluft during mechanical ventilation. Am J Respir Crit Care Med. 2013; 188(12): 1420-7.

[5] Bastia L, Engelberts D, Osada K, Katira BH, Damiani LF, Yoshida T, et al. Role of positive end-expiratory pressure and regional transpulmonary pressure in asymmetrical lung injury. Am J Respir Crit Care Med. 2021; 203(8): 969-76.

[6] Chen L, Del Sorbo L, Grieco DL, Shklar O, Junhasavasdikul D, Telias I, et al. Airway closure in acute respiratory distress syndrome: an underestimated and misinterpreted phenomenon. Am J Respir Crit Care Med. 2018; 197(1): 132-6.

[7] Gulati G, Novero A, Loring SH, Talmor D. Pleural pressure and optimal positive end-expiratory pressure based on esophageal pressure versus chest wall elastance: incompatible results*. Crit Care Med. 2013; 41(8): 1951-7.

[8] Yoshida T, Amato MBP, Grieco DL, Chen L, Lima CAS, Roldan R, et al. Esophageal manometry and regional transpulmonary pressure in lung injury. Am J Respir Crit Care Med. 2018; 197(8): 1018-26.

[9] Loring SH, O'Donnell CR, Behazin N, Malhotra A, Sarge T, Ritz R, et al. Esophageal pressures in acute lung injury: do they represent artifact or useful information about transpulmonary pressure, chest wall mechanics, and lung stress? J Appl Physiol (1985). 2010; 108(3): 515-22.

[10] Goligher EC, Jonkman AH, Dianti J, Vaporidi K, Beitler JR, Patel BK, et al. Clinical strategies for implementing lung and diaphragm-protective ventilation: avoiding insufficient and excessive effort. Intensive Care Med. 2020; 46(12): 2314-26.

[11] Goligher EC, Dres M, Patel BK, Sahetya SK, Beitler JR, Telias I, et al. Lung- and diaphragm-

protective ventilation. Am J Respir Crit Care Med. 2020; 202(7): 950-61.

[12] Fumagalli J, Berra L, Zhang C, Pirrone M, Santiago RRDS, Gomes S, et al. Transpulmonary pressure describes lung morphology during decremental positive end-expiratory pressure trials in obesity. Crit Care Med. 2017; 45(8): 1374-81.

[13] Talmor D, Sarge T, Malhotra A, O'Donnell CR, Ritz R, Lisbon A, et al. Mechanical ventilation guided by esophageal pressure in acute lung injury. N Engl J Med. 2008; 359(20): 2095-104.

[14] Beitler JR, Sarge T, Banner-Goodspeed VM, Gong MN, Cook D, Novack V, et al. Effect of titrating positive end-expiratory pressure (PEEP) with an esophageal pressure-guided strategy vs an empirical high PEEP-FiO_2 strategy on death and days free from mechanical ventilation among patients with acute respiratory distress syndrome: a randomized clinical trial. JAMA. 2019; 321(9): 846-57.

[15] Amato MBP, Meade MO, Slutsky AS, Brochard L, Costa ELV, Schoenfeld DA, et al. Driving pressure and survival in the acute respiratory distress syndrome. N Engl J Med. 2015; 372(8): 747-55.

[16] Chiumello D, Carlesso E, Brioni M, Cressoni M. Airway driving pressure and lung stress in ARDS patients. Crit Care. 2016; 22(20): 276.

[17] Chiumello D, Carlesso E, Cadringher P, Caironi P, Valenza F, Polli F, et al. Lung stress and strain during mechanical ventilation for acute respiratory distress syndrome. Am J Respir Crit Care Med. 2008; 178(4): 346-55.

[18] Protti A, Cressoni M, Santini A, Langer T, Mietto C, Febres D, et al. Lung stress and strain during mechanical ventilation: any safe threshold? Am J Respir Crit Care Med. 2011; 183(10): 1354-62.

[19] Cressoni M, Cadringher P, Chiurazzi C, Amini M, Gallazzi E, Marino A, et al. Lung inhomogeneity in patients with acute respiratory distress syndrome. Am J Respir Crit Care Med. 2014; 189(2): 149-58.

[20] Soundoulounaki S, Akoumianaki E, Kondili E, Pediaditis E, Prinianakis G, Vaporidi K, et al. Airway pressure morphology and respiratory muscle activity during end-inspiratory occlusions in pressure support ventilation. Crit Care. 2020; 24(1): 467.

[21] Mancebo J, Isabey D, Lorino H, Lofaso F, Lemaire F, Brochard L. Comparative effects of pressure support ventilation and intermittent positive pressure breathing (IPPB) in non-intubated healthy subjects. Eur Respir J. 1995; 8(11): 1901-9.

[22] Cabello B, Thille AW, Roche-Campo F, Brochard L, Gómez FJ, Mancebo J. Physiological comparison of three spontaneous breathing trials in difficult-to-wean patients. Intensive Care Med. 2010; 36(7): 1171-9.

[23] Jubran A, Tobin MJ. Pathophysiologic basis of acute respiratory distress in patients who fail a trial of weaning from mechanical ventilation. Am J Respir Crit Care Med. 1997; 155(3): 906-15.

[24] Vaporidi K, Soundoulounaki S, Papadakis E, Akoumianaki E, Kondili E, Georgopoulos D. Esophageal and transdiaphragmatic pressure swings as indices of inspiratory effort. Respir Physiol Neurobiol. 2021; 284: 103561.

[25] Umbrello M, Formenti P, Lusardi AC, Guanziroli M, Caccioppola A, Coppola S, et al. Oesophageal pressure and respiratory muscle ultrasonographic measurements indicate inspiratory effort during pressure support ventilation. Br J Anaesth. 2020; 125(1): e148-57.

[26] Georgopoulos D, Prinianakis G, Kondili E. Bedside waveforms interpretation as a tool to identify

patient-ventilator asynchronies. Intensive Care Med. 2006; 32(1): 34-47.

[27] Thille AW, Lyazidi A, Richard J-CM, Galia F, Brochard L. A bench study of intensive-care-unit ventilators: new versus old and turbine-based versus compressed gas-based ventilators. Intensive Care Med. 2009; 35(8): 1368-76.

[28] Vaporidi K, Babalis D, Chytas A, Lilitsis E, Kondili E, Amargianitakis V, et al. Clusters of ineffective efforts during mechanical ventilation: impact on outcome. Intensive Care Med. 2017; 43(2): 184-91.

[29] Akoumianaki E, Lyazidi A, Rey N, Matamis D, Perez-Martinez N, Giraud R, et al. Mechanical ventilation-induced reverse-triggered breaths: a frequently unrecognized form of neuromechanical coupling. Chest. 2013; 143(4): 927-38.

35 肺容积和容积二氧化碳图
Lung Volumes and Volumetric Capnography

Hong-liang Li, Jian-Xin Zhou, Lu Chen

35.1 引言

机械通气可以挽救生命,也可以产生继发性损伤和炎症,称为呼吸机诱发的肺损伤(ventilator-induced lung injury,VILI)。肺容积的评估对于了解每个患者的呼吸力学从而降低VILI的风险至关重要[1]。虽然潮气量(V_T)是常规监测的,但是其他容积指标,如呼气末肺容积(end-expiratory lung volume,EELV)和肺复张容积,值得更多的关注以提供更安全的通气模式[2-4]。另一方面,无效腔的测量是评估气体交换以优化呼吸机设置的基础。容量二氧化碳图提供了一种无创和连续的方法来床旁监测无效腔和通气的有效性。在本章中,我们将讨论一些有关肺容积和容积二氧化碳图的相关问题。

35.2 肺容积

35.2.1 为什么测量绝对肺容积具有临床意义

绝对肺容积的测量对于肺保护性通气具有重要的生理意义,尽管它尚未在常规实践中广泛应用。例如,急性呼吸窘迫综合征(acute respiratory distress syndrome,ARDS)

的一个关键特征是由于肺不张和实变而导致功能残气量的减少。在接受呼气末正压(positive end-expiratory pressure，PEEP)的患者中，功能性肺容积被定义为功能残气量与 PEEP 产生复张容积的总和，这反映了肺可以承受多少 V_T。评估功能性肺容积可以计算肺应变(V_T 与功能性肺容积的比值)，这表明肺形变与其原始状态相关。实验研究表明，应变是 VILI 的关键决定因素。临床试验也支持这一观点，因为在所有评估的呼吸力学参数中，应变替代参数(即驱动压)与生存率的相关性最强。

35.2.2　如何测量绝对肺容积

测量肺绝对容积主要有三种方法：① 最敏感的方法，比如，计算机断层成像(computed tomography，CT)的定量分析，这也显示了肺容积的区域分布。其基于一个体积像素的 X 射线衰减与该体素的物理密度之间的线性相关性。比如，密度为 −500 亨氏单位(Hounsfield unit，HU)，相当于体素一半由组织组成(其放射密度相当于水)，一半由气体组成。换句话说，可以通过 CT 值计算出任何给定体素(以及任何肺区域)的气体和组织量。然而，CT 也是最复杂和最耗时的方法。② 气体稀释技术，根据惰性气体(如氦气)平衡过程中的稀释浓度来估算肺体积。该技术通常用于肺功能检测实验室，但在 ICU 中实施过于复杂。③ Olegard 及其同事提出了一种改良的氮气洗脱/吸入技术，该技术基于 FiO_2 的阶梯变化，可以在不中断机械通气的情况下测量 EELV，并且已经有特定商用呼吸机可供使用。

35.2.3　如何测量肺容积变化

肺容积变化最常见的评估指标是 V_T，其计算方法为流量与时间的积分。因此，一个流量传感器对于评估 V_T 来说是必要的。一个现代的呼吸机通常配备有一个吸气传感器和嵌入在机器上的(远离患者端)呼气流量传感器。可靠测量呼出 V_T 需要评估管道中的漏气率和呼吸回路的顺应性。一些呼吸机还配备了一个近端流量传感器，放置在 Y 型管和气管插管之间，提供更好的准确性。虽然水蒸气和分泌物会降低其准确性，但近端流量传感器对儿科患者特别有用[5]。因为流量信号存在不可避免的偏差，都会在检测到新的呼吸开始时将 V_T 重置为零。当呼吸重叠发生时，这种技术操作会导致显著低估输送给患者的气体量。例如，在容量控制模式下，患者可能在常规呼吸时以 6 mL/kg 的潮气量进行通气，但当反向触发出现呼吸重叠时，实际潮气量可能达 12 mL/kg。在临床实践中应关注这个问题，以提供更好的肺保护性通气。

用流量传感器测量的 V_T 可以校准电阻抗断层成像(electrical impedance tomography，EIT)测量的呼吸阻抗变化。例如，呼吸系统的区域顺应性可以通过区域 V_T 除以驱动压来计算。通过 EIT，Yoshida 等[6]证实了 V_T 分布的呼吸摆动现象，强调了自主呼吸时肺依赖区存在潜在的过度牵拉：这不能通过监测"全局" V_T 来识别。

肺容积的另一个重要变化是由 PEEP 引起的。PEEP 引起的肺容积变化包含两个方面：已经打开的肺单位充气/过度充气和塌陷的肺单位复张[7,8]。我们将在下面的章节中介绍它们的测量。

35.2.4 如何使用计算机断层成像测量肺复张

评估肺复张最直观的方法是胸部CT,早前由Gattinoni等描述[9]。如先前章节所述,CT可以用来评估EELV。EELV的变化是两个PEEP水平之间EELV的差异。此外,肺组织的局部通气也可以通过CT来测量和分类。无通气肺组织的CT值为$-100\sim 100$ HU,通气不良肺组织为$-500\sim -101$ HU,通气良好肺组织为$-900\sim -501$ HU,过度膨胀肺组织为$-1\,000\sim -910$ HU[1]。根据区域通气水平的变化,EELV的改变可分为复张、充气和过度充气。然而,对复张的具体定义仍存在争论,通过CT有两种方法来定义肺复张:Gattinoni法[2]和Rouby法[10]。我们在表35.1中总结了它们的主要差异,这对临床实践很重要。在过去的三十年里,CT极大地提高了我们对由PEEP和俯卧位导致肺复张的理解[2,11]。尽管CT很有用,但它在临床实践中很少用于评估肺复张,可能是由于会带来辐射和转运的风险,以及耗时的定量分析。

表 35.1　Gattinoni 法和 Rouby 法在使用 CT 评估复张时的差异

	Gattinoni 法	Rouby 法
比较	基于体素	基于解剖分区
肺组织	非充气	非充气和充气不良
临界值	-100 HU	-500 HU
计算	组织重量变化[a]	气体体积变化
对比	类似统计学中的独立 t 检验,高 PEEP 的肺区域与低 PEEP 的区域进行非配对比较	类似统计学中的配对 t 检验,高 PEEP 肺区域与低 PEEP 区域进行配对比较

[a] 组织重量由组织体积获得,假设组织密度为 1 g/mL。

35.2.5 如何使用压力-容积曲线测量肺复张

与形态学方法(即CT)相比,基于力学的方法(使用多条压力-容积曲线),虽然直观性较差(无法直接观察肺复张),却是更可行的床旁评估方法。压力-容积曲线方法的基本原理是测量复张或去复张的容积,也就是在给定的静态压力下,测量两个压力-容积曲线之间的容积差。请注意,这两个压力-容积曲线是在两个PEEP水平分别生成的(图35.1),因此是从不同的EELV开始的。为了在相同的坐标轴上绘图进行比较,采用了前面提到的技术(即氮气洗脱/吸入技术)来测量EELV。此外,静态(弹性)压力可以通过使用低流速(即5 L/min)吸气来测量,其产生的气道阻力可以忽略不计。如果较高的PEEP产生显著的肺复张,在相同的弹性回缩力下,压力-容积曲线之间会有很大的容积偏移(图35.1a)。相比之下,如果几乎没有肺复张,容积差异就会很小(图35.1b)。压力-容积曲线虽然比CT方法更容易,但在常规实践中仍然很烦琐。

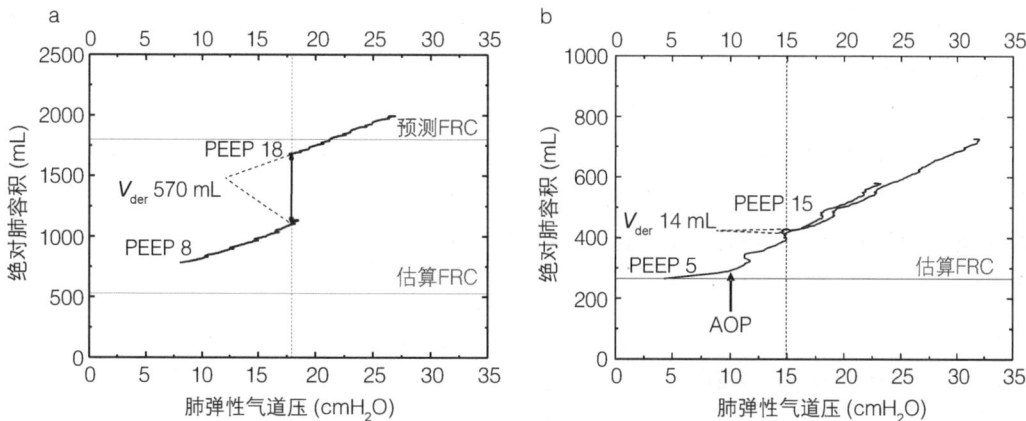

图35.1 通过多条压力-容积曲线来评估去复张的容积。曲线 a 是具有高可复张性的代表性患者,而曲线 b 则是低可复张性和气道闭合的患者。采用氮气洗脱/吸入技术测量肺的绝对容积。反映肺弹性的气道压是通过低流速(5 L/min)吸气来测量的。V_{der} 指的是去复张容积,通过相同弹性回缩力下(在曲线 a 为 18 cmH$_2$O;在曲线 b 为 15 cmH$_2$O)两条压力-容积曲线间的容积差计算。AOP 是指气道完全闭合患者开放气道所需的压力[25]。估算功能残气量(FRC)是通过撤除 PEEP 的方式来估算的,通过原 PEEP 水平下的呼气末肺容积减去呼出的 PEEP 诱导的肺容积得出。仰卧位时的预测功能残气量(FRC)是基于性别和身高进行预测的

35.2.6 如何测量肺复张-充气比

在最近的一项临床研究中,Chen 等[8]提出了一种单次呼吸方法在床旁测量的肺可复张性(图 35.2)。这一方法的基本原理衍生于多条压力-容积曲线的机制。此方法只需要

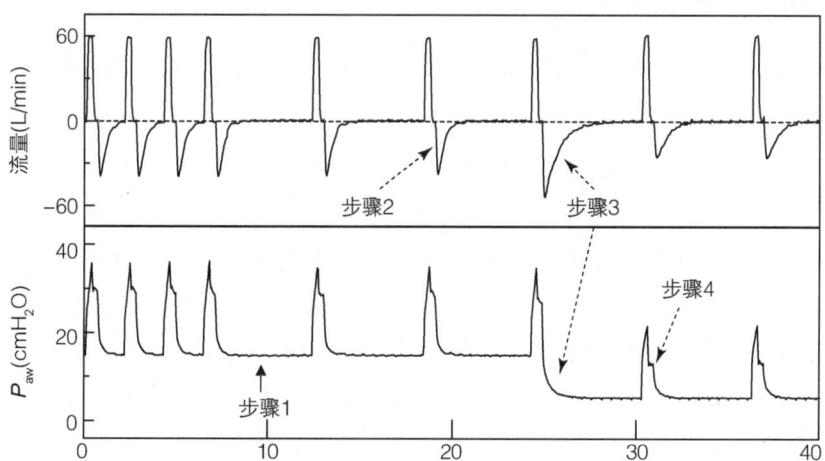

图35.2 通过单次呼吸法测量复张-充气比。测量步骤:① 将呼吸频率降低到 6~8 次/分,以最小化自动 PEEP;② 在一次或两次呼吸后,记录在高 PEEP 下呼出的潮气量(V_T);③ 将 PEEP 降低 10 cm H$_2$O(如从 15 cmH$_2$O 降低到 5 cmH$_2$O),并记录 PEEP 从高到低时的呼出 V_T;记录低 PEEP 时的平台压(P_{plat}),并恢复之前的呼吸机设置。然后可以将记录的数据输入在线计算器 https://crec.coemv.ca(提供视频演示)

在几次呼吸过程中降低PEEP,在床旁完成且只需要不到1分钟。作者还强调,萎陷肺单元复张的获益应该与已开放肺单元充气/过度充气的代价保持平衡,并由此提出了一个称为复张-充气比(recruitment-to-inflation, R/I)的指标[8]。R/I可以作为一个连续的变量来评估与充气相关的复张潜力(R/I值越高,复张潜力越大),也可以被离散化用于确定肺的可复张性(R/I≥0.5表示高度可复张性,R/I<0.5表示可复张性差)。由于测量R/I的简便性,即使医疗资源有限的环境中也可以使用,可应用于COVID-19导致的ARDS患者[12]。

35.3 容积二氧化碳图

35.3.1 什么是无效腔

无效腔是指潮气量中不参与气体交换的部分。纯无效腔指那些通气但无灌注的肺单位;换句话说,就是具有无限大通气/灌注(V/Q)的肺区域。然而,在临床实践中,区分纯无效腔和高V/Q(1<V/Q<∞)的肺单位是不切实际的。纯无效腔和高V/Q肺单位对二氧化碳(CO_2)的清除都有相似的作用,因此,它们被视为是等同的。生理无效腔(physiological dead space, VD_{phys})包括两个部分:① 传导气道(VD_{aw});② 灌注不良或无灌注的通气肺泡(VD_{alv})。在机械通气的患者中,气管插管和Y型回路间会产生额外的无效腔,如加热湿化器、细菌-病毒过滤器和连接器,这些无效腔应尽可能最小化。在本章中,我们将仪器相关无效腔作为VD_{aw}的一部分,除非另有说明。

35.3.2 如何计算无效腔

无效腔通常表示为单次呼吸的绝对容积,可以用1891年提出的Bohr公式计算,或用其重排公式:

$$VD_{phys} = \frac{P_{\bar{A}}CO_2 - P_{\bar{E}}CO_2}{P_{\bar{A}}CO_2} \times V_T \tag{35.1}$$

其中$P_{\bar{A}}CO_2$为肺泡中平均二氧化碳分压,$P_{\bar{E}}CO_2$是混合呼出气体中平均二氧化碳分压,V_T是潮气量。值得注意的是,Enghoff修正了Bohr公式,用动脉血中的二氧化碳分压代替$P_{\bar{A}}CO_2$。Enghoff的修正公式可以作为整体V/Q不匹配的指标,而不只是无效腔[13,14]。事实上,Enghoff的方法提供了来自肺泡-毛细血管膜两侧的信息,因此包括无效腔和肺内分流[13-15]。需要动脉血样本也使得Enghoff的方法无法用于无创、实时监测。因此,我们建议使用原始的Bohr方法来计算无效腔。

35.3.3 什么是二氧化碳图

二氧化碳图是指CO_2的浓度或分压随时间或容积变化的曲线图。基于时间的二氧化碳图在临床实践中主要用于监测呼气末二氧化碳分压($P_{ET}CO_2$)。请注意,即使观察到

呼气期间 CO_2 的平台分压，$P_{ET}CO_2$ 也不等于 P_ACO_2（计算无效腔所需的）。基于容积的二氧化碳图，或称为容积二氧化碳图整合了 CO_2 和容积信号，可绘制随呼气潮气量变化的 CO_2 浓度或分压曲线图。与基于时间的二氧化碳图不同，容积二氧化碳图提供了计算无效腔所需的所有信息。

35.3.4 什么是二氧化碳测定仪

二氧化碳测定仪是一种用于测量呼出气体中 CO_2 浓度的非侵入性设备。其设计是基于 CO_2 的特性：优先吸收特定波长（4.26 μm）的红外辐射。根据传感器位置的不同，二氧化碳测定仪可以分为两类。主流式二氧化碳测定仪在气管插管和 Y 型延长管之间使用红外传感器进行采样。旁流式二氧化碳测定仪广泛应用于手术室和重症监护室，可能是因为它是一次性使用且易于监测 $P_{ET}CO_2$。然而，旁流式二氧化碳测定仪的气流和 CO_2 浓度信号之间存在延迟，即使通过校正，也可能导致容积二氧化碳图形状出现一定程度的失真[16]。主流式二氧化碳测定仪可以快速准确地分析 CO_2 浓度，与主气流同步，因此更适合于测量无效腔。

35.3.5 如何应用容积二氧化碳图来计算无效腔

如图 35.3 所示，容量二氧化碳图的记录可分为三个阶段：Ⅰ阶段是来自气道和仪器的不含有 CO_2 的气体（如果仪器放置于 CO_2 传感器和患者之间）；Ⅱ阶段代表气道和肺泡之间的过渡气体；Ⅲ阶段是纯肺泡内气体。Ⅱ和Ⅲ阶段由这两段斜面延长线的交点区分。根据 Fowler 的理论[17]，Ⅱ阶段的拐点（即曲线曲率变化的点）被认为是气道-肺泡界面的

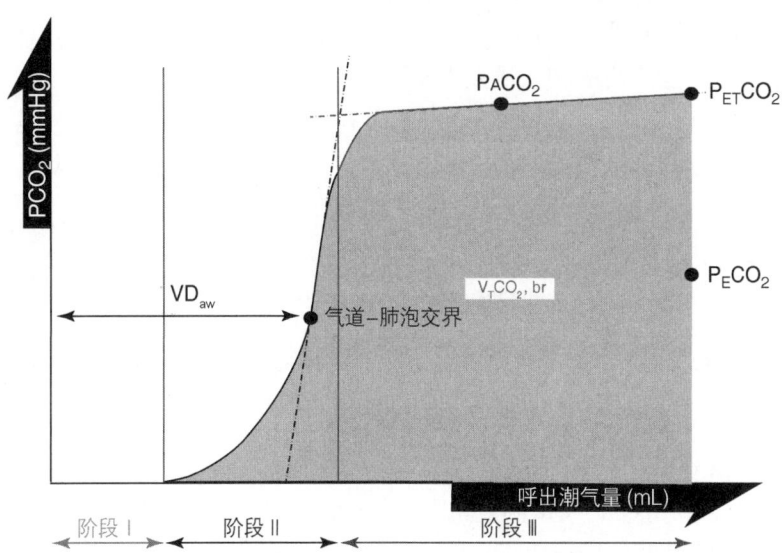

图 35.3 容积二氧化碳图测量无效腔示意图。PCO_2 是 CO_2 的分压。P_ACO_2 是肺泡气体中的平均 CO_2 分压，P_ECO_2 是混合呼出气体中的平均 CO_2 分压。$P_{ET}CO_2$ 是呼气末 CO_2 分压。$VTCO_2,br$ 是潮式呼吸中 CO_2 被清除的量（曲线下面积）。VD_{aw} 是气道无效腔的体积

标志。从呼气开始到此拐点所呼出的容积就是 VD_{aw}。CO_2-容积曲线下的面积代表被潮式呼吸所清除的 CO_2 总量(V_TCO_2,br),可以通过数值积分计算出来。$P_{\bar{E}}CO_2$ 可以通过 V_TCO_2,br 与 V_T 的比值乘以大气压来计算。在过去,计算无效腔中最具挑战性的部分是测量 $P_{\bar{A}}CO_2$。多亏 Fletcher 和 Jonson 的理论工作[14],以及 Tusman 的验证[18],我们现在可以利用气道-肺泡界面和 $P_{ET}CO_2$ 的中点对应的Ⅲ阶段曲线的点直接确定 $P_{\bar{A}}CO_2$。然后,将 $P_{\bar{A}}CO_2$ 和 $P_{ET}CO_2$ 的值插入 Bohr 公式中,可以计算出 VD_{phys}。获得 VD_{phys} 和 VD_{aw} 的值,我们最终可以计算出肺泡无效腔为:

$$VD_{alv} = VD_{phys} - VD_{aw} \tag{35.2}$$

显然,上述测量过程需要计算机协助;事实上,大多数研究使用的是定制的研究软件。与呼吸机集成的商业可用软件可以自动完成所有这些无效腔的测量,可能会便于床旁应用容积二氧化碳图。

35.3.6 临床意义

通过测量无效腔和其他容积参数,容积二氧化碳图在机械通气患者中提供了广泛的潜在临床应用价值[19]。例如,一些临床研究已经证明,在不同病因诱发的早期和晚期或者轻度和重度 ARDS 中,升高的 VD_{phys} 与病死率有很强的相关性[20,21]。事实上,VD_{phys} 与预后的关联比任何氧合衍生指标更强,突显了无效腔的预后价值。容量二氧化碳图可用于个体化设定呼吸机,也许最明显的应用是用于优化 V_T。在不同的容积二氧化碳图衍生参数中,Jonson 提出了一个效率指数,该指数直接反映与 CO_2 清除有关的通气效率[22]。此外,无效腔的测量可以帮助评估肺泡复张和过度膨胀,为滴定 PEEP 提供有用的信息[23]。它也可用于评估容量反应性和无创心输出量的测算[24]。尽管这些应用前景光明,但还需要进一步广泛的临床研究来验证。

(魏东坡,周芳庆 译)

参考文献

[1] Chen L, Brochard L. Lung volume assessment in acute respiratory distress syndrome. Curr Opin Crit Care. 2015; 21: 259 - 64.

[2] Gattinoni L, Caironi P, Cressoni M, Chiumello D, Ranieri VM, Quintel M, Russo S, Patroniti N, Cornejo R, Bugedo G. Lung recruitment in patients with the acute respiratory distress syndrome. N Engl J Med. 2006; 354: 1775 - 86.

[3] Maggiore SM, Jonson B, Richard JC, Jaber S, Lemaire F, Brochard L. Alveolar derecruitment at decremental positive end-expiratory pressure levels in acute lung injury: comparison with the lower inflection point, oxygenation, and compliance. Am J Respir Crit Care Med. 2001; 164: 795 - 801.

[4] Chiumello D, Carlesso E, Cadringher P, Caironi P, Valenza F, Polli F, Tallarini F, Cozzi P, Cressoni M, Colombo A, Marini JJ, Gattinoni L. Lung stress and strain during mechanical ventilation for acute respiratory distress syndrome. Am J Respir Crit Care Med. 2008; 178: 346 -

55.

[5] Cannon ML, Cornell J, Tripp-Hamel DS, Gentile MA, Hubble CL, Meliones JN, Cheifetz IM. Tidal volumes for ventilated infants should be determined with a pneumotachometer placed at the endotracheal tube. Am J Respir Crit Care Med. 2000; 162: 2109 - 12.

[6] Yoshida T, Torsani V, Gomes S, De Santis RR, Beraldo MA, Costa EL, Tucci MR, Zin WA, Kavanagh BP, Amato MB. Spontaneous effort causes occult pendelluft during mechanical ventilation. Am J Respir Crit Care Med. 2013; 188: 1420 - 7.

[7] Mauri T, Eronia N, Turrini C, Battistini M, Grasselli G, Rona R, Volta CA, Bellani G, Pesenti A. Bedside assessment of the effects of positive end-expiratory pressure on lung inflation and recruitment by the helium dilution technique and electrical impedance tomography. Intensive Care Med. 2016; 42: 1576 - 87.

[8] Chen L, Del Sorbo L, Grieco DL, Junhasavasdikul D, Rittayamai N, Soliman I, Sklar MC, Rauseo M, Ferguson ND, Fan E, Richard JM, Brochard L. Potential for lung recruitment estimated by the recruitment-to-inflation ratio in acute respiratory distress syndrome. A clinical trial. Am J Respir Crit Care Med. 2020; 201: 178 - 87.

[9] Gattinoni L, Mascheroni D, Torresin A, Marcolin R, Fumagalli R, Vesconi S, Rossi GP, Rossi F, Baglioni S, Bassi F, et al. Morphological response to positive end expiratory pressure in acute respiratory failure. Computerized tomography study. Intensive Care Med. 1986; 12: 137 - 42.

[10] Malbouisson LM, Muller JC, Constantin JM, Lu Q, Puybasset L, Rouby JJ, Group CTSAS. Computed tomography assessment of positive end-expiratory pressure-induced alveolar recruitment in patients with acute respiratory distress syndrome. Am J Respir Crit Care Med. 2001; 163: 1444 - 50.

[11] Cornejo RA, Diaz JC, Tobar EA, Bruhn AR, Ramos CA, Gonzalez RA, Repetto CA, Romero CM, Galvez LR, Llanos O, Arellano DH, Neira WR, Diaz GA, Zamorano AJ, Pereira GL. Effects of prone positioning on lung protection in patients with acute respiratory distress syndrome. Am J Respir Crit Care Med. 2013; 188: 440 - 8.

[12] Pan C, Chen L, Lu C, Zhang W, Xia JA, Sklar MC, Du B, Brochard L, Qiu H. Lung recruitability in COVID-19-associated acute respiratory distress syndrome: a single-center observational study. Am J Respir Crit Care Med. 2020; 201: 1294 - 7.

[13] Tusman G, Sipmann FS, Bohm SH. Rationale of dead space measurement by volumetric capnography. Anesth Analg. 2012; 114: 866 - 74.

[14] Fletcher R, Jonson B, Cumming G, Brew J. The concept of deadspace with special reference to the single breath test for carbon dioxide. Br J Anaesth. 1981; 53: 77 - 88.

[15] Wagner PD. Causes of a high physiological dead space in critically ill patients. Crit Care. 2008; 12: 148.

[16] Balogh AL, Petak F, Fodor GH, Tolnai J, Csorba Z, Babik B. Capnogram slope and ventilation dead space parameters: comparison of mainstream and sidestream techniques. Br J Anaesth. 2016; 117: 109 - 17.

[17] Fowler WS. Lung function studies; the respiratory dead space. Am J Phys. 1948; 154: 405 - 16.

[18] Tusman G, Sipmann FS, Borges JB, Hedenstierna G, Bohm SH. Validation of Bohr dead space measured by volumetric capnography. Intensive Care Med. 2011; 37: 870 - 4.

[19] Kreit JW. Volume capnography in the intensive care unit: potential clinical applications. Ann Am Thorac Soc. 2019; 16: 409 - 20.

[20] Nuckton TJ, Alonso JA, Kallet RH, Daniel BM, Pittet JF, Eisner MD, Matthay MA.

Pulmonary dead-space fraction as a risk factor for death in the acute respiratory distress syndrome. N Engl J Med. 2002; 346: 1281-6.

[21] Kallet RH, Zhuo H, Ho K, Lipnick MS, Gomez A, Matthay MA. Lung injury etiology and other factors influencing the relationship between dead-space fraction and mortality in ARDS. Respir Care. 2017; 62: 1241-8.

[22] Jonson B. Volumetric capnography for noninvasive monitoring of acute respiratory distress syndrome. Am J Respir Crit Care Med. 2018; 198: 396-8.

[23] Tusman G, Suarez-Sipmann F, Bohm SH, Pech T, Reissmann H, Meschino G, Scandurra A, Hedenstierna G. Monitoring dead space during recruitment and PEEP titration in an experimental model. Intensive Care Med. 2006; 32: 1863-71.

[24] Tusman G, Groisman I, Maidana GA, Scandurra A, Arca JM, Bohm SH, Suarez-Sipmann F. The sensitivity and specificity of pulmonary carbon dioxide elimination for noninvasive assessment of fluid responsiveness. Anesth Analg. 2016; 122: 1404-11.

[25] Chen L, Del Sorbo L, Grieco DL, Shklar O, Junhasavasdikul D, Telias I, Fan E, Brochard L. Airway closure in acute respiratory distress syndrome: an underestimated and misinterpreted phenomenon. Am J Respir Crit Care Med. 2018; 197: 132-6.

36 影像学监测

Radiological Monitoring

Jean-Michel Constantin, Elodie Baron, Bao Long Nguyen

36.1 引言

ICU 的肺部影像学检查是一个有争议的话题，通常是有意义的，但并不总是合理的。尽管床旁胸片检查（chest radiography, CRX）的使用几乎与重症医学一样久远，但超声技术的出现使其在很大程度上受到挑战。肺部 CT 仍然是评估肺部形态和急慢性肺损伤的金标准，但也受到无创技术如超声和常规 EIT 的挑战[1]。过去，ICU 医生认为每天的 CXR 对于评估肺部疾病的进展和监测常用留置导管（如中心静脉导管、鼻胃管、肺动脉导管、气管插管等）的状态是非常重要的。十多年来，科学论文已经表明常规每日 CXR 检查会增加医疗费用，不会改变临床实践，不再被推荐[2]。除此之外，在当代重症医学临床实践中许多以往进行每日 CXR 的理由不复存在。例如，现代呼吸机密切监测呼吸力学（平台压、顺应性和阻力），而无创传感器可以监测 CO_2 和氧合水平以指导临床管理。更重要的是，即时肺部超声已得到广泛应用，并可能在某些急性肺部疾病（如气胸）的诊断方面比 CXR 有更好的表现[3]。但比较常规和按需 CRX 的研究显示，这些研究中 CXR 的减少是由于上午系统性 CXR 的减少，在非计划性 CXR 方面没有差异[4]。这并不意味着 CXR 没有价值，而意味着应该避免常规 CXR，因为其附加值低。我们期望在疾病的哪个阶段通过影像技术得到什么信息？在 ICU 申请进行肺部影像检查之前，应该提出这些问题。我们将试着对这些情况做一个概述。

J.-M. Constantin (✉) · E. Baron · B. L. Nguyen
Sorbonne University, GRC29, AP-HP, DMU DREAM and Department of Anesthesiology and Critical Care, Pitie-Salpetriere Hospital, Paris, France
e-mail: jean-michel.constantin@aphp.fr

© The Author(s), under exclusive license to Springer Nature Switzerland AG 2022
G. Bellani (ed.), *Mechanical Ventilation from Pathophysiology to Clinical Evidence*, https://doi.org/10.1007/978-3-030-93401-9_36

36.2 我们能从 ICU 里的胸片检查中得到什么

36.2.1 肺水肿评估

肺水肿是 ICU 住院的一个常见原因,也是 ICU 住院期间的一个常见并发症。根据其病理生理特征可以将肺水肿分为两种类型:一种是充血性心力衰竭或液体过负荷引起的静水压性水肿,另一种是会引起急性呼吸窘迫综合征(acute respiratory distress syndrome,ARDS)的渗透性水肿。充血性心力衰竭的典型表现包括血管蒂的增宽和支气管周围血管充血,血管结构扩大和模糊不清,小叶间隔增厚(Kerley B 线)并进展为所谓的"蝙蝠翼状"肺泡水肿伴双肺门实变。此外,充血性心力衰竭的典型表现还包括心脏扩大和双侧胸腔积液[5]。各种肺部和肺部以外的疾病可能导致毛细血管壁的渗透性增加,从而导致非心源性肺水肿。从放射学角度看,区分静水压性和渗透性肺水肿往往是一个挑战。临床表现、心脏超声检查、阴影的分布及疾病进程是缩小鉴别诊断范围及区分心源性肺水肿与肺炎或 ARDS 的重要因素。此外,间质性肺炎或肺出血可表现出与间质性肺水肿难以区分的影像学表现,在这些情况下,只有 CT 才能诊断。

CXR 在评估 ARDS 的肺水肿程度和与时间或治疗干预相关的肺水肿变化方面可能更有意义。肺水肿影像评估(radiographic assessment of lung edema,RALE)评分被认为是评估 ARDS 患者肺水肿影像学程度的无创工具(图 36.1)[6]。RALE 评分提供了一个胸片上肺泡大小和密度的半定量测量方法,与通过人类移植供体肺的重量评估肺水肿的程度有很好的相关性。在 ARDSNet FACTT 研究中,基于患者入组时的 CXR,计算出

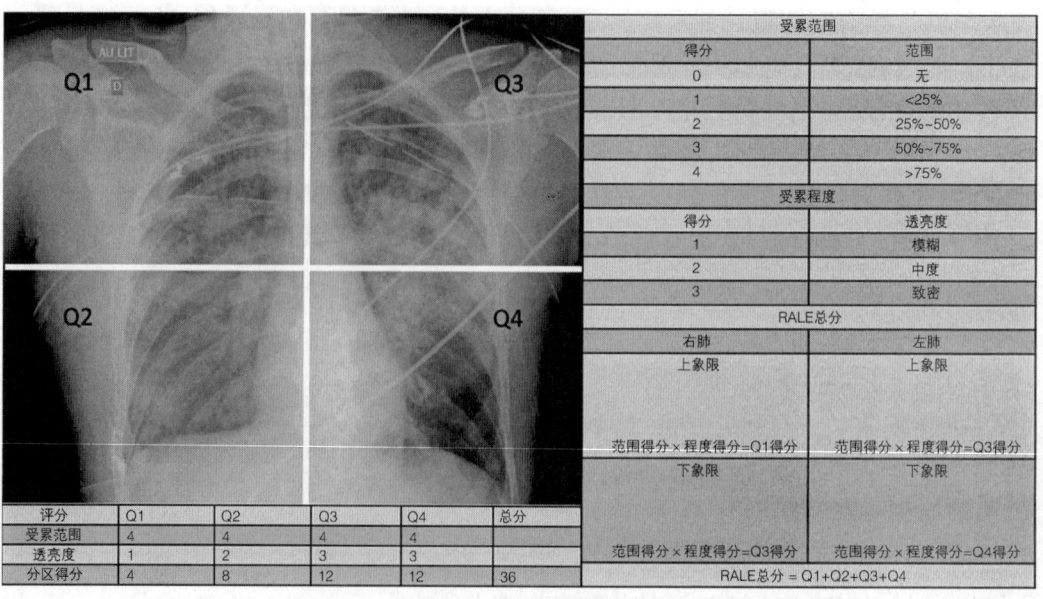

图 36.1 RALE 评分的定义和 ARDS 患者 RALE 评分的计算示例

的 RALE 评分与 ARDS 的严重程度和临床结局相关。在一项随机对照试验的回顾性分析中,ARDS 发病后第一天的 RALE 评分变化与生存率独立相关。因此,RALE 评分可能在床旁非常有用,也可作为 ARDS 临床试验中的替代终点[7]。

36.2.2　定位监测和(或)治疗设备

(1) 中心静脉导管:理想情况下,中心静脉导管的尖端应恰好在右心房上方,位于上腔静脉末端。大约 10% 的对照组出现了位移。气胸是最常见的并发症,大约 6% 的患者会发生,锁骨下入路比颈内入路中更常见[8]。尽管如此,CXR 并不是评估气胸的更准确的工具,初始正常的 CXR 并不能排除迟发性气胸的发生。如果患者在置管后数小时或数天出现呼吸恶化,应怀疑是迟发性气胸。

(2) 胸腔引流管:胸腔引流管的最佳位置取决于其适应证——是用于引流气胸还是胸腔积液,并取决于气体或液体积聚的范围和位置。胸腔引流管的侧孔应该置于胸膜腔内。即使可以使用肺部超声来评估胸腔积液量和(或)局部解剖结构,在置管后仍建议进行 CXR 检查以确定引流管的位置、评估引流的效果并排除相关的并发症[8]。胸腔引流管的移位包括导管位于叶间裂、肺实质、胸壁甚至是腹部。

(3) 鼻胃管:鼻胃管的最佳位置取决于其预期用途。如果用于喂养,其尖端应在胃腔内或胃腔远端(幽门后)以减少误吸的风险。所有的侧口(在离胃管尖端几厘米处)都应该留置在胃里以避免误吸。鼻胃管移位很罕见,但如果发生了,而在临床上没有被发现,则可能是致命的。在插入鼻胃管后,强烈建议至少在输注肠内营养之前进行 CXR 以确认导管的正确位置。鼻胃管最常见的位移包括尖端向上盘旋在口咽、食管或胃中。

(4) CXR 可用于所有其他设备,如肺动脉导管、主动脉球囊、气管导管等。必须根据患者病情和团队的专业知识仔细评估 CXR 替代超声的好处。

36.2.3　胸腔积液

胸腔积液在 ICU 机械通气的患者中非常常见(超过 60%),可以是漏出液、渗出液或血液。胸腔积液的典型影像学表现是基底混浊不透明、没有支气管充气征、膈肌轮廓消失,以及侧方肋膈角变钝。CXR 对胸腔积液的检测灵敏度低,虽然特异性好,但无法评估胸膜腔积液量。肺部超声检查是评估胸腔积液以及指导穿刺和胸腔引流更有效的工具。气胸常见于创伤患者,但也可能是医源性的,出现在穿刺插管或通气患者发生气压伤后[3]。虽然 CRX 对于诊断完全性的气胸较为明确,但如果是部分气胸和(或)前部气胸,CRX 的敏感性就会下降。肺部超声检查可能在这种情况下更敏感,但有时可能只有通过 CT 才能够确诊气胸。

36.2.4　肺炎

医院获得性肺炎是 ICU 患者的一个常见问题,特别是那些使用呼吸机和患有 ARDS 的患者[9]。肺炎的诊断通常是困难的,无论是临床上还是影像学上。肺实质的气腔阴影是肺炎的特征,但这些阴影也可能存在于肺不张、误吸、出血或肺水肿中。支持肺炎诊断的典型影像学特征是胸部非重力依赖性区出现斑片状实变区域或界限不清的阴影,通常是多灶性的且没有容积减少。支气管充气征是肺炎的典型表现,但并不特异。数日内出现阻射影的影像学变化是肺炎渗出的典型表现,与水肿不同——水肿的阴影在治疗后数小时内就会出现变化。虽然 CXR 的特异性较低,但对于这种难以确诊的疾病而言,它仍是一种有价值的诊断工具[3]。

36.3 机械通气患者何时需要 CT 检查

CT 极大地改变了人们对 ARDS 病理生理过程的理解,并更好地描述了通气丧失和实变的区域分布[10,11]。CT 既可以允许放射科医生进行可视化评估,也可以允许基于计算机的定量分析。事实上,CT 创建了一个图像,其中每个体素都被赋予了一个 CT 值,基于其衰减 X 线的能力,以−1 000~0 HU 的统一尺度将其标准化处理,分别对应于 X 线在空气和水中的衰减[12]。CT 的定量分析主要用于研究,以评估对呼气末正压(positive end expiratory pressure,PEEP)或体位改变的肺可复张性[13]。这些方法不仅耗时,而且需要特定的软件和高水平的专业知识。为了将研究工具转化为临床实践,最好能通过机器学习算法来标准化和自动化分析,如将腹部 CT 应用于肌肉减少症的评估[14]。

在临床实践中通过 CT,可以在 ARDS 早期阶段可视化评估肺部形态,此外,还可以将患者分为局灶性或非局灶性 ARDS(图 36.2)[15]。这两种表型的 ARDS 对 PEEP、肺复张手法和俯卧位的反应不同[16]。最初,"CT 评估 ARDS 研究组"建立了三种通气不足分布模式:局灶性(通气不足主要在下叶背侧部分)、弥漫性(全肺通气不足和实变,通常为双侧),以及斑片状(健康肺区域存在弥漫性 CT 衰减)[17]。然而,在过去的 10 年中,为了简化,将表现为弥漫性或斑块状通气不足的患者归类为非局灶性,因为对 PEEP 的反应和肺上皮损伤的生物标志物在这两种模式之间没有区别[18]。从生理学的角度来看,根据这些表型设置呼吸机参数是有意义的,但可能因为很难准确地根据肺部形态对患者进行分类,因此在随机对照试验中未能降低病死率[19]。这是一个支持基于自动算法进行分类,或者评估两种不同压力下两次不同 CT 中肺形态的变化,以提高医生分类准确性的论据。

在 ARDS 的病程中,CT 仍然是评估机械通气相关并发症或疾病进展的最佳工具。气胸是由气压伤、肺炎、脓胸或肺纤维化引起的。肺纤维化是 ARDS 的主要并发症,可能导致严重的后果。从呼吸力学或 CXR 的角度来看,肺炎和肺纤维化之间的鉴别诊断具有挑战性。遗憾的是,目前还缺乏有效的治疗干预措施。ARDS 相关肺纤维化的诊断金标准仍然是开放性肺活检和组织学检查,但这种手段是有创性的,而且难以反复进行;对于低氧血症的 ARDS 患者,大多数情况下是不可行的。肺纤维化时,CT 可突显肺实质条带、结构扭曲病灶、肺间隔增厚、牵拉性支气管扩张,有时可见蜂窝状改变(图 36.3)[20]。当肺部生理学的变化无法用 ARDS 的自然病程来解释时,重复进行 CT 可能是有意义的。但是每次都必须根据结果的预期相关性、患者院内转运和辐射暴露的风险来评估利益-风险的平衡。

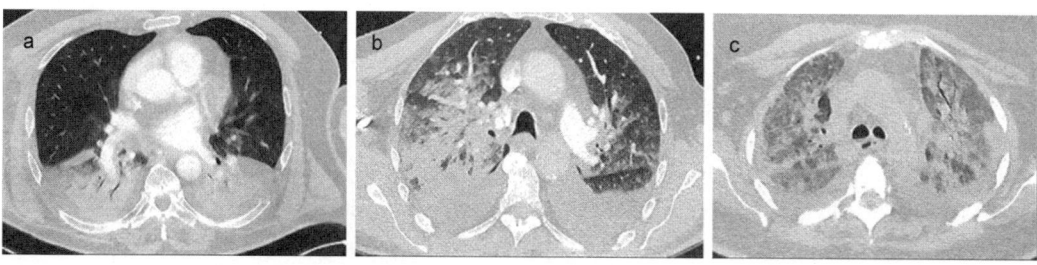

图 36.2　3 例 ARDS 患者的 CT，局灶性（a）和非局灶性（b，c），PaO_2/FiO_2 相似，为 (115 ± 3) mmHg

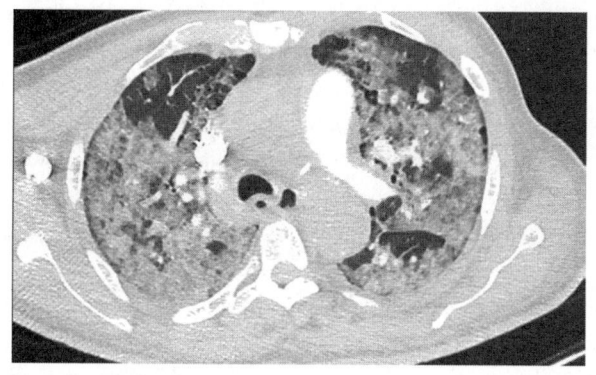

图 36.3　1 例 COVID-19 相关 ARDS 患者，静态顺应性在 2 天内恶化，CT 显示早期肺纤维化表现：小叶间隔增厚，牵拉性支气管扩张

36.4　总结

监测机械通气的 ICU 患者是 ICU 团队的日常挑战。自从肺部超声和无创技术（如 EIT）出现后，监测的模式已经发生了改变，从高成本、低收益的常规 CXR 转向有针对性的、能帮医生解决问题的按需检查。CXR 不应该被忽视，因为它对通气监测仍然是有用的。CT 仍然是评估肺部形态和机械通气患者并发症的金标准。在正确的时间进行正确的检查以支持临床的判断，保证了高效的监测，这对危重症患者的医疗质量至关重要。

（魏东坡，周芳庆　译）

参考文献

[1] Eronia N, Mauri T, Maffezzini E, et al. Bedside selection of positive end-expiratory pressure by electrical impedance tomography in hypoxemic patients: a feasibility study. Ann Intensive Care. 2017；7：1-10.

[2] Maley JH, Stevens JP. Low-value diagnostic imaging in the intensive care unit. JAMA Intern Med. 2020；180：1368-9.

[3] Lichtenstein D, Goldstein I, Mourgeon E, Cluzel P, Grenier P, Rouby J-J. Comparative diagnostic performances of auscultation, chest radiography, and lung ultrasonography in acute respiratory distress syndrome. Anesthesiology. 2004; 100: 9-15.

[4] Hejblum G, Chalumeau-Lemoine L, Ioos V, Boëlle P-Y, Salomon L, Simon T, Vibert J-F, Guidet B. Comparison of routine and on-demand prescription of chest radiographs in mechanically ventilated adults: a multicentre, cluster-randomised, two-period crossover study. Lancet. 2009; 374: 1687-93.

[5] Lohan R. Thoracic imaging, basic to advanced. 2019. p. 173-94.

[6] Warren MA, Zhao Z, Koyama T, Bastarache JA, Shaver CM, Semler MW, Rice TW, Matthay MA, Calfee CS, Ware LB. Severity scoring of lung oedema on the chest radiograph is associated with clinical outcomes in ARDS. Thorax. 2018; 73(9): 840-6.

[7] Jabaudon M, Audard J, Pereira B, et al. Early changes over time in the radiographic assessment of lung edema score are associated with survival in ARDS. Chest. 2020; 158: 2394-403.

[8] Baratella E, Marrocchio C, Bozzato AM, Roman-Pognuz E, Cova MA. Chest X-ray in intensive care unit patients: what there is to know about thoracic devices. Diagn Interv Radiol. 2021; 27: 633-8.

[9] American Thoracic Society, Infectious Diseases Society of America. Guidelines for the management of adults with hospital-acquired, ventilator-associated, and healthcare-associated pneumonia. Am J Respir Crit Care Med. 2005; 171(4): 388-416.

[10] Bellani G, Rouby J-J, Constantin J-M, Pesenti A. Looking closer at acute respiratory distress syndrome: the role of advanced imaging techniques. Curr Opin Crit Care. 2017; 23: 30-7.

[11] Constantin J. Lung imaging in patients with acute respiratory distress syndrome: from an understanding of pathophysiology to bedside monitoring. Minerva Anestesiol. 2013; 79(2): 176-84.

[12] Puybasset L, Cluzel P, Chao N, Slutsky A, Coriat P, Rouby J. A computed tomography scan assessment of regional lung volume in acute lung injury. Am J Respir Crit Care Med. 1998; 158: 1644.

[13] Malbuisson L, Muller J-C, Constantin J-M, Lu Q, Puybasset L, Rouby J-J, Group the CSAS. Computed tomography assessment of positive end-expiratory pressure-induced alveolar recruitment in patients with acute respiratory distress syndrome. Am J Resp Crit Care. 2001; 163: 1444-50.

[14] Burns JE, Yao J, Chalhoub D, Chen JJ, Summers RM. A machine learning algorithm to estimate sarcopenia on abdominal CT. Acad Radiol. 2020; 27: 311-20.

[15] Mrozek S, Jabaudon M, Jaber S, et al. Elevated plasma levels of sRAGE are associated with nonfocal CT-based lung imaging in patients with ARDS: a prospective multicenter study. Chest. 2016; 150: 998-1007.

[16] Gattinoni L, Caironi P, Cressoni M, Chiumello D, Ranieri V, Quintel M, Russo S, Patroniti N, Cornejo R, Bugedo G. Lung recruitment in patients with the acute respiratory distress syndrome. N Engl J Med. 2006; 354: 1775.

[17] Rouby J, Puybasset L, Cluzel P, Richecoeur J, Lu Q, Grenier P. Regional distribution of gas and tissue in acute respiratory distress syndrome. II. Physiological correlations and definition of an ARDS Severity Score. Intensive Care Med. 2000; 26: 1046-56.

[18] Constantin J, Jaber S, Futier E, Cayot-Constantin S, Verny-Pic M, Jung B, Bailly A, Guerin R, Bazin J. Respiratory effects of different recruitment maneuvers in acute respiratory distress syndrome. Crit Care. 2008; 12: R50.

[19] Constantin J-M, Jabaudon M, Lefrant J-Y, et al. Personalised mechanical ventilation tailored to lung morphology versus low positive end-expiratory pressure for patients with acute respiratory distress syndrome in France (the LIVE study): a multicentre, single-blind, randomised controlled trial. Lancet Resp Med. 2019; 7: 870 - 80.

[20] Hamon A, Scemama U, Bourenne J, et al. Chest CT scan and alveolar procollagen III to predict lung fibroproliferation in acute respiratory distress syndrome. Ann Intensive Care. 2019; 9: 42.

第五部分
教育资源

37 机械通气的教学：在线资源和模拟教学

Teaching Mechanical Ventilation: Online Resources and Simulation

Thomas Piraino

37.1 引言

机械通气的目的、目标可以用多种书面形式来叙述、教学。机械通气的不同模式及其操作的细节也可以被叙述。然而，要真正理解机械通气应用于患者的复杂性，如气道阻力、呼吸系统顺应性及患者努力等具体情况和条件对其的影响，最好是以可视化的方式在患者床旁或者模拟情境中进行教学。下面将提供机械通气学习和教学的资源。

37.2 在线资源和应用

以下在线资源使用不同方式进行机械通气概念的教学，但不是模拟工具，包括主要聚焦于机械通气的手机应用、博客和在线课程。

37.2.1 通气辅助的标准化课程

克利夫兰医学中心的呼吸和危重症医学激励培训项目研发了一套标准化系统，用于教授基础机械通气知识。这个项目被称作通气辅助的标准化课程（Standardized Education for Ventilatory Assistance, SEVA）。课程包含入门级课程，以及进阶的大师级课程。所有的课程都是免费的，可以从 https://mylearning.ccf.org/login/index.php 访问。

37.2.2 iVentilate 应用

iVentilates 应用由 SimVA 医疗集团开发，这个应用通过将截图、视频、病例及其他等

T. Piraino (✉)
Department of Anesthesia, Division of Critical Care, McMaster University, Hamilton, ON, Canada

© The Author(s), under exclusive license to Springer Nature Switzerland AG 2022
G. Bellani (ed.), *Mechanical Ventilation from Pathophysiology to Clinical Evidence*, https://doi.org/10.1007/978-3-030-93401-9_37

相结合的方式来帮助医学专家们提高自己对机械通气的认识。它链接了与每个主题相关的研究,还包括用于床旁评估的各种计算器。该应用可以从 AppStore、Google Play Store 中免费获得。更多的信息可以从 https://www.sim-va.com 获取。

37.2.3 多伦多机械通气卓越中心

机械通气卓越中心(Centre of Excellence in Mechanical Ventilation,CoEMV)是一个在线博客,发布与机械通气监测、识别和分类人-机不同步相关新概念的文章、访谈和述评。该博客可以免费浏览、订阅邮件更新。http://coemv.ca。

37.3 机械通气模拟教学

在机械通气教学中,最有用的工具之一是附带有病例描述的呼吸机波形截图。许多呼吸机在设计时就内置了截屏工具,可以对屏幕截图并可以导出为图片文件。截图和录像的局限在于他们仅是回顾性的案例,学习者不能自己调整参数来观察其对患者-呼吸机的交互作用及对呼吸机波形的影响。因此,模拟工具已成为机械通气深入教学的首选方法。现有多种模拟方法,价格差异巨大。简单的软件,包括应用程序、Excel 表格和网站,不需要呼吸机或者特定的设备,只需要电脑或者平板电脑就可以模拟从基础到复杂的情境进行教学。

37.3.1 软件模拟的选择

37.3.1.1 呼吸机分析模拟界面

Robert L. Chatburn、MHHS、RRT-NPS、FAARC 使用 Microsoft Excel 开发了一个高级的脚本,该脚本在教育者中广泛传播(图 37.1)。它有三种最为广泛使用的模式可供选择,分别为:容量控制(VC-CMV)、压力控制(PC-CMV)和压力支持(PC-CSV)模式,所有与通气有关的设置都可以调整,并且变化以图形形式直观地显示出来。此外,可以调整患者变量,如气道阻力、顺应性和患者努力以显示其对呼吸机波形的影响。这个模拟程序的独特之处在于患者努力可以通过努力的强度、时长甚至努力的延迟来定制,从而展示可视的不同步,如反向触发、无效努力、吸-呼切换过早和延迟。除了模拟图形外,该程序还有许多其他资源,包括公式、模式分类示例和市面上现有呼吸机模式的比较。该程序可以从此下载:https://1drv.ms/x/s!AuFakBJODC3Dgtlhw03JXi8I2dzTTA?e=6u86gP。

37.3.1.2 VentSim

VentSim 是由 Sami Safadi 博士创建的在线交互式模拟网站,该网站模拟常见通气模式下患者-呼吸机的交互作用。与上文提到的 Microsoft Excel 脚本相似,该网站用户可以通过增加或去除自主呼吸努力和改变患者的特征,如顺应性、气道阻力、患者努力(P_{mus})、中枢驱动时长和增加患者努力的延迟来演示人-机不同步的所有形式。它有一个交互式模拟模式,在这一模式中屏幕像呼吸机一样输出波形(图 37.2a)。此外,还有其他

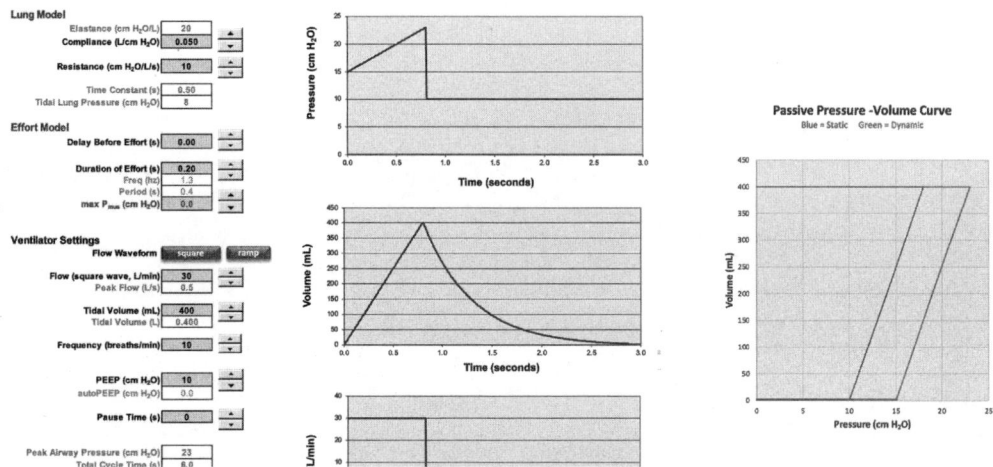

图 37.1 呼吸机分析模拟界面（SIVA）运行截图。由 Robert L. Chatburn，MHHS，RRT‐NPS，FAARC 研发

图形特征，如压力-容积环、流速-容积环和不同模式静态波形的分析，还可以同屏比较波形差异（图 37.2b）。此交互式模拟器可以模拟增加无效腔通气量后患者酸碱平衡的变化，以及随后对呼吸机呼吸频率和潮气量调整的反应。VentSim 可以免费使用，但是需要注册并且通过邮件认证。更多信息以及注册信息可以从 https://ventsim.cc 获得。

37.3.1.3 XLung

XLung 是由巴西的 Marcelo Alcantara Holand 博士设计的在线模拟软件。这个模拟器有很多模式可选择，可以完全控制包括患者特征和努力在内的所有参数。许多预设和生理参数（如无效腔及分流）都可以调整，屏幕上的血气指标会随着呼吸机参数（包括呼吸频率、潮气量和 PEEP）的调整而变化（图 37.3a）。当一个模拟案例被设置好后，这套设置可以被其他人导出使用，这使它成为教育者的重要资源。其具备完整的图形界面，通过可视化的波形展示呼吸机调整的结果（图 37.3b）。该模拟器可以免费尝试，但后续使用和访问所有功能需要订阅。该网站也提供了一些资源和信息，包括可以免费在线观看的视频讲座。https://xlung.net/en。

37.3.2 硬件模拟选项

37.3.2.1 模拟肺和呼吸模拟器

使用真实（而非虚拟）的呼吸机模拟机械通气需要应用设备来模拟患者的肺部，同时还要能控制模拟患者的呼吸模式。在某些情况下，教学或模拟中不需要评估患者的呼吸做功。由两侧被硬质塑料（模拟胸壁）包裹的可充气材料构成的模拟肺只需连接到呼吸机回路上，从而模拟被动呼气。教学时，应选择带有可调节顺应性和阻力的模拟肺，以演示呼吸力学的变化。但是如果模拟的目的是展示完整的人-机交互作用，则需要呼吸模拟设备和相应软件。IngMar Medical 是模拟肺和硬件模拟器的热门制造商。其生产了带有可

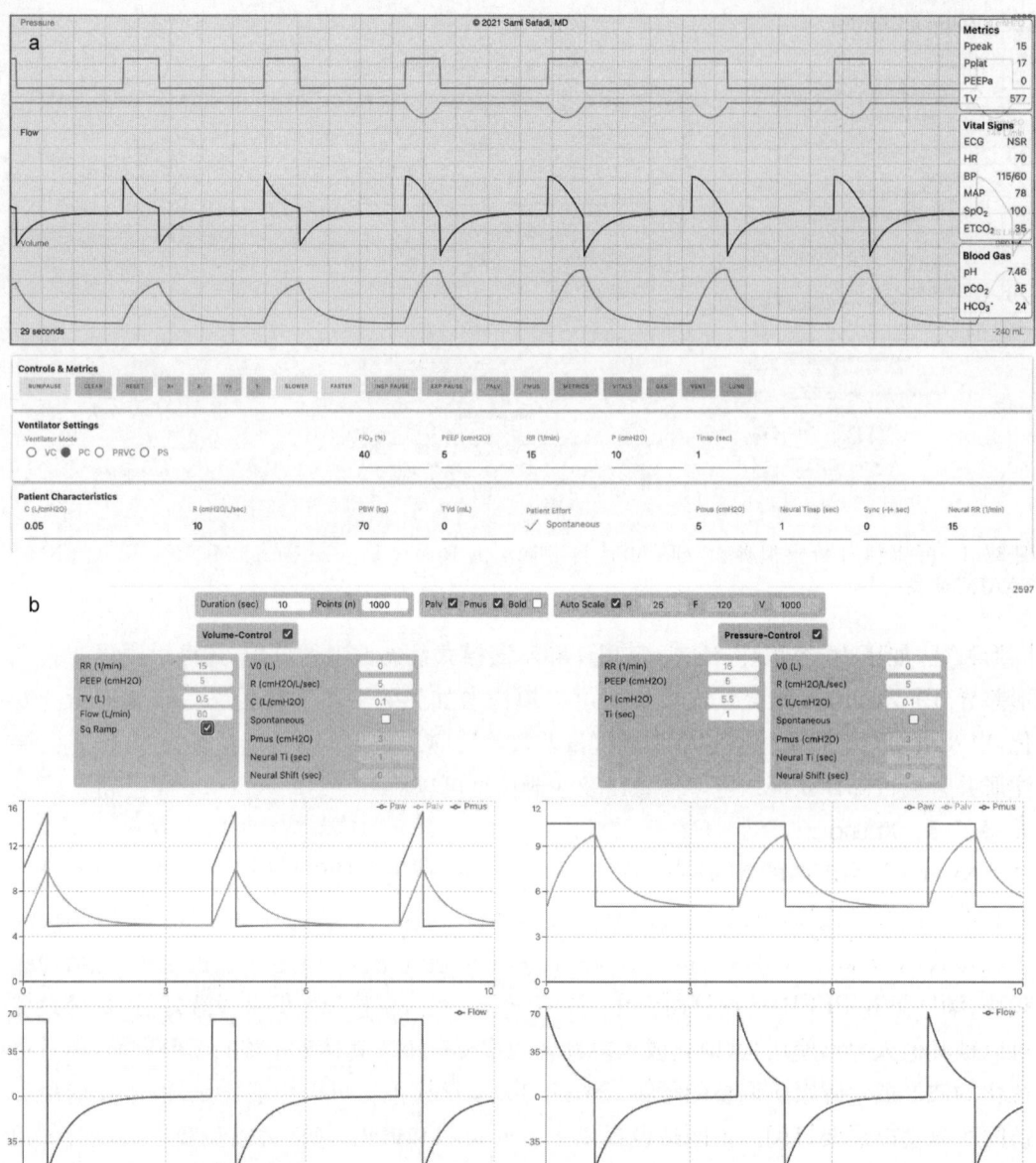

图 37.2 a. VentSim 在线软件的交互部分的截图；b. VentSim 在线软件的同屏比较截图

调阻力和顺应性的简单模拟肺，以及最常见的高级呼吸模拟器 ASL5000。ASL5000 包括运行复杂模拟会话所需的硬件和软件。可以实时创建、保存或修改临床情境。另一个热门的呼吸模拟器制造商是 neosim AG，他们也有各种人形模拟设备可用于模拟。

使用上述硬件创建在线教学资源时，需要使用视频捕捉设备来记录呼吸机屏幕的视频输出。

37.3.3 成功模拟教学活动的设置

在教学活动中加入模拟内容的首要目标，是希望参加人员能够掌握管理和应对模拟

37 机械通气的教学：在线资源和模拟教学

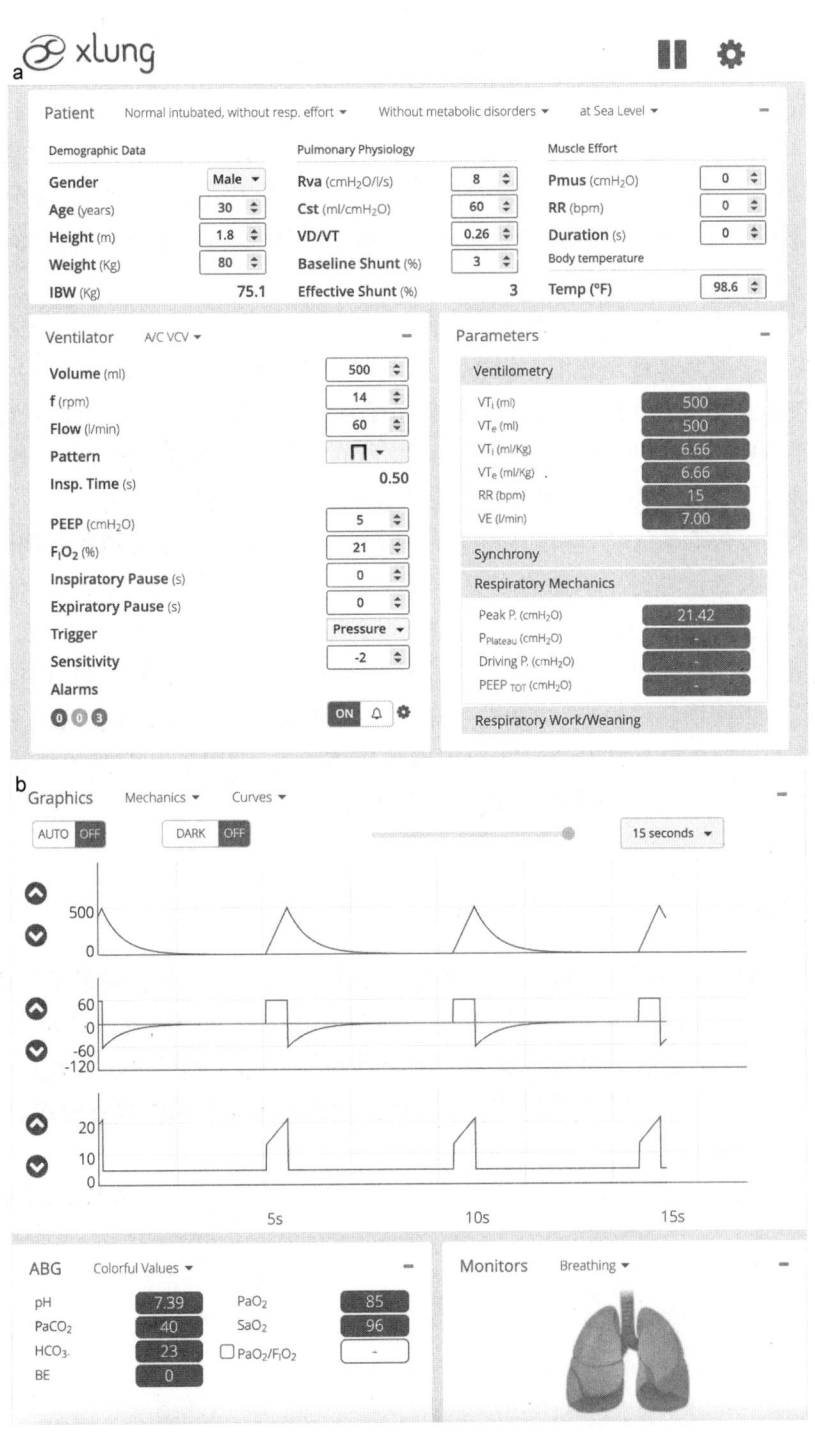

图 37.3　a. XLung 模拟软件截图，演示可调整的患者特征和呼吸机设置；b. XLung 模拟软件呼吸机波形截图

临床情境的技术或措施。这通常需要对临床案例或情境有一个大体的了解或介绍,还需要一些背景信息,以了解为什么该主题值得关注。运用模拟教学的机械通气课程或活动可以从会议讨论风格的介绍开始,按照传统结构化的方法(回答"什么""为什么""何时"等一系列问题)来进行。例如,如果一个模拟教学主题是讨论被称为无效努力的人-机不同步现象,结构化的教学方法是首先回答什么是无效努力,为什么它们对患者的临床病程很重要,何时最为常见。教学活动的模拟部分可以用一个案例情境继续进行,先介绍患者的情况(临床表现,既往病史,当前问题等),然后通过模拟让学习者亲身参与,在问题出现时进行识别和(或)纠正。

虽然实际的呼吸机并不是必须的(先前提到的其他选项可能已足够),但使用实际设备进行模拟教学通常是最理想的。设备制造商通常愿意提供设备(如呼吸机),因为这可以让新用户体验他们的产品。然而,要模拟呼吸或将其投影到大屏幕上以便所有观众都能看到,可能需要额外的资源,这些资源并不是所有设备供应商都能提供的。机械通气研究实验室通常配备呼吸模拟器,且往往能提供参与教学活动的优秀资源。

为了让学习效率最大化,应该让学生有机会来识别、解释情境模拟所呈现的结果,并根据他们所掌握的信息提出需要的改变。随后执行这些提议,观察结果,并对他们的措施提供反馈(无论是正确还是错误)。在实际操作呼吸机时,对于大型教学活动来说,从时间管理角度,学生代表执行提议更为理想。对于小型教学活动,让所有人亲自操作呼吸机是理想的方式。当使用软件模拟(计算机屏幕,而非呼吸机)时,使用键盘更改数字或在计算机屏幕上拖动鼠标指针的体验与试图模拟的临床体验并不相同,让学员操作也不会提供相同的益处,因此让所有人进行操作也不是必要的。

37.4 总结

机械通气的教学最好是通过介绍呼吸机的功能,以及可用的各种设置来完成,这大多可以通过书面形式完成。为了获得机械通气的经验并学习处理更复杂的情况和患者特征,实战经验是非常宝贵的,但很多复杂临床场景并不常见。为了教授所有人-机交互作用的内容,我们通常应用临床情境模拟,并且这已成为越来越普遍的教育形式。

(李慧敏,王伟琴 译)

38 案例教学：机械通气控制模式

Vignettes: Controlled Mechanical Ventilation

Matteo Pozzi, Giacomo Bellani, Emanuele Rezoagli

38.1 引言

在接下来的两章（"案例教学：机械通气控制模式"和"案例教学：机械通气辅助模式"）中，我们收集了 24 个临床案例，都是 ICU 医师在日常临床工作中可能面临的关于通气管理的两种主要临床情况的一些典型例子。

这两章的目的是向重症医学科医生提供直接的建议，关于：
(1) 如何在床边解读呼吸机波形的变化。
(2) 如何提供可用信息以优化机械通气，以及被动和主动通气患者的人-机交互作用。

38.2 临床案例

首先，我们展示了十个控制通气模式下的呼吸机场景，描述了如何解读和改善呼吸机设置和监测，以优化机械通气。所描述的设置包括容量控制和压力控制模式下进行控制性通气的呼吸机条件，使用的呼吸监测方法包括食管压测量和压力-容积环。此外，我们报告了可以更好理解危重症患者机械通气的新方法，如气道闭合、复张/充气和胸外压迫时床旁肺过度膨胀的检测。

临床案例 38.1 在容量控制和压力控制通气中气道驱动压和阻力的测量

驱动压是指在容量控制通气中，输送潮气量时克服肺和胸壁的弹性回缩力使其扩张的驱动力[1]。驱动压的计算方法为平台压（通过吸气阻断操作测得，如 A 和 B 中的左侧灰色区域所示）减去总呼气末正压（PEEPtot，通过呼气阻断操作测得，如图右侧的深灰色区域所示）。气道阻力等于气道峰压（P_{peak}）和平台压（P_{plat}）的差值除以吸气流量。在 B 中，尽管与 A 具有相同的气道阻力，但由于 A 中更高的吸气流速，P_{peak} 和 P_{plat} 在 A 中明显更高。

驱动压的测量在压力控制模式下同样可以进行。在 C 和 D 中，尽管驱动压相同，但 C 比 D 的气道阻力更大[2]，且吸气峰流速更大。E 可见吸气流速降为零，这意味着弹性回缩力与吸气末气道压相平衡。P_{aw}=气道压，Insp=吸气，Exp=呼气。

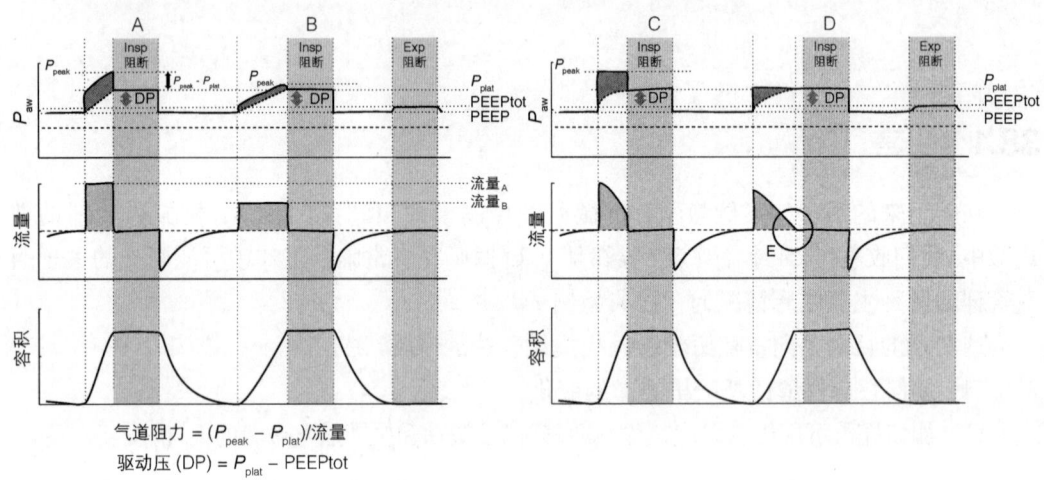

临床案例 38.2　容量控制通气时的肺牵张指数

在容量控制通气中，压力曲线随着时间推移的形状可以用公式 $P_{aw}=a\times t^b+c$ 进行拟合。指数 b 被称为肺牵张指数（stress index），可以帮助定制 ARDS 患者的肺保护性通气策略[3]。牵张指数<1 表明可能存在潮式肺复张（A）。牵张指数>1 则表示可能存在过度膨胀（C）。在该图中，PEEP 的增加可以将牵张指数从<1（A）移动到 1（B），这表示呼吸

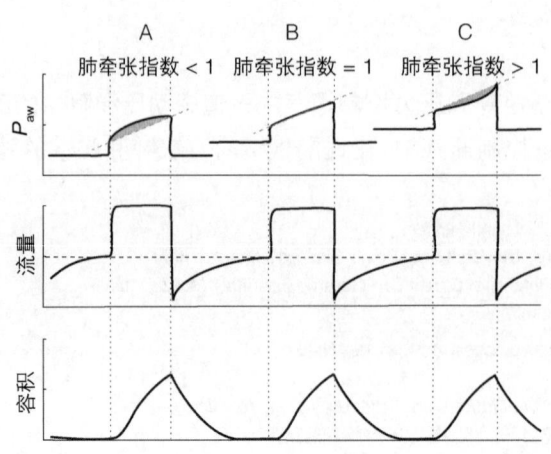

机输送的恒定气流与气道压力的增加呈线性关系。PEEP 的进一步增加可能会导致牵张指数>1(C)。一些学者提议使用牵张指数作为指导 PEEP 滴定的指标[4]。P_{aw} =气道压。

临床案例 38.3　压力控制通气：吸气时间对吸气流量波形和潮气量的影响

下图代表控制机械通气在压力控制模式时的典型波形。在 A 中，气道压增加的时间不足以使气道压(P_{aw})和肺泡压之间达到平衡。如果进行吸气阻断，气道压和肺泡压将平衡，并得出此时的平台压(P_{plat})。增加吸气时间可以使吸气流量归零(从 D 到 F)，因为气道压与肺泡压相平衡。这导致与 A 相比，B 中的潮气量增加(从 E 到 G)。在 C 中，吸气时间进一步增加，然而这并不能进一步使肺充气(H)，因为吸气流量已经达到零。与 B 一样，平台压与峰压没有差异，也不需要进行吸气阻断(如案例 38.1 中所示)。

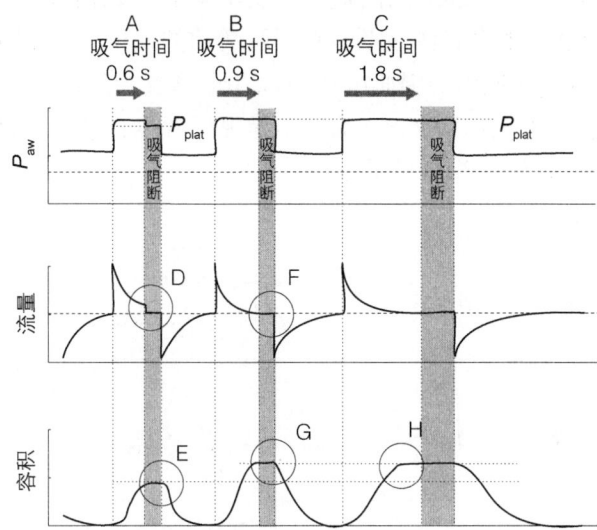

临床案例 38.4　容量辅助控制通气中的人-机不同步：流量不同步

该图展示了流量不同步。吸气流量设置低于患者的需求[即食管压(P_{es})明显下降]，因此由于呼吸机旨在保持恒定的吸气流量，吸气时气道压(P_{aw})比"被动"吸气时(虚线)低。

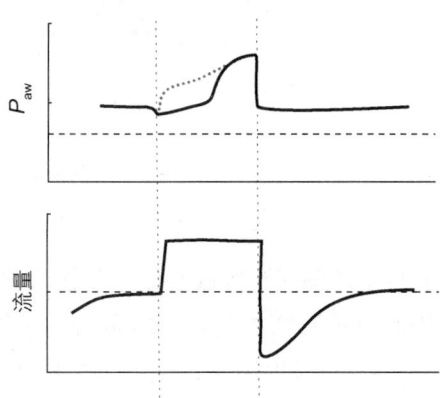

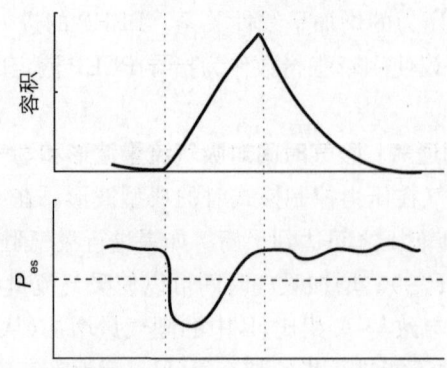

临床案例 38.5　控制通气中的人-机不同步（触发不同步）：反向触发

反向触发是控制通气中强制性呼吸引起膈肌活动的现象[5]。如图所示，患者的吸气努力[如随之发生在灰色区域内的膈肌电活动（EAdi）和食管压波动 P_{es}—B]仅在强制呼吸开始后才产生。这意味着患者的吸气动作不是由患者本身触发，而相反地由呼吸机触发，因此被称为"反向"触发。P_{aw}=气道压。

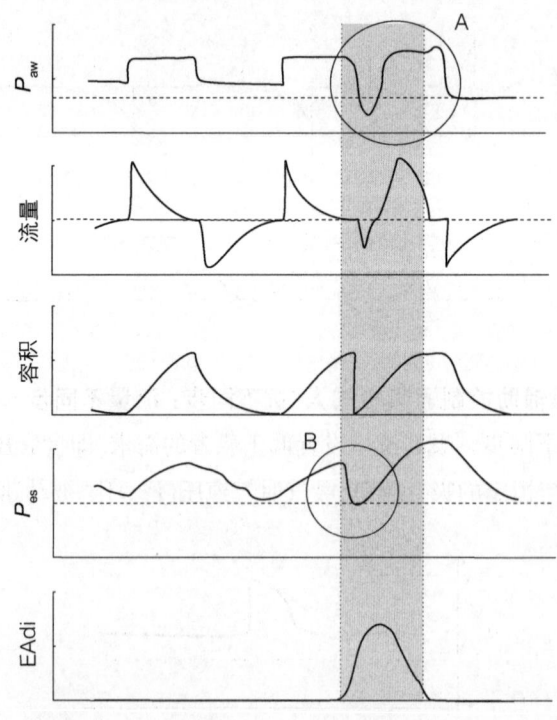

临床案例 38.6　容量控制通气中跨肺压和呼吸系统顺应性分段的测量

食管压（P_{es}）的变化与胸腔内压密切相关，因此，食管压被用作测量胸腔内压的替代指标。胸腔内压的测量是有意义的，因为它可以估算肺的膨胀压（即跨肺压，P_L）。呼吸系统压力之间的关系为：P_L＝气道压(P_{aw})＋P_{es}[6]。

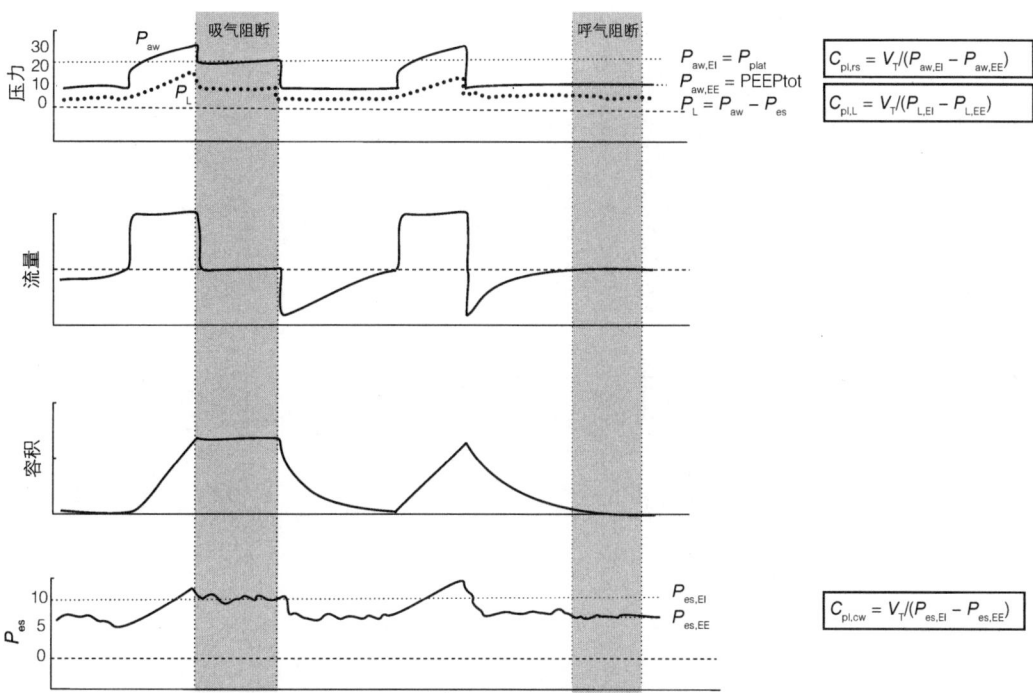

在容量控制通气中，潮气量(V_T)是设定好的，肺扩张的驱动压等于呼吸系统驱动压与胸壁驱动压的差值。

气道驱动压等于平台压和总 PEEP(PEEPtot)的差值，这两个压力值分别通过吸气末阻断(即左侧的灰色区域，$P_{aw,EI}$)和呼气末阻断(即右侧的灰色区域，$P_{aw,EE}$)测得。呼吸系统总顺应性($C_{pl,rs}$)等于潮气量与气道驱动压(即 $P_{aw,EI}-P_{aw,EE}$)的比值。

同样地，扩张胸廓的驱动压等于在吸气末阻断(即左侧的灰色区域，$P_{es,EI}$)和呼气末阻断(即右侧的灰色区域，$P_{es,EE}$)时测得的吸气末食管压和呼气末食管压的差值。胸壁顺应性($C_{pl,cw}$)等于潮气量与胸壁驱动压(即 $P_{es,EI}-P_{es,EE}$)的比值。

跨肺平台压和 PEEP 分别等于吸气末阻断时(即 $P_{L,EI}$)和呼气末阻断(即 $P_{L,EE}$)时气道压与 P_{es} 之间的差值。跨肺平台压和 PEEP 之间的差值就是跨肺驱动压(即 $P_{L,EI}-P_{L,EE}$)。肺顺应性(即跨肺顺应性，$C_{pl,L}$)为潮气量与跨肺驱动压的比值。

临床案例 38.7　容量控制机械通气中，PEEP 滴定对高胸腔内压患者的作用

高胸腔内压(如肥胖)患者[7]与瘦体型患者[8]相比，胸壁的压力-容积曲线向右移。因此，PEEP 的增加(从 A 到 B)使得呼气末气道压高于呼气末食管压。一些学者主张在 PEEP 滴定时监测食管压，以使得呼气末跨肺压大于 0 cmH_2O[7]。如果这种方法能使肺不张区域复张，那么将会得到更低的驱动压。

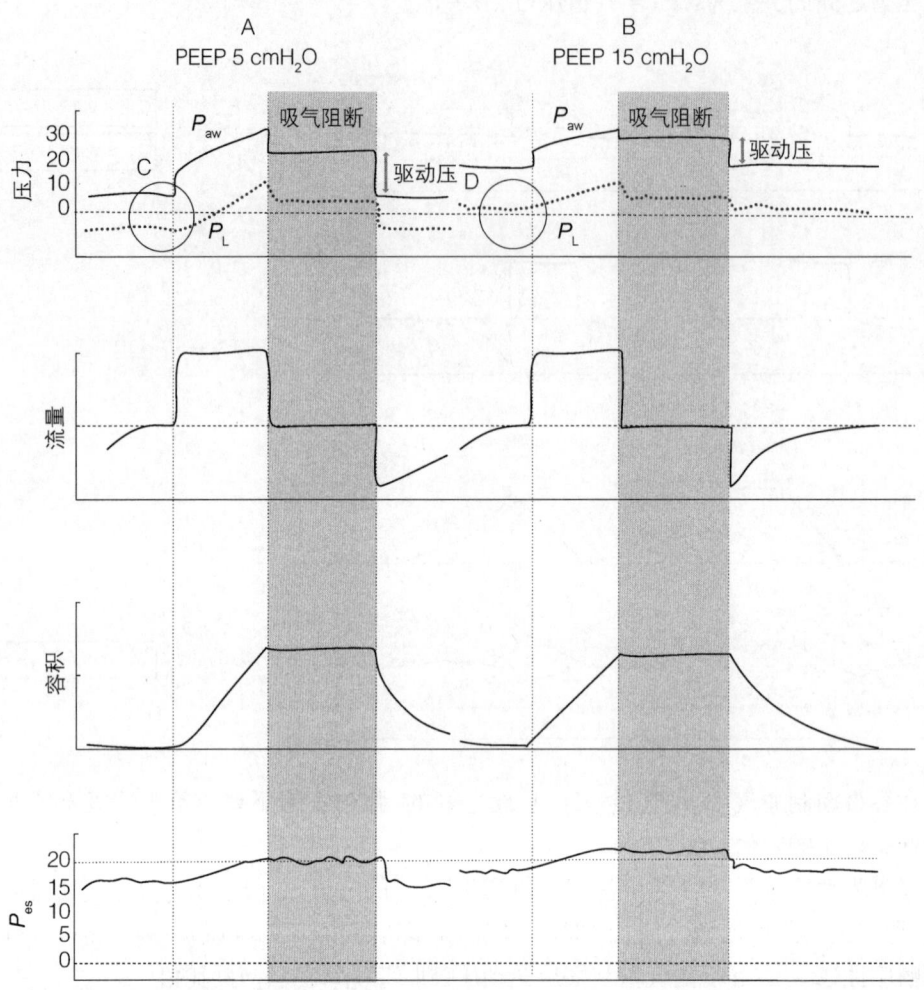

临床案例 38.8　容量控制机械通气中的气道闭合

最近在 ARDS 患者中报道了这种现象可能会干扰呼吸力学评估[9]。在容量控制通气[10]中,当没有吸气气流产生潮气量时(B)气道压力(P_{aw})可能会出现初始的大幅上升(A)。这种气道压的双斜率波形也是食管压(P_{es})的初始变化(C)的典型表现。在排除呼气阻断产生的内源性 PEEP 后,在缓慢充气的情况下气道压波形可能揭示了气道闭合的存在。具体而言,气道压曲线斜率的变化点可确定"气道开放压"(AOP),其对应于气流开始扩张肺泡的点(D)。在右下角的放大方框中,通过呼吸系统的压力-容积曲线可以确定气道闭合的存在,根据呼吸系统顺应性,AOP 为产生的肺泡通气量(即 Y 轴)随着压力水平增加(即 X 轴)而出现变化的拐点。在 E 中,与缓慢通气的起始点相比,容量增加的延迟进一步证实了气道闭合的存在。

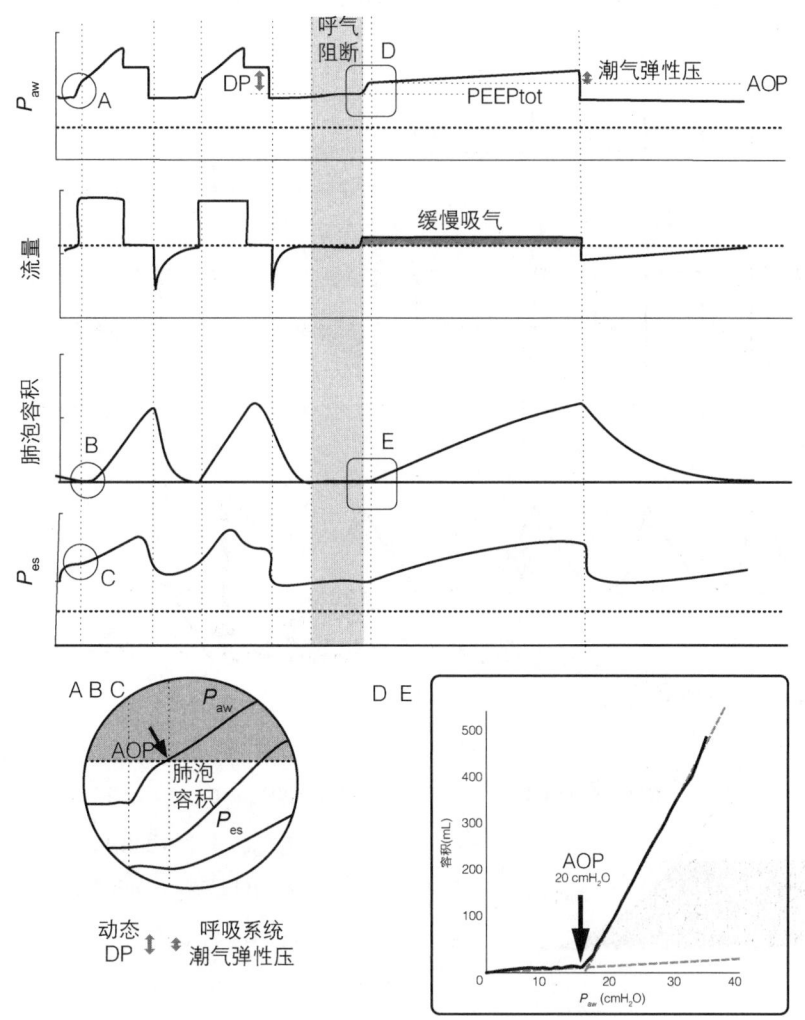

临床案例 38.9　容量控制通气中的复张/充气

ARDS 患者肺可复张的量化可能与设置 PEEP 和优化通气相关。在床旁使用单次呼吸法计算复张/充气近期被提出用于描述肺的可复张性[11]。确定采用两个水平的 PEEP [即低 PEEP($PEEP_{LOW}$)和高 PEEP($PEEP_{HIGH}$)]。首先,降低呼吸频率以避免内源性 PEEP 的存在(A)。然后,将 PEEP 从高水平突然降低至低水平(B),获得的总呼气量(V_E)由设置的潮气量(V_T)和松弛容量($V_{Relaxation}$)(C)组成。$V_{Relaxation}$ 可根据 $PEEP_{HIGH}$ 到 $PEEP_{LOW}$ 呼出时的容积得出。它由预测的呼出 V_T(predicted exhaled V_T)和因复张增加的潮气量(V_{rec})(D)组成,预测呼出 V_T 可以估算为在 $PEEP_{LOW}$ 下肺顺应性($C_{PEEP,\,LOW}$)与高 PEEP 和低 PEEP 之间的差值($PEEP_{HIGH}-PEEP_{LOW}$)的乘积。V_{rec} 根据压力变化(即 $PEEP_{HIGH}-PEEP_{LOW}$)标准化,得出复张潮气量的顺应性(C_{rec})。复张/充气(R/I)是利用 C_{rec} 与在 $PEEP_{LOW}$ 下计算出的顺应性(即 $PEEP_{LOW}$ 时呼吸系统的顺应性 $C_{PEEP,\,LOW}$)之比。在气道开放压存在的情况下，必须将气道陷闭考虑到 R/I 值的计算中。

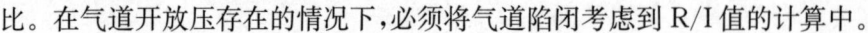

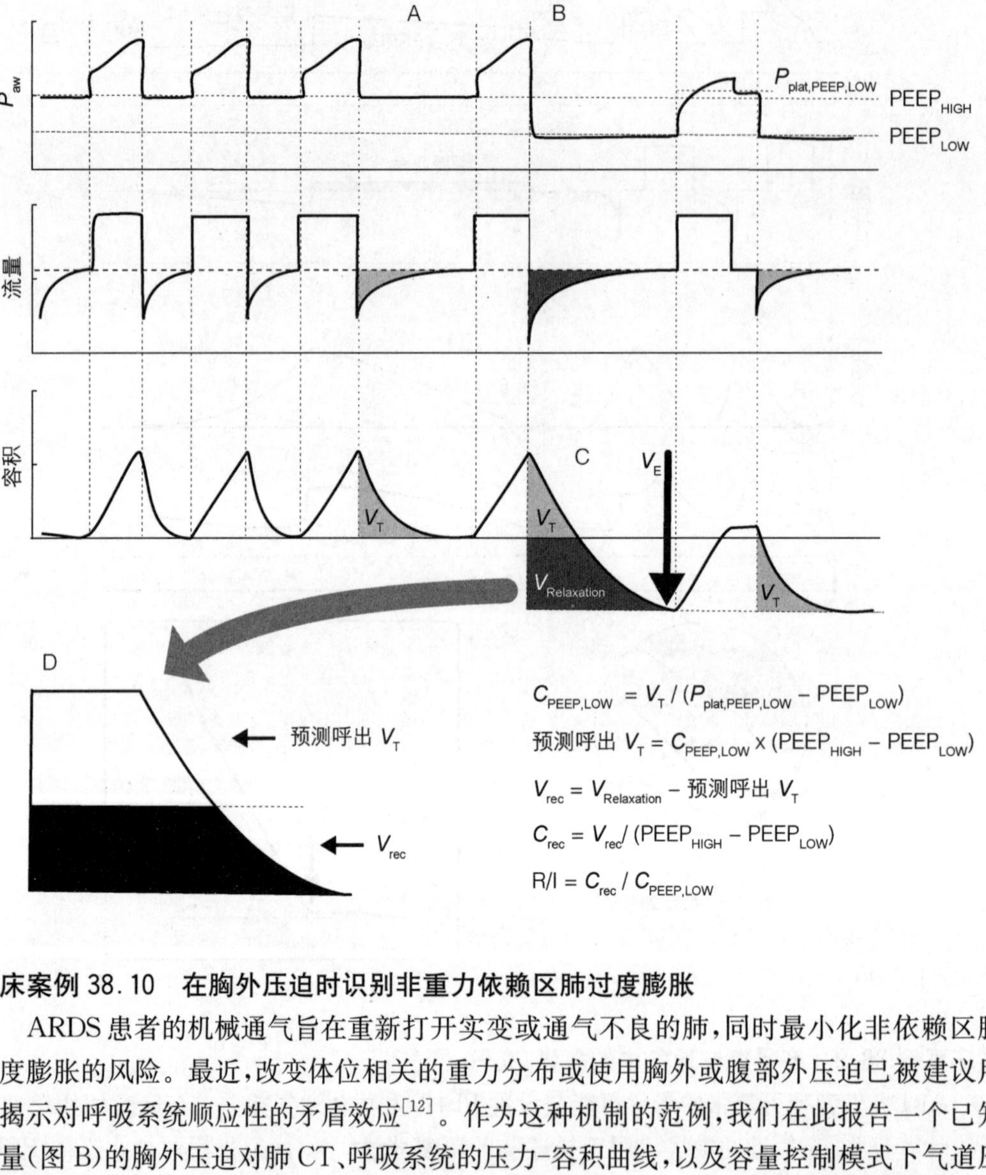
A
B
P_{aw}
$P_{plat,PEEP,LOW}$
$PEEP_{HIGH}$
$PEEP_{LOW}$
流量
容积
C
V_E
V_T
$V_{Relaxation}$
D
预测呼出 V_T
V_{rec}
$C_{PEEP,LOW} = V_T / (P_{plat,PEEP,LOW} - PEEP_{LOW})$
预测呼出 $V_T = C_{PEEP,LOW} \times (PEEP_{HIGH} - PEEP_{LOW})$
$V_{rec} = V_{Relaxation}$ − 预测呼出 V_T
$C_{rec} = V_{rec} / (PEEP_{HIGH} - PEEP_{LOW})$
$R/I = C_{rec} / C_{PEEP,LOW}$

临床案例 38.10　在胸外压迫时识别非重力依赖区肺过度膨胀

ARDS 患者的机械通气旨在重新打开实变或通气不良的肺，同时最小化非依赖区肺过度膨胀的风险。最近，改变体位相关的重力分布或使用胸外或腹部外压迫已被建议用于揭示对呼吸系统顺应性的矛盾效应[12]。作为这种机制的范例，我们在此报告一个已知重量(图 B)的胸外压迫对肺 CT、呼吸系统的压力-容积曲线，以及容量控制模式下气道压波形的作用，并将其与无胸外压迫的情况(A)进行比较。胸外压迫通过减少非依赖区肺过度膨胀，降低了呼气末肺容积。这可以通过呼吸机上平台压及相应驱动压的下降体现出来。此外，牵张指数(stress index)在给予胸外压迫之前大于 1(A)，当等于 1 时表明在呼吸机提供恒定吸气流速的情况下，压力的线性增加得到恢复。可能的机制是胸壁(CW)的压力-容积曲线右移，随之整个呼吸系统(RS)的压力-容积曲线也向右移动，使得潮式通气位于呼吸系统压力-容积曲线的较陡峭部分，从而在容量控制通气下降低驱动压。这个操作提示，当胸外压迫时出现平台压下降，可能需要降低 PEEP[13]。PEEP，呼气末正压；P_{plat}，平台压；V_T，潮气量。

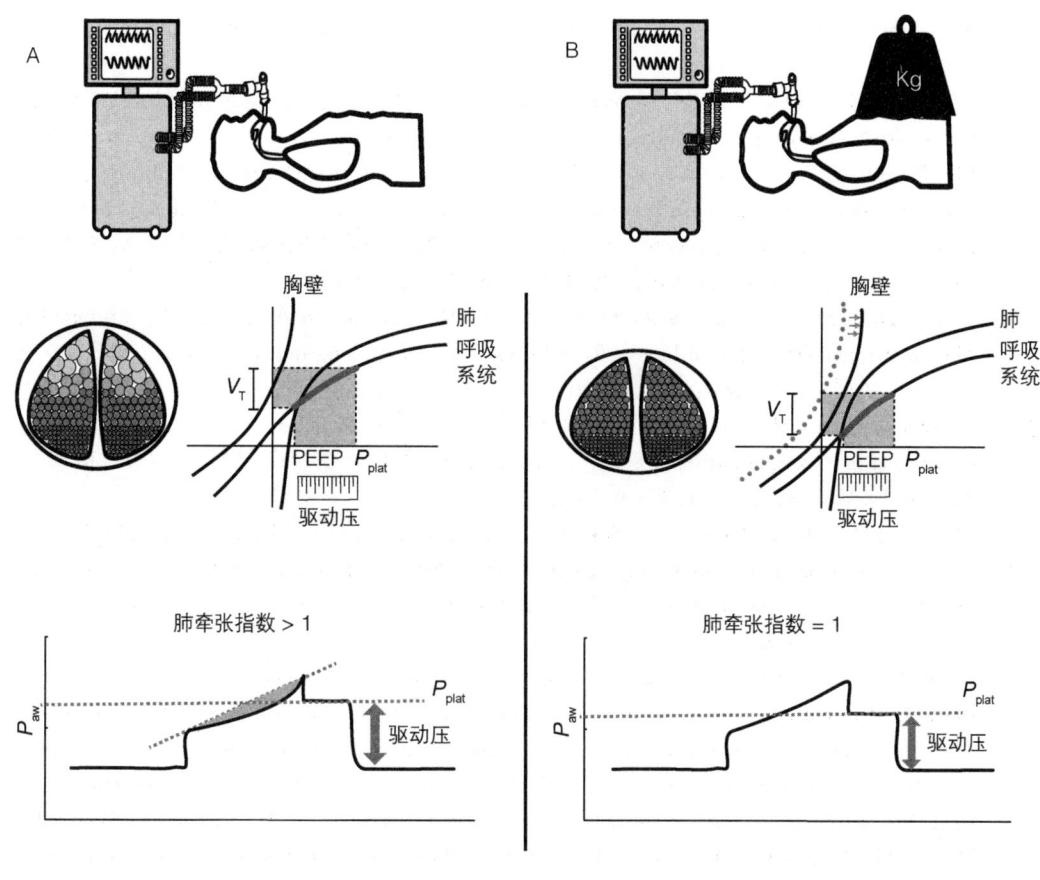

(李慧敏,王伟琴 译)

参考文献

[1] Amato MB, Meade MO, Slutsky AS, Brochard L, Costa EL, Schoenfeld DA, Stewart TE, Briel M, Talmor D, Mercat A, Richard JC, Carvalho CR, Brower RG. Driving pressure and survival in the acute respiratory distress syndrome. N Engl J Med. 2015; 372(8): 747-55. https://doi.org/10.1056/NEJMsa1410639.

[2] Hess DR. Respiratory mechanics in mechanically ventilated patients. Respir Care. 2014; 59(11): 1773-94. https://doi.org/10.4187/respcare.03410.

[3] Grasso S, Terragni P, Mascia L, Fanelli V, Quintel M, Herrmann P, Hedenstierna G, Slutsky AS, Ranieri VM. Airway pressure-time curve profile (stress index) detects tidal recruitment/hyperinflation in experimental acute lung injury. Crit Care Med. 2004; 32(4): 1018-27. https://doi.org/10.1097/01.ccm.0000120059.94009.ad.

[4] Grasso S, Stripoli T, De Michele M, Bruno F, Moschetta M, Angelelli G, Munno I, Ruggiero V, Anaclerio R, Cafarelli A, Driessen B, Fiore T. ARDSnet ventilatory protocol and alveolar hyperinflation: role of positive end-expiratory pressure. Am J Respir Crit Care Med. 2007; 176(8): 761-7. https://doi.org/10.1164/rccm.200702-193OC.

[5] Akoumianaki E, Lyazidi A, Rey N, Matamis D, Perez-Martinez N, Giraud R, Mancebo J, Brochard L, Richard JM. Mechanical ventilation-induced reverse-triggered breaths: a frequently

unrecognized form of neuromechanical coupling. Chest. 2013; 143(4): 927 – 38. https://doi.org/10.1378/chest.12-1817.

[6] Akoumianaki E, Maggiore SM, Valenza F, Bellani G, Jubran A, Loring SH, Pelosi P, Talmor D, Grasso S, Chiumello D, Guérin C, Patroniti N, Ranieri VM, Gattinoni L, Nava S, Terragni PP, Pesenti A, Tobin M, Mancebo J, Brochard L. PLUG Working Group (Acute Respiratory Failure Section of the European Society of Intensive Care Medicine). The application of esophageal pressure measurement in patients with respiratory failure. Am J Respir Crit Care Med. 2014; 189(5): 520 – 31. https://doi.org/10.1164/rccm.201312-2193CI.

[7] Talmor D, Sarge T, Malhotra A, O'Donnell CR, Ritz R, Lisbon A, Novack V, Loring SH. Mechanical ventilation guided by esophageal pressure in acute lung injury. N Engl J Med. 2008; 359(20): 2095 – 104. https://doi.org/10.1056/NEJMoa0708638.

[8] Behazin N, Jones SB, Cohen RI, Loring SH. Respiratory restriction and elevated pleural and esophageal pressures in morbid obesity. J Appl Physiol (1985). 2010; 108(1): 212 – 8. https://doi.org/10.1152/japplphysiol.91356.2008.

[9] Chen L, Del Sorbo L, Grieco DL, Shklar O, Junhasavasdikul D, Telias I, Fan E, Brochard L. Airway closure in acute respiratory distress syndrome: an underestimated and misinterpreted phenomenon. Am J Respir Crit Care Med. 2018; 197(1): 132 – 6. https://doi.org/10.1164/rccm.201702-0388LE.

[10] Grieco DL, Anzellotti GM, Russo A, Bongiovanni F, Costantini B, D'Indinosante M, Varone F, Cavallaro F, Tortorella L, Polidori L, Romanò B, Gallotta V, Dell'Anna AM, Sollazzi L, Scambia G, Conti G, Antonelli M. Airway closure during surgical pneumoperitoneum in obese patients. Anesthesiology. 2019; 131(1): 58 – 73. https://doi.org/10.1097/ALN.0000000000002662.

[11] Chen L, Del Sorbo L, Grieco DL, Junhasavasdikul D, Rittayamai N, Soliman I, Sklar MC, Rauseo M, Ferguson ND, Fan E, Richard JM, Brochard L. Potential for lung recruitment estimated by the recruitment-to-inflation ratio in acute respiratory distress syndrome. A clinical trial. Am J Respir Crit Care Med. 2020; 201(2): 178 – 87. https://doi.org/10.1164/rccm.201902-0334OC.

[12] Rezoagli E, Bastia L, Grassi A, Chieregato A, Langer T, Grasselli G, Caironi P, Pradella A, Santini A, Protti A, Fumagalli R, Foti G, Bellani G. Paradoxical effect of chest wall compression on respiratory system compliance: a multicenter case series of patients with ARDS, with multimodal assessment. Chest. 2021; 160(4): 1335 – 9. https://doi.org/10.1016/j.chest.2021.05.057.

[13] Rezoagli E, Bellani G. How I set up positive end-expiratory pressure: evidence- and physiology-based! Crit Care. 2019; 23(1): 412. https://doi.org/10.1186/s13054-019-2695-z.

39 案例教学：机械通气辅助模式

Vignettes: Assisted Mechanical Ventilation

Matteo Pozzi, Giacomo Bellani, Emanuele Rezoagli

39.1 引言

在本章中，我们将重点关注存在自主呼吸的患者在压力支持呼吸或 NAVA 模式通气期间的 14 种辅助通气情境、人-机不同步，以及包括膈肌电活动在内的多种肺部监测方法。

临床案例 39.1　患者吸气努力对吸气流量波形的作用

下图显示了吸气努力增加时流量波形的变化，如食管压（P_{es}）波形中 A 到 C。尽管食

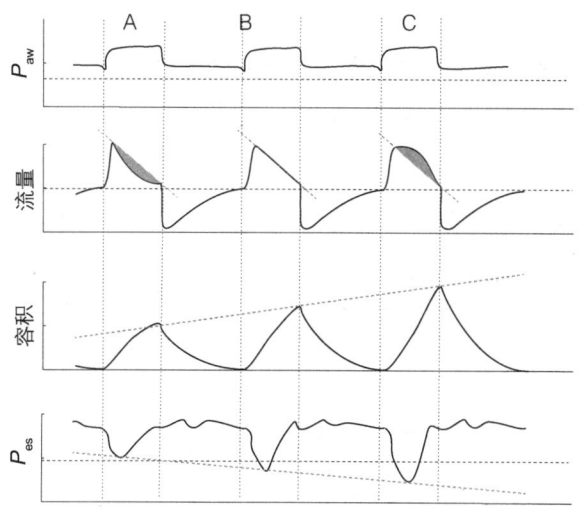

管压振幅波动增加,但气道压(P_{aw})并不会如预期发生显著变化。相反地,为了维持相同水平的气道吸气压,呼吸机会输送不同的吸气流量,从而使得流量波形的形态变得更加凸起;相应地,潮气量增加。

临床案例39.2　通过 P0.1 监测患者的吸气努力

P0.1是气道闭塞时,患者在吸气努力最初100 ms所产生的压力,可以合理地评估没有镇静及神经功能障碍气管插管患者的吸气驱动[1]。在强烈吸气努力的情况下,P0.1将更高。气道压力(P_{aw})的下降斜率越大,导致前100 ms内气道压的下降幅度越大,P0.1值更高。如果吸气努力较弱,则P0.1值将变低。如B和C所示,气道压下降得越平缓,前100 ms内气道压的降低越少,即P0.1值更低。

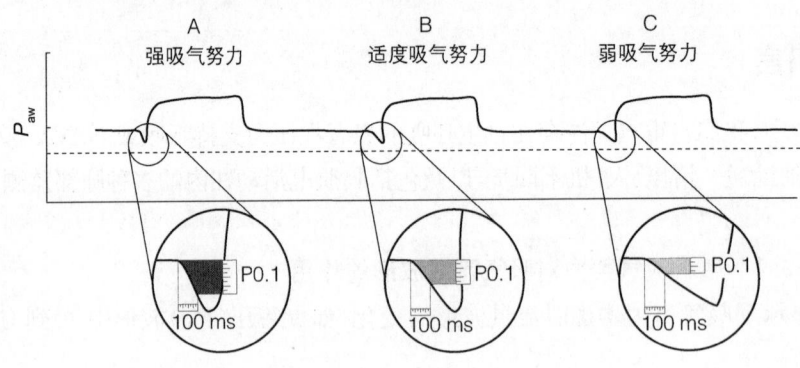

临床案例39.3　压力支持通气中平台压和驱动压的测量

下图显示了在压力支持(PS)模式下,患者吸气努力低(A)或高(B)时平台压力(P_{plat})

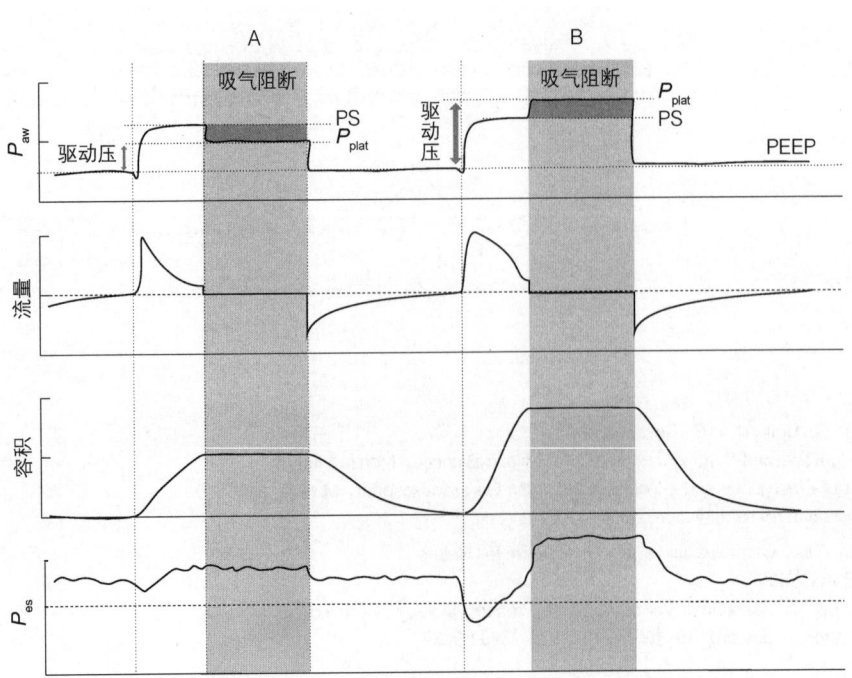

的测量。平台压是在吸气末阻断期间测量的,平台压减去总呼气末正压(PEEP)可以计算出驱动压。在 A 中,在吸气结束时的吸气努力可以忽略不计[即食管压(P_{es})振幅最小]。相反地,在 B 中,吸气努力在患者吸气相快结束时仍然存在(即 P_{es} 有明显下降),因此在气道阻断时,平台压可理解为压力支持加上吸气肌在松弛时释放的压力。两个图中驱动压(DP)的测量值均为平台压与 PEEP 之差[2]。P_{aw}=气道压。

临床案例 39.4 压力支持通气中患者努力的量化

患者的吸气努力可以在吸气末阻断或呼气阻断期间被量化[3]。在 A 中,吸气保持期间增加的压力被称为压力肌肉指数(Pressure Muscle Index,PMI),可量化吸气肌放松时的吸气努力。吸气末阻断期间的压力(左侧的灰色区域)是压力支持(pressure support,PS)通气模式中测得的平台压(P_{plat})[4]。呼气阻断期间测得的气道压变化(ΔP_{occ},右侧的灰色区域)反映了吸气肌压力(P_{mus}),可以根据以下公式计算:$P_{mus}=-3/4\times\Delta P_{occ}$[5]。与 A 相比,在 B 中我们进行吸气和呼气阻断操作来量化患者努力显示出更低的 P_{mus}。PEEP=呼气末正压。

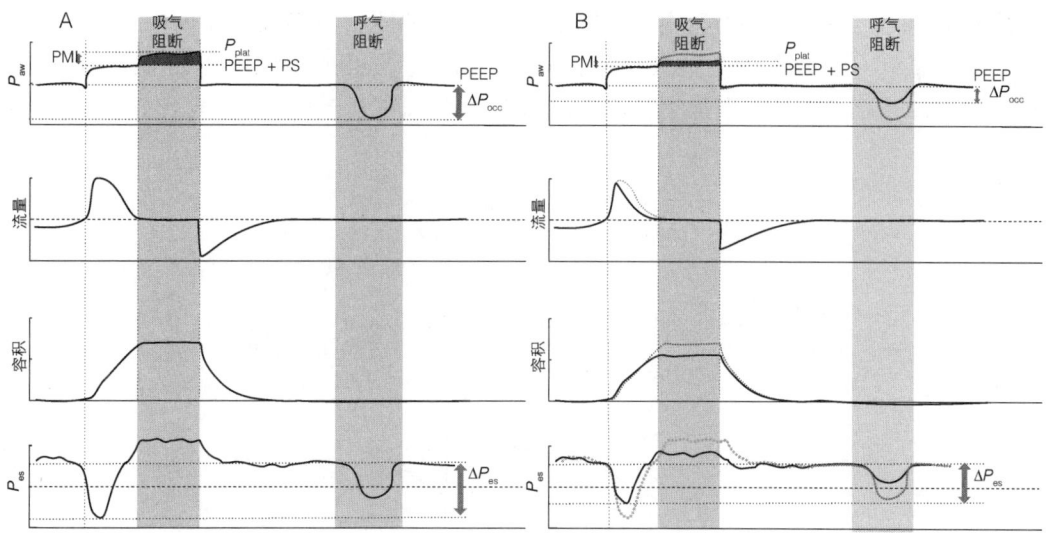

临床案例 39.5 吸气负压或最大吸气压的测量

下图展示了吸气负压(negative inspiratory force,NIF)的测量,NIF 也被称作最大吸气压(maximum inspiratory pressure,MIP)[6]。为了进行这个操作,医生必须在进行呼气阻断操作前提前告知患者需要持续约 25~30 秒。患者需要进行连续吸气努力以产生最大吸气压。在进行长时间的呼气阻断时,气道压(P_{aw})或食管压(P_{es})波形的最大振幅被视为 NIF。在尝试拔管时,推荐 NIF 值高于 30 cmH_2O。PEEP=呼气末正压。

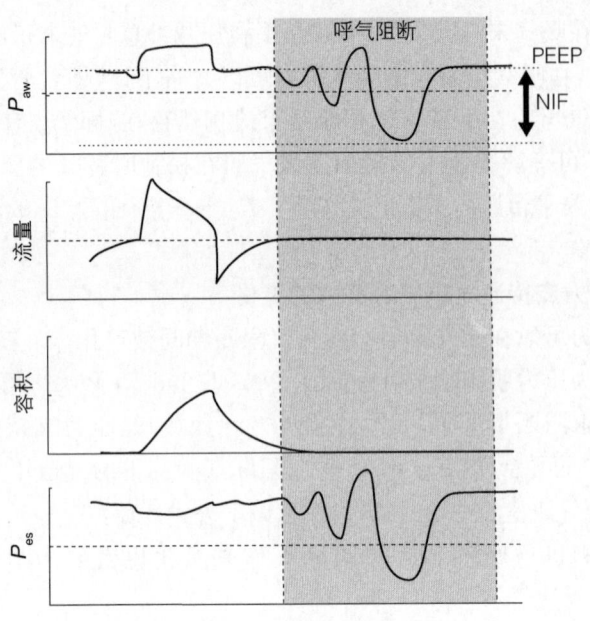

临床案例 39.6 压力支持通气中的通气不同步（触发不同步）：自动触发

下图展示了自动触发，是指患者无吸气努力的情况下，由呼吸机触发的呼吸。在这个例子中，自动触发（C）可以不需要神经信号（E）[即膈肌电活动（EAdi）]或者食管压（P_{es}）

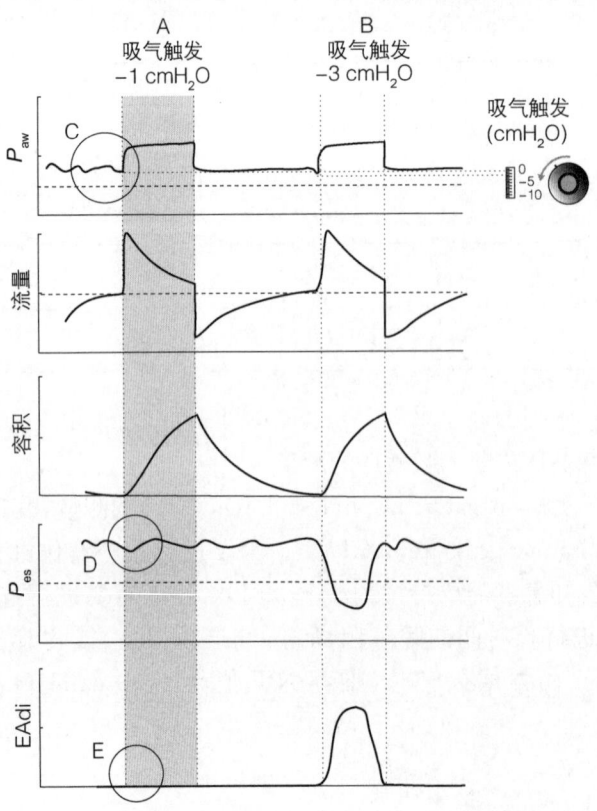

的变化(D)而触发。然而,如 A 所示,由于吸气触发过于敏感,呼吸机仍会输送气体。降低吸气触发的灵敏度可以避免呼吸机在患者没有吸气努力时输送气体(B)。P_{aw} = 气道压。

临床病例 39.7　压力支持通气中的通气不同步(触发不同步):延迟触发

下图展示了延迟触发。当吸气触发设置不恰当时,患者可能需要更大的吸气努力来让呼吸机输送吸气气流(A)。在这种情境下,膈肌电活动(EAdi, E)和食管压(P_{es}, D)开始偏移(即灰色区域),但呼吸机未输送吸气气流(C)。只有当患者的努力达到一定的压力阈值(至少 6 cmH_2O)时,吸气周期才会开始。在 B 中,吸气触发后 P_{aw} 降低 2 cmH_2O 呼吸机就开始输送吸气气流以快速响应患者的需求。P_{aw} = 气道压,EAdi = 膈肌电活动。

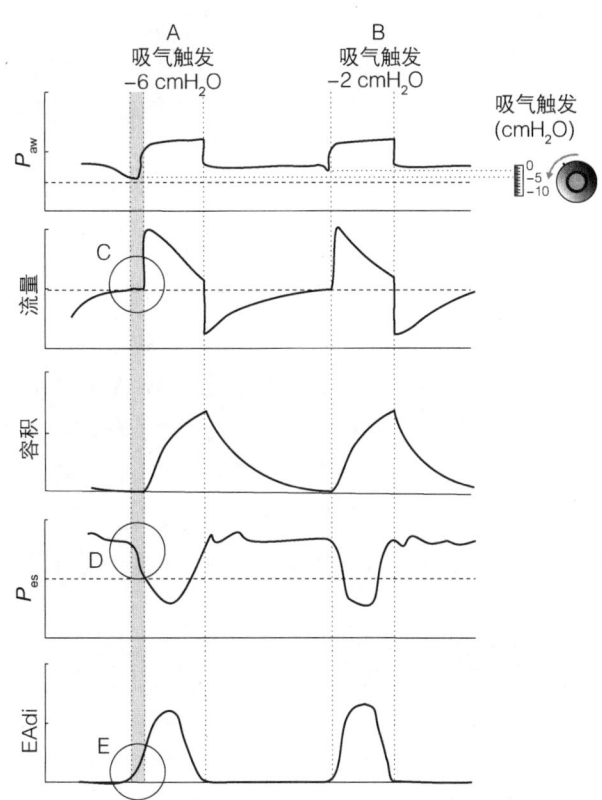

临床案例 39.8　压力支持通气中的通气不同步(触发不同步):无效触发和不达标努力

下图展示了无效和不达标努力。如果吸气努力不足以打开吸气阀(即灰色区域),呼吸机就不会输送吸气气流。这通常发生在设置的吸气触发压力太高的情况下(即 −6 cmH_2O, A)。这种不同步通常被称为无效触发。在 B 中,吸气触发设置为 −2 cmH_2O,这是患者在吸气期间很容易达到的压力,可使呼吸机输送的气体与患者需求相匹配。如果患者努力在气流量未到 0 时的呼气相开始,或者在存在动态过度充气引起的内源性呼气末正压(PEEP)时开始,即使吸气触发设置为 −2 cmH_2O,呼吸机也不能确保同时开始一个新的吸气周期。这种不同步在慢性阻塞性肺疾病的患者中很常见,他们往往在呼气相开始吸气。P_{aw}=气道压,P_{es}=食管压,EAdi=膈肌电活动。

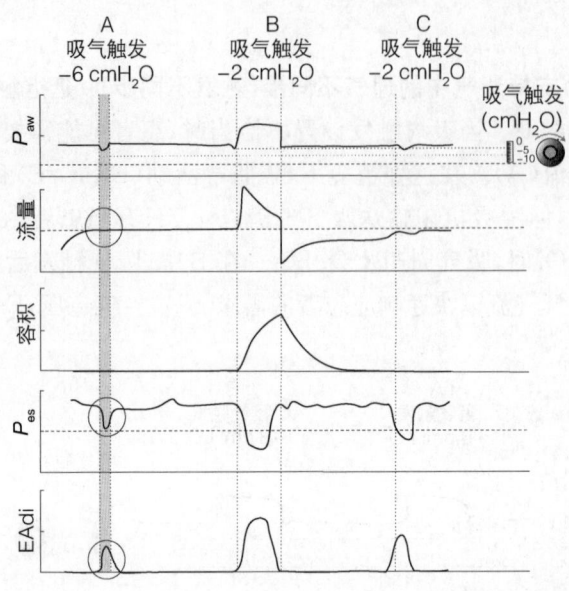

临床案例 39.9 压力支持通气中的通气不同步(终止不同步):提前切换和双重触发[7,8]

在下图 A 中,在深大的吸气努力下,提前吸-呼切换后会出现双重触发。将呼气切换设置在吸气峰流速(peak inspiratory flow,PIF)的百分比较高处,切换至呼气后患者仍然可以通过足够强的吸气努力再次触发吸气。灰色区域中食管压波形的下降表明患者仍处于呼吸周期的吸气相。在 B 中,将呼气切换降低到 PIF 的 30%。食管压(P_{es})仍在呼气开始时处于下降状态,但不足以触发吸气,只反映为呼气流速的偏移。在 C 中,将呼气触发设置在 PIF 的 10%处,提前吸-呼切换的问题随之解决。P_{aw}=气道压。

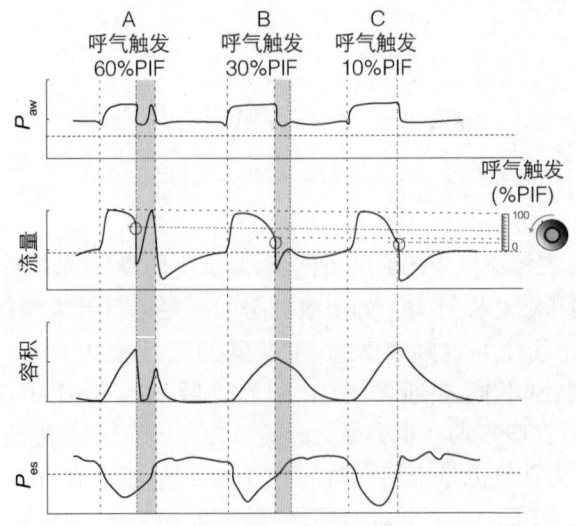

临床案例 39.10　压力支持通气中的通气不同步(终止不同步)：延迟切换

下图展示了延迟循环。将呼气切换设置在 PIF 的百分比较低时，如 A 中食管压波形中所示，此时患者已经终止吸气努力。在 B 中，呼气切换被设置在更高的 PIF 百分比上，这使得患者吸气努力的结束和呼气相的开始(即切换)同步进行。P_{aw}=气道压。

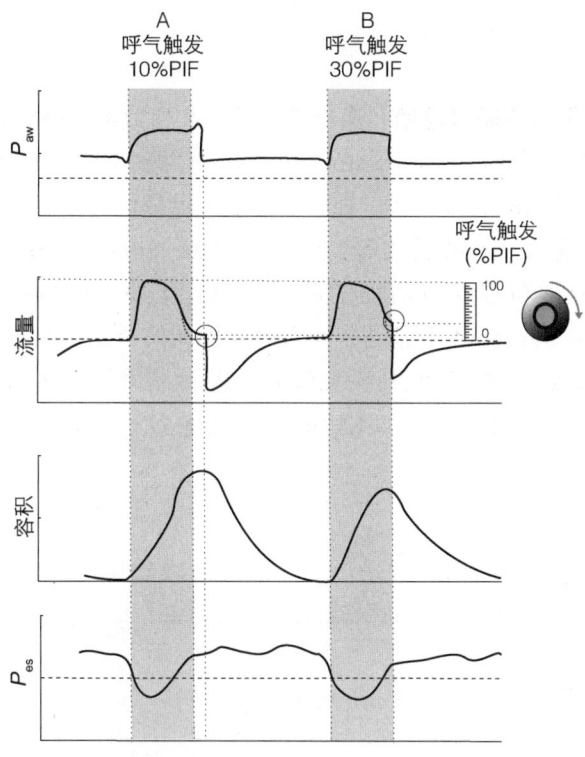

临床案例 39.11　辅助通气中内源性 PEEP 的测量

在内源性 PEEP 存在的情况下，需要付出额外的努力克服它，才能开始吸气。这可以在下图中左侧的灰色区域中看出，食管压(P_{es})或膈肌电活动(EAdi)(autoEAdi)(B)的初始下降时，没有产生吸气气流(A)。autoEAdi (AB)是在吸气相由膈肌产生的初始电活动，这部分电活动在触发吸气之前被"浪费"在对抗呼吸系统的呼气弹性阻力上[9]。P_{aw}=气道压。

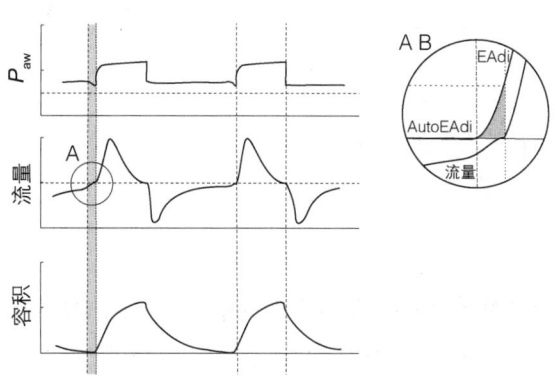

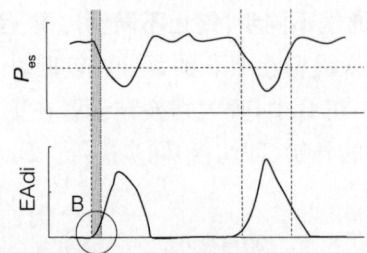

临床案例 39.12 神经调节通气辅助和通过 P_{musc}/EAdi 指数量化神经力学效率

下图展示了神经调节通气辅助（neurally adjusted ventilatory assist，NAVA），即一种基于膈肌神经触发的辅助通气模式。神经活动信号以微伏表示。下图显示三种以相同辅助水平（NAVA 增益）下不同的患者努力（即不同的膈肌电活动幅度，EAdi）为特征的不同呼吸。气道压的波形与神经电活动的波形相似。此外，可以通过 P_{musc}/EAdi 指数（Pressure P_{musc}/EAdi Index，PEI）估算出患者呼吸模式的神经力学效率。PEI 值为呼气阻塞操作时的吸气肌压，量化为气道压变化（ΔP_{aw}，A）或食管压变化（ΔP_{es}，B）和激活这些肌纤维的电活动（C）之间的耦合[10]。PEI 值越高，神经力学效率越高。P_{aw} = 气道压力，P_{es} = 食管压。

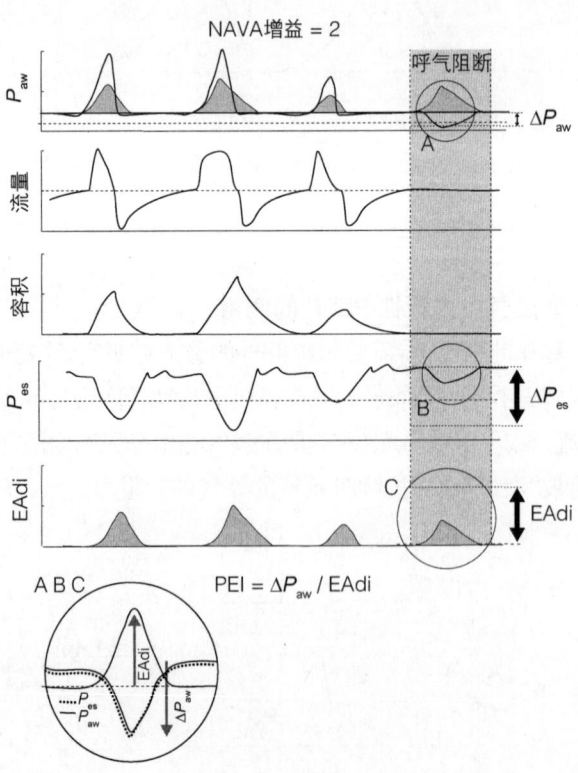

临床案例 39.13 辅助通气模式：神经调节通气辅助与压力支持通气

A 展示了 NAVA 期间气道压力（P_{aw}）、流量、潮气量和膈肌电活动（EAdi）波形。B 展示了压力支持通气期间的相应波形。在 NAVA 期间,患者根据的 EAdi 的高低接受由呼吸机产生更高或更低的压力。因此,NAVA 被认为是一种比例通气模式,因为呼吸支持的程度会根据患者的需求(即 EAdi)而变化,即吸气流量会根据 EAdi 的不同而变化(A)。相反,在压力支持通气期间,呼吸机输送的压力在每次呼吸中保持不变,即使患者的神经活动(即 EAdi)有不同变化,吸气流量也只会略微改变(B)[11]。

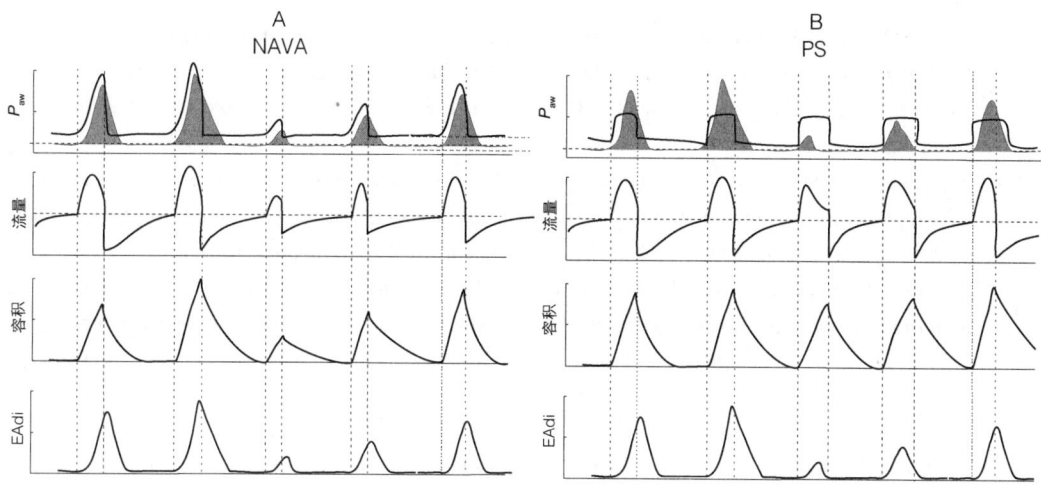

临床案例 39.14　压力支持通气中吸气努力对跨肺压的作用

下图展示了气道压、流量、潮气量和食管压(P_{es})。图像左侧描绘了气道压(P_{aw})。跨肺压(PL)通过 P_{aw} 与 P_{es} 的差值估算。灰色区域表示吸气末阻断时气道平台压和食管平台压的测量,继而获取跨肺平台压。由于患者吸气努力缓和,P_{es} 波动有限(左侧),因此平台跨肺压较低。相反,在图右侧,患者的吸气努力比之前剧烈,表现为 P_{es} 更大的下降幅

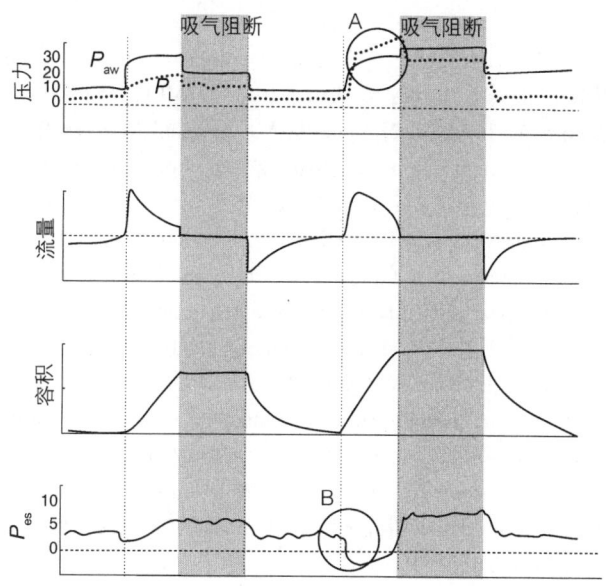

度。因此,跨肺平台压将更高,并使肺部更容易发生患者自戕性肺损伤(patient self-inflicted lung injury, P – SILI)[12]。

(李慧敏,王伟琴 译)

参考文献

[1] Alberti A, Gallo F, Fongaro A, Valenti S, Rossi A. P0.1 is a useful parameter in setting the level of pressure support ventilation. Intensive Care Med. 1995; 21: 547 – 53.

[2] Bellani G, Grassi A, Sosio S, Foti G. Plateau and driving pressure in the presence of spontaneous breathing. Intensive Care Med. 2019; 45(1): 97 – 8. https://doi.org/10.1007/s00134-018-5311-9.

[3] Teggia-Droghi M, Grassi A, Rezoagli E, Pozzi M, Foti G, Patroniti N, Bellani G. Comparison of two approaches to estimate driving pressure during assisted ventilation. Am J Respir Crit Care Med. 2020; 202(11): 1595 – 8. https://doi.org/10.1164/rccm.202004-1281LE.

[4] Foti G, Cereda M, Banfi G, Pelosi P, Fumagalli R, Pesenti A. End-inspiratory airway occlusion: a method to assess the pressure developed by inspiratory muscles in patients with acute lung injury undergoing pressure support. Am J Respir Crit Care Med. 1997; 156(4 Pt 1): 1210 – 6. https://doi.org/10.1164/ajrccm.156.4.96-02031.

[5] Bertoni M, Telias I, Urner M, Long M, Del Sorbo L, Fan E, Sinderby C, Beck J, Liu L, Qiu H, Wong J, Slutsky AS, Ferguson ND, Brochard LJ, Goligher EC. A novel non-invasive method to detect excessively high respiratory effort and dynamic transpulmonary driving pressure during mechanical ventilation. Crit Care. 2019; 23(1): 346. https://doi.org/10.1186/s13054-019-2617-0.

[6] Sclauser Pessoa IM, Franco Parreira V, Fregonezi GA, Sheel AW, Chung F, Reid WD. Reference values for maximal inspiratory pressure: a systematic review. Can Respir J. 2014; 21(1): 43 – 50. https://doi.org/10.1155/2014/982374.

[7] Pham T, Telias I, Piraino T, Yoshida T, Brochard LJ. Asynchrony consequences and management. Crit Care Clin. 2018; 34(3): 325 – 41. https://doi.org/10.1016/j.ccc.2018.03.008.

[8] Dres M, Rittayamai N, Brochard L. Monitoring patient-ventilator asynchrony. Curr Opin Crit Care. 2016; 22(3): 246 – 53. https://doi.org/10.1097/MCC.0000000000000307.

[9] Bellani G, Coppadoro A, Patroniti N, Turella M, Arrigoni Marocco S, Grasselli G, Mauri T, Pesenti A. Clinical assessment of auto-positive end-expiratory pressure by diaphragmatic electrical activity during pressure support and neurally adjusted ventilatory assist. Anesthesiology. 2014; 121(3): 563 – 71. https://doi.org/10.1097/ALN.0000000000000371.

[10] Bellani G, Mauri T, Coppadoro A, Grasselli G, Patroniti N, Spadaro S, Sala V, Foti G, Pesenti A. Estimation of patient's inspiratory effort from the electrical activity of the diaphragm. Crit Care Med. 2013; 41(6): 1483 – 91. https://doi.org/10.1097/CCM.0b013e31827caba0.

[11] Patroniti N, Bellani G, Saccavino E, Zanella A, Grasselli G, Isgrò S, Milan M, Foti G, Pesenti A. Respiratory pattern during neurally adjusted ventilatory assist in acute respiratory failure patients. Intensive Care Med. 2012; 38(2): 230 – 9. https://doi.org/10.1007/s00134-011-2433-8.

[12] Brochard L, Slutsky A, Pesenti A. Mechanical ventilation to minimize progression of lung injury in acute respiratory failure. Am J Respir Crit Care Med. 2017; 195(4): 438 – 42. https://doi.org/10.1164/rccm.201605-1081CP.

彩色插图

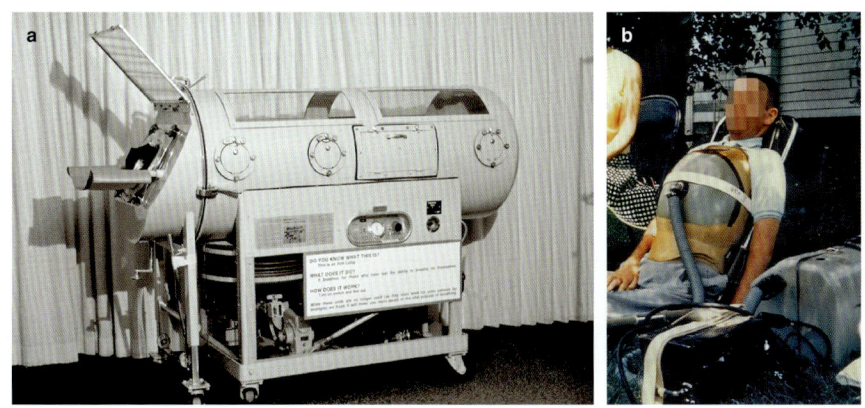

图2.2 a. 梅奥医学中心展示的一台负压通气机(铁肺)。b. 一名梅奥医学中心患者使用的便携式铁肺(龟壳)

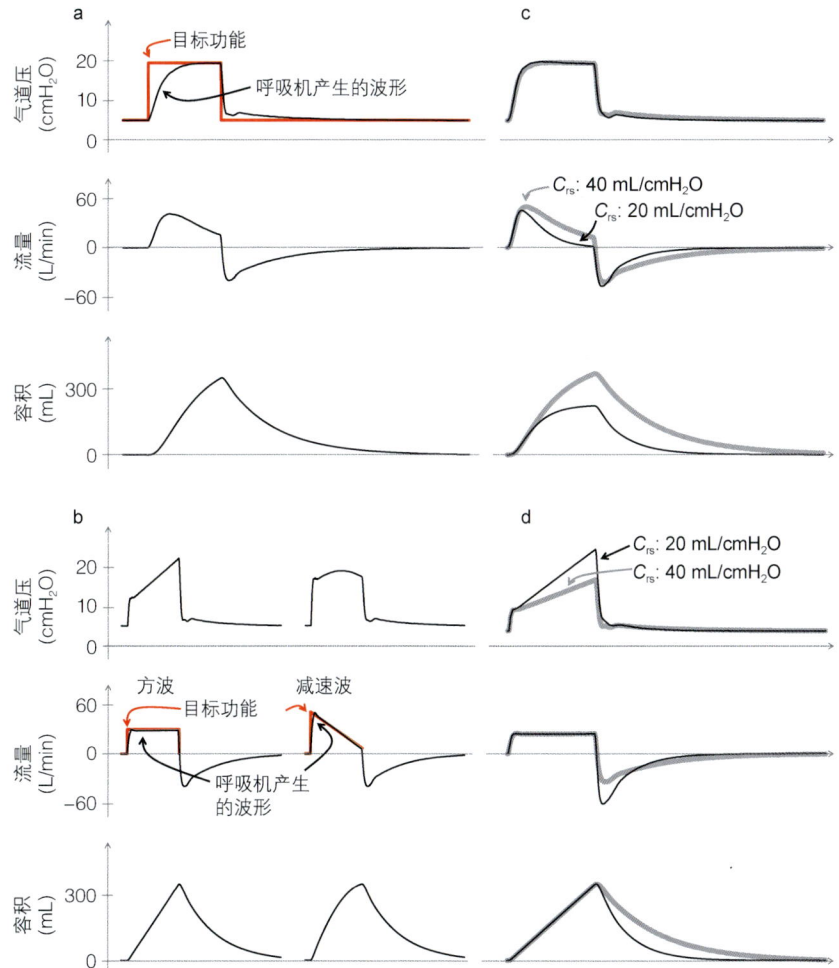

图4.1 气道压力(P_{aw})、流量和容量波形在压力控制通气模式(PCV，a)和容量控制通气模式(VCV，b)过程中的表现。红色的线代表每种模式下的目标参数。c和d分别说明了在压力控制和容量控制模式下呼吸系统顺应性(C_{rs})变化的影响。在PCV(c)中，C_{rs}的下降减少了输送的潮气量。相反，在VCV(d)中，尽管C_{rs}有变化，但潮气量是相似的；然而，P_{aw}与C_{rs}呈反向变化

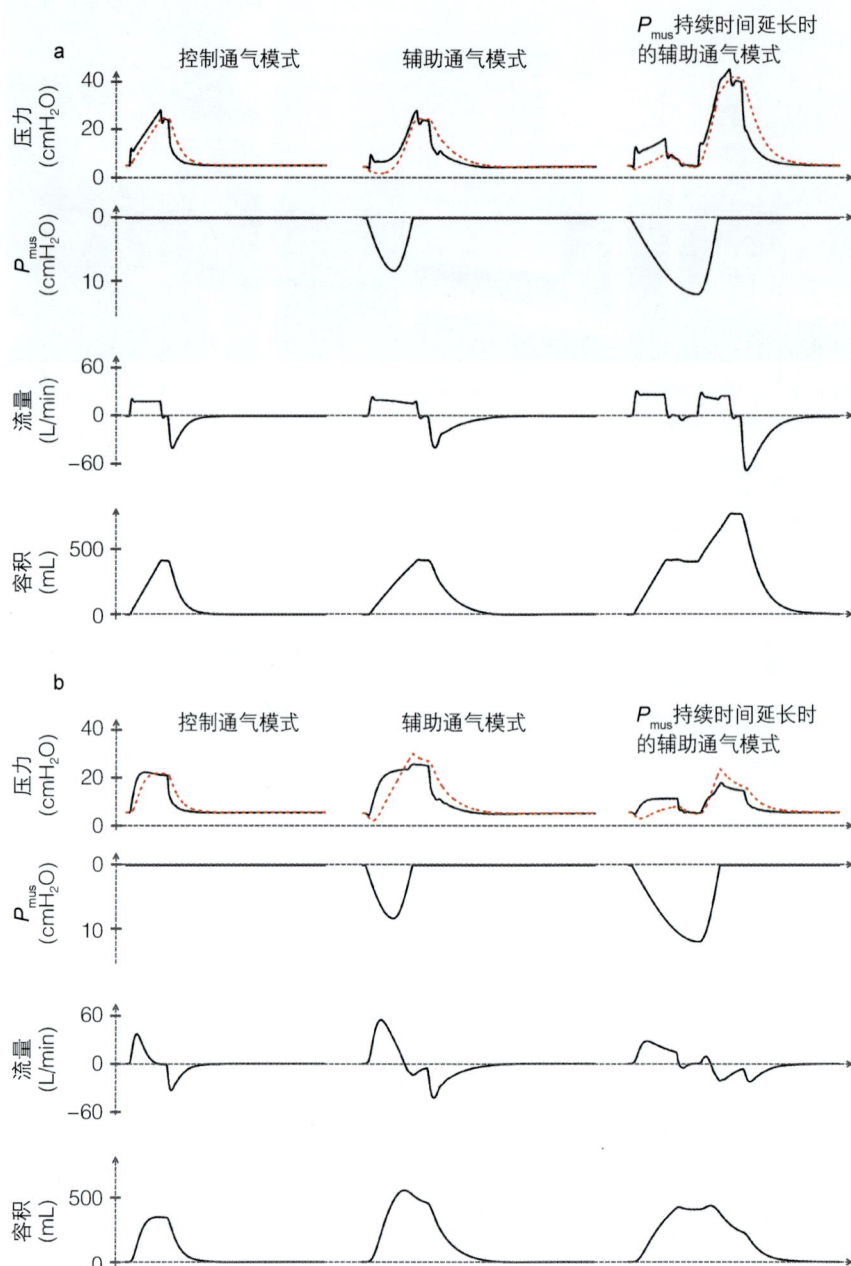

图 4.2 在辅助通气/控制通气（A/C）时使用容量控制通气模式（VCV，a）和压力控制通气模式（PCV，b）的气道压、肺泡压（红色虚线）、肌肉压力（P_{mus}）、流量和容量波形。请注意，在 VCV 中，辅助通气时气道压下降，吸气流量和容量恒定。流量受限可能导致呼吸不耐受，被定义为"流量饥饿"，增加了双重触发的风险。相反，与完全控制通气相比，辅助通气 PCV 引起吸气流量增加，同时肺泡压力升高。P_{mus} 长于设定的吸气时间可能会导致双重触发不同步（a 和 b 中右侧的图）。注意在固定的 P_{mus} 下 VCV 和 PCV 之间的"叠加"潮气量的差异；真正的潮气量是通过连续吸气周期中的流量-时间波形积分来计算的

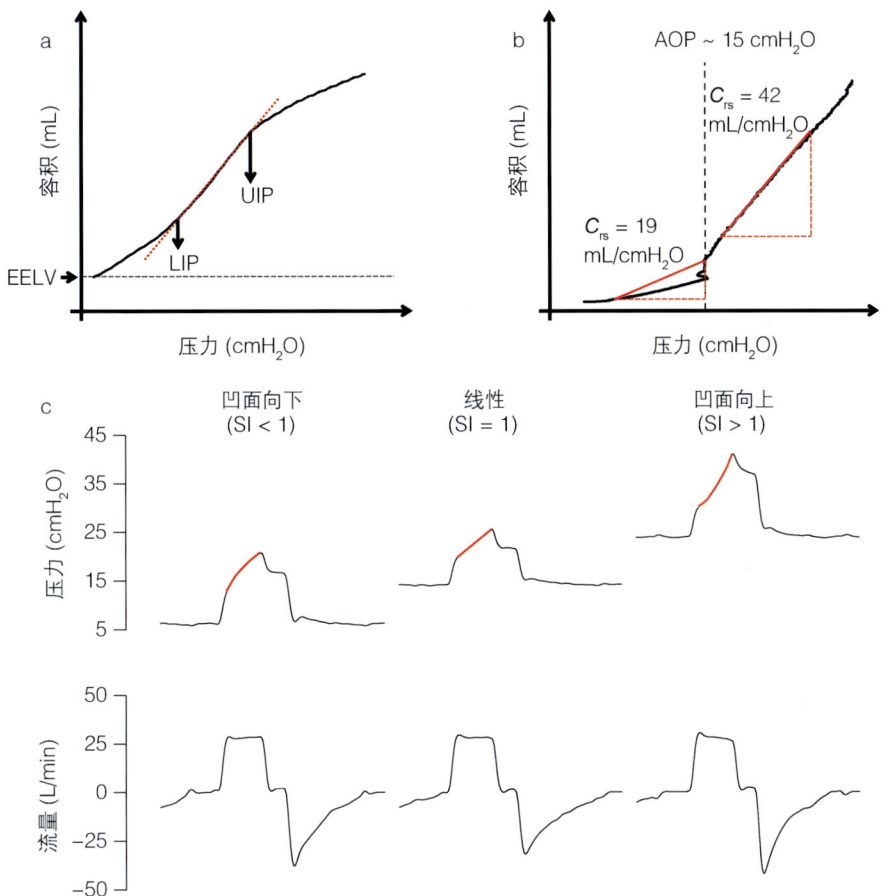

图 4.4　a. 急性呼吸窘迫综合征（ARDS）模型的压力-容积曲线。下拐点（LIP）和上拐点（UIP）定义为曲线开始偏离最大顺应线（红色虚线）的地方。b. 气道陷闭模型的低流量压力-容积曲线。注意压力-容积曲线起始段有一个极小的斜率，随后在压力达到气道开放压（AOP）（约 15 cmH$_2$O）以上后出现顺应性的突然改变。气道陷闭现象可导致呼吸系统顺应性（C_{rs}）计算错误。c. 吸气流量固定时动态压力-时间曲线示意图。左图为凹面向下（牵张指数 SI<1），表示呼吸时有塌陷的肺泡复张。中间图中压力与时间呈线性关系（SI=1），提示无肺复张或过度膨胀。右图，凹面向上（SI>1），表示呼吸时存在肺泡过度膨胀。EELV，呼气末肺容积

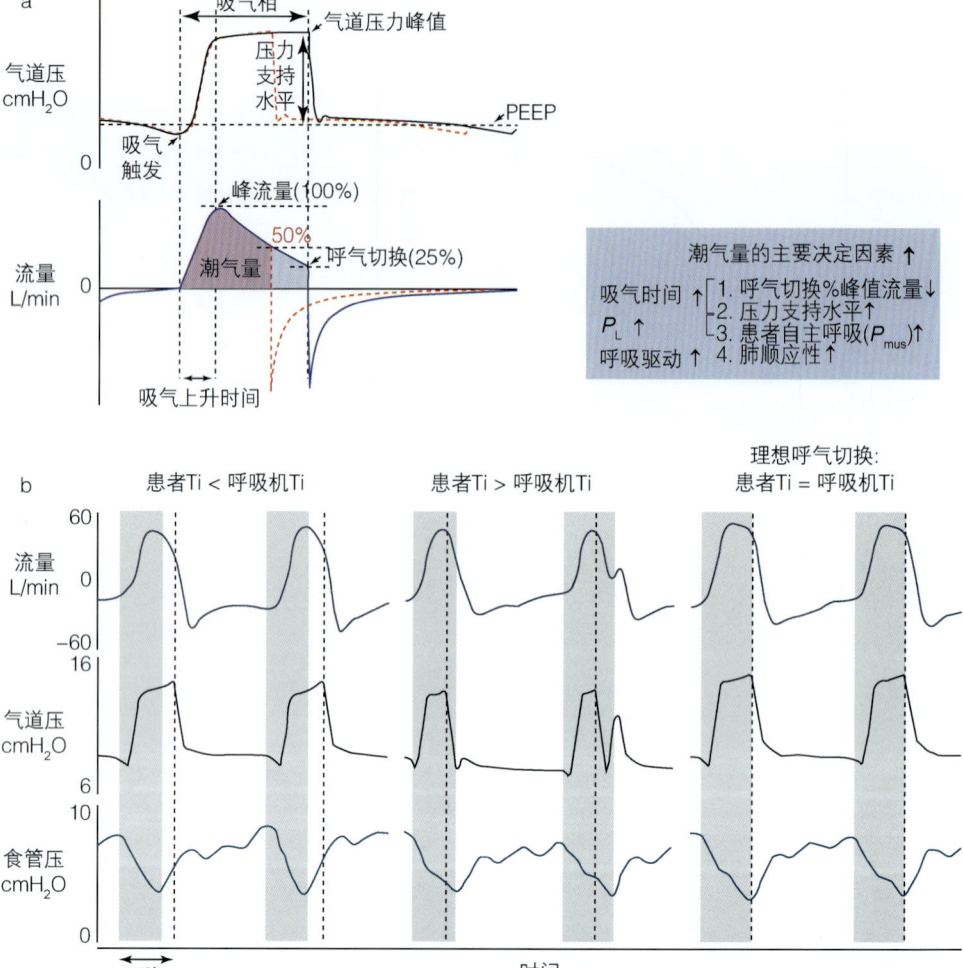

图 5.1 压力支持通气工作原理及呼吸机吸气时间与患者吸气时间的关系。a. 压力支持通气模式下基本参数包括气道压力(P_{aw})、流量(Flow),以及单纯调整呼气切换设置(比如增加%峰值流量)对潮气量的影响。压力支持水平:设置的支持压力,即每次触发由呼吸机提供的高于 PEEP 的压力。吸气上升时间:从吸气开始到吸气峰值流量(也是气道峰压)的时间。通过增加%峰值流量(红色的虚线部分)来调整呼气切换可缩短呼吸机吸气时间(Ti),从而降低潮气量。在压力支持模式中,潮气量由呼吸机设置的参数(如呼气切换及压力支持水平)及患者自身因素(如患者呼吸肌压力及呼吸系统顺应性)共同决定。压力支持水平和呼吸肌压力共同决定了跨肺驱动压(P_L),而呼气切换及压力支持水平主要决定呼吸机 Ti,还受到患者吸气努力的强度及时机的影响。b. 显示了压力支持通气模式下呼吸机 Ti 与患者 Ti 不匹配情况(左图及中间图),以及呼气切换设置匹配患者 Ti 的例子(右图)。垂直虚线:呼吸机吸气周期末的呼气切换点。灰色区域:患者 Ti,将食管压力(P_{es})的最低点定义为患者吸气结束,说明不同呼气切换设置的效果。需要注意的是,患者吸气时间的确切定义存在争议

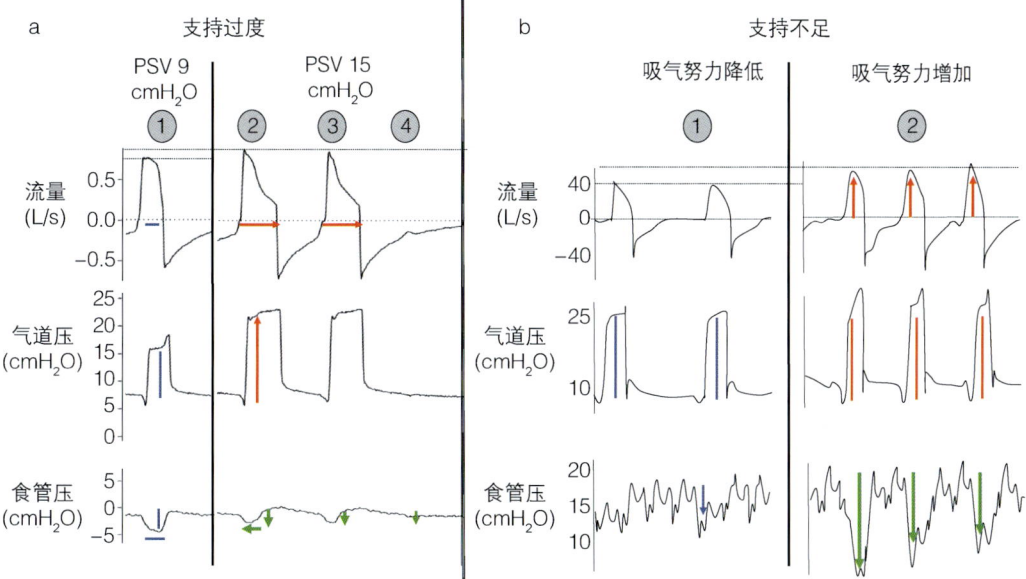

图 5.2 PSV 模式下支持过度和支持不足的机制和生理后果。a. 同一患者不同压力支持水平下流量、气道压(P_{aw})和食管压(P_{eso})波形图,左侧①中压力支持水平较低(支持压力=9 cmH$_2$O),右侧②③④中压力支持水平更高(支持压力=15 cmH$_2$O)。提高支持水平会引起吸气峰值流量、吸气时间(②中红色箭头)和潮气量(未显示)增加。增加辅助力度可以减少大多数患者的吸气力度和时间(食管压变化幅度更小、时间更短,②③中绿色箭头)。过度辅助会导致无效吸气,在呼吸机呼气相微小吸气努力(④绿色箭头)不足以触发呼吸机送气。b. 低吸气努力(左侧①)和吸气努力增加情况下(右侧②)患者的吸气峰值流量、气道压(P_{aw})和食管压(P_{eso})波形图,吸气努力增加可发生在新发感染导致代谢需求增加的情况下。在 PSV 模式下,即使患者付出更大的吸气努力,支持水平仍然保持不变。更高的吸气努力会导致食管压力的下降幅度(绿色箭头)增加,同时也会导致更高的峰值流量(红色箭头)和更高的潮气量(未显示),并在气道压曲线中(红线)表现为流量饥饿。辅助不足可能导致过高呼吸驱动持续存在,对肺和膈肌产生不利影响。PSV,压力支持通气

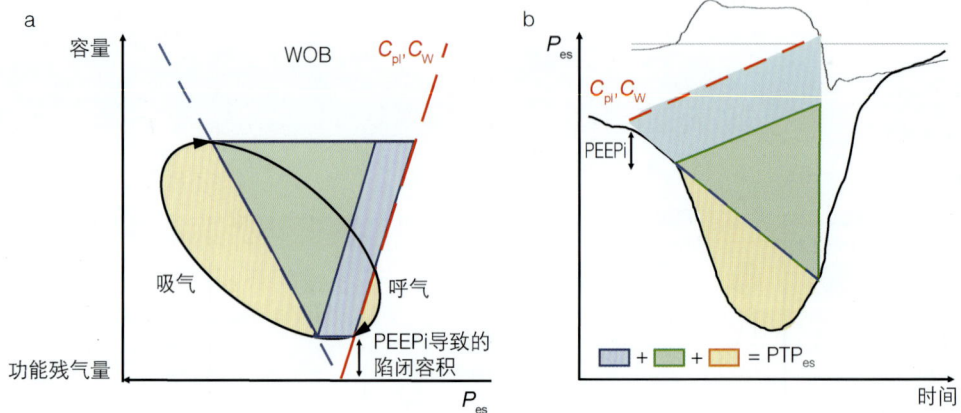

图6.1　左图展示了以食管压力和肺容积绘制的坎贝尔图。内源性PEEP(PEEPi)是指在没有吸入任何气体的情况下产生的压力。呼吸做功(WOB)是吸气肌压力(P_{mus})的积分。红色虚线表示胸壁的被动回弹力。WOB有三个组成部分：阻力(吸气阶段的黄色区域)、弹性回缩力(绿色区域)和PEEPi(蓝色区域)。呼气期的黄色小区域代表主动呼气WOB。右图示压力-时间乘积(PTP)，即P_{mus}在吸气时间内的面积。作为WOB，PTP同样由三种成分组成：阻力(黄色)，弹性回缩力(绿色)和PEEPi(蓝色)。PTP是在吸气阶段计算的，即在两个零气流点之间。流量-时间曲线显示在P_{es}上方。C_{pl}, C_W：胸壁顺应性

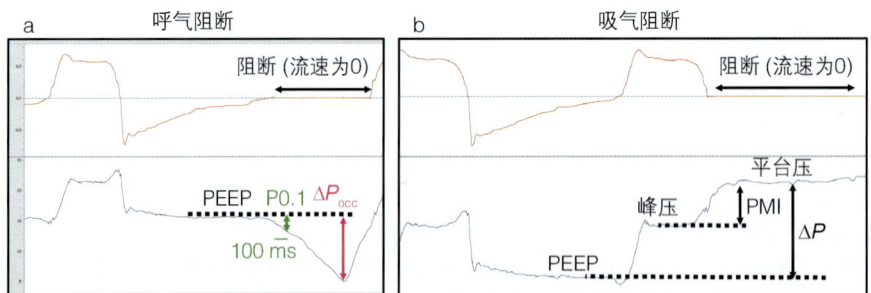

图6.2　a. 显示在压力支持通气期间进行的呼气末阻断。粉色的呼气末气道阻断压力变化(ΔP_{occ})为PEEP和气道压最低点之间的差值。绿色的P0.1是在呼气末气道阻断期间，前100 ms内所产生的压力下降。b. 显示在压力支持通气期间进行的吸气末阻断。其间气道压稳定，气流为零，因此可以得到平台压的值。来自吸气末阻断的测量值有：平台压、压力肌肉指数(PMI=平台压-气道峰压)、驱动压(ΔP)

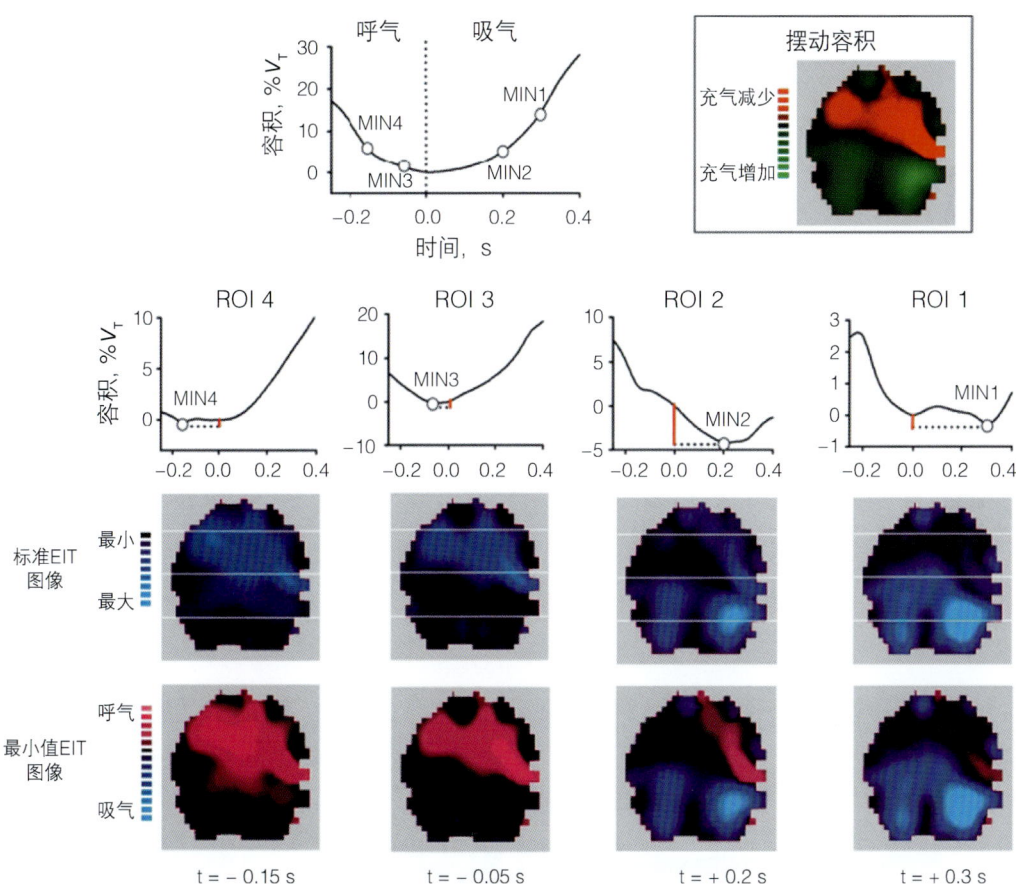

图 6.4 撤机试验中的钟摆现象：观察到不同区域之间的不同步,背侧关注区域(ROI 3 和 ROI4)在呼气时显示出最小阻抗值(局部呼气),而腹侧区域(ROI1 和 ROI2)则在吸气时显示出最小阻抗值(吸气时最容易通气)。因此,一些进入 ROI 3 和 ROI4 的气体(红色)来自 ROI 1 和 ROI2；当背侧 ROI 开始吸气,腹侧 ROI 仍在呼气时(紫色区域)。摆动的气体从腹侧向背侧肺区域移动(方框图)。ROI,感兴趣区域(获得授权转载于参考文献[46])

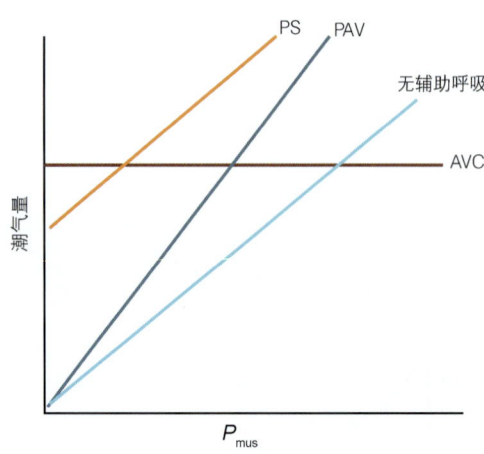

图 8.2 患者吸气努力(P_{mus})与潮气量(V_T)的关系。无辅助呼吸(浅蓝色线)、PS(橙色线)、AVC(棕色线)和 PAV+(蓝色线)。无辅助呼吸时,P_{mus} 增加将导致 V_T 呈线性增加。在 AVC 中,输送的预设 V_T 与患者的吸气努力无关,且 $P_{mus_{peak}} - V_T$ 的斜率始终为零。在 PS 中,触发后,呼吸系统会承受预先设置的压力(无论 $P_{mus_{peak}}$ 是多少),从而导致相较于无辅助的 $P_{mus} - V_T$ 曲线平行上移。而在 PAV+ 情况下,V_T 与 P_{mus} 呈正比,因为当改变辅助百分比时,$P_{mus} - V_T$ 关系的斜率也会随之改变。在 PS 和 AVC(而非 PAV+)中,即便在 $P_{mus_{peak}}$ 非常低的情况下,仍有可能产生较高的 V_T

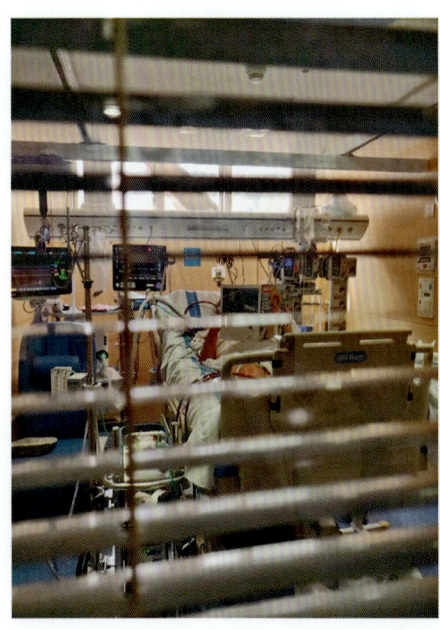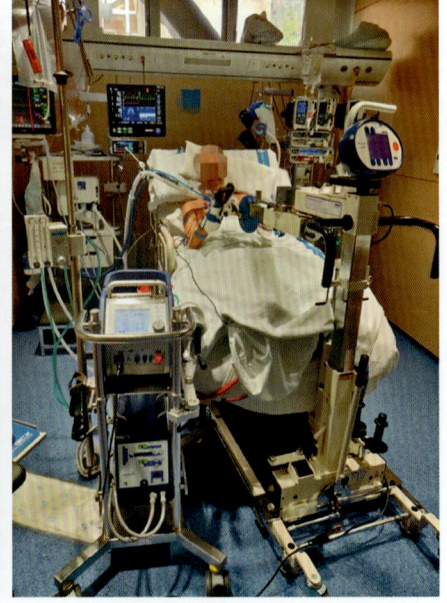

图 11.1 ECMO 支持下的康复治疗。由 Jordi Riera MD PhD 提供,并获得了患者的许可

表 11.2 基本 ECMO 流程、命名、监测，以及与 ECMO 支持可能相关的主要机械并发症；同时也包括与 V-V 体外循环支持的生理学和病理生理学相关的一些典型的情景

ECMO 流程及核查表 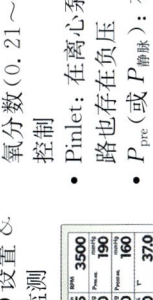	开发并实施标准化 ECMO 流程，并制定清晰定义团队角色/责任的流程/核查表，重点关注 • 插管和 ECMO 启动 • 直接灌注/组装、报警设置与监测 • 并发症预防、早期识别与故障排除 • 患者管理、床旁护理和康复 • 出凝血的管理 • 跨院内 ECMO 紧急情况下的管路更换 • ECMO 拆机 • 临床评估主要不良事件 • ECMO 项目评估	ECMO 设置 & 监测 (设置面板图: RPM 4.5 / 3500, Pvenous -50, Parterial 190, ΔP 30, SvO₂ 70 / 160, T 37.0) • 泵速 (RPM)：根据前负荷和后负荷产生 EBF，通过流量计以 LPM 读数显示 EBF • 扫气流量 (SGF) 或新鲜气体流量 (FGF)：气体流入向膜肺 (ML) 的流量，以 LPM 读数 • 设备氧分数 (FdO₂) 或扫描气中的氧分数 (FsO₂): SGF 的氧分数 (0.21~1)，由气体/氧气混合器或气体调节器控制 • Pinlet：在离心泵入口处的负压；排水插管和排水插管管路也存在负压 • P_{pre}（或 $P_{静脉}$）：在 ML 入口处的正压 • P_{post}（或 $P_{动脉}$）：在 ML 出口处的正压，$P_{post} < P_{pre}$ • ΔP：ML 入口/出口之间的压力梯度，计算为 $\Delta P = P_{pre} - P_{post}$。$\Delta P/EBF$ 表示 ML 阻力 • $S_{pre}O_2$：在 ML 入口处的氧饱和度 • $S_{post}O_2$：在 ML 出口处的氧饱和度
引流不足 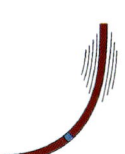	引流不足或引流失败是在血液流经至引流导管时，出现了血管内压力与导管压力的不匹配，这可能是由于过度负压引起，插管开孔部分堵塞，暂时性血流阻塞，出现了血流量与 ECMO 流量的不匹配，从而出现 ECMO 导管的振动或摆动（"抖管"） 鉴别诊断 • 绝对/相对低血容量状态 • 增加的 IBP 或 CVP（张力性气胸、心包填塞、AIH） • 咳嗽、人-机对抗和躁动 • ECMO 导管的阻塞	气体可能进入 ECMO 循环，产生微小气泡甚至导致离心泵失压的大规模气体栓塞，进而形成"气锁"。如果在循环的负压侧发生任何断开或通过中心静脉导管的开放端口，大气中的空气可能被吸入。此外，如果血液暴露于过度负压下，还可能产生气泡

续表

再循环	高度氧合的血液从回流管返回至机体[在ECMO中被称为再循环分数（RF）=再循环血流（RBF）/体外血流（EBF）]，RF升高不利于气体交换，导致体外循环的效率降低。如果转泵速度增加并且管道之间的距离减少，可使RF增高，引流导管中的血液颜色（富氧血的颜色）与回流导管中的血液颜色（较红血液的颜色）看起来很相似	
回流受阻	由于出口端对离心泵的阻碍而导致血液回流阻力增加。阻碍可能是泵内在的（如凝血）或外在的（如管路弯曲，压缩，张力性气胸压迫），并且可能发生在回流管，中心静脉或血管内，增加了ΔP（膜肺内部的压差）。回流阻碍损害了EBF对体外生命体质（ECLS）的效率	
管路断裂	管路断裂：如果发生在泵前，会导致失血。如果发生在泵后，会导致空气进入；体外循环中的任何主要组件的空气进入，ECMO以防止进一步的空气进入/失血，并处理管路破裂/更换组件；否则，ECLS会突然中断	
意外脱管	ECMO插管/接头的意外移除或显著位移。 • 如果是引流导管，空气会通过导管进入循环系统 • 如果是回流导管，则会导致失血性休克。两种情况下，脱离部位都会发生大量血液丢失。意外脱管需要紧急停止ECMO。体外生命支持系统会突然中断	
泵故障	泵故障发生在离心泵（CP）无法提供EBF时；EBF的缺失导致支持丧失。CP可能因涉及泵头的并发症（脱落，血栓形成或大量空气栓塞）或受控制台、驱动单元故障（电源丧失和电池耗尽，电子/机械故障）而失败	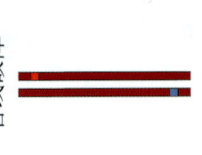
膜肺&气体管线故障	• 凝血块/血栓和纤维蛋白沉积的渐进性或急性形成减少了ML内用于体外气体交换的可用面积，损害了血液氧合/二氧化碳清除的效果，凝血块，血栓和纤维蛋白可通过亮光照射膜肺发现（"手电筒测试"）。由于更高的阻力影响EBF：P_{pre}增加而P_{post}减少，增加了ΔP，此外，如果ML内部有广泛的血栓形成，可能会出现系统性凝血或溶血 • 任何影响提供FGF到ML的气体管线问题（不适当的FGF/FdO₂设置，意外断开连接，气源耗尽）都会损害ML的气体交换功能，水分可能在气体纤维膜内聚集，减少体外二氧化碳去除，需要定期清除（"吹膜"）	

ECMO，体外膜肺氧合；RPM，每分钟转速；CP(s)，离心泵；EBF，体外血流量；FGF，新鲜气流量；LPM，L/min；SGF，换气流量；FdO₂，设备氧浓度；FsO₂，换气氧浓度；ECLS，体外生命支持；IAP，腹腔压；IAH，腹腔高压；PTX，气胸；ITP，胸腔压；ML，膜肺（人工肺）；V-V，静脉-静脉；RF，回流分数；RBF，回流血流量；CVL，中心静脉导管

注意：关于如何预防、早期发现和处理ECLS的机械并发症的详细讨论超出了本章的范围。

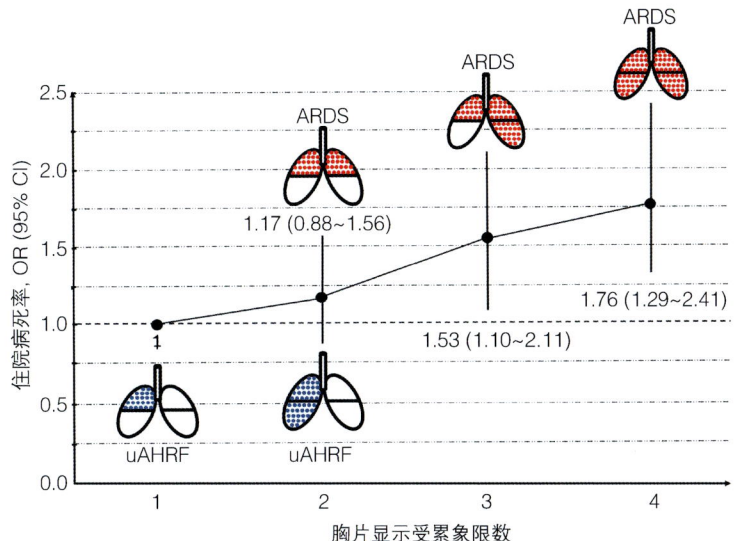

图 14.2 LUNG SAFE 队列研究中校正后的 AHRF 患者的住院死亡风险。呼吸衰竭患者可能表现为单侧浸润[AHRF(蓝点)]或双侧浸润[ARDS(红点)]。基于单侧或双侧分布,2 个象限出现浸润可分别被定义为 AHRF 或 ARDS。与仅存在一个象限浸润相比,肺浸润象限数量增加(即 2 个以上)与死亡风险逐渐增加相关。根据基线特征、合并症、是否伴随心力衰竭、ARDS 的危险因素、通气变量和地缘经济校正了 95％ 置信区间的比值比(OR),比值比和 95％ 置信区间用点和误差线表示,使用单象限浸润作为参照。图中数据来自 Pham et al. Eur Resp Journal[6]

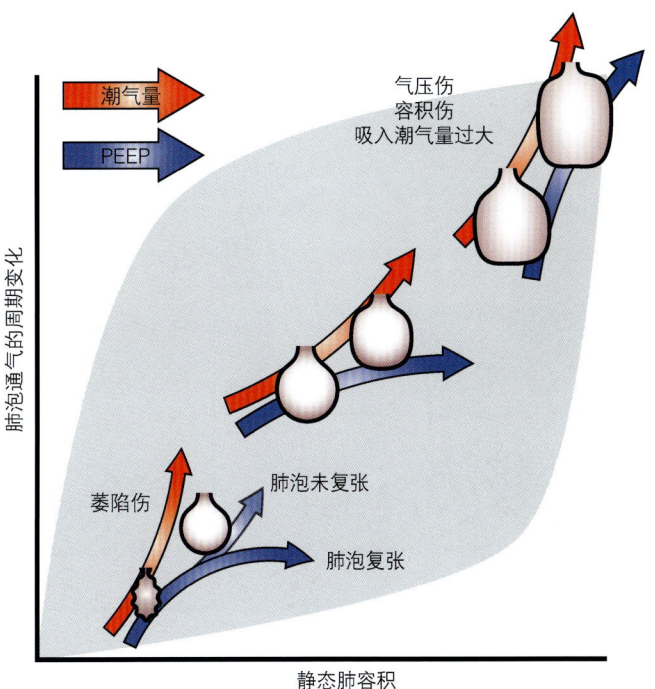

图 15.2 潮气量和 PEEP 的作用。成对的肺泡代表呼气末和吸气末肺泡充气情况。在受伤的肺中,通气设置对静态肺容积和肺泡通气周期性变化的影响取决于先前的充气情况和损伤的性质。所谓的可复张肺可能对 PEEP 有更好的反应,从而有利于静态体积的增加和通气周期肺泡变化的减少

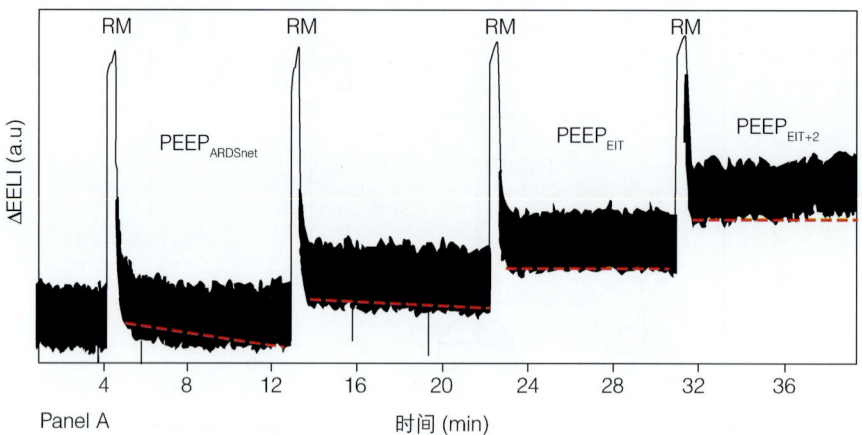

图 17.1 该图显示了 EIT 监测下呼气末正压(PEEP)变化中穿插"诊断性"肺复张手法(RM)时肺容量的变化。PEEP 水平保持不变后的第一次 RM,通过增加的呼气末肺容积(EELV),提示存在肺泡复张。然而,该 PEEP 水平不能阻止肺泡塌陷,故 EELV 又回到了基线水平。增加(2+2)cmH₂O 的 PEEP 可以保持肺复张后肺泡的稳定性(根据知识共享许可协议改编自参考文献[34])

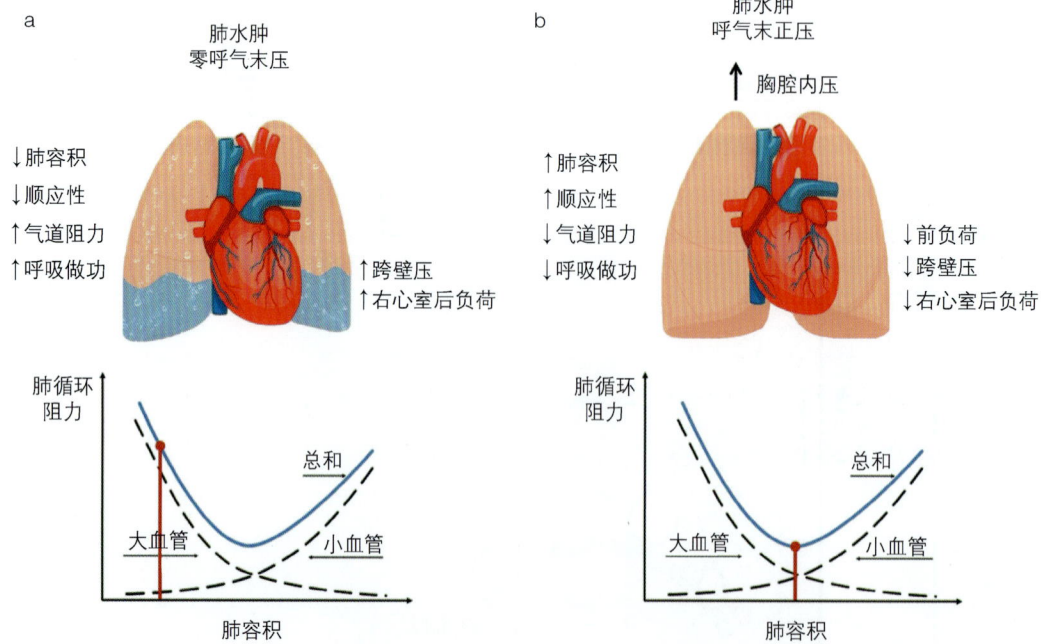

图 19.1 a. 心源性肺水肿时呼吸衰竭的病理生理机制。b. 气道正压通气对呼吸力学和血流动力学的生理效应。ZEEP,零呼气末压;PEEP,呼气末正压;ITP,胸腔内压;RV,右心室;PVR,肺循环阻力

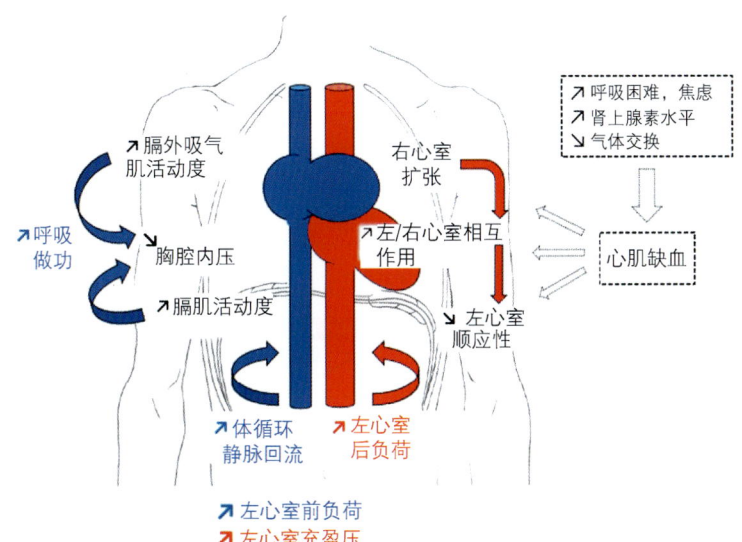

图 22.2 撤机致肺水肿（weaning induced pulmonary oedema，WIPO）的机制。因为心血管和呼吸系统之间的密切相互作用，所有这些机制都可能在慢性阻塞性肺疾病患者中加剧。胸内压降低主要的诱发因素是由机械通气（胸内正压）转为自主呼吸（胸内负压）。静脉回流增加，可能会导致右心室扩张和右/左心室相互作用。胸内压力的降低也会导致左心室后负荷的增加（左心室必须克服胸内压力的下降，才能将血液从胸腔泵出）。此外，还可能发生心肌缺血，使左心室功能恶化。这些机制均可引起 WIPO，导致肺水肿和自主呼吸试验失败。图片来源：Ann. Intensive Care 11，99(2021)

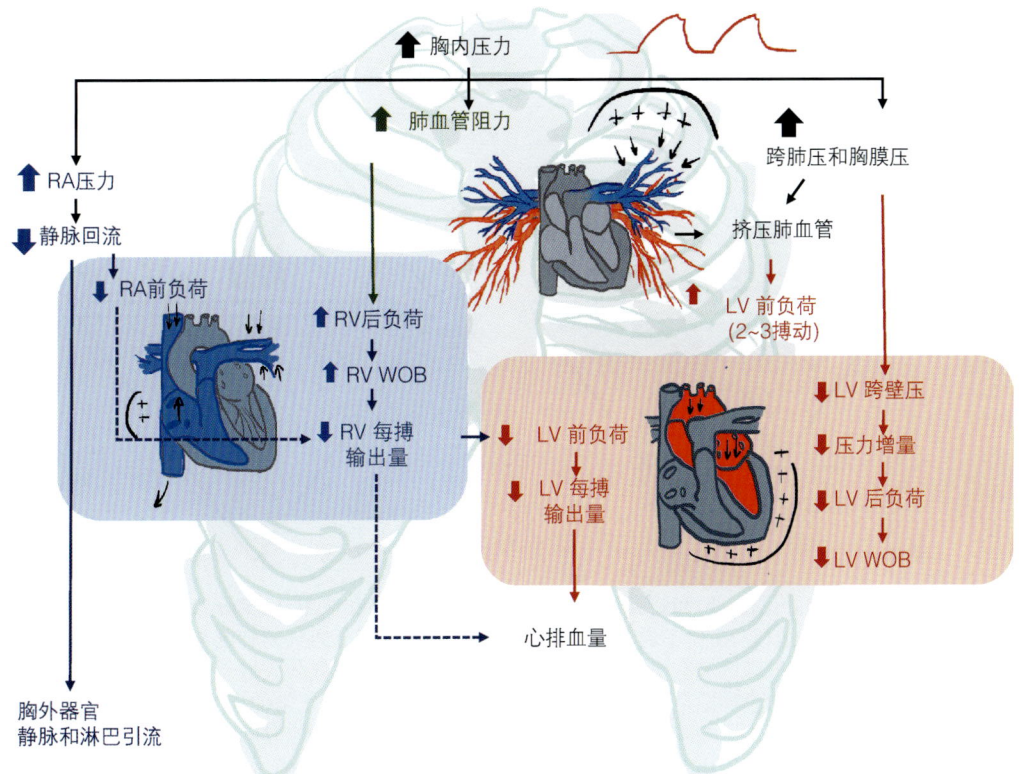

图 25.2 正压机械通气时的心肺交互作用。RA，右心房；RV，右心室；LV，左心室

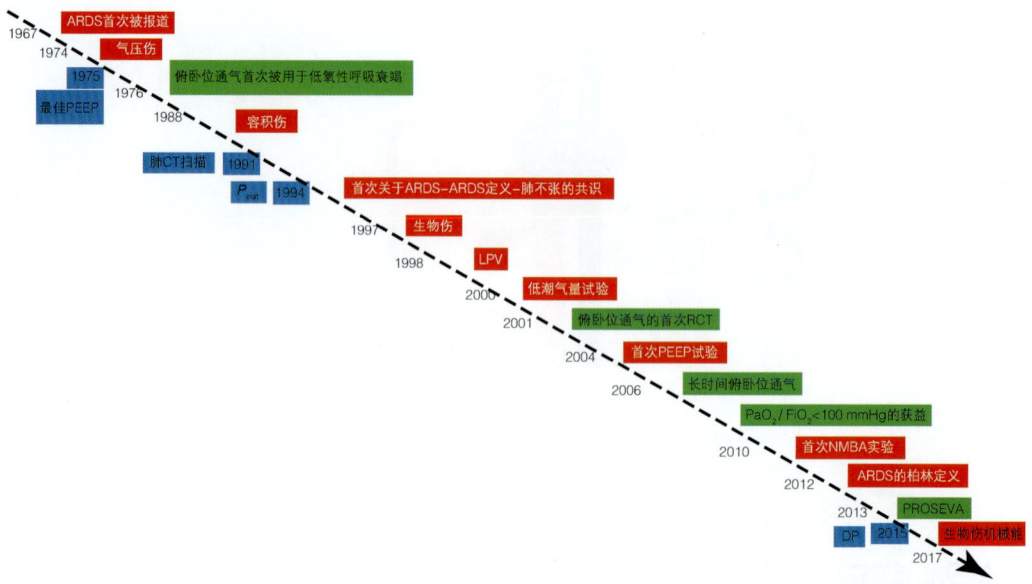

图 29.1 急性呼吸窘迫综合征管理的主要进展时间轴(未按比例显示)。红框表示机械通气,蓝框表示生理监测,绿框表示俯卧位。P_{plat},平台压;LPV,肺保护性通气;PEEP,呼气末正压;DP,驱动压;RCT,随机对照试验;NMBA,神经肌肉阻滞剂

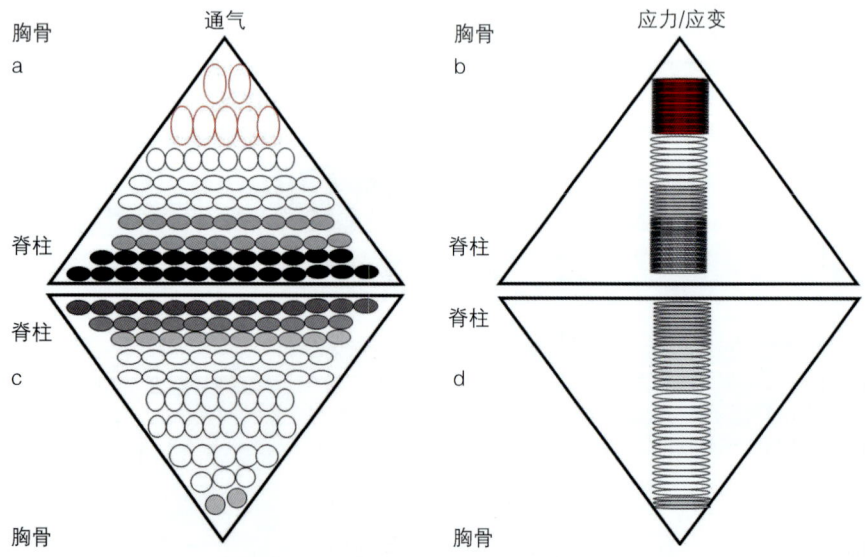

图 29.2 仰卧位(a,b)和俯卧位(c,d)的 ARDS 肺通气和应力/应变分布示意图。黑色椭圆是肺无效腔,由于不通气而无应力。灰色椭圆为部分通气的肺区域。靠近肺无效腔的部分通气肺区域有很高的应力,而距离较远的部分通气肺区域承受较低但高于正常的应力。白色椭圆是正常通气的肺区域,即婴儿肺,承受正常的应力。最后,红色空心椭圆是过度膨胀的肺区域,存在着较高应力。当转向俯卧位时肺复张并且减少了过度膨胀。整个肺的压力/应变降低,在肺内的分布更加均匀

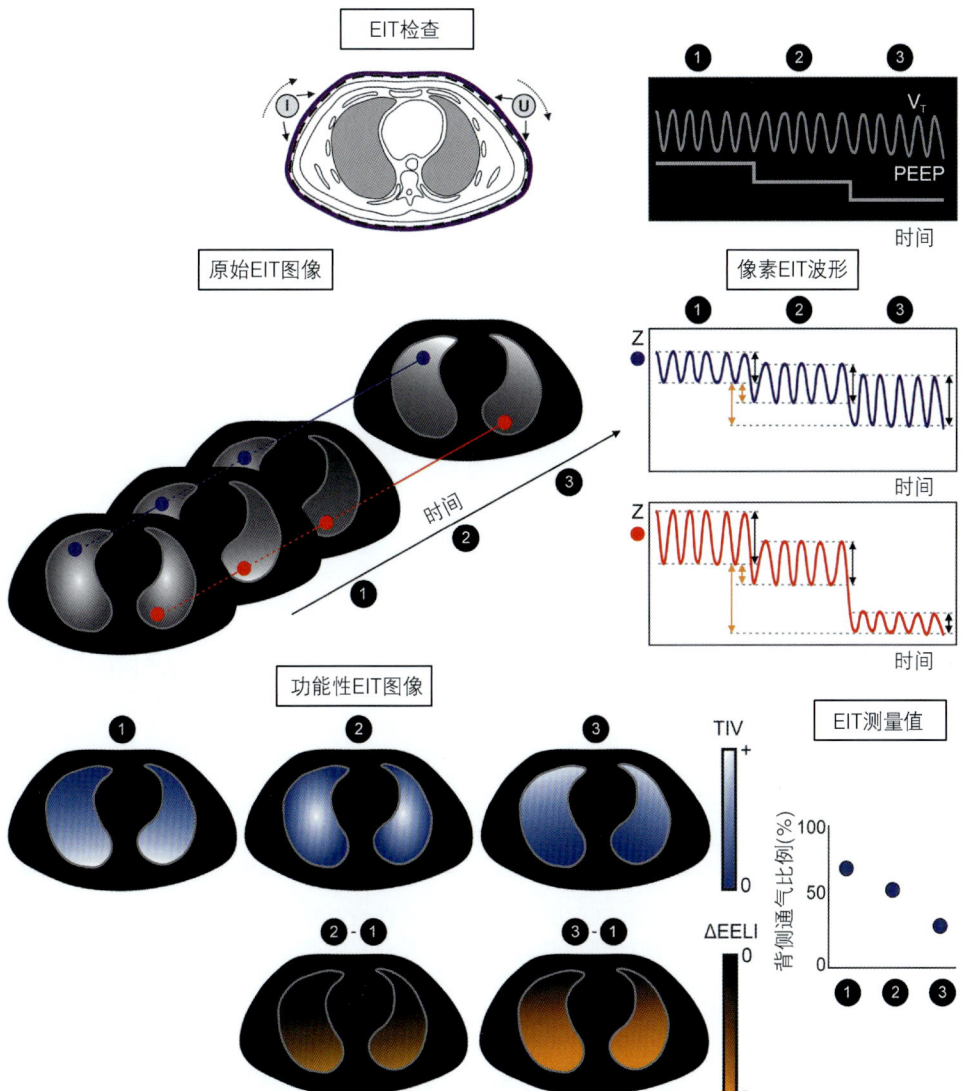

图 33.1 电阻抗断层成像(EIT)的测量原理和 EIT 数据采集和分析的不同步骤。在 EIT 检查期间(左上角),一个集成电极的 EIT 条带作为接口(带有短黑条的紫色线)被放置在胸壁周围。所有电极依次经历快速施加短暂且微小的交流电流(I)和测量施加的电流产生的电压(U)差这两个过程。EIT 数据可以在机械通气过程中获得,如在三个呼气末正压(PEEP)水平下进行恒定潮气量(V_T)的通气过程中(右上)。原始 EIT 数据产生了一系列原始 EIT 图像(左中)。其中,两个图像被标记出来,一个在右肺的非重力依赖区(蓝色),另一个在左肺的重力依赖区(红色)。区域像素阻抗(Z)波形(右中)显示了在三个不同 PEEP 时选定像素的周期阻抗变化(TIV)(黑色箭头)。第一个和其他两个 PEEP 水平间的呼气末肺阻抗(ΔEELI)的变化也被显示出来(橙色箭头)。所有像素中 TIV 和 ΔEELI 的计算值可以绘制在各自的位置上,从而生成两种不同类型的功能性 EIT 图像(左下)。顶部的蓝白色图像显示了 V_T 的空间分布,底部的黑橙色图像显示了呼气末肺容积的区域性下降。在功能图像中得到的值可以用于计算 EIT 相关定量指标。例如,测量背侧肺通气比例,即背侧 TIV 相对于整个图像的占比。图中给出了它在三个 PEEP 时的值(右下)

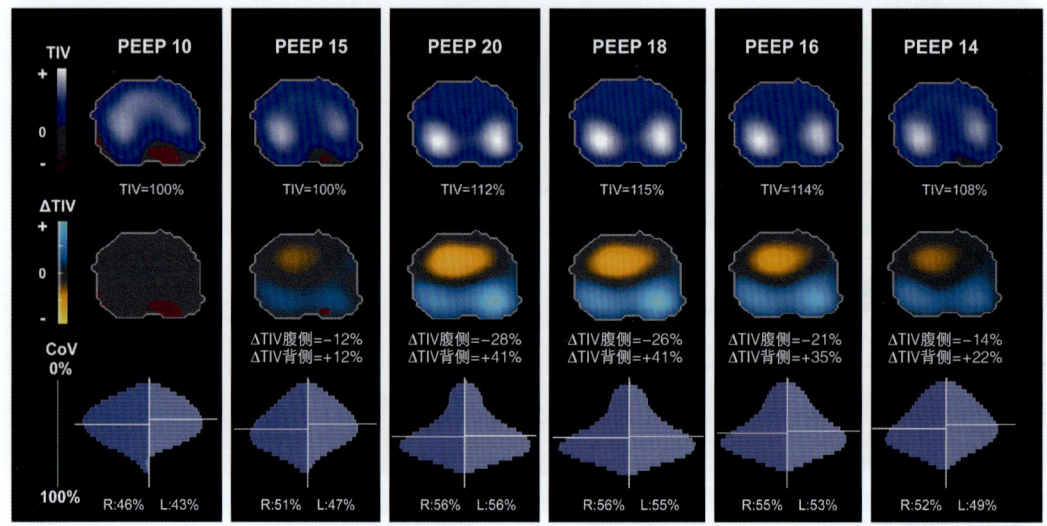

图 33.3　使用 EIT 分析采用俯卧位的 COVID-19 相关 ARDS 患者的区域肺通气。检查也如图 33.2 所示，在呼气末正压(PEEP)的两次增加和四个递减步骤的完整过程中进行。在功能性 EIT 图像上区域周期性阻抗变化(TIV)(上)显示了胸部横断面中的潮气量分布。通气区域以白色和蓝色表示，图像下面的数字给出了 TIV 值，以 10 cmH$_2$O PEEP 时 TIV 初始值为基线按比例显示的全局 TIV 值总和。与初始最低 PEEP 值相比，展示区域 TIV 变化(ΔTIV)(中)的功能性 EIT 图像显示了各个 PEEP 值下通气的局部增加(浅蓝色区域)和减少(橙色区域)。图像下面的数字说明了与操作开始时的初始 TIV 分布相比，肺腹侧和背侧区域的 TIV 相对变化。通气分布图(下)显示了左、右肺的区域通气分布。每个图中的白色水平线表示通气中心(CoV)的位置，对应的值绘制在每个图像的下面。数值小于 50% 意味着通气分布偏向腹侧区域。CoV，通气中心(引自参考文献[2])

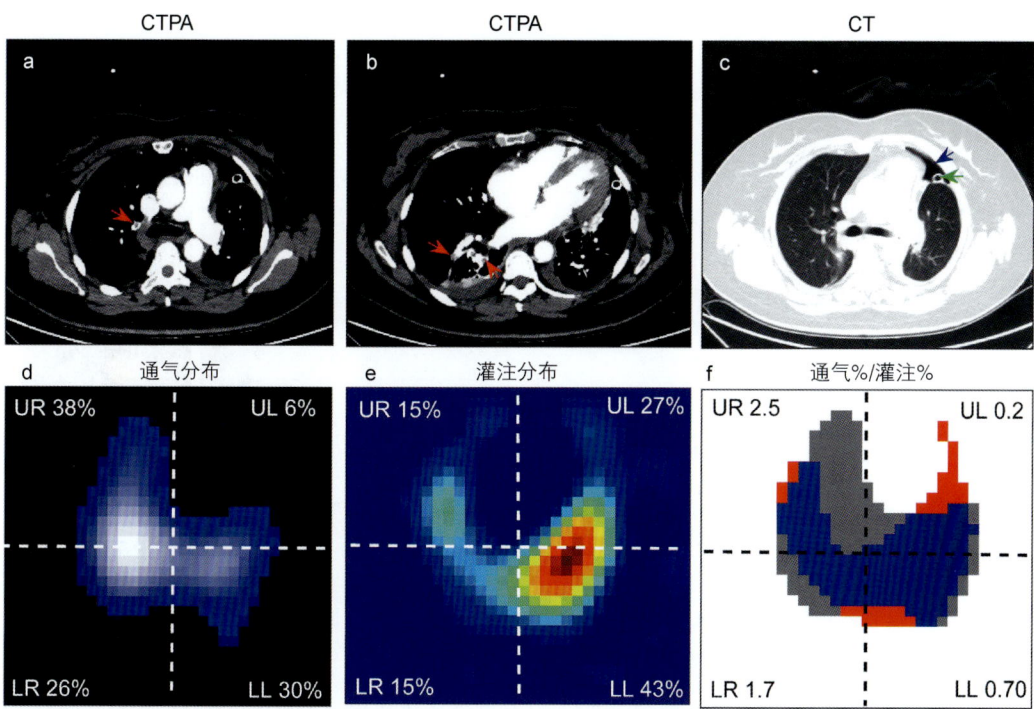

图 33.4　47 岁的仰卧位女性在胸部手术后 1 天进行了计算机断层成像(CT)、CT 肺动脉造影(CTPA)和电阻抗断层成像(EIT),显示了通气和灌注受损。CTPA 显示右肺动脉分支有多个栓塞(a 和 b 中的红色箭头)。CT 发现左腹侧有少量气胸(c 中的蓝色箭头)。胸腔内可见引流管(绿色箭头)。通气分布的功能性 EIT 图像(d)显示深蓝色为低通气区域,白色为高通气区域。图像四个角中的值给出了相应象限中的通气百分比。灌注分布的功能性 EIT 图像中红色为高灌注区域,蓝色为低灌注区域(e)。图像四个角中的值给出了相应象限的灌注百分比。显示区域通气/灌注分布的功能 EIT 图像(f)中:灰色为高通气和低灌注区域(像素点对应的区域有通气而无灌注),红色为低通气和高灌注区域(像素点对应的区域有灌注而无通气),蓝色为良好的通气/灌注匹配(像素点对应的区域在通气和灌注这两个方面都有良好表现)。每个象限显示的区域通气/灌注对应于相应象限的通气分布(以％显示)超过灌注分布(以％显示)的值。LL,左下肺;LR,右下肺;UL,左上肺;UR,右上肺(经美国胸科学会许可,转载自参考文献[3]。版权所有:© 2021 美国胸科学会。保留所有权利)

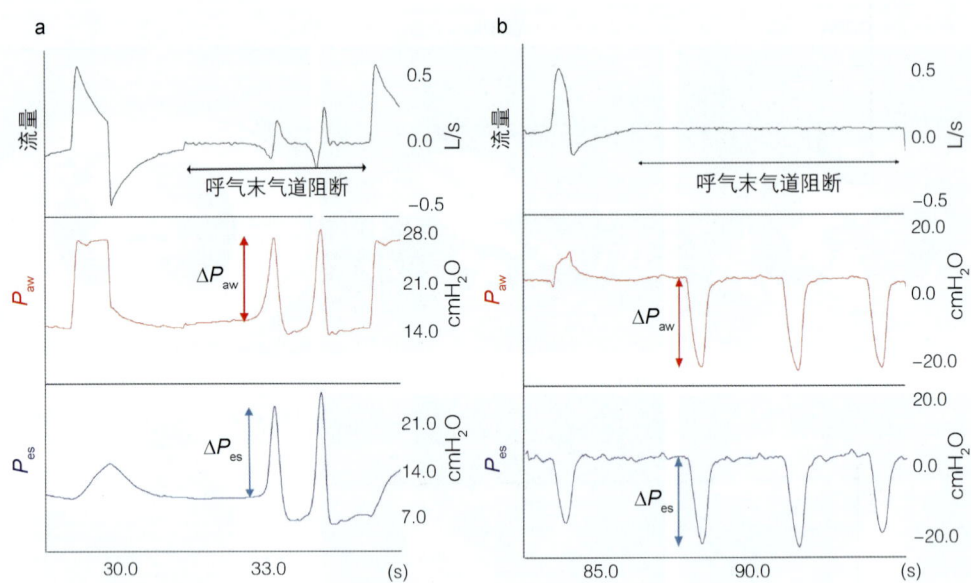

图 34.1 食管导管的放置及气囊填充和位置的评估。食管导管像鼻胃管一样放置,经鼻或经口,通常深度为 40~55 厘米。远端部分连接到压力传感器上,用空气对气囊充气。气囊在食管中的位置可通过 P_{es} 波形中出现呼吸与心脏搏动波形来确定。气囊充气包括以下步骤:① 使气囊完全放气,以精确计算充气体积;② 通过短暂的断开连接使其与大气压平衡;③ 充入允许的最大气体量(根据每种气囊的具体规定),以均匀地展开气囊;④ 放气至推荐的气体量。优化充气量可以进一步通过逐步(0.5 mL)注入气囊来实现,选择与 P_{es} 潮气量最大波动相关的最低体积。随后,通过比较呼气末气道阻断时的 P_{aw} 波形和 P_{es} 波形来确定气囊的正确位置:在肺容积不变的情况下,跨肺压不变,因此 P_{es} 的变化应该等于 P_{aw} 的变化,反之亦然。理想情况下,$\Delta P_{es}/\Delta P_{aw}$ 应该接近 1,但 0.8~1.2 也是可接受的。本图从上到下依次为,气流量、气道压(P_{aw})和食管压(P_{es})随时间的波形图。a. 在控制模式下,胸部施加两次轻柔的压力会在 P_{aw} 和 P_{es} 中产生相似的正向压力波动(红色和蓝色箭头)。b. 在辅助模式下(此处为压力支持),在呼气末阻断期间,患者对抗阻断气道的吸气努力在气道压和食管压中产生相似的负向压力波动(红色和蓝色箭头)

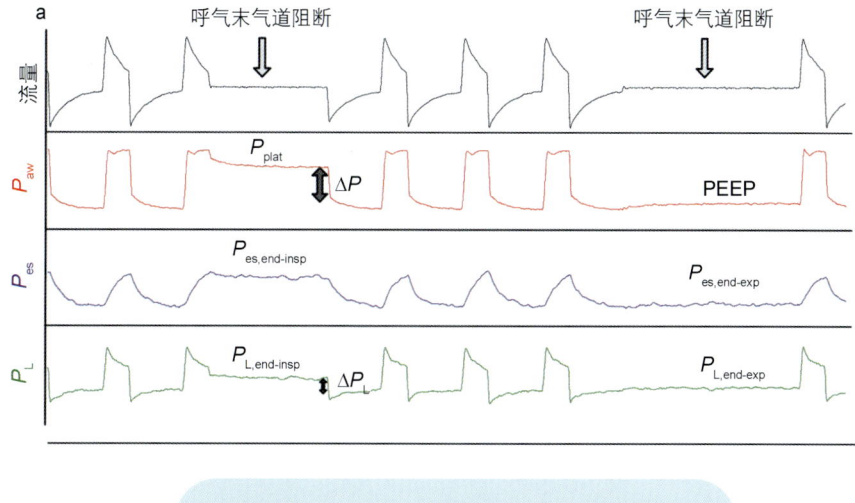

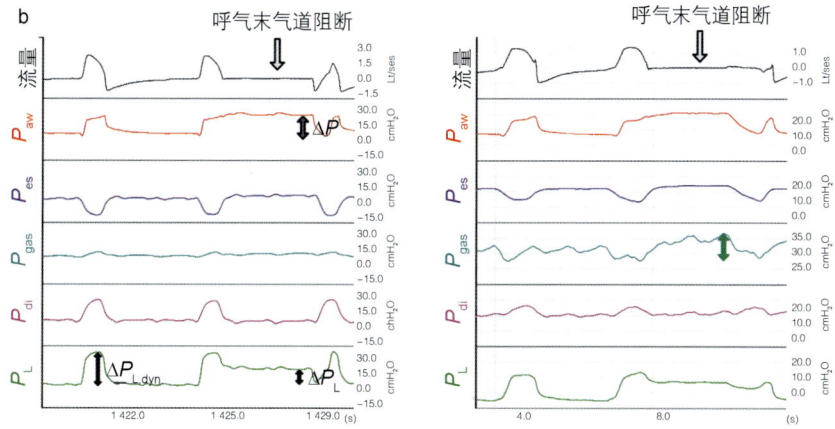

图34.2 控制性通气（a）和辅助性通气（b）期间的跨肺压和肺部力学计算。a. 从上到下依次为：被动通气患者的流量、气道压（P_{aw}）、食管压（P_{es}）和跨肺压（P_L）随时间变化的波形图。P_L 通过计算 P_{aw} 和 P_{es} 间的差值得出。图中可见吸气末和呼气末气道阻断的操作。在气道阻断期间假设所有的气道都是开放的，此时 P_{alv} 与 P_{aw} 达到平衡。因此，在没有呼吸肌活动的情况下，吸气末的 P_{aw}（P_{plat}）和呼气末阻断时的 P_{aw}（PEEP）被认为分别近似于吸气末和呼气末的静态 P_{alv}。肺的弹性回缩力（流量为零时的 P_L）是肺在高于功能残气量时的不同肺容积时所克服的实际压力。如图所示，使用 P_{es} 的绝对值可以计算静态吸气末 P_L（$P_{L,end-insp}$）和呼气末 P_L（$P_{L,end-exp}$）。呼吸系统的驱动压（ΔP）可通过 P_{plat} 和 PEEP 的差值计算得出，呼吸系统的弹性（E_{rs}）为 ΔP 与 V_T 的比值。如图所示，P_{es} 的计算允许将 E_{rs} 拆分为肺弹性（E_L）和胸壁弹性（E_{CW}）。ΔP_L 称为跨肺驱动压，反映了 V_T 引起的肺应力变化。跨肺压也可以用 P_{aw} 乘以 E_L 与 E_{rs} 之比（弹性推导法）进行计算。因此，该方法只需要 P_{es} 的变化值，而不需要绝对值。b. 从上到下依次为：辅助通气患者在压力支持期间的流量、气道压（P_{aw}）、食管压（P_{es}）、胃内压（P_{gas}）、跨膈压（P_{di}）和动态跨肺压（P_L）随时间变化的波形图。通过 P_{gas} 减去 P_{es} 来计算跨膈压。通过吸气末阻断以测量静态吸气末气道压（P_{plat}）和跨肺压（$P_{L,end-insp}$）。b 左侧图中，无呼吸肌收缩保证了测量 P_{plat} 和 ΔP 的可靠性；而在右侧图中，呼气肌收缩，表现为呼气末 P_{gas} 升高（绿色箭头），P_{plat} 和 ΔP 的测量是无效的

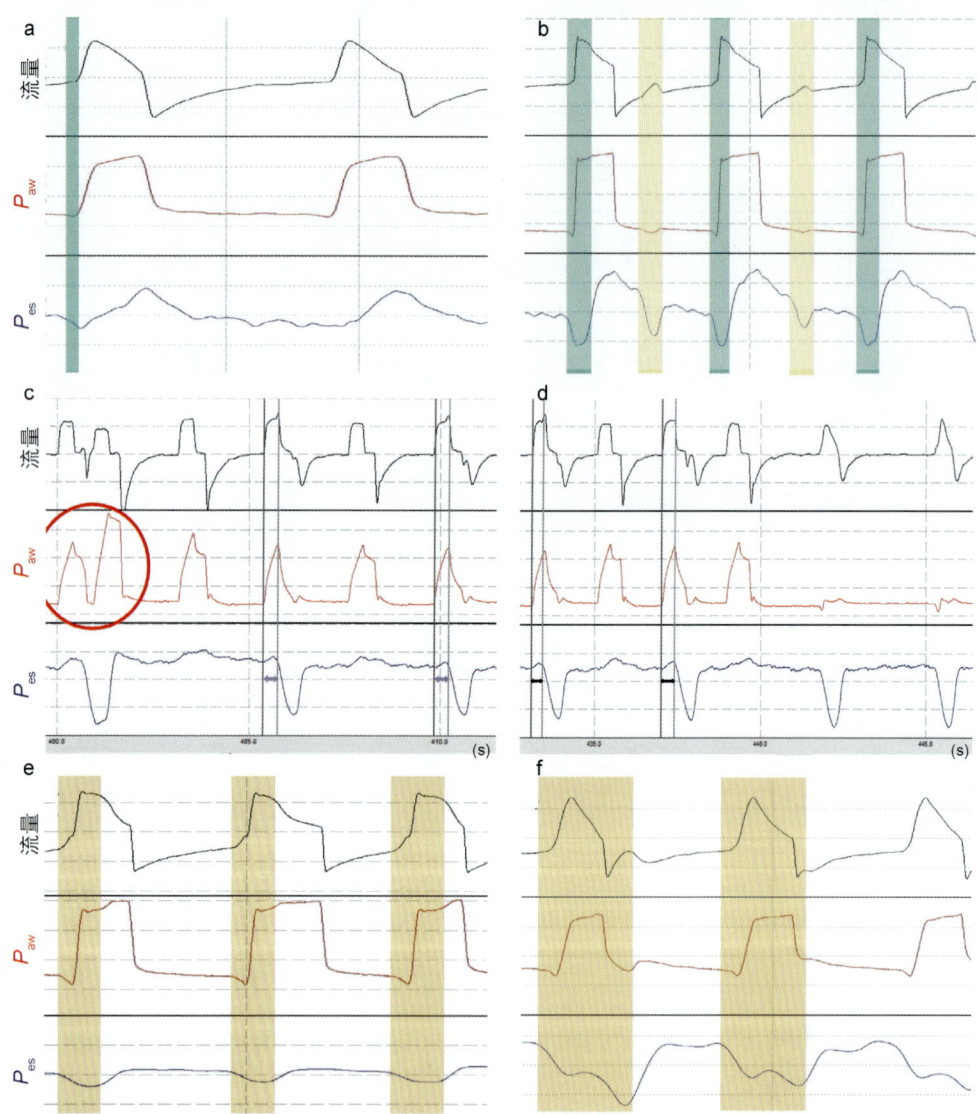

图 34.4 识别不同步现象。从上到下依次为：流量、气道压(P_{aw})和食管压(P_{es})随时间变化的波形图。a. 触发延迟和自动触发：在压力支持模式下，患者小幅努力会触发第一次呼吸，随后吸气肌放松，表现为P_{es}上移（与被动通气一样）。触发延迟（显示为蓝色）为120毫秒，在这种情况下，几乎与患者努力时间一样长。第二次呼吸是自动触发的呼吸，因为在P_{es}波形中没检测到任何努力。这种自动触发在P_{aw}波形中无法识别。b. 高水平压力支持下的无效努力：患者的努力可以在P_{es}波形上识别出来，第一、第三和第六次努力触发了呼吸机送气（显示为蓝色），而第二和第四次努力是无效的（显示为黄色）。呼气流速波形的轻度变形表明存在无效努力，但P_{es}波形可以更清楚地识别患者的努力。c. 辅助容量控制通气中的呼吸叠加和夹带（反向触发）：延伸到机器呼气时间的吸气努力触发了呼吸机送第二次的叠加呼吸，增加了潮气量带来的应力（红圈）。这种患者努力可能是夹带的结果，其特征是与机器呼吸（紫色箭头）保持稳定的时间关系，可以使用P_{es}波形进行测量。d. 在控制模式下的自发努力可与夹带表现相似，可以通过与机器呼吸缺乏稳定的时间关系（黑色箭头）和CPAP试验中存在吸气努力进行区分。e, f. 机器和中枢吸气时间不匹配：在压力支持模式下，中枢吸气时间（显示为橙色）可能比机器吸气时间短，表现为吸-呼切换延迟(e)；也可能比机械时间长，表现为吸-呼切换过早(f)

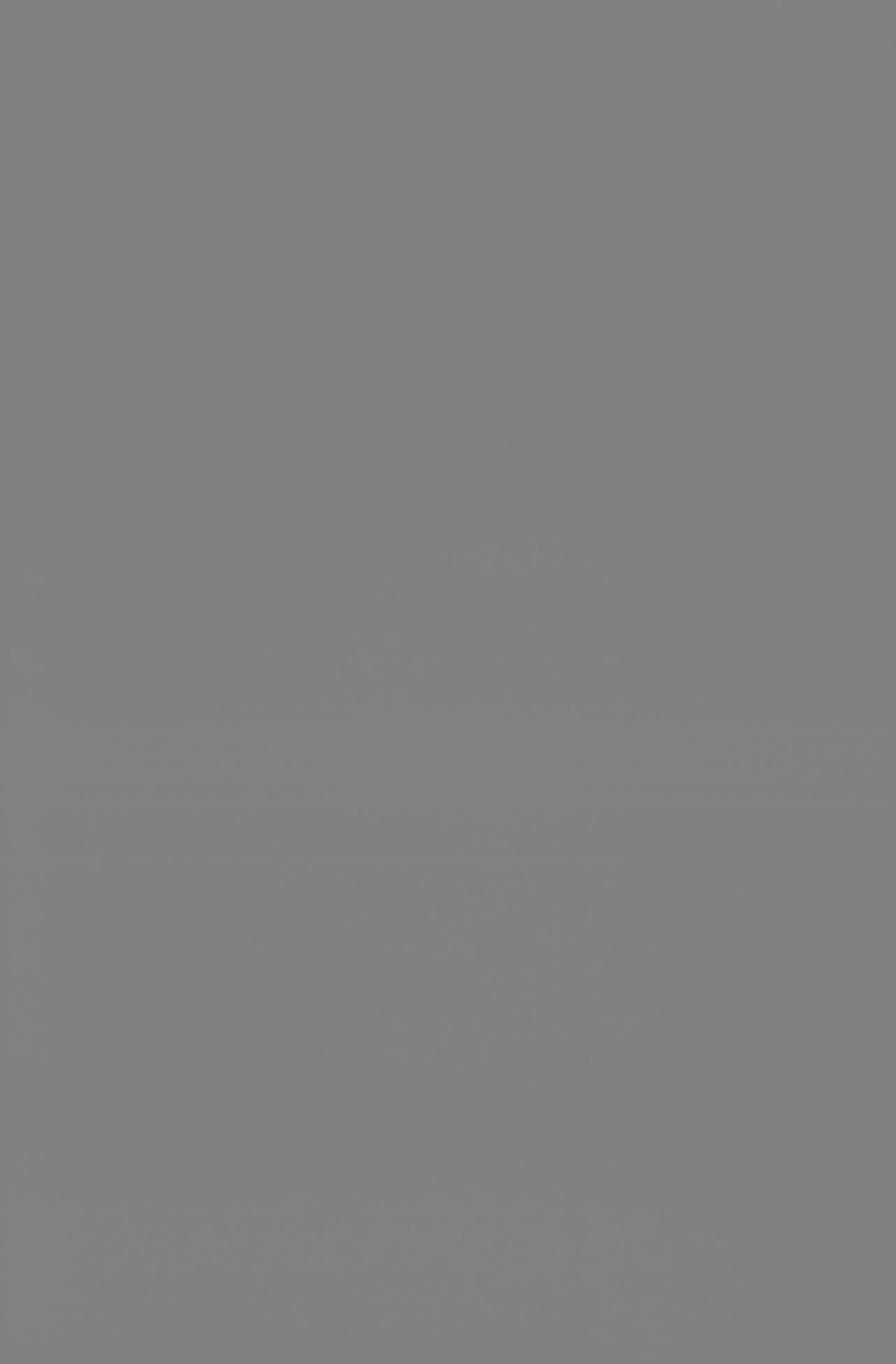